Advanced Reconstruction Foot and Ankle

American Academy of Orthopaedic Surgeons

Advanced Reconstruction Foot and Ankle

Edited by

James A. Nunley, MD
Professor and Vice Chairman
Division of Orthopaedic Surgery
Department of Surgery
Duke University Medical Center
Durham, North Carolina

Glenn B. Pfeffer, MD
Assistant Clinical Professor
Department of Orthopaedic Surgery
University of California
San Francisco, California

Roy W. Sanders, MD
Clinical Professor of Orthopaedic Surgery
University of South Florida School of Medicine
Florida Orthopaedic Institute
Tampa, Florida

Elly Trepman, MD
Associate Professor, Section of Orthopaedic Surgery
Department of Surgery
University of Manitoba
Winnipeg, Manitoba
Canada

Developed by the
American Orthopaedic Foot and Ankle Society

Published by the
American Academy of Orthopaedic Surgeons
6300 North River Road
Rosemont, IL 60018

Advanced Reconstruction Foot and Ankle

American Academy of Orthopaedic Surgeons

First Edition

ISBN 0-89203-314-2

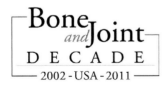

Acknowledgments

Contributors

Robert S. Adelaar, MD
Professor of Surgery
Chairman, Department of Orthopedics
Medical College of Virginia
Virginia Commonwealth University
Richmond, Virginia

Ian J. Alexander, MD
Clinical Associate Professor of Orthopaedic Surgery
Department of Orthopaedic Surgery
Northeastern Ohio University College of Medicine
Akron, Ohio

John G. Anderson, MD
Assistant Clinical Professor
Department of Surgery
Michigan State University College of Human Medicine
Grand Rapids, Michigan

Robert B. Anderson, MD
Chief, Foot and Ankle Service
Carolinas Medical Center
Miller Orthopaedic Clinic
Charlotte, North Carolina

Christopher E. Attinger, MD
Director, Wound Healing Clinic
Professor, Plastic and Orthopedic Surgery
Georgetown University Hospital
Washington, DC

Judith F. Baumhauer, MD
Associate Professor of Orthopaedic Surgery
Chief, Division of Foot and Ankle Surgery
Department of Orthopaedic Surgery
University of Rochester School of Medicine and Dentistry
Rochester, New York

John A. Bergfeld, MD
Director, Cleveland Clinic Sports Health
Department of Orthopaedic Surgery
Cleveland Clinic Foundation
Cleveland, Ohio

Gregory C. Berlet, MD
Orthopaedic Foot and Ankle Center
Columbus, Ohio

James L. Beskin, MD
Assistant Clinical Professor of Orthopedics
Tulane University
New Orleans, Louisiana
Peachtree Orthopedic Clinic
Atlanta, Georgia

Donald R. Bohay, MD
Assistant Clinical Professor
Department of Orthopaedic Surgery
Michigan State University College of Human Medicine
Grand Rapids, Michigan

Michael J. Botte, MD
Head, Section of Neuromuscular Reconstructive Surgery and Rehabilitation
Division of Orthopaedic Surgery
Scripps Clinic
La Jolla, California

Matison L. Boyer, MD
Department of Orthopaedics
Orthopaedic Specialists of Charleston
Charleston, South Carolina

James W. Brodsky, MD
Clinical Professor of Orthopaedic Surgery
University of Texas Southwestern Medical School
Baylor University Medical Center
Dallas, Texas

Jason H. Calhoun, MD
Professor and Chairman
The John Sealy Distinguished Centennial Chair in Rehabilitation Sciences
Department of Orthopaedics and Rehabilitation
The University of Texas Medical Branch
Galveston, Texas

Thomas O. Clanton, MD
Professor and Chairman
Department of Orthopaedic Surgery
The University of Texas Health Science Center at Houston Medical School
Houston, Texas

Michael P. Clare, MD
Assistant Professor of Orthopaedic Surgery
Department of Orthopaedic Surgery
University of Nebraska Medical Center
Omaha, Nebraska

Richard J. Claridge, MD, FRCS
Assistant Professor of Orthopaedic
  Surgery
Division of Orthopaedic Surgery
Mayo Medical School
Consultant in Orthopaedics
Mayo Clinic Scottsdale
Scottsdale, Arizona

J. Chris Coetzee, MD, FRCSC
Assistant Professor, Foot and Ankle
  Division
Department of Orthopaedic Surgery
University of Minnesota
Minneapolis, Minnesota

Stephen F. Conti, MD
Director, Division of Foot and Ankle
  Surgery
Human Motion Center
Allegheny General Hospital
Pittsburgh, Pennsylvania

Michael J. Coughlin, MD
Director, Idaho Foot and Ankle
  Fellowship
Clinical Professor of Orthopedic
  Surgery
Oregon Health Sciences University
Boise, Idaho

Andrea Cracchiolo III, MD
Professor of Orthopaedic Surgery
Department of Orthopaedic Surgery
UCLA Medical Center
Los Angeles, California

Timothy R. Daniels, MD, FRCSC
Assistant Professor
Department of Orthopaedic Surgery
University of Toronto
Toronto, Ontario

W. Hodges Davis, MD
Director, Foot and Ankle Center
Miller Orthopaedic Clinic
Charlotte, North Carolina

Jonathan T. Deland, MD
Chief, Foot and Ankle Center
The Hospital for Special Surgery
New York, New York

Brian G. Donley, MD
Director, Research and Education
Section of Foot and Ankle
Department of Orthopaedic Surgery
Cleveland Clinic Foundation
Cleveland, Ohio

Mark E. Easley, MD
Assistant Professor
Division of Orthopaedic Surgery
Duke University Medical Center
Durham, North Carolina

Richard D. Ferkel, MD
Director of Sports Medicine
  Fellowship and Attending Surgeon
Southern California Orthopedic
  Institute
Van Nuys, California

Adolph S. Flemister, Jr, MD
Assistant Professor of Orthopaedics
Department of Orthopaedics
University of Rochester School of
  Medicine and Dentistry
Rochester, New York

Paul T. Fortin, MD
Department of Orthopaedic Surgery
William Beaumont Hospital
Royal Oak, Michigan

Carol C. Frey, MD
Assistant Clinical Professor of
  Orthopaedic Surgery
University of California at Los
  Angeles
Director, Orthopaedic Foot and
  Ankle Surgery
West Coast Sports Performance
Manhattan Beach, California

Jessica Galina, MD
Foot and Ankle Fellow
Department of Orthopaedics
Mount Sinai Hospital
New York, New York

John S. Gould, MD
Clinical Professor of Orthopaedic
  Surgery
University of South Alabama
Director, Foot and Ankle Fellowship
  Program
American Sports Medicine Institute
Alabama Sports Medicine
  Orthopaedic Center
Birmingham, Alabama

George J. Haidukewych, MD
Director, Orthopedic Trauma Service
Consultant, Department of
  Orthopedic Surgery
Mayo Clinic
Rochester, Minnesota

William G. Hamilton, MD
Clinical Professor of Orthopaedic
  Surgery
Columbia University College of
  Physicians and Surgeons
Senior Attending Orthopaedic
  Surgeon
St. Lukes Roosevelt Hospital Center
New York, New York

Keith A. Heier, MD
Metrocrest Orthopedics and Sports
  Medicine
Trinity Medical Center
Dallas, Texas

Christoph Heitmann, MD
Division of Plastic, Reconstructive,
  Maxillofacial and Oral Surgery
Duke University Medical Center
Durham, North Carolina

Beat Hintermann, MD
Associate Professor
Head, Division of Orthopaedic
  Trauma
Orthopaedic Department
University of Basel, Kantonsspital
Basel, Switzerland

David J. Inda, MD
Foot and Ankle Fellow
Orthopaedic Department
The Hospital for Special Surgery
New York, New York

William C. James III, MD
Fellow, Foot and Ankle Service
Miller Orthopaedic Clinic
Charlotte, North Carolina

Jeffrey E. Johnson, MD
Associate Professor
Chief, Foot and Ankle Service
Department of Orthopaedic Surgery
Barnes-Jewish Hospital at
    Washington University School
    of Medicine
St. Louis, Missouri

Paul J. Juliano, MD
Associate Professor of Orthopedic
    Surgery
Pennsylvania State College of
    Medicine
Milton S. Hershey Medical Center
Hershey, Pennsylvania

Todd A. Kile, MD
Chair, Division of Foot and Ankle
    Surgery
Assistant Professor of Orthopedic
    Surgery
Department of Orthopedic Surgery
Mayo Clinic Scottsdale
Scottsdale, Arizona

Richard T. Laughlin, MD
Associate Professor of Orthopaedic
    Surgery
Department of Orthopaedic Surgery
Wright State University School of
    Medicine
Dayton, Ohio

Simon Lee, MD
Assistant Professor
Department of Orthopaedic Surgery
Rush-Presbyterian-St. Luke's Medical
    Center
Chicago, Illinois

Thomas H. Lee, MD
Orthopedic Foot and Ankle Center
Columbus, Ohio

Efraim D. Leibner, MD, PhD
Assistant Professor
Department of Orthopaedic Surgery
Hadassah Medical Center
Jerusalem, Israel

Lawrence Scott Levin, MD
Professor, Division of Plastic,
    Reconstructive, Maxillofacial and
    Oral Surgery
Duke University Medical Center
Durham, North Carolina

Lowell D. Lutter, MD
Director, Orthopaedic Foot and
    Ankle Center
St. Paul, Minnesota

Roger A. Mann, MD
Director, Foot Fellowship
University of California
Oakland, California

Richard M. Marks, MD
Assistant Professor
Director, Division of Foot and Ankle
    Surgery
Department of Orthopaedic Surgery
Medical College of Wisconsin
Milwaukee, Wisconsin

John E. McDermott, MD
Department of Orthopaedic Surgery
Swedish Medical Center in
    Providence
Seattle, Washington

William C. McGarvey, MD
Assistant Professor of Orthopaedic
    Surgery
Chief of Foot and Ankle Surgery
Department of Orthopaedic Surgery
University of Texas Health Science
    Center at Houston Medical School
Houston, Texas

Mark S. Myerson, MD
Director Foot and Ankle Service
Mercy Hospital
Baltimore, Maryland

Gregory P. Nowinski, MD
William Beaumont Hospital
Troy, Michigan

James A. Nunley, MD
Professor and Vice Chairman
Division of Orthopaedic Surgery
Department of Surgery
Duke University Medical Center
Durham, North Carolina

Martin J. O'Malley, MD
Assistant Professor of Orthopaedics
Cornell University Medical College
Assistant Attending Orthopaedic
    Surgeon
The Hospital for Special Surgery
New York, New York

Walter J. Pedowitz, MD
Clinical Professor of Orthopedic
    Surgery
Department of Orthopaedic Surgery
Columbia University
New York, New York

Jiun-Rong Peng, MD
Foot and Ankle Specialist
Orthopaedic Specialty Institute
    Medical Group of Orange County
Orange, California

Glenn B. Pfeffer, MD
Assistant Clinical Professor
Department of Orthopaedic Surgery
University of California
San Francisco, California

Michael S. Pinzur, MD
Professor of Orthopaedic Surgery and
    Rehabilitation
Department of Orthopaedic Surgery
    and Rehabilitation
Loyola University Medical Center
Maywood, Illinois

George E. Quill, Jr, MD
Assistant Clinical Professor
Department of Orthopaedic Surgery
University of Louisville School of
    Medicine
Louisville, Kentucky

E. Greer Richardson, MD
Professor of Orthopedic Surgery
Department of Orthopedics
University of Tennessee, Campbell
    Clinic
Memphis, Tennessee

Pascal F. Rippstein, MD
Head, Department for Foot and
    Ankle Surgery
Schulthess Clinic
Zurich, Switzerland

Michael M. Romash, MD
Orthopedic Foot and Ankle Center of
Hampton Roads
Sports Medicine and Orthopedic
Center, Inc.
Chesapeake, Virginia

G. James Sammarco, MD
Volunteer Professor
Department of Orthopaedic Surgery
University of Cincinnati School of
Medicine
Cincinnati, Ohio

Roy W. Sanders, MD
Clinical Professor of Orthopaedic
Surgery
University of South Florida School of
Medicine
Florida Orthopaedic Institute
Tampa, Florida

Andrew K. Sands, MD
Section Chief, Foot and Ankle
Surgery
Department of Orthopedic Surgery
Saint Vincent Medical Center
New York, New York

Lew C. Schon, MD
Attending Physician
Director, Foot and Ankle Services
Department of Orthopaedic Surgery
Union Memorial Hospital
Baltimore, Maryland

Pierce E. Scranton, Jr, MD
Orthopaedics International, LTD PS
Seattle, Washington

Michael J. Shereff, MD
Clinical Professor
Department of Orthopaedic Surgery
Medical University of South Carolina
Charleston, South Carolina

Douglas G. Smith, MD
Associate Professor
Director, Prosthetics Research Study
Department of Orthopaedic Surgery
University of Washington
Seattle, Washington

**Heidi Multhopp Stephens,
MD, MBA**
Department of Orthopaedic Surgery
Foot and Ankle Section
University of South Florida School of
Medicine
Tampa, Florida

James W. Stone, MD
Department of Orthopaedic Surgery
Medical College of Wisconsin
Milwaukee, Wisconsin

Eric J. Strauss
Cornell University Medical Center
New York, New York

David B. Thordarson, MD
Professor of Orthopaedics
Chief, Foot and Ankle Trauma and
Reconstructive Surgery
Keck School of Medicine
University of Southern California
Los Angeles, California

Elly Trepman, MD
Associate Professor, Section of
Orthopaedic Surgery
Department of Surgery
University of Manitoba
Winnipeg, Manitoba, Canada

Saul G. Trevino, MD
Professor and Chief
Division of Foot, Ankle, and
Infections
Department of Orthopaedics and
Rehabilitation
The University of Texas Medical
Branch
Galveston, Texas

Norman S. Turner, MD
Consultant, Orthopedic Surgery
Mayo Clinic
Rochester, Minnesota

Arthur K. Walling, MD
Director, Foot and Ankle
Fellowships
Clinical Professor of Orthopaedic
Surgery
Florida Orthopaedic Institute
Tampa, Florida

Keith L. Wapner, MD
Clinical Professor of Orthopedic
Surgery
University of Pennsylvania
Adjunct Professor of Orthopaedic
Surgery
Drexel University Medical School
Philadelphia, Pennsylvania

Troy S. Watson, MD
Director, Foot and Ankle Institute
Desert Orthopaedic Center
Las Vegas, Nevada

Foreword

The American Academy of Orthopaedics has a long history of developing educational materials with the specialty societies. One of the best examples of this collaboration is the *Orthopaedic Knowledge Update* (OKU) specialty series. The first volume, *Orthopaedic Knowledge Update Foot and Ankle*, was published 10 years ago to great acclaim and is now in its third edition. Clearly, general orthopaedists and specialists alike recognize the tremendous value of educational materials developed in this cooperative manner. The OKU specialty volumes are among the most popular of our publications.

I am pleased to see the Academy once again working with the American Orthopaedic Foot and Ankle Society (AOFAS) on a collaborative project. *Advanced Reconstruction Foot and Ankle* is the first truly "technique oriented" text published by the Academy. When members of the AOFAS approached the Academy with the idea for developing this innovative text, the Board was eager to listen. The AOFAS saw a need for its members and for general orthopaedists who have asked for this type of publication. Glenn Pfeffer, MD, James Nunley, MD, Roy Sanders, MD, and Elly Trepman, MD, the volume's editors, along with the Academy's Publications Department, developed a text that will prove invaluable to the busy practitioner.

The synergies achieved with collaborative relationships are evident in our work environment; they are also important in our professional development. We look to one another not only for vision but also for realism and efficiency. The efforts put forth by both organizations on this project have resulted in exactly the right balance of vision with a heavy dose of practicality. All of our members will benefit from this venture. Congratulations to the editors and their authors on this exciting new text.

James H. Herndon, MD, MBA
President
American Academy of Orthopaedic Surgeons

Preface

Advanced Reconstruction Foot and Ankle is the first in a new series of technique-focused textbooks developed specifically to address the challenges of complex orthopaedic problems and their complications. Each volume will be dedicated to a specific area of orthopaedics to (1) provide in-depth coverage of a wide variety of topics in a particular subspecialty area and (2) present several options with detailed illustrations for treating each problem. *Advanced Reconstruction* is a natural outgrowth of the *Orthopaedic Knowledge Update* specialty series. The latter continues to be a valuable review of current practice and emerging developments, whereas *Advanced Reconstruction* reflects the demand for a more detailed, focused, and practical approach to complex orthopaedic evaluation and treatments. This volume on foot and ankle surgery is intended for both the general orthopaedist who needs to stay current with advanced care and the foot and ankle subspecialist who demands a state-of-the-art subspecialty textbook that delivers expert direction in a concise and accessible format. The chapters in this volume are authored by recognized experts in foot and ankle surgery; they present many options for treatment of each problem, but the highlight of each chapter is the author's personal choice and rationale for selecting a specific treatment.

Advanced Reconstruction Foot and Ankle is a collaborative effort between the American Orthopaedic Foot and Ankle Society (AOFAS) and the American Academy of Orthopaedic Surgeons (AAOS) and draws on the individual talents of each organization. Each chapter is detailed and technique oriented. You will notice that there are few citations; this was intentional because the content emphasizes the practical, cutting-edge experience and opinion of the author rather than a general review of the literature. Each chapter is formatted in the same way so that you can access the information quickly and easily.

We also wish to thank Brian Donley, MD, and William McGarvey, MD, along with the faculty of Advanced Techniques in Foot and Ankle Surgery. The CD-ROM that accompanies this text shows a number of procedures detailed in the chapters of *Advanced Reconstruction* and were presented at the course. Note that these video demonstrations may differ from information presented in the text. We thank the faculty who donated their materials for the CD-ROM.

We want especially to thank the Boards of the AAOS and the AOFAS for their support of the *Advanced Reconstruction* series. This project exemplifies the great benefits of close collaboration between the AAOS and the specialty societies. We also thank Lynne Shindoll, Managing Editor, and Joan Abern, Senior Editor, for without their exhaustive efforts this text would not have been possible. Also to be thanked are the staff of the Production Department, Mary Steermann, Sophie Tosta, and David Stanley, for ensuring that an enormously complex art program was produced with such high quality. Reid Stanton and Ray Moore of the Electronic Media Department have our thanks for their work on the CD-ROM that accompanies this book. It has been a privilege to work with them. We hope that this volume, and the rest of the series of *Advanced Reconstruction*, will become an essential component of your orthopaedic library.

Glenn B. Pfeffer, MD
James A. Nunley, MD
Roy W. Sanders, MD
Elly Trepman, MD

Table of Contents

Section 6   Athletic Injuries— *James A. Nunley, MD*

SECTION 1
Problems of the Great Toe

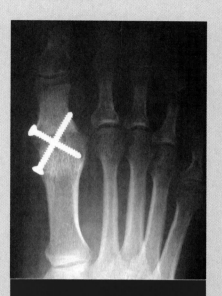

James A. Nunley, MD
Editor

Hallux Valgus With Increased Distal Metatarsal Articular Angle

Michael J. Coughlin, MD

◼ Definition of the Problem

Patient Presentation

Patients who present with a hallux valgus deformity most commonly report pain over a prominent medial eminence, a widened forefoot, and incompatibility with shoe wear; often a history of bunion deformities is noted in other members of the family. However, the underlying radiographic findings may differentiate a hallux valgus deformity that is characterized by a congruent metatarsophalangeal (MTP) joint articulation; this less common type of hallux valgus frequently requires a unique approach to treatment.

To understand the notion of the distal metatarsal angle (DMAA) and its association with hallux valgus, it is important to understand the basic anatomy of the first MTP joint. This MTP joint is stabilized circumferentially by a capsular ligamentous complex on the dorsal, medial, and lateral aspects. On the plantar surface, the medial and lateral sesamoids, enclosed within the tendons of the flexor hallucis brevis, give stability and strength to the plantar capsule. The intrinsic and extrinsic muscles that encircle the MTP joint provide for dorsiflexion and plantar flexion of the toe and stabilize the joint in a mediolateral plane. The first and second metatarsals diverge at their distal extent, normally at an angle of 9° or less; this constitutes the 1-2 intermetatar-

sal angle. The alignment of the hallux and the first metatarsal at their articulation is measured by the hallux valgus angle; the alignment of the distal and proximal phalanges is quantitated by the hallux interphalangeal angle (**Figure 1**).

The proximal phalanx of the hallux articulates with the distal articular surface of the first metatarsal. Both surfaces are covered by a cartilage surface, which is concave on the phalangeal surface and convex on the metatarsal surface. Although it initially might be assumed that these articular surfaces are positioned perpendicular to the longitudinal axis of the proximal phalanx and first metatarsal shaft, that is rarely the case. Frequently there is a slight valgus inclination at the MTP joint, which typifies the normal appearance of the foot as it fits in a toe box that is slightly pointed. Under normal circumstances the great toe is not perfectly straight, and thus, by definition, a hallux valgus angle of less than 15° is considered normal.

When the concept of joint congruity is discussed in relationship to the hallux MTP joint, it is the alignment of the articular surfaces that must be examined. In the case of a normal first ray, with no hallux valgus deformity, the base of the proximal phalanx is aligned concentrically with the first metatarsal head articular surface. This alignment is basically a congruent articulation that may remain congruent for the person's lifetime. However, with the passage of time, a

dynamic hallux valgus deformity develops in some people.

In a dynamic hallux valgus deformity, the base of the proximal phalanx subluxates in a lateral direction as it virtually slides off of the articular surface of the first metatarsal head. This subluxation rarely occurs in a rapid or dramatic fashion but typically develops slowly over a period of years. It begins with mild deviation and, in some cases, progresses to a substantial deformity characterized by a marked increase in the hallux valgus angle and the 1-2 intermetatarsal angle. This condition, characterized as a subluxated hallux valgus deformity, is by far the most common situation seen in adults. This joint relationship can also be described as incongruent or nonconcentric because the articular surfaces have migrated from their original congruent or aligned position to their incongruent or misaligned position. The deformity is described as dynamic because it progresses with time; the hallux can actually deviate more, although improvement or reduction in the deformity rarely if ever occurs.

In contradistinction to the subluxated or incongruent hallux valgus deformity, a congruent hallux valgus deformity may be observed (**Figure 2**). These deformities are decidedly less common, occurring in probably 5% of those with hallux valgus, although they have been noted to occur with increased frequency in adolescent hallux valgus deformities and in men with hallux valgus. What typifies

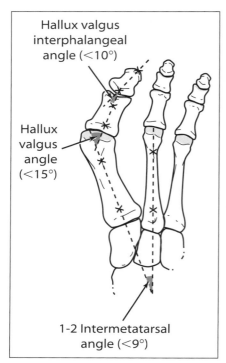

Hallux valgus interphalangeal angle (<10°)

Hallux valgus angle (<15°)

1-2 Intermetatarsal angle (<9°)

Figure 1 The hallux valgus and 1-2 intermetatarsal angles are formed by the intersection of the diaphyseal axes of the proximal phalanx, first metatarsal, and second metatarsal. The interphalangeal angle is formed by the axis of the distal phalanx (reference points at the tip of the phalanx and the center of the proximal articular surface) and the axis of the proximal phalanx. (Reproduced with permission from Coughlin MJ: Hallux valgus in men: Effect of the distal metatarsal articular angle on hallux valgus correction. *Foot Ankle Int* 1997;18:463-470.)

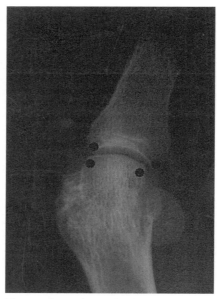

Figure 2 Radiograph demonstrating a congruent hallux valgus deformity. (The marks identify the medial and lateral extent of the articular surface.)

a congruent hallux valgus deformity is the concentric relationship of the corresponding articular surfaces. The deformity is static and rarely progresses because the hallux valgus is a result of the angular relationship of the articular surfaces to the long axis of the phalanx and first metatarsal and not of subluxation at the MTP joint. Thus, in younger patients with hallux valgus, a congruent deformity is more often the underlying cause of the hallux valgus. Although this deformity rarely progresses, the patient's age at presentation depends on when symptoms develop.

All hallux valgus deformities are quantitated by measuring the hallux valgus angle, the hallux interphalangeal angle, and the 1-2 intermetatarsal angle; however, the analysis of a congruent deformity requires estimation of the angulation of the respective articular surfaces. The major deformity typically occurs at the distal articular surface of the first metatarsal. The DMAA defines the relationship of the articular surface of the distal metatarsal to the longitudinal axis of the first metatarsal (**Figure 3**, *A*). A DMAA of less than 6° is considered normal. The proximal phalangeal articular angle (PPAA) defines the relationship of the articular surface of the proximal aspect of the proximal phalanx to the longitudinal axis of the proximal phalanx. A PPAA of less than 10° is considered normal (**Figure 3**, *B*). Whereas it is relatively easy to obtain angular measurements while evaluating a hallux valgus deformity, estimating the medial and lateral extent of the metatarsal articular surface can be difficult, especially in the younger patient. The reliability of this analysis depends on the experience of

the physician, and the angular measurements sometimes may be accurately estimated only at the time of surgical correction. Nonetheless, in many circumstances careful inspection of the radiographs of all hallux valgus deformities will uncover an increased DMAA that may otherwise have not been noticed.

Physical Examination

The history and physical examination of a patient with a hallux valgus deformity should include an in-depth family history and a history of shoe wear, injury, and any factors that may influence the onset of progression of a hallux valgus deformity. A positive family history is associated with a higher incidence of a congruent deformity. Typically, constricting shoe wear is not a factor in the progression of deformity; however, it may lead to discomfort and eventual medical evaluation. A history of early onset of a bunion and the development of a bunion deformity in a man typically is associated with an increased risk of a congruent hallux valgus deformity.

The physical examination should include evaluation of the patient in both standing and sitting positions. Frequently, the deformity is accentuated with the patient standing. Attention should be directed to the posture of the forefoot and hindfoot and to ankle motion. Pes planus, pes cavus, metatarsus adductus, and a contracted Achilles tendon are no more common in patients with hallux valgus than in the general population; nonetheless, patients should be evaluated for these problems because they may require other treatment. Assessment of the mobility of the metatarsocuneiform joint is also part of the evaluation process because, in a small percentage of patients with a congruent hallux valgus deformity, metatarsocuneiform hypermobility must be addressed as well.

The forefoot is examined for any lateral forefoot or lesser toe deformi-

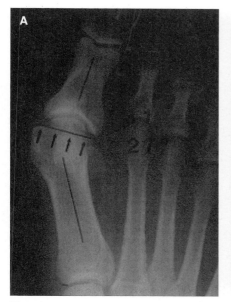

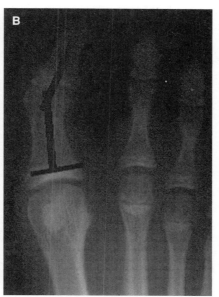

Figure 3 Representative examples of DMAA and PPAA. **A,** Congruent hallux valgus deformity with a hallux valgus angle of 31° and DMAA of 27°. Almost all of the hallux valgus is caused by the DMAA. **B,** Hallux valgus interphalangeus with angulation at the proximal phalanx. (Reproduced with permission from Mann R, Coughlin M: Adult hallux valgus, in Coughlin M, Mann R (eds): *Surgery of the Foot and Ankle,* ed 7. St. Louis, MO, Mosby, 1999, pp 150-269.)

ties and for callosities; the neurovascular status of the foot is examined as well. Attention is then directed to the first ray, which is inspected for alignment and motion. The magnitude of valgus of both the distal and proximal phalanx is quantitated, and pronation of the hallux is noted. Passive dorsiflexion and plantar flexion are noted. Then the great toe is deviated into a corrected alignment with the metatarsal articular surface, and range of motion is again evaluated. This provocative test is performed to determine if passive range of motion is decreased when the articular surfaces are realigned. In the presence of a congruent articulation, motion is often decreased. In the presence of a subluxated articulation, motion often does not diminish.

Weight-bearing AP and lateral radiographs are obtained to evaluate the hallux valgus deformity. Axes of the first and second metatarsals, the proximal and distal phalanges of the hallux, and the DMAA are drawn to analyze the deformity.

Differential Diagnosis
- Mild, moderate, or severely subluxated deformity
- Metatarsocuneiform hypermobility
- Degenerative arthritis of the MTP joint

Additional Work-Up
Rarely are hematologic or chemistry studies needed before bunion surgery unless there is an underlying medical problem. On occasion, further evaluation of the hallux valgus deformity to assess the MTP articulation necessitates CT or MRI. Adding air or contrast media may assist in defining the extent and shape of the articular cartilage.

───────■

■ The Solutions

Treatment Options and Rationale
For mild congruent hallux valgus deformities, the DMAA is not greatly in-

creased. By definition, a mild deformity is characterized by a hallux valgus angle less than or equal to 20°. Thus, a distal metatarsal osteotomy usually will suffice for correcting the DMAA and the angular deformity of the first ray. Choices to be considered are the chevron osteotomy, a distal closing wedge osteotomy (Reverdin), Mitchell osteotomy, and Scarf osteotomy. There are numerous other variations; however, these techniques are probably the most commonly used. A major consideration, however, is that all these osteotomies do not change the MTP articulation but rather achieve correction by a periarticular osteotomy. A distal soft-tissue realignment in the presence of a congruent deformity will create an incongruent articulation that may be at risk for joint stiffness, degenerative arthritis, or recurrence. Sometimes recurrence may be dramatic and rapid, within weeks or months after surgery (**Figure 4**). It is beyond the scope of this chapter to provide a step-by-step description of the surgical procedures; however, diagrammatic descriptions are helpful to understand the principles of specific procedures.

For moderate congruent hallux valgus deformities, the magnitude of the DMAA may vary from greater than 20° to less than or equal to 40°, and much if not all of the hallux valgus deformity can be attributed to this angulation. A Scarf osteotomy (**Figure 5**) or a biplanar chevron osteotomy (**Figure 6**) often will be adequate to correct the lower moderate deformities, but these osteotomies are underpowered for greater deformities. A closing wedge distal metaphyseal osteotomy can achieve greater correction in these instances. As the 1-2 intermetatarsal angle increases, a proximal osteotomy may be necessary; options include but are not exclusive to an opening wedge cuneiform osteotomy or a proximal first metatarsal osteotomy (opening wedge,

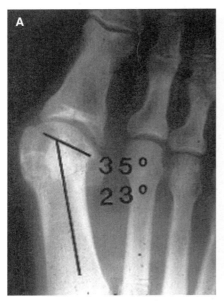
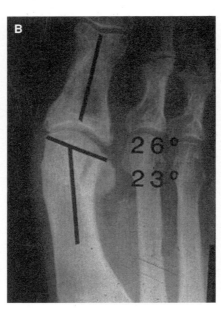
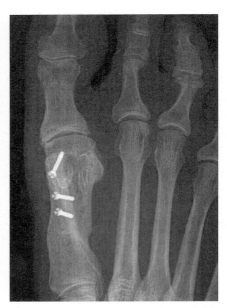

Figure 4   A, Preoperative radiograph demonstrating congruent hallux valgus deformity (hallux valgus angle = 35°, DMAA = 23°). **B,** Postoperative radiograph demonstrating recurrence (hallux valgus angle = 26°, DMAA = 23°). With a soft-tissue realignment, the DMAA limits the angular correction.

Figure 5   Postoperative AP radiograph following Scarf osteotomy. (Courtesy of P. Rippstein, MD)

closing wedge, crescentic). Often, an element of hallux valgus interphalangeus is present with moderate and severe deformities, and a closing wedge phalangeal osteotomy (Akin) may be considered as well.

In severe congruent hallux valgus deformities, the hallux valgus angle is greater than 40°, and much if not all of the deformity is a result of the increased DMAA. Surgical options remain similar to those for high moderate deformities. On occasion, there may be an element of further subluxation superimposed on a sloped distal metatarsal articular surface. In this situation, a capsulorrhaphy may also be a component of the surgical repair.

Author's Preferred Treatment and Rationale

The armamentarium of a foot and ankle surgeon should include several procedures with which to correct the underlying pathology associated with a congruent hallux valgus deformity. For hallux valgus interphalangeus, a closing wedge phalangeal osteotomy is frequently a component of any of

these other first ray realignment procedures. This closing wedge osteotomy may be in the proximal or distal metaphysis, depending on the location of the major phalangeal misalignment.

For a mild and low moderate deformity with a DMAA of 25° or less, a chevron osteotomy or a biplanar osteotomy is a reliable means of correcting the DMAA. Double and triple first ray osteotomies are preferable for correcting upper moderate and severe deformities and are used depending on the amount of correction necessary (**Figure 7**). A closing wedge distal metaphyseal osteotomy can be performed to correct a large amount of the increased DMAA. A proximal crescentic osteotomy can be performed to obtain a large correction of the increased 1-2 intermetatarsal angle. A phalangeal osteotomy can be performed to correct an increased interphalangeal deformity. Usually internal fixation is achieved with buried Kirschner wires that are removed 6 weeks after surgery.

Ambulation is allowed in a postoperative shoe, walking boot, or below knee cast, depending on the stability of the osteotomies, security of internal fixation, and reliability of the patient. Care must also be taken during any surgical exposure, certainly in the first ray when multiple osteotomies are performed, to minimize excess surgical dissection to prevent devascularization of bone. A lateral MTP joint release is not performed in association with a closing wedge distal metatarsal osteotomy; when multiple osteotomies are performed in the first ray, care is taken to leave an extensive soft-tissue bridge on the intervening tissue to minimize the chance of vascular compromise that will affect ultimate bone healing.

Management of Complications

Complications after surgical correction of a hallux valgus deformity are numerous and include wound healing problems, osseous delayed unions and nonunions, nerve injuries, and a host of other expected and unexpected

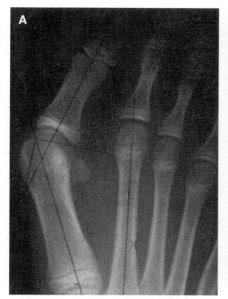

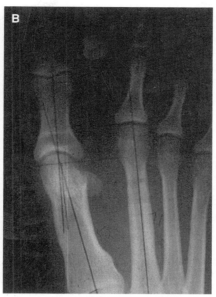

Figure 6 Biplanar chevron osteotomy. **A,** Preoperative radiograph demonstrating congruent hallux valgus deformity. **B,** Radiograph following phalangeal, biplanar distal chevron and proximal crescentic osteotomies.

problems. The main complications particular to a congruent MTP joint with hallux valgus are undercorrection, recurrence, osteonecrosis, and malunion.

Undercorrection can occur when an underpowered procedure is used for correction. For example, a chevron osteotomy is not very likely to achieve total correction of a severe

deformity. Analysis of the reasons for undercorrection will enable the physician to plan the salvage procedure, which may be a revision with periarticular osteotomies, or an MTP fusion may be a final solution. Recurrence is more often associated with failure to recognize the underlying congruent joint and may develop if the magnitude of the articular slope is underestimated. In this situation, a revision with periarticular osteotomies again may be the route of salvage. Osteonecrosis can occur after a procedure in which the vascular supply to the metatarsal head or the base of the proximal phalanx has been disrupted. It also can occur following attempts to salvage a failed correction, and a patient should be advised about the risks of salvage surgery. Usually the salvage following osteonecrosis is an MTP fusion. Malunion is probably one of the most significant risks when multiple first ray osteotomies are performed. Kirschner wire fixation usually is adequate, but external immobilization may be necessary if the osteotomy has

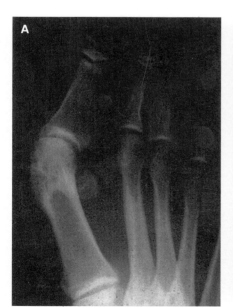

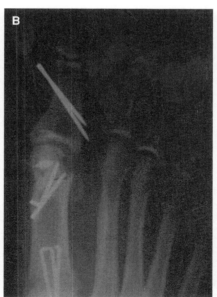

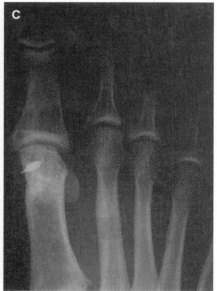

Figure 7 Multiple first ray osteotomies. **A,** Preoperative radiograph demonstrating recurrent hallux valgus deformity with substantial DMAA. **B,** Intraoperative radiograph demonstrating phalangeal, distal metatarsal, and proximal metatarsal osteotomies. **C,** At long-term follow-up, a suture anchor that was used to repair a medial capsular tear is shown. Alignment is acceptable. (Reproduced with permission from Mann R, Coughlin M: Adult hallux valgus, in Coughlin M, Mann R (eds): *Surgery of the Foot and Ankle*, ed 7. St. Louis, MO, Mosby, 1999, pp 150-269.)

questionable stability or patient reliability is in doubt. A malunion may actually result in an acceptable outcome; however, if over- or undercorrection results in an unacceptable outcome, a correctional osteotomy may be considered. It is usually wise to wait several months before proceeding with correctional osteotomies to decrease the chance of osteonecrosis, delayed union, or wound healing problems. ━━━■

References

Coughlin M, Carlson R: Treatment of hallux valgus with an increased distal metatarsal articular angle: Evaluation of double and triple first ray osteotomies. *Foot Ankle Int* 1999;20:762-770.

Coughlin M, Freund E: The reliability of angular measurements in hallux valgus deformities. *Foot Ankle Int* 2001;22:369-379.

Coughlin M, Saltzman C, Nunley J: Angular measurements in the evaluation of hallux valgus deformities: A report of the ad hoc committee of the American Orthopaedic Foot and Ankle Society on Angular Measurements. *Foot Ankle Int* 2002;23:68-74.

Mann R, Coughlin M: Adult hallux valgus, in Coughlin M, Mann R (eds): *Surgery of the Foot and Ankle*, ed 7. St Louis, MO, Mosby, 1999, pp 150-269.

Coding

ICD-9 CODE
735.0   Acquired deformities of toe, Hallux valgus (acquired)

CPT CODES
28292   Correction, hallux valgus (bunion), with or without sesamoidectomy; Keller, McBride or Mayo type procedure

28296   Correction, hallux valgus (bunion) with or without sesamoidectomy; with metatarsal osteotomy (eg, Mitchell, chevron, or concentric type procedures)

28297   Correction, hallux valgus (bunion) with or without sesamoidectomy; Lapidus type procedure

28298   Correction, hallux valgus (bunion) with or without sesamoidectomy; by phalanx osteotomy

28299   Correction, hallux valgus (bunion) with or without sesamoidectomy; by double osteotomy

Stiffness After Bunion Surgery
Arthur K. Walling, MD

Definition of the Problem

Patient Presentation

So many corrective bunion procedures are performed that there is a potential for complications even when the surgery is performed by an experienced surgeon under well-planned and meticulous conditions. Although many complications are possible after bunion surgery, symptomatic postoperative stiffness is rare. However, a symptomatic decrease in the range of motion in the metatarsophalangeal (MTP) joint is so common that all patients should be advised that they may lose flexibility in the joint following surgery. Because unrealistic expectations often lead patients to believe the procedure has failed, it is imperative to include loss of joint motion as a potential outcome of bunion surgery.

Causes of symptomatic postoperative stiffness include infection, inappropriate surgical procedure, osteonecrosis, and fibrosis of the joint. A deep postoperative infection can certainly lead to marked fibrosis or degenerative arthritis within the joint. Selection of an inappropriate procedure to correct the pathology producing the bunion can result in stiffness as well. The deformity of

patients with significant metatarsus primus varus can be overcorrected to the point that a negative intermetatarsal angle develops. This overcorrection brings the metatarsal head into excessive lateral deviation such that the articular surface of the first metatarsal is sloped laterally. This slope can produce an incongruent joint that may be painful, and degenerative changes can develop, leading to increased stiffness (**Figure 1**). Stiffness can also result from converting an unrecognized congruent joint to an incongruent one. In this situ-

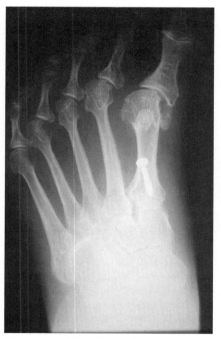

Figure 1 AP radiograph shows hallux varus and arthritic changes secondary to overcorrection of the intermetatarsal angle and overplication of the medial capsule.

ation, the incongruency may lead to arthrosis and decreased motion. If there is significant arthrosis in the joint before surgery, realignment can lead to stiffness. Over imbrication of the medial capsule in an attempt to better position the hallux may also result in decreased motion through the MTP joint. The obvious way to avoid these problems is to select the proper initial procedure.

Osteonecrosis of the metatarsal head is another cause of stiffness. Although the true incidence of osteonecrosis is extremely difficult to determine, there is no question that it does occur. However, development of osteonecrosis does not necessarily mean that the joint will become symptomatic.

Occasionally, following hallux valgus correction, fibrosis of the joint results in decreased first MTP motion and pain.

Physical Examination

The most obvious finding is decreased range of motion within the first MTP joint with accompanying pain. Appropriate radiographs will usually identify incongruencies, arthrosis, or osteonecrosis. If no joint abnormality is identified, capsular joint contracture should be suspected as the cause of the restricted motion.

Differential Diagnosis
- Deep infection
- Osteonecrosis

Additional Work-up

If infection in the joint is suspected, an erythrocyte sedimentation rate or a

C-reactive protein may be used as a screening procedure. Generally, it is better to consider aspiration of the joint and/or thin needle biopsy of bone if deep infection is suspected. MRI could be used, but it would rarely be beneficial in the postoperative situation.

———————————■

■ The Solutions

Treatment Options and Rationale

Treatment goals for patients with postoperative joint stiffness include

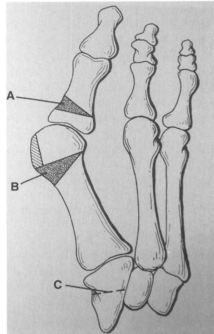

Figure 2 Multiple first ray osteotomies can be used to achieve extra-articular correction of a hallux valgus deformity, especially with an increased DMAA. They can also be used to salvage over- or undercorrection when arthrosis is not present. A = Closing wedge osteotomy of the phalanx. B = Closing wedge osteotomy of distal first metatarsal. C = Opening wedge osteotomy of the first cuneiform. (Reproduced with permission from Mann RA, Coughlin MJ: Juvenile hallux valgus, in Coughlin MJ, Mann RA (eds): *Surgery of the Foot and Ankle*, ed 7. St. Louis, MO, Mosby, 1999, p 311.)

decreasing pain, possibly correcting any deformity, and increasing function. Nonsurgical treatment includes nonsteroidal anti-inflammatory medications, if tolerated, and attempts at shoe modification to limit excursion through the MTP joint. An insole with a Morton's extension allows mobility from shoe to shoe. The addition of an extended steel or fiberglass shank to the sole is another effective way of decreasing pressure through the joint.

Surgical treatment consists of corrective osteotomies, capsular release, interpositional capsular arthroplasty, resection arthroplasty (Keller), or arthrodesis, depending on the pathology responsible for the stiffness.

Author's Preferred Treatment and Rationale

If stiffness is secondary to incongruency of the joint and no arthrosis has developed, correction of the incongruency may be considered. The incongruency may be corrected when

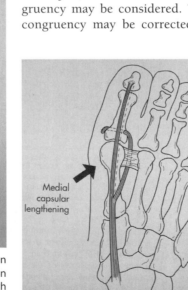

Figure 3 When hallux varus occurs without joint arthrosis, medial capsular release with partial extensor hallucis longus tendon transfer provides excellent correction. (Reproduced with permission from Mann RA, Coughlin MJ: Adult hallux valgus, in Coughlin MJ, Mann RA (eds): *Surgery of the Foot and Ankle*, ed 7. St. Louis, MO, Mosby, 1999, pp 150-269.)

the intermetatarsal angle has been overcorrected, resulting in lateral tilt of the distal metatarsal articular surface. In this case a distal soft-tissue release is performed, and the proximal metatarsal malunion is corrected to restore the normal relationship between the metatarsal head and the proximal phalanx. The other situation in which a corrective osteotomy may be useful is when an unrecognized congruent joint with a high distal metatarsal articular angle has been improperly corrected, resulting in an incongruent joint (**Figure 2**). In this instance, distal soft-tissue release is coupled with a closing wedge distal metatarsal osteotomy to reestablish congruency.

As mentioned earlier, only rarely does symptomatic stiffness in which there is no obvious cause for the fibrosis occur following hallux valgus correction. In this instance, no obvious incongruity or arthrosis is visible on radiographs, and joint motion is restricted to the point of pain. To be symptomatic, motion usually is restricted to less than 10° to 15° of dorsiflexion at the MTP joint. In my experience, the most common denominator in this unusual situation is pain out of proportion to the procedure and a patient's lack of willingness to begin active joint mobilization. If excessive stiffness is detected early in the postoperative course, the joint should be mobilized sooner than usual in an attempt to prevent the situation from becoming worse. If seen later, vigorous physical therapy, consisting of active assisted and passive manipulation, should be instituted in an attempt to mobilize the joint. Usually this therapy will result in at least enough improvement in dorsiflexion to make the toe functional.

In the 5 years from 1996 to 2001, I performed approximately 180 hallux valgus procedures. Among these I could identify only three patients who had residual postoperative stiffness

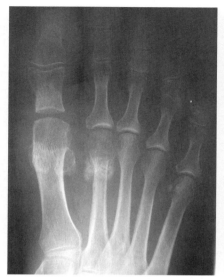

Figure 4 Stress fractures of the second and (eventually) third metatarsals developed in a young, active patient who was treated with Keller resection arthroplasty.

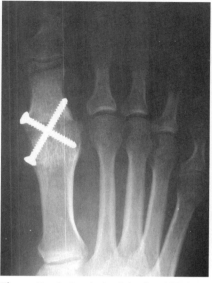

Figure 5 Arthrodesis of the first MTP joint using two 3.5-mm compression screws with one screw placed proximal to distal and the other placed distal to proximal.

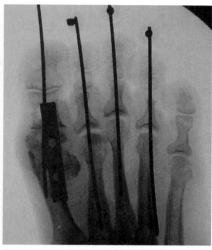

Figure 6 Arthrodesis of the first MTP joint for a failed Silastic implant using an interpositional tricortical bone graft to restore length and a dorsal plate to add stability.

that did not respond to physical therapy and remained symptomatic enough that repeat surgery was offered in an attempt to improve range of motion. Two patients had distal chevron procedures, and one patient had a proximal crescentic osteotomy and distal soft-tissue release. Their average dorsiflexion was 12°. At the time of surgery the dorsal and plantar capsule was released, including the plantar plate. There was mild fibrosis but no real intra-articular adhesions were noted. Intraoperative motion was increased by an average of 20°. Aggressive range-of-motion exercises were begun immediately following the surgery. Most of the regained motion was retained (± 5°), and all three patients felt that the second surgery was beneficial from the standpoint of both pain relief and functional improvement.

In patients who have only mild first MTP arthrosis and whose valgus deformity can be corrected, interpositional arthroplasty may be an option instead of arthrodesis. In this procedure, a portion of joint capsule, extensor hallucis brevis tendon, or both is interpositioned between the degenerated articular surfaces to preserve the joint space and allow motion (**Figure 3**). It is imperative to advise the patient that this procedure may result in more stiffness, pain, and dissatisfaction that may ultimately require a fusion.

Keller resection arthroplasty remains a possible option for the postoperatively stiff first MTP joint. Historically this is recommended only for patients who are elderly, otherwise disabled, or have a less demanding lifestyle. The Keller procedure is frequently complicated by dorsal displacement of the hallux and transfer metatarsalgia (**Figure 4**). Avoidance of excessive proximal phalanx resection and reattachment of the plantar tendon attachments may reduce the complications, but I personally do not use this option often and believe that patient selection is paramount.

For all other situations in which postoperative stiffness is related to first MTP arthritis, the primary salvage method is arthrodesis. To some extent the surgical approach is dictated by previous surgical incisions, but when at all possible I prefer a dorsal incision. I create opposing flat surfaces for apposition, although the option of ball-and-socket preparation has been advocated as being easier for adjustment of position. Optimal position is 15° of valgus and 10° to 15° of dorsiflexion in relation to the plantar aspect of the foot. Two 3.5-mm lag screws are usually sufficient for fixation (**Figure 5**). A dorsal plate also may be added for additional fixation. Fusion rates with this technique approach 96%. Postoperatively, patients are allowed to bear weight as tolerated in a postoperative wooden shoe for 6 to 8 weeks.

Management of Complications
For any of the joint-preserving procedures that fail, the best salvage remains arthrodesis. Salvage of the Keller resection arthroplasty is more difficult because of the loss of length of the proximal phalanx. Because of this, and to reestablish normal weight bearing through the first ray, it may be necessary to add an interpositional bone graft to the arthrodesis (**Figure 6**).

The primary complications from arthrodesis are nonunion, malunion, and degenerative arthrosis of the interphalangeal joint of the great toe. Often a nonunion will actually result in a pseudarthrosis that is not painful and requires no treatment. Symptomatic nonunions or malunions require repositioning and refusion.

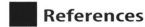

References

Mann RA, Coughlin MJ: Adult hallux valgus, in Coughlin MJ, Mann RA (eds): *Surgery of the Foot and Ankle*, ed 7. St. Louis, MO, Mosby, 1999, pp 150-269.

Richardson EG: Complications after hallux valgus surgery. *Instr Course Lect* 1999;48:331-342.

Sammarco GJ, Idusuyi OB: Complications after surgery of the hallux. *Clin Orthop* 2001;391:59-71.

Trnka HJ: Arthrodesis procedures for salvage of the hallux metatarsophalangeal joint. *Foot Ankle Clin* 2000;5:673-686.

Coding

ICD-9 CODES

715.97 Osteoarthrosis, unspecified whether generalized or localized, ankle and foot

735.0 Acquired deformities of toe, Hallux valgus (acquired)

735.1 Acquired deformities of toe, Hallux varus (acquired)

CPT CODES

28270 Capsulotomy; metatarsophalangeal joint, with or without tenorrhaphy, each joint (separate procedure)

28292 Correction, hallux valgus (bunion), with or without sesamoidectomy; Keller, McBride or Mayo type procedure

28306 Osteotomy, with or without lengthening, shortening or angular correction, metatarsal; first metatarsal

28322 Repair nonunion or malunion; metatarsal, with or without bone graft (includes obtaining graft)

28750 Arthrodesis, great toe; metatarsophalangeal joint

Hallux Varus

Mark S. Myerson, MD

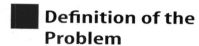

Definition of the Problem

Patient Presentation

Usually, hallux varus occurs following procedures for the correction of hallux valgus. Although idiopathic hallux varus and deformity of the hallux may occur after trauma, rheumatologic conditions, and generalized ligamentous laxity, most hallux varus occurs following attempted correction of hallux valgus deformity.

Following bunion surgery, patients may present either early (within a few weeks) or late (several months) with a varus deviation of the great toe. The deformity may be mild and not noticeable with shoe wear or may be severe and prevent normal shoe wear.

Hallux varus following bunionectomy is the result of interruption of the conjoint tendon of the lateral head of the flexor hallucis brevis (FHB) and the adductor hallucis and, therefore, is usually a result of excessive lateral soft-tissue release with or without sesamoidectomy (**Figure 1**). It can, however, occur as a result of excessive tightening of the medial capsulorrhaphy or following a malunion of the first metatarsal osteotomy, whether this osteotomy is performed proximally or distally. Excessive removal of the medial eminence with exostectomy can lead to medial subluxation of the tibial sesamoid with imbalance and hallux varus.

Physical Examination

The examination focuses on the static and dynamic function of the hallux and the forefoot. Specifically, evaluation should focus on whether the deformity affects the hallux alone, or if there are secondary changes in the lesser toes. Usually in long-standing cases, the lesser toes will follow the position of the hallux, drifting into a varus, adducted position. The range of motion of both the hallux metatarsophalangeal (MTP) and interphalangeal (IP) joints are checked. Is there a fixed contracture at either of these joints? Is there crepitus to range of motion? Is a fixed deformity of the hallux present, or is it flexible, and reducible to the neutral position? Is there any pain under the MTP joint, indicating possible sesamoid pathology? Weight-bearing radiographs of both feet are obtained. No additional imaging studies are necessary, unless there is evidence of osteonecrosis of the metatarsal head, in which case MRI may be obtained.

Differential Diagnosis
None

Additional Work-up
No additional work-up is required.

———————————■

The Solutions

Treatment Options and Rationale
The type of treatment is determined by the flexibility of the MTP and IP joints. With muscle imbalance of the FHB and the extensor hallucis brevis (EHB), as well as the abductor and adductor hallucis, the deformity will gradually increase. This increase leads to a wide spectrum of pathologies, including fixed deformity of the MTP and IP joints with or without arthritis of the MTP joint. Fortunately, the IP joint remains flexible for most hallux varus deformities. Over time, however, with increasing imbalance of the FHB and EHB, a contracture of the IP joint will occur (**Figure 2**). If a rigid contracture or arthritis of the IP joint is present, an arthrodesis of this joint is necessary because manipulation or release of the joint contracture is not successful. Once an arthrodesis of the IP joint is performed, the MTP joint must be corrected either dynamically with a tendon transfer or statically by restoring ligament stability with a tenodesis.

Maintaining MTP joint mobility is ideal, but not always possible, because arthritis or rigid deformity of this joint may be present. In the presence of an extremely rigid deformity with contracture of the MTP joint, both in varus and extension, the likelihood of attaining soft-tissue balance using a tendon transfer is unlikely. In these cases, an arthrodesis of the MTP joint is preferable. However, a resection arthroplasty of the MTP joint can be considered for some patients. Arthrodesis of the MTP joint is a good salvage procedure, but it should not be performed if the IP joint is de-

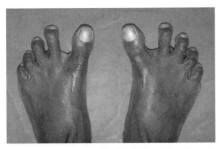

Figure 1 Bilateral hallux varus developed following a distal soft-tissue release with sesamoidectomy and medial exostectomy for correction of hallux valgus.

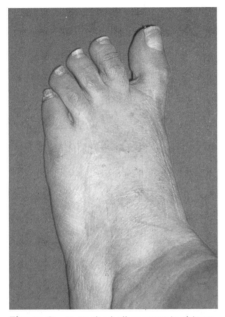

Figure 2 Note the hallux varus in this patient is associated with dorsal extension contracture of the MTP joint, as well as a flexion contracture of the IP joint.

formed. This situation presents a difficult treatment decision in the occasional patient who presents with arthritis of the MTP joint and rigid contracture of the IP joint. Addition of an arthrodesis of the IP joint to an arthrodesis of the MTP joint is not the ideal procedure because it results in significant rigidity and problems with toe-off. For these patients, an arthrodesis of the IP joint can be combined with a resection arthroplasty of the MTP joint.

Wherever possible, therefore, tendon transfer should be used to correct the deformity. As noted, tendon transfer is contraindicated if either arthritis or rigidity of the MTP joint is present; deformity of the first metatarsal is another contraindication to tendon transfer alone. For example, some patients with hallux varus have a malunion of the first metatarsal, either from a distal or proximal metatarsal osteotomy, and an MTP joint that remains fairly flexible. Usually, there is overcorrection of the metatarsal with a negative intermetatarsal angle, which leads to medial subluxation of the MTP joint and hallux varus. If the malunion of the first metatarsal is left uncorrected, it is unlikely that tendon transfer can result in adequate maintenance of soft-tissue balance. Correction of the metatarsal alignment with osteotomy must then be performed in conjunction with a tendon transfer.

Not all patients with hallux varus will undergo surgical correction. Deformity that has been present for many years, remains flexible, and is more of a cosmetic concern for the patient very often does not require surgical correction. It is surprising that slight varus positioning of the hallux, which is noted radiographically but not clinically, is quite well accepted and tolerated by patients. Some patients may experience very slight pressure on the medial aspect of the hallux with shoe wear but provided this pressure is not progressive, it is rarely necessary to correct this type of deformity.

Author's Preferred Treatment and Rationale

I divide the surgical approach into those procedures that primarily address the soft tissues (abductor hallucis release, tendon transfer, or tenodesis), the bone (first metatarsal osteotomy, hallux proximal phalangeal osteotomy), or the joint (arthrodesis of the IP joint and arthrodesis or resection arthroplasty of the

MTP joint). Whenever soft-tissue procedures (tendon transfer or tenodesis) are performed, it is imperative that there is balance of both ligaments with muscle balance about the hallux MTP joint. Therefore, the abductor hallucis tendon should be lengthened and a medial capsulotomy performed in conjunction with the lateral stabilizing procedure. In rare situations in which symptomatic hallux varus is diagnosed immediately postoperatively and can be determined to be caused by excessive bandaging or overplication of the capsule medially, simple release of the capsulorrhaphy may be sufficient. For all other situations, tendon and soft-tissue balancing is required.

ARTHRODESIS AND RESECTION ARTHROPLASTY

For correction of rigid deformity, I prefer arthrodesis, and occasionally, either because of a fixed, contracted IP joint or patient preference, resection arthroplasty of the base of the proximal phalanx. If either of these procedures is performed, further soft-tissue balancing usually is not required.

For the resection arthroplasty, the cut of the base of the proximal phalanx must be vertical. The surgeon should be careful with the plane of the cut to prevent any further inadvertent dorsiflexion of the MTP joint, and the varus deformity can be addressed by making the cut perpendicular to the long axis of the proximal phalanx with a very slight valgus inclination. This arthroplasty needs to be performed in conjunction with complete release of the medial joint contracture.

Arthrodesis of the MTP joint can be performed according to the surgeon's preference. However, because of the aberrant position of the metatarsal head, the prior medial exostectomy, and the malunion of the first metatarsal, arthrodesis needs to be performed very carefully. I have found that it is quite difficult to accurately position the hallux as a result of various deformities about the MTP joint.

The normal landmarks for positioning the phalanx on the first metatarsal cannot always be followed, and it often is easier to use the clinical position of the hallux to guide the final position for the arthrodesis.

TENDON TRANSFERS

Various tendon transfers are available for correction of dynamic deformity. These are indicated by the presence of flexible IP and MTP joints. The use of the entire extensor hallucis longus (EHL) tendon in conjunction with arthrodesis of the IP joint has been described; this is a good procedure when an arthrodesis of the IP joint is performed. However, when the IP joint is flexible, it is unnecessary to fuse the joint, and in this instance, either a portion of the EHL (a split transfer of the EHL) or a transfer using the EHB is performed.

It is important to distinguish a tendon transfer, which has the potential for dynamic correction of deformity, from a tenodesis in which the tendon is used as a static device to replace a torn ligament. Both apply to the EHL and EHB transfer. One of the problems I have experienced with the split EHL transfer is that when the tendon is split from proximal to distal and the lateral half of the tendon used for the transfer, the medial half of the EHL never retains adequate tension. There is no way to avoid this imbalance and loss of tension in the tendon. Shortening the medial half of the tendon further weakens an already compromised tendon, leading to dorsiflexion weakness. An alternative would be to use the EHL in a tenodesis procedure by splitting the tendon from distal to proximal in the same way that the EHB tenodesis is performed. Gen-

erally, it is preferable to maintain the EHL intact, and in the presence of flexible IP and MTP joints, I prefer to use the EHB in a tenodesis procedure. From a technical standpoint, the EHB tenodesis can be performed almost identically to the EHL tenodesis.

Through a dorsal longitudinal incision, lateral to the EHL tendon, the EHB tendon is identified and carefully dissected from the EHL and extensor retinaculum. Proximally, the EHB is transected just distal to the musculotendinous junction at the level of the base of the first metatarsal. A careful dissection is performed distal to the MTP joint by releasing the extensor hood dorsally. If there is concern about overrelease of the EHB or if the distal attachment of the EHB is tenuous, a suture can be inserted to maintain its attachment to the extensor hood. A No. 2-0 suture is inserted on the tip of the EHB using a fine needle, and this curved needle is then passed under the deep transverse metatarsal ligament from distal to proximal. A curved tapered needle (an aneurysm needle) works well here. It is not absolutely necessary to pass the tendon under the deep transverse metatarsal ligament, and any firm tether from scar tissue in the first web space is sufficient.

A drill hole is then made from medial to lateral in the distal neck of the first metatarsal, and the tendon is passed through the drill hole and secured under tension. Before tightening the tendon, adequate balance must be restored. I prefer to see that the hallux is lying in a neutral position after release of the medial capsule and contracted abductor tendon. A Z-lengthening of the abductor tendon can be performed. There is always sufficient

length of the EHB tendon to suture it back down over the dorsal periosteum; a nonresorbable suture should be used.

The EHL tenodesis is performed in exactly the same manner. There is usually more available tendon from the split EHL, and the tendon can be passed back onto itself over the dorsal surface of the metatarsal following passage through the drill hole. It should not be necessary to fix the MTP joint with a Kirschner wire during surgery. Adequate balance should have been restored with the tendon transfer or tenodesis.

I like to use taping to maintain the hallux in an overcorrected position with slight valgus for 2 months. Patients are allowed to bear weight immediately after this procedure while wearing a postoperative walking shoe. After 4 weeks patients are allowed to use a stiff-soled shoe. Toe-off with bending of the MTP joint should not be allowed for 8 weeks.

Management of Complications

The most common complications of correction of hallux varus using tendon transfer is recurrence of deformity. Usually, the patient is asymptomatic since the deformity has been improved; however, this may not necessarily be the case. If the patient is symptomatic, then repeat tendon transfer is unlikely to work, and either an arthrodesis or arthroplasty of the MTP joint would be necessary. The latter two alternatives also apply if arthritis in the MTP joint occurs. If an arthrodesis of the IP joint has already been performed, then an arthroplasty of the MTP joint is preferable.

References

Johnson KA, Spiegl PV: Extensor hallucis longus transfer for hallux varus deformity. *J Bone Joint Surg Am* 1984;66:681-686.

Myerson MS, Komenda GA: Results of hallux varus correction using an extensor hallucis brevis tenodesis. *Foot Ankle Int* 1996;17:21-27.

Skalley TC, Myerson MS: The operative treatment of acquired hallux varus. *Clin Orthop* 1994;306:183-191.

Coding

ICD-9 CODES

718.47   Contracture of joint, ankle and foot

719.07   Effusion of joint, ankle and foot

719.77   Difficulty in walking, ankle and foot

735.1   Hallux varus (acquired)

CPT CODES

27690   Transfer or transplant of single tendon

28292   Arthroplasty, hallux metatarsophalangeal joint

28750   Arthrodesis, great toe; metatarsophalangeal joint

28755   Arthrodesis, great toe; interphalangeal joint

Malunion of a Proximal First Metatarsal Osteotomy

Roger A. Mann, MD

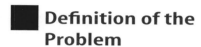

Definition of the Problem

Patient Presentation

Whenever an osteotomy is created, the potential for a malunion exists, whether it is in the foot or any other extremity. This malunion may occur because the osteotomy was biomechanically unsound, because a technical problem developed, or because of the patient's biology. Because the foot is a weight-bearing structure, a malunion often is symptomatic as a result of altered weight bearing of the first metatarsal and the resultant transfer metatarsalgia.

The foot may be able to compensate for a malunion if there is an adequate range of motion of the first metatarsophalangeal (MTP) joint. The windlass mechanism depresses the first metatarsal head during terminal stance, and weight is transferred from the metatarsal area to the hallux, further unloading the metatarsal heads, especially the second and third heads. If the deformity is too severe or if the patient has lost dorsiflexion at the MTP joint, thereby negating the effect of the windlass mechanism, weight is transferred to the lesser metatarsal heads, particularly the second and third heads, resulting in transfer metatarsalgia.

If a patient presents reporting lesser metatarsal pain following hallux valgus surgery, the orthopaedist should suspect either a problem with the first metatarsal (ie, excessive el-evation and/or shortening) or loss of motion of the first MTP joint. If the patient presents with a hallux varus deformity, it may be the result of an overcorrection of the metatarsal shaft or, possibly, a problem with the distal soft-tissue repair. A recurrent hallux valgus may be the result of insufficient correction of the first metatarsal or, possibly, of failure of the distal soft-tissue procedure.

Physical Examination

The general alignment of the toes and the foot is observed with the patient bearing weight. The range of motion of the first MTP joint is evaluated with the patient seated and is compared with that of the first MTP joint on the contralateral foot. Areas of pain, particularly beneath the first metatarsal head, may indicate incomplete correction of the sesamoids or possible injury of the plantar-medial cutaneous nerve. If a varus deformity is present, the orthopaedist should note whether it is a transverse plane deformity (ie, only varus) or whether it has a cock-up component, making it both a transverse plane and sagittal plane deformity. The rigidity of the deformity also needs to be determined because an easily corrected deformity may be treated with an extensor hallucis longus tendon transfer and medial release, whereas a rigid varus deformity may require an arthrodesis. If there is a recurrent hallux valgus deformity, the orthopaedist should check for the integrity of the medial joint capsule and palpate the metatarsal heads to determine whether the intermetatarsal angle is increased.

The plantar aspect of the foot is carefully evaluated for the presence of diffuse callus formation beneath the second and possibly the third metatarsal heads. Firmly palpating the metatarsal heads usually will reveal whether the first metatarsal is excessively elevated or shortened as a cause for the metatarsalgia. If there is sesamoid pain, the patient tends to roll the foot to the lateral side creating what might be called a pseudotransfer lesion beneath the fifth metatarsal head.

Differential Diagnosis

None

Additional Work-up

Weight-bearing radiographs of the foot are essential to evaluate the etiology of the malunion.

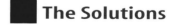

The Solutions

Treatment Options and Rationale

The treatment options depend on the nature of the deformity. The first consideration, however, is whether the first MTP joint is still functional and, if so, the type of corrective procedure that would be worthwhile. Nonsurgical management should always be considered, typically an accommodative orthosis to unload the metatarsal heads. The support is placed just proximal to the metatarsal heads to unload them and, in some cases, a Morton's extension, which is a pad underneath the first metatarsal to increase its area of weight bearing, is added.

If the first MTP joint is not functional as a result of arthritis or, possibly, an anatomic problem (eg, too much metatarsal head excised), then an arthrodesis of the first MTP joint may be adequate, although the metatarsal deformity occasionally may need to be corrected as well.

SAGITTAL PLANE DEFORMITY

When a sagittal plane deformity is caused by dorsiflexion of the metatarsal, a plantar flexion osteotomy can be performed. An alternative method of treatment would be to do a plantar flexion closing wedge or a dorsiflexion opening wedge osteotomy. Either of these techniques can be successful, although the former tends to shorten the metatarsal somewhat, and the latter requires a bone graft. It is for this reason that I prefer the crescentic osteotomy (**Figure 1**).

TRANSVERSE PLANE DEFORMITY

If the transverse plane deformity is caused by overcorrection of the intermetatarsal angle, which results in a hallux varus deformity and/or painful tibial sesamoid resulting from medial subluxation, a proximal osteotomy can be performed. It is important to establish whether or not the first MTP joint is still functional. If it is not functional, then sometimes the simplest way to manage the problem is to do an arthrodesis of the first MTP joint rather than correct the intermetatarsal angle. If, however, the first MTP joint is functional, then a corrective osteotomy bringing the metatarsal out of its excessive lateral deviation into a more anatomic alignment and correcting the soft tissues around the MTP

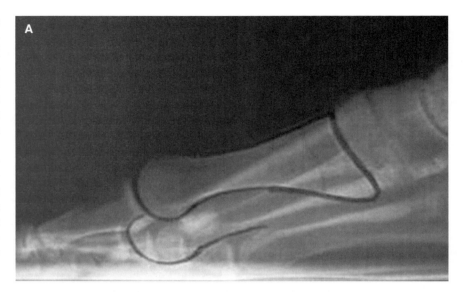

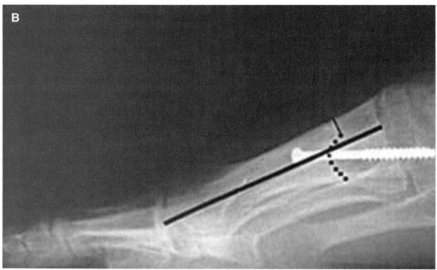

Figure 1 Preoperative (**A**) and postoperative (**B**) radiographs show correction of dorsiflexion of the first metatarsal. Note that the screw usually is removed after the osteotomy has healed. (Reproduced with permission from Mann RA, Coughlin MJ: Adult hallux valgus, in Mann RA, Coughlin MJ (eds): *Surgery of the Foot and Ankle*, ed 7. St. Louis, MO, Mosby, 1999, pp 150–269.)

joint can solve the problem satisfactorily (**Figure 2**).

SHORTENING OF THE METATARSAL

Shortening of the metatarsal is a difficult problem because lengthening the first metatarsal is a technically difficult procedure that has a high complication rate. It is very tempting to place a block of bone in a shortened metatarsal, but the soft-

tissue envelope has usually been significantly scarred, making this procedure very difficult and possibly leading to angulation at the graft site (**Figure 3**).

SHORTENING OF THE METATARSAL ASSOCIATED WITH DORSIFLEXION

Although this is an unusual combination of deformity, the clinical

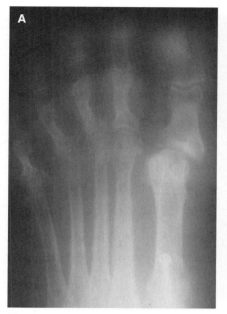

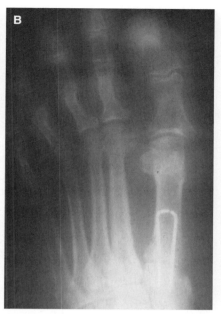

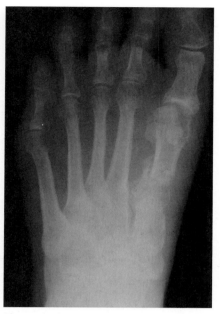

Figure 2 **A,** Postoperative radiograph demonstrating excessive lateral displacement of the first metatarsal resulting in a hallux varus deformity. **B,** Revision surgery with removal of the screw and realignment of the osteotomy site. Pin fixation was used because of lack of strength of the metatarsal bone. The medial joint capsule was also revised.

Figure 3 Excessive shortening and dorsiflexion following a hallux valgus repair with a proximal metatarsal osteotomy.

problem is that of a metatarsalgia because of the lack of weight bearing by the first metatarsal. In this situation, a plantar flexion osteotomy of the malunion site can be performed, followed by an arthrodesis of the first MTP joint to increase the length of the first metatarsal. A lengthening procedure could be attempted, but it would not be my first choice for treatment of this difficult problem (**Figure 4**).

Author's Preferred Treatment and Rationale

SAGITTAL PLANE DEFORMITY

When the sagittal plane deformity is caused by dorsiflexion of the metatarsal, I prefer to create a crescentic osteotomy in the transverse plane along the plantar two thirds of the first metatarsal and then create a dorsal osteotomy to mobilize the osteotomy site. In this way, the first metatarsal literally can be rolled down into proper alignment without sacrificing length. This procedure creates a very stable osteotomy that usually corrects the problem.

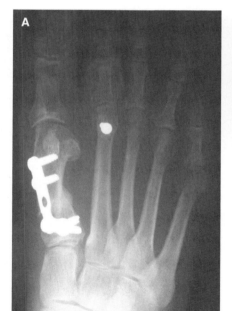

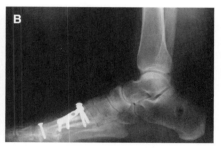

Figure 4 Correction of a malunion. **A,** The nonunion was curetted and bone grafted with local bone from the calcaneus, and a small plate was applied for rigid fixation. **B,** Lateral view demonstrates that correction of the dorsiflexion angulation was also present. Note the bone graft site in the calcaneus.

TRANSVERSE PLANE DEFORMITY

Again I favor a crescentic osteotomy because the degree of correction can be accurately controlled and the osteotomy site stabilized with either a single screw or a small plate. A complete distal soft-tissue procedure will need to be added to this procedure to correct the hallux varus.

If the transverse plane deformity

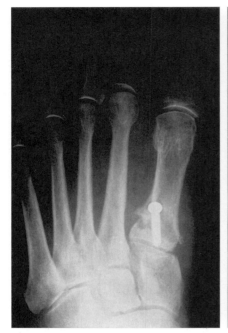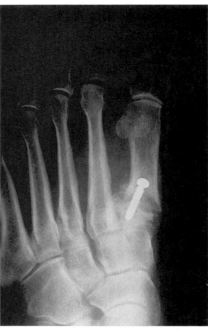

Figure 5   Nonunion of a proximal crescentic osteotomy. (Reproduced with permission from Mann RA, Coughlin MJ: Adult hallux valgus, in Mann RA, Coughlin MJ (eds): *Surgery of the Foot and Ankle*, ed 6. St. Louis, MO, Mosby, 1993.)

was caused by an increase in the intermetatarsal angle resulting from lack of correction at the time of the index procedure, a complete revision of the procedure can be performed and usually is successful. This revision would include a distal soft-tissue procedure and a proximal crescentic osteotomy. However, the orthopaedist must approach this revision cautiously because if the intermetatarsal angle failed to correct the first time, as sometimes happens, particularly in large male patients, it may not be possible to correct the in-

termetatarsal angle the second time either. For some reason, some feet seem "too rigid," making correction of the intermetatarsal angle almost impossible. In this situation, an arthrodesis may be the best solution.

SHORTENING OF THE METATARSAL

If the shortening is not too severe and the problem is a transfer metatarsalgia beneath the second and third metatarsals, a distal metatarsal osteotomy of metatarsals two and three might be considered to help to realign the meta-

tarsal arch. If, however, the shortening is too great, an arthrodesis of the first MTP joint sometimes will produce lengthening of the first ray (by adding the proximal phalanx to the length of the metatarsal), increasing its weight-bearing capacity and unloading the lesser metatarsals. As a general rule, I prefer to either shorten the second and third metatarsals or arthrodese the first MTP joint rather than carry out a lengthening procedure.

NONUNION

A nonunion of a proximal osteotomy site without deformity can occur, although it is uncommon. My initial treatment would be to place the patient into a short leg cast for 2 or 3 months in an attempt to obtain union, but if this fails, then the nonunion will need to be repaired.

Repair of a nonunion in this area consists of exploring the area of nonunion and débriding it if necessary. I prefer to obtain a local bone graft from the calcaneus and pack it into the defect. Some type of internal fixation such as a small plate or screws is essential. This method of treatment is usually adequate to produce a union (**Figure 5**).

Management of Complications
None

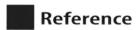

Reference

Mann RA, Coughlin MJ: Adult hallux valgus, in Mann RA, Coughlin MJ (eds): *Surgery of the Foot and Ankle*, ed 7. St. Louis, MO, Mosby, 1999, pp. 150-269.

Coding

ICD-9 CODES

735.0   Hallux valgus (acquired)

735.1   Hallux varus (acquired)

CPT CODES

28292   Correction, hallux valgus (bunion), with or without sesamoidectomy; Keller, McBride or Mayo type procedure

28296   Correction, hallux valgus (bunion), with or without sesamoidectomy; with metatarsal osteotomy (eg, Mitchell, Chevron, or concentric type procedures)

28306   Osteotomy, with or without lengthening, shortening or angular correction, metatarsal; first metatarsal

Complications of Distal Metatarsal Osteotomy

E. Greer Richardson, MD

▮ Definition of the Problem

Patient Presentation

The most often reported complications after distal metatarsal osteotomy are malunion with transfer metatarsalgia, recurrence of deformity, osteonecrosis with arthrosis, nonunion, and infection.

Patients with a dorsiflexion malunion of a distal metatarsal osteotomy (**Figure 1**) usually present 6 months or more after surgery reporting of pain beneath the second metatarsal head that was not present preoperatively, decreased flexion of the first metatarsophalangeal (MTP) joint, and a callus beneath the second metatarsal head.

Patients with osteonecrosis of the first metatarsal head usually present with a decreasing range of motion of the first MTP joint within 6 months postoperatively, although motion had been improving in the first few weeks or months after surgery. In addition, low to moderate grade unresolving pain is present at the first MTP joint and pericapsularly.

Patients with nonunion of a distal metatarsal osteotomy present with pain with ambulation, as well as lateral column overload from weight shifting. Patients with an infection usually have generalized pain, swelling, and fever.

Physical Examination

Physical examination of a patient with malunion shows loss of flexion of the first MTP joint past neutral, approximately 40° of dorsiflexion, and difficulty placing the pulp of the hallux flat on the floor when standing.

Weight-bearing AP and lateral radiographs of the involved foot reveal 5 to 7 mm of shortening of the first metatarsal on the AP view compared with preoperative measurements (**Figure 1**). Alternatively, dorsiflexion of the distal fragment of the osteotomy may be seen with no evidence of osteonecrosis (**Figure 2**).

A patient with osteonecrosis has decreased range of motion of the first MTP joint, mild to moderate pericapsular tenderness at the joint, and slight swelling that appears as capsular thickening rather than an effusion. The most likely diagnosis will be osteonecrosis of the capital fragment. AP, lateral, and oblique radiographs should be obtained. For the first 3 to 4 months after surgery, serial radiographs for osteonecrosis can be disturbing. Subchondral cysts, sclerosis, and slight joint space narrowing may be present initially, only to resolve completely in 3 to 6 months (**Figures 3** and **4**). This radiographic presentation is common, whereas frank osteonecrosis is uncommon.

A patient with a nonunion shifts weight from the painful first metatarsal head area to the lesser metatarsal heads as well as the midfoot. This shifting can be observed in the gait. There is tenderness at the osteotomy site as well as pericapsular tenderness if a reactive synovitis has developed.

In addition, there may be tenderness beneath the second and third metatarsal heads, as well as lateral midfoot tenderness in the area of the cuboid bone. Symptoms in areas other than that of the first metatarsal osteotomy are due to weight shifting. There may be swelling and warmth over the distal metatarsal and first MTP joint as a result of nonunion and micromotion. This symptom may mimic sepsis as nonunions elsewhere often do. A stress fracture may develop in the area of the cuboid.

Superficial infection generally produces local cellulitis and some lymphangitis. The skin over the involved area may be red and warm, but joint motion usually does not cause pain, and fever usually is not present. Oral antibiotics usually are effective in eradicating superficial infection.

Osteomyelitis of the first metatarsal is the most serious infection following a distal metatarsal osteotomy. It may be difficult to diagnose. AP, lateral, and oblique radiographs focusing on the first MTP joint area are essential.

Differential Diagnosis

- Vasomotor dystrophy
- Dorsiflexion malunion
- First metatarsal shortening
- Osteonecrosis
- Nonunion
- Infection

Additional Work-up

For malunion, a Harris footprint reveals decreased weight bearing beneath the

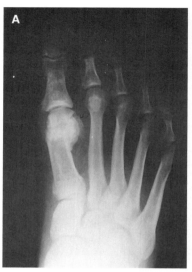

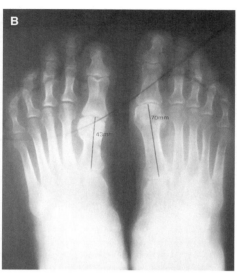

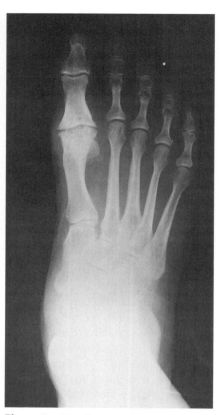

Figure 1 **A,** Shortening of 7 mm after dorsiflexion malunion of chevron distal metatarsal osteotomy; the patient also had transfer metatarsalgia. **B,** Marked shortening after chevron osteotomy in which no internal fixation was used.

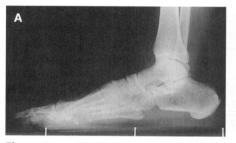

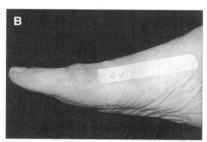

Figure 2 **A,** Dorsiflexion malunion after chevron distal metatarsal osteotomy. **B,** Note the dorsal bunion; the patient also had metatarsalgia.

Figure 3 AP radiograph showing osteonecrosis after chevron osteotomy with secondary degenerative joint disease of the first MTP joint.

first metatarsal head and hallucal pulp and increased weight bearing beneath the second metatarsal head.

Plain radiographs should be all that are needed to diagnosis osteonecrosis of the first metatarsal head after osteotomy but cannot be depended on until 4 to 6 months postoperatively. Internal fixation may reduce the reliability of MRI to diagnose osteonecrosis, even if bioabsorbable pins are used. In addition, what may appear as simple mottling of the first metatarsal head on plain radiographs may appear as frank osteonecrosis on MRI if the study is done too early.

A combination of various scintigraphic techniques (eg, bone scan, gallium scan, white blood cell labeled scan) may be required to diagnose an infection. MRI may be useful if internal fixation is not present. Infection with bioabsorbable screw fixation is particularly troublesome because the entire track of the screw may need to be débrided, and the relatively large area of bone resection can compromise bony stability.

■

The Solutions

Treatment Options and Rationale
The surgical solution to malunion of the capital fragment is to reposition it into normal alignment in the transverse and sagittal planes and maintain length (ie, avoid further shortening). This procedure will allow the first metatarsal head to resume bearing its share of the weight of the forefoot. If the length of the first metatarsal cannot be restored to normal and its position improved sufficiently by the osteotomy to unload the second metatarsal, then a second metatarsal shortening osteotomy can be combined with the first metatarsal repositioning osteotomy. Before any surgical correction, a trial of metatarsal pads or bars is recommended.

Osteonecrosis of the first metatarsal head is not an "all-or-none" complication. Most commonly, osteonecrosis is segmental, limited in area, and of no major long-term consequence. Many patients can be treated successfully with simple activity and shoe modifications. However, if there is fragmentation and collapse of a large part of the first metatarsal head accompanied by severe symptoms, the following treatment options are available: (1) arthrodesis of the first MTP joint with interpositional corticocancellous bone graft and stable internal fixation, (2) resection arthroplasty (Keller procedure), (3) interpositional capsular arthroplasty, and (4) total joint arthroplasty.

Treatment of a distal osteotomy nonunion includes excision of the pseudarthrosis followed by bone grafting and compression fixation, with care taken not to displace or additionally shorten the metatarsal. If joint degeneration is present, an arthrodesis or resection arthroplasty is indicated.

The treatment of infection depends on the stage of the infection. If only cellulitis is present without abscess or bone involvement, rest, elevation of the extremity, and an oral broad-spectrum antibiotic should be adequate treatment. If, however, fluctuation is present, indicating abscess formation, pyarthrosis and osteomyelitis must be considered. Drainage of an abscess, removal of any internal fixation, appropriate cultures, and antibiotic treatment, as well as consulta-

tion with an infectious disease specialist, may be required.

Author's Preferred Treatment and Rationale

Malunion is a most difficult problem because invariably there is enough shortening associated with the dorsiflexion malunion that any repositioning osteotomy is likely to produce further shortening, albeit of a small degree, that will negate the benefit of repositioning the first metatarsal head in normal sagittal plane alignment. Therefore, if a repeat osteotomy is done, I prefer a semicircular configuration using a medial skin and capsular approach with a medial (transverse plane) osteotomy, 1.2 to 1.7 cm proximal to the medial articular surface of the first metatarsal head, and stable pin fixation (**Figure 5**). The distal fragment is rotated plantarward and internally fixed with one or two Kirschner wires or bioabsorbable pins. The capsule is imbricated medially to prevent recurrent hallux valgus, and a dressing is applied that buttresses the capsular repair. A short leg nonwalking cast is worn for 3 weeks, followed by a short leg walking cast for another 3 weeks. At that time (6 weeks after surgery), motion is begun at the first MTP joint, and a protective removable

short leg walker boot is worn another 6 weeks.

If the malunion is in varus (articular surface of first metatarsal angled medially past neutral alignment with the first metatarsal shaft) or in valgus (lateral angulation of the capital fragment), I also use a semicircular rotational osteotomy to correct the deformity. This osteotomy allows correction of multiplanar deformities. Internal fixation is, of course, essential.

If the repositioning osteotomy does not correct the second metatarsal head overload, an arthrodesis of the first MTP joint with a plantar condylectomy of the second metatarsal head is my preferred treatment. Shortening osteotomies of the second and third metatarsals, with or without surgical correction of the first metatarsal malunion, have been reported to redistribute lesser metatarsal head pressures.

I encourage patients with osteonecrosis to wait as long as their symptoms will allow, while protecting the first MTP joint in a full-length 1/16-in thick steel shank in a rockerbottom shoe. The joint may retain enough range of motion that the patient will accept this compromised result if the motion is not too painful, or (more likely) the joint will progres-

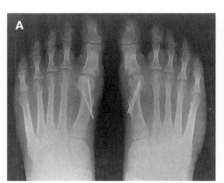 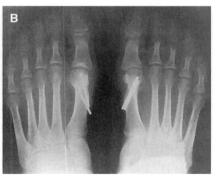 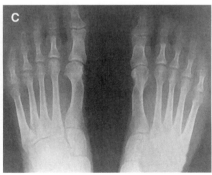

Figure 4   A, AP radiograph obtained 6 weeks after surgery shows severe mottling of both metatarsal heads and a subchondral lucency involving 75% of the right metatarsal head and 50% of the left metatarsal head. **B,** At 6 months after surgery, the subchondral lucency and mottling have resolved. A focal lucency is present at the pin tip in the right metatarsal head. **C,** At 33 months after surgery, both metatarsal heads appear relatively normal. (Reproduced with permission from Thomas RL, Espinosa FJ, Richardson EG: Radiographic changes in the first metatarsal head after distal chevron osteotomy combined with lateral release through a plantar approach. *Foot Ankle Int* 1994;15:285-292.)

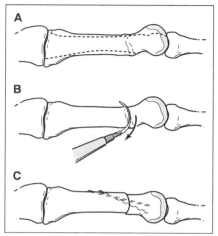

Figure 5 **A,** Dorsal malunion after osteotomy. **B,** The hemispherical osteotomy is created with a curved blade or a 2.5-mm drill and osteotome. **C,** The osteotomy is fixed with one or two Kirschner wires or a bioabsorbable pin. (Reproduced with permission from Myerson M: Metatarsal osteotomy, in Myerson M (ed): *Current Therapy in Foot and Ankle Surgery*. St. Louis, Mosby-Year Book, 1993.)

sively lose motion until the pain resolves.

The surgical options I prefer depend on the age and functional demands of the patient. I set an arbitrary age of younger than 50 years for patients to whom I recommend arthrodesis with interpositional bone graft, stable fixation, and prolonged immobilization (8 weeks in a non–weight-bearing short leg cast and 8 weeks in a weight-bearing short leg cast). This arbitrary age is chosen with the assumption that patients at or younger than age 50 years will be at their height of activity and that patients older than age 50 years will have decreased activity.

For patients younger than age 50 years who reject arthrodesis and

patients older than age 50 years, I recommend a Keller resection arthroplasty. This is a compromised recommendation, but I believe it offers more likelihood of at least marginal success than do the synthetic interpositional arthroplasties (capsular or rubber) or total joint arthroplasty. This is not a routine Keller procedure. Some degree of arthrofibrosis is helpful to give soft-tissue capsular stability. Therefore, the first metatarsal is manually displaced as far laterally (toward the second toe) as possible, while the hallux is aligned straight to the metatarsal and held with two intramedullary 0.062-in Kirschner wires drilled antegrade through the tip of the hallux and then retrograde into the first metatarsal. A firm purse-string medial capsulorrhaphy is done after internal fixation. The pins are left in place for 4 to 6 weeks.

I ask the patient to wait 9 to 12 months with prolonged period(s) of cast immobilization before surgically treating a nonunion of the distal first metatarsal. There are two reasons for this prolonged waiting. Bony union may occur much later than anticipated or a firm fibrous union may develop, which will decrease the patient's symptoms sufficiently to avoid surgery.

If surgical correction becomes necessary, I prefer to débride the area of nonunion and fill the gap with cancellous bone graft and a small cortical strut component to maintain length. Bone graft material can be harvested from the medial aspect of the calcaneal tuberosity or the medial supramalleolar area of the tibia. The smallest curets available should be used when débriding the nonunion to avoid removal of too much bone from the capital fragment. Screw fixation

with a lag technique for compression should be used if sufficient bone is available for firm purchase.

Management of Complications

For cellulitis alone, rest, elevation, and antibiotic treatment are sufficient. For abscess formation within the first 3 weeks after surgery, I drain the area of fluctuation, obtain aerobic and anaerobic skin cultures and sensitivities, leave the wound open, and place the patient on bed rest with bathroom privileges only (no weight bearing on the injured foot). I prescribe a broad-spectrum oral antibiotic that covers *Staphylococcus epidermis* and *S aureus*.

If an abscess or any other sign of deep infection is present at 3 or more weeks after surgery, I assume a bone infection is present, order a bone scan with technetium Tc 99m to confirm my suspicion, but do not delay débridement even if the scan is not diagnostic of osteomyelitis. The capsule is opened, internal fixation is removed, bone and soft-tissue cultures are obtained, and any obviously involved bone is débrided. The capsule is closed, the skin is left open, and intravenous antibiotics are begun under the supervision of an infectious disease specialist. The skin and subcutaneous portions of the wound heal by tertiary intention. A splint or removable cast boot that extends to the toes is used to immobilize the foot and ankle. No weight bearing is allowed until there is union of the osteotomy. With lengthy antibiotic treatment, no weight bearing, and immobilization, a good result should be obtained.

References

Kitaoka HB, Patzer GL: Arthrodesis versus resection arthroplasty for failed hallux valgus operations. *Clin Orthop* 1998;347:208-214.

Lehman DE: Salvage of complications of hallux valgus surgery. *Foot Ankle Clin* 2003;8:15-35.

Richardson EG: Complications after hallux valgus surgery. *Instr Course Lect* 1999;48:331-342.

Sammarco GJ, Idusuyi OB: Complications after surgery of the hallux. *Clin Orthop* 2001;391:59-71.

Trnka HJ: Arthodesis procedures for salvage of the hallux metatarsophalangeal joint. *Foot Ankle Clin* 2000;5:673-686.

Coding

ICD-9 CODES

733.49   Other aseptic necrosis of bone

733.81   Other disorders of bone and cartilage, Malunion and nonunion of fracture, Malunion of fracture

733.82   Other disorders of bone and cartilage, Malunion and nonunion of fracture, Nonunion of fracture

CPT CODES

28292   Keller, McBride, or Mayo type procedure

28293   Resection of joint with implaint

28306   Osteotomy, with or without lengthening, shortening or angular correction, metatarsal; first metatarsal

28750   Arthrodesis, great toe; metatarsophalangeal joint

The Short First Metatarsal After Hallux Valgus Surgery

James A. Nunley, MD

◼ Definition of the Problem

Patient Presentation

Shortening of the first metatarsal is a complication of hallux valgus surgery that can produce serious secondary consequences. The first and second metatarsals usually are approximately equal in length. Nevertheless, there is a significant incidence of patients whose second metatarsal is longer than the first metatarsal. When symptomatic hallux valgus develops in these patients, if the surgical procedure involves a first metatarsal osteotomy, further shortening can occur because the length of the first metatarsal is certainly shortened in all osteotomies except the proximal oblique metatarsal osteotomy, as described by Nunley and McKibbin. Shortening of the first metatarsal usually is asymptomatic because it frequently involves only the thickness of the saw blade, as in a chevron osteotomy. However, with the proximal crescentic or proximal closing wedge osteotomy, or with a Ludloff type of oblique osteotomy, significant shortening can occur as a result of malunion. In addition, nonunion with resorption at

the osteotomy site can lead to a greater difference in length between the first and second metatarsals.

Many patients who present for bunion surgery have second metatarsal overload with a plantar callus and pain. I believe this problem is caused by failure of weight bearing on the first ray. If hallux valgus surgery further compromises the apparent discrepancy, second metatarsal overload with metatarsalgia and pain can persist or be exacerbated by the bunion surgery.

Physical Examination

Examination findings are fairly obvious. Inspection of the plantar surface may reveal a callus or intractable plantar keratosis under the second metatarsal head. When the patient is standing, the tip of

the great toe will be shorter than the second toe, a finding that suggests this problem. Range of motion should be assessed at the first tarsal metatarsal and the first metatarsophalangeal (MTP) joint. Previous skin incisions must also be noted.

Differential Diagnosis

None

Additional Work-up

Radiographs will clearly demonstrate the abnormality. Gait analysis or Harris Mat impression will demonstrate overload at the second metatarsal and poor weight transfer on the first ray.

———————◼

The author or the departments with which he is affiliated have received something of value from a commercial or other party related directly or indirectly to the subject of this chapter.

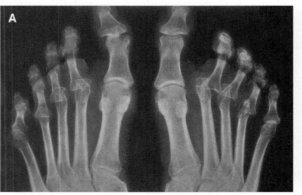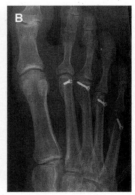

Figure 1 Rheumatoid arthritis and dislocation of the lesser MTP joints. **A**, AP radiograph. Although the patient does not have a short first metatarsal, the principle of osteotomy of the second through fifth metatarsals with oblique osteotomies is well illustrated. **B**, Postoperative radiograph shows reduction of dislocated MTP joints and restoration of a normal transverse arch to the foot with oblique osteotomies of the second through fifth metatarsals with screw fixation. (Courtesy of Pascal Rippstein, MD, Zurich, Switzerland)

■ The Solutions

Treatment Options and Rationale

Under normal circumstances, second metatarsal overload frequently can be treated using orthoses. If, however, use of an orthotic device fails, the physician is left with two options. The first would be to perform shortening osteotomies of the second, third, and sometimes fourth and fifth metatarsals (**Figure 1**). The second option is to consider lengthening of the first metatarsal. I prefer to lengthen the first metatarsal rather than jeopardizing the normal anatomy of the lesser MTP joints. Several articles address lengthening of the metatarsals, but these generally focus on congenital abnormalities and usually involve the lesser metatarsals. To my knowledge, there is no literature describing lengthening of the first metatarsal exclusively for either malunion or shortening that occurs after bunion surgery.

Patients who present with a short first metatarsal radiographically and who have a plantar callus with pain at the second and third MTP joints are initially evaluated for tightness of the Achilles tendon, which may exacerbate the condition, as may an unstable second MTP joint. A customized orthotic device, which will cushion the area beneath the metatarsals that are overloaded and increase pressure under the first metatarsal, is always the first form of treatment. In most cases this treatment is successful; however, in some patients an orthosis is insufficient, and pain persists. In these patients, I recommend lengthening of the first metatarsal (**Figure 2**). The surgery is done as an outpatient procedure with the patient under regional anesthesia. In all of the lengthening procedures I have done to date, shortening has been in the line of the first metatarsal and there has been no need for angular correction. Usually, there is a need to simultaneously

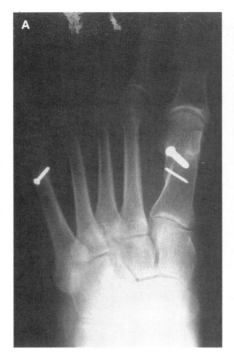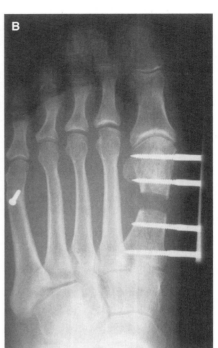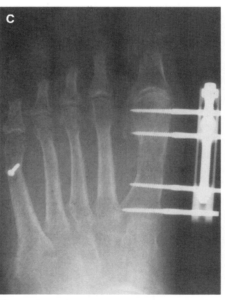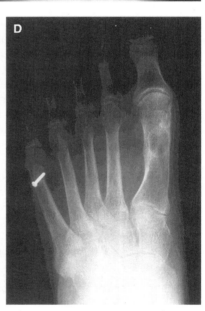

Figure 2 **A**, Preoperative AP radiograph of a patient who underwent osteotomy of the first metatarsal for hallux valgus and osteotomy of the fifth metatarsal for bunionette deformity who has severe incapacitating pain under the second metatarsal head and shortening of the first metatarsal. **B**, AP radiograph obtained 1 week postoperatively shows the osteotomy of the first metatarsal and application of the lengthening external fixator. **C**, AP radiograph obtained 3 months postoperatively shows lengthening of the first metatarsal equal to the second metatarsal. **D**, After removal of the external fixator, the length of the first metatarsal has been restored, as has the position of the sesamoids and overall alignment.

reposition the metatarsal head in the plantar direction. This can easily be accomplished with great toe lengthening.

Author's Preferred Treatment and Rationale

With the patient adequately anesthetized, a unilateral single planar external fixator that will allow gradual distraction (Orthofix M-100, Orthofix, Huntersville, NC) is applied. Initial drill holes are made with 1.5-mm Kirschner wires, and then four self-tapping pins with 3-mm diameter shaft and 3- to 2.5-mm tapered threads are inserted. All pins should be inserted in line with the long axis of the metatarsal.

A transverse osteotomy between the second and third screws is performed with a mini sagittal saw and cooling with normal saline irrigating solution. The periosteum is cut and minimally stripped on either side of the bone with a sharp periosteal elevator. The osteotomy is complete, and the external fixator is tightened. No distraction is permitted at this point, and the skin is closed with simple sutures.

One week after surgery, radio-graphic imaging is obtained as a control, and the distraction lengthening is initiated. The device is turned one quarter turn four times a day to equal 1 mm of lengthening per day, the rate and rhythm defined by Ilizarov as ideal for distraction lengthening.

Patients are not to bear weight until lengthening is complete. Once the first and second metatarsals are of equal length, partial weight bearing increasing to full weight bearing is allowed with the external fixator still in place. Mineralization of the lengthened metatarsal follows. It is important during the lengthening period for patients to maintain passive range of motion at the MTP joint. It also is imperative to examine the foot radiographically and watch for possible subluxation or dislocation of the MTP joint. This problem has not occurred in my series but has been reported with congenital short metatarsals. The external fixator is not removed until complete consolidation of the distracted metatarsal is seen radiographically.

Management of Complications

To date the results have been excellent. All patients have been able to obtain a first metatarsal that is equal in length to the second metatarsal. No angular malalignment, pin tract infection, or deep infection has occurred as a result of distraction lengthening. No secondary bone grafting has been necessary despite the fact that our patients range in age from 22 to 60 years. The cosmetic result has been excellent, and in all patients the second metatarsal overload with metatarsalgia has resolved as a result of lengthening the first metatarsal.

——————————■

■ References

Choudhury SN, Kitaoka HB, Peterson HA: Metatarsal lengthening: Case report and review of literature. *Foot Ankle Int* 1997;18:739-745.

Ilizarov GA: Clinical application of the tension-stress effect for limb lengthening. *Clin Orthop* 1990;250:8-26.

Magnan B, Bragantini A, Regis D, Bartolozzi P: Metatarsal lengthening by callotasis during the growth phase. *J Bone Joint Surg Br* 1995;77:602-607.

Saxby T, Nunley JA: Metatarsal lengthening by distraction osteogenesis: A report of two cases. *Foot Ankle* 1992;13:536-539.

Takakura Y, Tanaka Y, Fujii T, Tamai S: Lengthening of short great toes by callus distraction. *J Bone Joint Surg Br* 1997;79:955-958.

Coding

ICD-9 CODES

996.4 Mechanical complication of internal orthopedic device, implant, and graft

996.67 Infection and inflammatory reaction due to internal prosthetic device, implant, and graft, Due to other internal orthopedic device, implant, and graft

998.59 Postoperative infection, other

998.83 Other specified complication of procedures, not elsewhere classified, non-healing surgical wound

CPT CODES

20690 Application of a uniplane (pins or wires in one plane), unilateral, external fixation system

28306 Osteotomy, with or without lengthening, shortening or angular correction, metatarsal; first metatarsal

The Lapidus Procedure for Correction of Moderate and Severe Metatarsus Primus Varus and Hallux Valgus Deformities

J. Chris Coetzee, MD, FRCSC

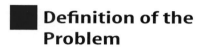

Definition of the Problem

Patient Presentation

Patients who might benefit from a Lapidus procedure (arthrodesis of the first tarsometatarsal [TMT] joint) typically are middle-aged or older women with long-standing and increasing metatarsus primus varus and hallux valgus in whom nonsurgical management has failed. Patients often will present with hypermobility of the first ray and associated abnormalities, including a pronated hallux that often is accompanied by an overload callus under the second and third metatarsal heads and the medial border of the foot at the level of the first metatarsal.

Physical Examination

The metatarsus primus varus and hallux valgus deformities are usually clearly visible in severe cases. Evaluating the patient's footwear often gives a good indication of the severity of the problem. With severe deformities, the bunion causes a typical bulging area on the medial aspect of the shoe. There are often signs of a medial eminence bursa.

In the patient with hypermobility of the medial ray, there is an apparent loss of the medial longitudinal arch with weight bearing. As with most forefoot disorders, the surgeon should assess the gastrocnemius-soleus complex for ex-

cessive tightness, which may contribute to the deformity (**Figure 1**).

Hypermobility of the first ray has been implicated as one of the contributing causes of a progressive hallux valgus deformity and, as such, is an ideal indication for the Lapidus procedure. At present, however, neither the definition of hypermobility nor a precise technique for its measurement has gained wide acceptance. The technique currently used for measurement of hypermobility is somewhat subjective and consists of evaluating sagittal motion of the first metatarsal relative to the second metatarsal with the foot in a neutral position. Medial column motion can occur primarily at the TMT joint or include the naviculocuneiform and intercuneiform joints.

The normal range of dorsal excursion of the first ray is about 4°, with combined plantar-dorsal excursion of about 8°. Hypermobility is quantified as more than 6° of dorsal and more than 13° of combined excursion.

The simplest method of measurement is manual determination of plantar flexion and dorsiflexion of the first ray against a stable lateral foot. A zero marker is placed on the second metatarsal neck, and with the lesser metatarsals stabilized, the first metatarsal is taken through its plantar and dorsal excursion. Measuring the excursion of the first metatarsal in relation to the second will give a crude measurement of mobility. To make it truly reliable, the length of the meta-

tarsal has to be taken into account as well (**Figure 2**).

Hypermobility in the transverse plane may facilitate a progressive varus deformity along with attenuation or laxity of other supportive structures. It can be evaluated grossly with the metatarsal squeeze test. Alternatives include performing a Coleman block test and obtaining weight-bearing lateral radiographs. Various mechanical devices also could be used for this measurement; however, it still remains somewhat subjective.

Plantar keratosis beneath the second and third metatarsal heads can indicate lesser metatarsal overload resulting from first ray instability. This indication is most reliable if the length of the first metatarsal is almost equal to that of the second metatarsal, and if the sesamoids are not dislocated. First ray hypermobility also can be a contributing cause of second metatarsophalangeal (MTP) synovitis and pain. A short first ray and dislocated sesamoids make it impossible to attribute lesser metatarsal skin calluses to first ray hypermobility alone. The presence of a dorsal bunion on weight bearing could also be a clinical indicator of hypermobility.

Radiographic signs of hypermobility may include cortical hypertrophy of the second ray, widening in the intercuneiform space, and an increased medial slope of the first metatarsocuneiform joint. The position and angle of the x-ray beam cause a great deal of variance in the slope and to de-

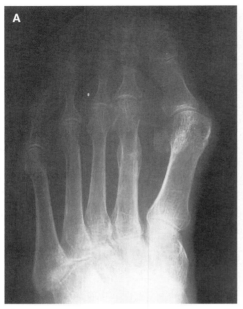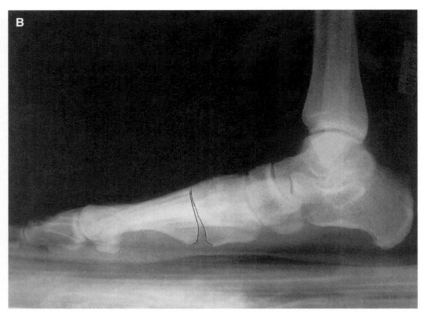

Figure 1 **A,** Weight-bearing AP radiograph shows the wide first IM angle and a healed stress fracture of the second metatarsal that could result from medial ray instability. **B,** Weight-bearing lateral view shows obvious widening over the plantar aspect of the first TMT joint resulting from instability.

rive any clinical benefit, the AP radiograph must be taken in a standardized fashion. The metatarsal squeeze test will provide an estimate of the transverse motion of the first metatarsal.

Differential Diagnosis
- Primary hallux valgus and metatarsus primus varus without hypermobility
- Rheumatoid or other arthritic condition causing hypermobility
- Hallux rigidus with a hallux valgus deformity
- Muscle imbalance secondary to a neuromuscular disorder

Additional Work-up
There is no additional work-up.

The Solutions

Treatment Options and Rationale
Although metatarsus primus varus and hallux valgus deformities consti-tute a common forefoot problem, there continues to be controversy as to the best treatment. The nonsurgical treatment option is shoe modification. Comfortable shoes with a low heel and a high, wide toe box are the mainstay of treatment. Bunion pads and various orthotics might aid in relieving pain and discomfort but are not successful in correcting bony malalignment.

Various surgical options are available for moderate and severe hallux valgus deformities. Over 150 operations have been described in the literature for correction of hallux valgus, and most have satisfactory results. The choice of procedure depends on the surgeon's comfort level, experience, and philosophy. The proximal first metatarsal osteotomy, which could be a concentric or wedge osteotomy, has about the same ability to correct the severe deformities and the same predictability of outcome as the Lapidus procedure. Shaft osteotomies, including the Ludloff and Scarf, have less power for correcting deformities in multiple planes than more proxi-mal osteotomies. The osteotomy chosen is usually a matter of the surgeon's preference. The Lapidus procedure could be the most powerful and reliable in obtaining correction, but it is not without complications. Because of its power in correcting severe deformities in multiple planes it is the author's preferred method of treating severe deformities. Fusion of the MTP joint is predictable and reliable, but it is not preferred by most patients with good, pain-free range of motion of the great toe.

Author's Preferred Treatment and Rationale
The Lapidus procedure is one of the alternatives for treating moderate and severe metatarsus primus varus and hallux valgus deformities. Correction of the first ray in the sagittal and transverse planes, along with the stabilization of the hypermobile first ray has been a powerful tool. Combination with adjuvant procedures has broadened the indications for the Lapidus procedure. In patients with severe deformity or intercuneiform laxity, the

first metatarsal also could be fused to the base of the second metatarsal.

INDICATIONS AND CONTRAINDICATIONS

Indications include hypermobility of the first ray with associated secondary findings (second metatarsal overload, second MTP joint synovitis, and dorsal bunion), severe metatarsus primus varus with an intermetatarsal (IM) angle of more than 18°, and revision of failed hallux valgus surgery. It is important to note that these patients do not necessarily have a significant increase in the IM angle. If the hypermobility is mainly in the sagittal plane, there could be a moderate IM angle (12° to 18°) but significant symptoms.

Contraindications include open physes, first MTP arthritis, an excessively short first ray, and severe ligamentous laxity.

SURGICAL PROCEDURE

The extensor hallucis longus is used as the landmark for the incision. The first and second TMT joints are exposed in the interval between the extensor hallucis longus and the extensor hallucis brevis through a 6-cm incision. The first TMT joint and the medial aspect of the second metatarsal are exposed and denuded of articular cartilage. To limit shortening of the metatarsal, the articular cartilage alone is removed with small osteotomes and curets. A small lamina spreader is an invaluable tool for opening the joint wide enough to allow removal of cartilage from even the most plantar surfaces of the metatarsal and cuneiform. The absence of this cartilage will ensure the surgeon's ability to slightly plantar flex the first ray during the reduction and fixation.

The adductor hallucis tendon is released through a 2-cm incision in the first web space. In severe deformities, the lateral first MTP joint capsule could be perforated longitudinally to allow the sesamoids to reduce. This step is followed by a standard medial procedure to remove the medial eminence from the metatarsal head.

Reducing the first metatarsal parallel to the second metatarsal now closes the IM gap. The first metatarsal is slightly plantar flexed, and rotation is confirmed. A 4.0- or 3.5-mm gliding cortical screw is then inserted from the cuneiform into the first metatarsal. A second screw can be either from the metatarsocuneiform or first metatarsal into the base of the second metatarsal. This option is used to close the IM gap securely in patients with severe deformities and in patients with obvious hypermobility.

A standard first MTP closure is now done to reduce the sesamoids, and local bone graft from the cuneiform is packed in any defects at the TMT or IM joints. An Akin osteotomy of the proximal phalanges is added if necessary. The tourniquet is deflated, and the wounds are closed.

The foot is immobilized in a fiberglass great toe spica cast for 2 weeks. The sutures are then removed, and a second slipper cast is applied for an additional 4 to 6 weeks. The patient should not bear weight or at most be allowed heel-touch weight bearing for 6 weeks. If radiographs taken 6 weeks postoperatively show satisfactory progression of the fusion, the cast is removed and physical therapy is begun. Sports or fairly vigorous activities are not recommended for at least 3 months. Swimming and bicycling are the ideal activities to start with as soon as range of motion and confidence allow.

Management of Complications

The Lapidus procedure unfortunately carries a fairly high complication rate. Major complications include nonunion, shortening of the first ray, and malunion, usually with dorsal elevation of the metatarsal. Minor complications include the long period of immobilization needed to ensure arthrodesis, the extended period in which weight bearing is not allowed,

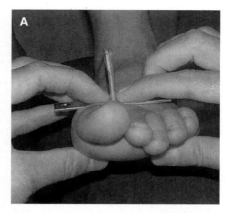

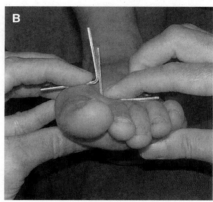

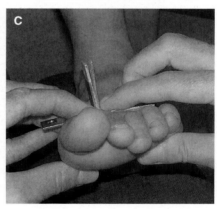

Figure 2 **A,** Forefoot in a neutral position. **B,** Maximum dorsiflexion of the first ray in relation to the second. Distance measured in millimeters. **C,** Maximum plantar flexion of the first ray.

superficial nerve injuries, and injury of the dorsalis pedis artery.

Nonunion of the first TMT fusion is the most problematic complication. The reported nonunion rate at this joint is between 2% and 10% for unilateral and up to 33% for bilateral

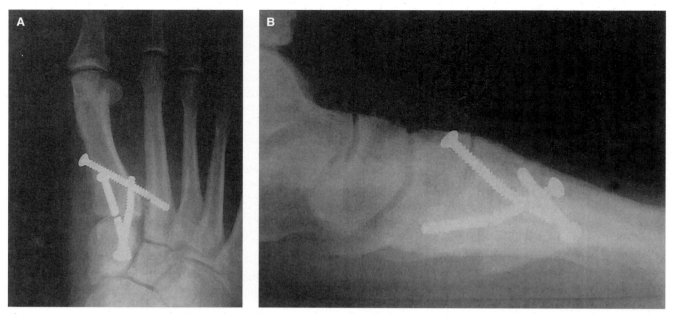

Figure 3 **A,** AP view showing nonunion of Lapidus fusion and recurrence of IM angle. **B,** Lateral view showing nonunion of Lapidus fusion.

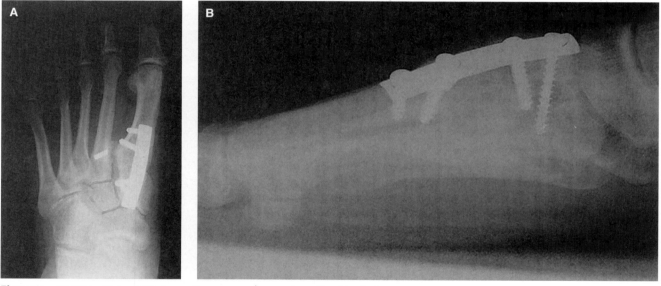

Figure 4 AP **(A)** and lateral **(B)** views after salvage of nonunion of Lapidus fusion.

procedures. Therefore, doing bilateral Lapidus procedures in one sitting is not recommended. The high nonunion rate is believed to be a result of the orientation of the joint perpendicular to the weight-bearing axis of the foot. This orientation results in a shear force across the joint, whereas most of the shaft osteotomies result in a compression force caused by the horizontal plane of the osteotomy. It also requires the foot treated with a Lapidus procedure to be immobilized and weight protected for much longer than feet treated with most of the other hallux valgus procedures (**Figures 3** and **4**).

The nonunion rate can be reduced by meticulous surgical technique. Adequate subchondral bone has to be exposed. Exposure can be done either by multiple subchondral perforations with a small diameter drill or "crushing" of the subchondral plate with an osteotome.

The Lapidus procedure is not indicated if the first ray is more than 1.5 cm shorter than the second unless the lesser metatarsals are shortened during the procedure with either a Weil or shaft osteotomy. Shortening of the first metatarsal could lead to transfer metatarsalgia and should be avoided. In patients with a short first metatarsal, only the cartilage is removed to limit further shortening of the metatarsal. In patients with a long first metatarsal, a small laterally based wedge could be removed from the medial cuneiform to help reduction at the TMT joint. A small plantar-based wedge also is removed from the TMT joint to ensure plantar flexion of the metatarsal before inserting screws.

Dorsal malunion is usually the result of inadequate removal of cartilage and bone from the plantar aspect of the TMT joint. The joint is about 30-mm deep and sometimes is difficult to visualize all the way to the plantar base. It is advisable to use a mini lamina spreader to open the joint to allow proper removal of the plantar cartilage.

The dorsalis pedis artery enters the first IM space about 1 to 1.5 cm distal to the TMT joint. Overzealous dissection could compromise the artery.

References

Glasoe WM, Allen MK, Saltzman CL: First ray dorsal mobility in relation to hallux valgus deformity and first intermetatarsal angle. *Foot Ankle Int* 2001;22:98-101.

Lapidus PW: Operative correction of the metatarsus varus primus in hallux valgus. *Surg Gynecol Obstet* 1934;58:183-191.

Mann RA, Coughlin MJ: Adult hallux valgus, in Coughlin MJ, Mann RA (eds): *Surgery of the Foot and Ankle*, ed 7. St. Louis, MO, Mosby, 1999, pp 150-269.

Myerson MS, Badekas A: Hypermobility of the first ray. *Foot Ankle Clin* 2000;5:469-484.

Sangeorzan BJ, Hansen ST Jr: Modified Lapidus procedure for hallux valgus. *Foot Ankle* 1989; 9:262-266.

Coding

ICD-9 CODES

727.1   Other disorders of synovium, tendon, and bursa, Bunion

735.9   Unspecified acquired deformity of toe

CPT CODES

28290   Correction, hallux valgus (bunion), with or without sesamoidectomy; simple exostectomy (eg, Silver type procedure)

28297   Correction, hallux valgus (bunion), with or without sesamoidectomy; Lapidus type procedure

CPT copyright © 2003 by the American Medical Association. All Rights Reserved.

Hallux Rigidus: Cheilectomy and Arthrodesis

Paul J. Juliano, MD

▮ Definition of the Problem

Patient Presentation

Hallux rigidus is a common condition of the first metatarsophalangeal (MTP) joint that occurs second only to hallux valgus. This condition has been recognized as a clinical entity for over 100 years. The presentation of patients with hallux rigidus is variable; some present with pain, dorsal swelling of the hallux, and negative radiographic features, while others have rather significant radiographic findings and relatively little pain. Patients may report neuritic-type symptoms, with the dorsal bony prominence causing a compression neurapraxia of the terminal branch of the superficial peroneal nerve.

Shoe fit can be a problem, with redness and callus over the dorsal aspect of the interphalangeal joint that results from the obligatory flexion of the interphalangeal joint to avoid con-

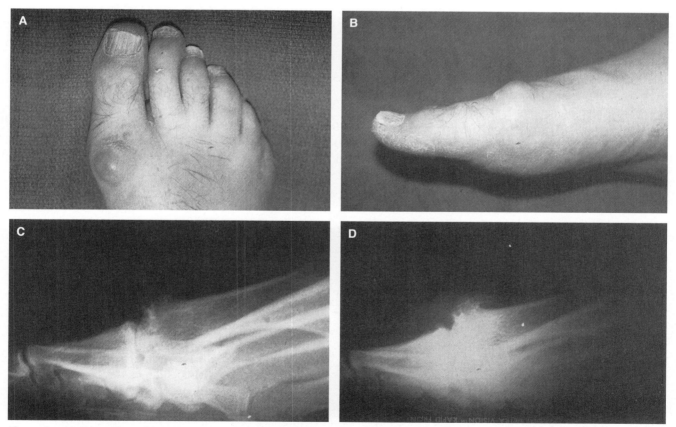

Figure 1 AP **(A)** and lateral **(B)** clinical photographs of a large dorsal prominence in a patient with hallux rigidus. **C,** Lateral radiograph of the same patient shows the large dorsal osteophyte. **D,** Use of a hot lamp may improve visualization of the osteophyte. (Reproduced with permission from Morton GA: Hallux rigidus, in Myerson MS (ed): *Foot and Ankle Disorders.* Philadelphia, PA, WB Saunders, 2000, pp 289-307.)

tact of the painful hallux MTP joint osteophytes. Another common complaint is dorsal foot pain and tendinitis subsequent to the patient loading the lateral border of the affected foot while avoiding contact of the hallux MTP joint. Patients also report difficulty wearing elevated heels and ascending inclined planes. Symptoms frequently worsen over time. There may be an oblique crease on top of the patient's toe box, instead of the usual transverse crease. This crease is caused by an immobile first MTP joint. Symptoms develop gradually, usually months to years. The patient may relate an acute or chronic event, especially if there is acute dorsiflexion stress causing a fracture of the dorsal osteophyte.

Physical Examination

The physical examination usually reveals a dorsal prominence, or "dorsal bunion," over the first MTP joint with callus or redness over this area, secondary to pressure from the shoe (**Figure 1**). There may be a Tinel's sign dorsally from pressure on the terminal branch of the superficial peroneal nerve. The presence of a dorsal osteophyte is not obligatory for the initial diagnosis. The pathognomonic finding is lack of dorsiflexion and limited motion of the MTP joint, or "hallux

limitus." (Normal walking requires 15° of dorsiflexion.) The patient usually retains plantar flexion until the very late stages of arthrosis. Typically, another expected finding is a painful clavi (corn) at the interphalangeal joint with restricted dorsiflexion. Compensatory lateral loading of the forefoot results in the lateral wear of the shoe, and the usual transverse oblique crease on the dorsum of the shoe becomes oblique as a result of the immobile first MTP joint. It is impossible for most patients to rise up on their toes. Patients may have a positive grind test, and a portion of the osteophyte may break loose contributing to crepitance and locking of the joint. The orthopaedist must be careful when patients principally report lateral foot pain with tibialis anterior tendinitis. This symptom frequently indicates pain in the first MTP joint, and as a result the initial office visit may be focused on the compensatory complaints while missing the pathology in the first MTP joint. Thus, a complete physical examination is essential.

Differential Diagnosis

- Gout, pseudogout
- Proliferative synovial disease; rheumatoid arthritis, seronegative arthropathy

- Posttraumatic degenerative joint disease
- Sequelae of severe hallux valgus
- Turf toe
- Osteochondrosis of the first MTP joint

Additional Work-up

Weight-bearing AP, lateral, and oblique radiographs should be obtained. The AP view is obtained with the x-ray tube angled 15° cephalad, minimizing the overlap of the proximal phalanges. In general, patients with hallux rigidus have a "squared off" joint or a more congruous joint. In mild hallux rigidus, the joint space is maintained with bony proliferation. As the process progresses from moderate to severe, the arthrosis begins dorsally and then progresses in plantarly. These changes are best viewed on the lateral radiograph (**Figure 2**). In general, bone scans and MRI are not required routinely. A bone scan would show increased uptake. MRI could possibly show an osteochondral defect, especially in the adolescent population, or a plantar plate injury. However, MRI is not part of the routine work-up for hallux rigidus.

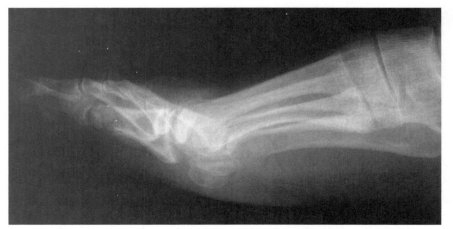

Figure 2   Lateral radiograph shows the beginning of dorsal joint destruction and a dorsal osteophyte.

■ The Solutions

Treatment Options and Rationale

Nonsurgical treatment is always indicated in the initial stages of hallux rigidus. Patients can use nonsteroidal anti-inflammatory drugs and shoe modifications, specifically a shoe with a wide and deep toe box and a stiff sole (shank) along its entire length. Orthotics, which stiffen the shoe, are a good idea. However, they may require too much room and frequently crowd the toe box. A steel or composite carbon fiber shank that is built into the sole of the shoe does not use valuable room. In addition to these shoe modifications, a rocker-bottom sole or metatarsal bar can be added to decrease the sagittal plane bending of the hallux during the toe-off phase of gait. Most of these modifications have a low degree of patient acceptance. For the sake of completeness these nonsurgical options are offered to and discussed with a patient before contemplating surgery. Intra-articular steroid injections are used by some; however, for the most part they provide only temporary relief and should be used judiciously. Repeated injections may accelerate the degenerative process.

Surgical management falls into two broad categories: joint sparing and arthrodesis. The most common joint sparing procedure is a dorsal cheilectomy. This procedure can be termed a "remodeling arthroplasty." Cheilectomy alone or in conjunction with a periarticular osteotomy (either a dorsal wedge phalangeal osteotomy or a dorsal wedge metatarsal osteotomy) has remained the most popular solution for mild to moderate hallux rigidus. An arthroscopic débridement of the MTP joint is considered for osteochondral defects and mildly arthritic conditions. The resection arthroplasty is another motion sparing, although not joint sparing, procedure. Options include the Keller procedure or the interposition arthroplasty as described by Hamilton.

The motion sparing procedures also include joint arthroplasty. This includes single or double Silastic implants with or without metal grommets, ball-and-socket metallic hemiarthroplasty, and finally the total metallic joint arthroplasty. The above options represent the spectrum of treatment of hallux rigidus. In the next section, I will describe my algorithm for treatment.

Author's Preferred Treatment and Rationale

Once the history and physical examination have been completed, I focus on patient expectations because these dictate the options for treatment. I usually select one of three options. (1) Cheilectomy is for young, active patients who report pain walking uphill, playing tennis, or playing golf and is my preferred treatment of stages 1 and 2 hallux rigidus. (2) Hallux MTP joint fusion is my preferred surgical treatment of stage 3 disease. (3) Finally, I consider an interposition arthroplasty as an alternative to fusion for patients whose activity goals do not necessitate a propulsive gait and/or those who refuse to undergo an arthrodesis.

Cheilectomy is not a difficult operation. I frequently perform this surgery with an ankle block alone or with conscious sedation. I make a dorsal medial incision over the MTP joint with the nerve and the extensor hallucis longus tendon protected and split the capsule longitudinally. I usually can get Hohman retractors around either side of the metatarsal head. This step exposes the dorsal osteophyte adequately. I then use a chisel to remove the dorsal one fifth to one third of the metatarsal (**Figure 3**). The preoperative motion is usually neutral to slight dorsiflexion of the hallux MTP joint. After adequate resection, joint motion should approach 80° to 90°; however, the patient will not retain this motion in the long term. Care is taken to remove osteophytes from the proximal phalanx at the same time. I use bone wax for hemostasis. I do not typically perform a dorsiflexion osteotomy of the proximal phalanx; however, I would consider it if the patient was a sprinter and needed slightly extra dorsiflexion. Most poor results can be

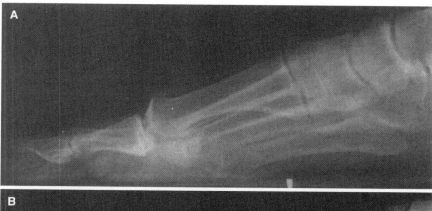
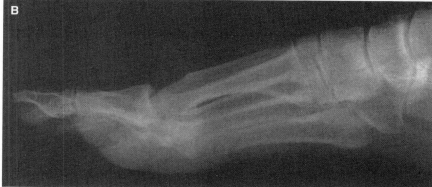

Figure 3 Preoperative (**A**) and postoperative (**B**) lateral radiographs show the amount of bone removed from the dorsum of the metatarsal head when performing a cheilectomy. (Reproduced with permission from Graves S: Hallux rigidus: Treatment of cheilectomy, in Myerson MS (ed): *Current Therapy in Foot and Ankle Surgery*. Philadelphia, PA, WB Saunders, 1993, pp 74-80.)

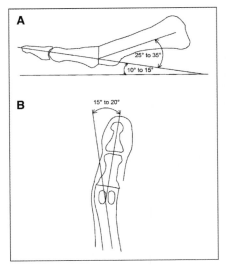

Figure 4 **A,** Lateral view of first MTP joint arthrodesis with 25° to 35° of dorsiflexion with respect to the plane of the foot. **B,** AP view of a first MTP arthrodesis with 15° to 20° of valgus with respect to the first metatarsal. (Reproduced from Katcherian DA: Pathology of the first ray, in Mizel MS (ed): *Orthopaedic Knowledge Update: Foot and Ankle 2.* Rosemont, IL, American Academy of Orthopaedic Surgeons, 1998, pp 151-161.)

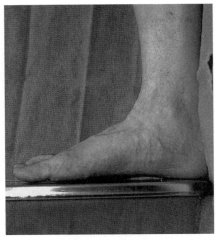

Figure 5 The foot is placed against the irrigation pan with the ankle in neutral position. In this photograph, the great toe should be set in more dorsiflexion to be parallel with the lesser toes. (Reproduced with permission from Holmes GB: Problems of the adult foot: Forefoot, in Gould JS, Thompson FM, Cracchiolo A III, et al (eds): *Operative Foot Surgery.* Philadelphia, PA, WB Saunders, 1994, pp 23-27.)

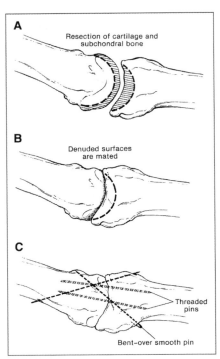

Figure 6 Arthrodesis of the first MTP joint. **A,** The articular surface is denuded to subchondral bone. The architecture is preserved. **B,** The denuded surfaces are mated. **C,** The arthrodesis is fixed with crossed pins or screws. (Reproduced with permission from Holmes GB: Problems of the adult foot: Forefoot, in Gould JS, Thompson FM, Cracchiolo A III, et al (eds): *Operative Foot Surgery.* Philadelphia, PA, WB Saunders, 1994, pp 23-27.)

correlated with inadequate resection of bone.

The positive aspect of cheilectomy is that the patient does not have to wait for bony healing; only soft-tissue healing is needed. Thus, it is a very attractive solution for a healthy patient who wants to return to sports as soon as possible. More restrictions are involved in the postoperative course of the osteotomy, including prolonged use of a postoperative shoe. It is very important to counsel the patient preoperatively that the joint will not be normal and that motion obtained at surgery will not be maintained. Patients should be made aware that the mechanical block has been removed dorsally and that this block is typically the source of their pain.

In more advanced disease, when the patient has a positive grind test and the radiographs show that the degenerative changes are from dorsal to plantar, I advise the patient that my treatment of choice is MTP joint arthrodesis.

Multiple techniques have been described for performing MTP joint arthrodesis. The "cone and cup" technique has the greatest surface area of bone-to-bone contact and perhaps is the most attractive with respect to bone healing. This procedure can be difficult technically because the surgeon gets only one chance to do it right. If the cuts are inaccurate when fashioning the cone and cup, the toe is essentially in an irreversible malposition. My preferred method of hallux MTP joint fusion is a capsular incision similar to the one described for cheilectomy, except that it is extended proximally and distally. The articular surface is exposed, whatever articular surface is remaining is removed, and the remaining joint is denuded to subchondral bone. It is then drilled with multiple 1.5-mm drill holes to expose bleeding bony surfaces. I then place the great toe in the position for fusion (which is ideally 15° of dorsiflexion with respect to the floor, 15° of valgus, neutral rotation, and 30° to 40° of dorsiflexion with respect to the first meta-

tarsal; **Figure 4**). I also denude the sesamoid apparatus and include these in the fusion mass. If the sesamoids are large and it appears that they may cause an intractable plantar keratosis, I will then consider excising them prophylactically.

Obtaining proper position of the toe during MTP joint arthrodesis can be difficult for the surgeon who rarely performs this type of surgery. A goniometer or a large straight edge, such as an irrigation pan, can be used on the plantar surface of the foot as a guide. The proper amount of dorsiflexion of the hallux should be equal to that of the lesser toes and metatarsals with respect to the irrigation pan (**Figure 5**). This is my primary method of judging a position. By leaving the normal ar-

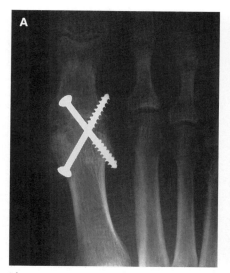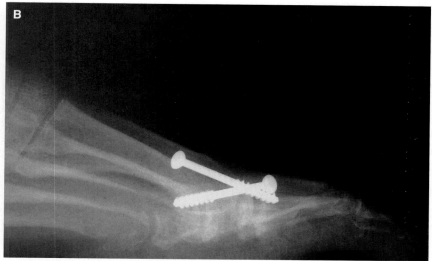

Figure 7 **A,** AP radiograph showing hallux MTP arthrodesis using the crossed screw technique. **B,** Lateral radiograph showing the same.

chitecture (and not doing a cone and cup), the surgeon can simply match up the denuded articular surfaces and "reduce" the joint in the proper position (**Figure 6**). This method usually gives a perfect positioning of the toe in MTP joint arthrodesis.

My preferred method of fixation is two crossed small fragment screws (**Figure 7**). I drill the initial holes from the inside out. I take care not to cross the screws at the same point across the joint because it may gap the arthrodesis (just as an orthopaedist would not want to cross the screws in a fracture plane during fixation). Frequently, depending on the bone quality, the surgeon may need to use only one screw and augment with terminally threaded Steinmann pins.

I am currently using terminally threaded 2-mm guide wires from the Synthes 7.0-mm cannulated screw system (Synthes, Monmouth, CO) in lieu of fully threaded Kirshner wires. This choice facilitates removal of the pins in clinic. It is difficult at times to construct optimal fixation for the hallux MTP joint. The tension band is the most biomechanically sound construct. Unfortunately, the tension side of the MTP joint is the plantar surface,

and there is no good approach to place a tension band on the plantar surface of the hallux MTP joint and avoid the sesamoid apparatus. If the need arises, fixation can be supplemented with the addition of a small fragment plate dorsally. My postoperative routine is protected weight bearing in a fracture boot for 6 to 12 weeks. The patient can advance to footwear as tolerated when radiographic union has occurred.

Management of Complications

Causes of nonunion could be patient noncompliance, errors in surgical technique or procedure selection, biologic issues, and hardware failure. The postoperative routine for hallux MTP joint fusion is limited weight bearing in a walker boot or cast for 6 weeks, followed by weight bearing as tolerated in an open-toe or stiff-soled shoe. If the patient uses tobacco or if the surgery is a revision, more restriction on weight bearing may be added and simultaneous electrical stimulation may be considered. Avoiding the surgery until the patient quits smoking is an optimal but frequently unrealistic option. Complications related to surgical technique can be reduced by avoiding crossing the

screws at the same level and ensuring that there is enough fixation so that there is no micromotion to prevent the fusion mass from consolidating. If the terminally threaded Kirschner wires do not provide enough fixation, a dorsal plate-and-screw construct can add stability even though it is not placed on the tension side.

Biologic problems include infection, tobacco use, and systemic illnesses. Patients frequently come to the orthopaedist with great toe pain as a result of silicone synovitis. In this instance, the implant must be removed. If a propulsive gait is required, then a structural tricortical interposition bone graft often is required. This construct requires a dorsal plate and sometimes intramedullary fixation with threaded Steinmann pins.

Malunion can frequently be adjusted with wedge osteotomy, depending on the plane of the deformity. Excessive dorsiflexion requires an opening wedge osteotomy; excessive valgus could be corrected with a closing wedge osteotomy from the medial side, such as an Akin osteotomy.

References

Easley ME, Davis WH, Anderson RB: Intermediate to long term follow-up of medial approach dorsal cheilectomy for hallux rigidus. *Foot Ankle Int* 1999;20:147-152.

Coughlin MJ, Shurnas PS: Hallux rigidus: Grading and long-term results of operative treatment. *J Bone Joint Surg Am* 2003;85:2072-2088.

Hamilton WG, O'Malley MJ, Thompson FM, et al: Capsular interposition arthroplasty for severe hallux rigidus. *Foot Ankle Int* 1997;18:68-70.

Lau JT, Daniels TR: Outcomes following cheilectomy and interpositional arthroplasty in hallux rigidus. *Foot Ankle Int* 2001;22:462-470.

Myerson MS, Schon LC, McGuigan FX, Oznur A: Result of arthrodesis of the hallux metatarsophalangeal joint using bone graft for restoration of length. *Foot Ankle Int* 2000;21:297-306.

Smith RW, Katchis SD, Ayson LC: Outcomes in hallux rigidus patients treated nonoperatively: A long term follow-up study. *Foot Ankle Int* 2000;21:906-913.

Coding

ICD-9 CODE

735.2   Acquired deformities of toe, Hallux rigidus

CPT CODES

20902   Bone graft, any donor area; major or large

28289   Hallux rigidus correction with cheilectomy, debridement and capsular release of the first metatarsophalangeal joint

28750   Arthrodesis, great toe; metatarsophalangeal joint

Hallux Rigidus: Extra-articular Osteotomies

Stephen F. Conti, MD

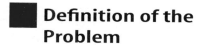 Definition of the Problem

Patient Presentation

Hallux rigidus is characterized by the gradual onset of pain and limited dorsiflexion of the metatarsophalangeal (MTP) joint with minimal involvement of the metatarsosesamoid articulations. The symptoms associated with hallux rigidus include the gradual onset of pain at the MTP joint of the great toe, especially dorsally. Patients often notice a dorsal or dorsomedial exostosis that may be confused with a bunion deformity. The discomfort may be exacerbated by activities such as squatting that require dorsiflexion of the first MTP joint. Shoes with flexible soles that bend at the MTP joint may apply pressure on the dorsal portion of the joint, causing additional discomfort.

Physical Examination

Although it is focused on the first MTP joint, physical examination must include a complete biomechanical evaluation of the entire lower extremity. Pertinent findings will include range of motion of the MTP joint in relation to the first metatarsal as well as to the plantar aspect of the foot (or floor). Dorsiflexion is limited, although range of motion often is normal during plantar flexion. Forced dorsiflexion will elicit pain in the dorsal aspect of the joint, whereas forced plantar flexion may cause discomfort as the capsule is stretched over the osteophytes. Tenderness should be noted in the dorsal aspect of the joint but not over the sesamoids. Interphalangeal joint range of motion should be assessed, with particular attention to joint hyperextension and palpable crepitus. Increased mobility of the first tarsometatarsal joint or medial column of the foot and the degree of forefoot varus in a subtalar neutral hindfoot position should be noted. The overall structure of the foot, whether pronated or supinated, is recorded. In addition, heel cord tightness should be assessed with the Silverskjold test. In the later stages of the disease, with either severe discomfort with any attempted dorsiflexion or with a hallux in a fixed position of plantar flexion, the patient may tend to walk on the outer edge of the foot.

Radiographic evaluation includes weight-bearing AP and lateral views, as well as non–weight-bearing oblique and metatarsal head or sesamoid views. Osteophyte formation on the dorsal, medial, and lateral aspects of the first metatarsal head and proximal phalanx is typical. Narrowing of the joint space, flattening of the first metatarsal head, and subchondral sclerosis and cyst formation are common findings as well. A plantar flexed position of the hallux (hallux flexus) with apparent elevation of the first metatarsal from the floor (metatarsus elevatus) has been described. Whether this is a primary manifestation of the deformity that leads to the arthritic changes in the first MTP joint or is secondary to osteophyte formation and subsequent lack of dorsiflexion in the first MTP joint remains controversial. The degree of arthritic changes is best evaluated on the lateral view because the overlying osteophytes may obscure accurate evaluation of the AP view. Particular attention must be paid to the inferior half of the MTP joint on the lateral view to assess for the degree of joint space narrowing.

Three stages of limited motion in the first MTP joint are recognized. Different authors describe these conditions differently. Hattrup and Johnson describe the following three stages of hallux rigidus: stage 1, dorsal osteophytes with no joint space narrowing; stage 2, dorsal osteophytes with less than 50% narrowing of the first MTP joint; and stage 3, periarticular osteophytes with complete joint space collapse and subchondral cyst formation at the first MTP joint.

Differential Diagnosis

- Inflammatory arthritides such as rheumatoid arthritis
- Osteochondral lesions of the metatarsal head
- Osteonecrosis of the metatarsal head

Additional Work-up

Additional testing is rarely needed in the diagnosis of hallux rigidus. MRI is occasionally useful to evaluate the degree of metatarsosesamoid arthrosis or to evaluate an osteochondral lesion that may be the source of pain. Bone scan has been shown to be unreliable in the evaluation of sesamoid disease and should not be used to determine the degree of metatarsosesamoid arthritis.

The Solutions

Treatment Options and Rationale

Treatment options are varied but initially are divided into nonsurgical and surgical. Determining the appropriate options depends on the etiology of the disease, patient complaints, physical examination, and radiographic stage of the hallux rigidus deformity. Nonsurgical options include weight loss, activity modification, nonsteroidal anti-inflammatory medications, and appropriate orthoses and shoe modifications. Physical therapy may be implemented to stretch contracted heel cords and plantar intrinsic muscles. Orthosis options range from simple arch supports for feet with a

pronation deformity to rigid Morton's extensions to arch supports with medial forefoot posting that ends at the sesamoid and a rigid extension distally to limit dorsiflexion of the hallux. Shoe options range from thin, stiff carbon fiber or metal plates to rigid rocker soles and extra-depth footwear. Other nonsurgical options are described in chapter 10.

Surgical options include intra-articular procedures and extra-articular osteotomies. Intra-articular procedures of cheilectomy, Keller arthroplasty, and arthrodesis were discussed in the preceding chapter. This chapter will focus on extra-articular osteotomies.

The first MTP joint consists of the first metatarsal head, the base of the proximal phalanx, the sesamoid grooves, and the sesamoids. Although it was first believed to be a simple hinge joint, it clearly is a gliding hinge joint with surface vectors tangential to the articular surface through its full range of motion. In the presence of certain biomechanical abnormalities,

these surface vectors become compressive in the dorsal aspect of the metatarsal head, leading to articular cartilage overload, damage, and osteophyte formation. A concept often discussed in the literature is that of hallux limitus, defined as a first MTP joint that lacks sufficient dorsiflexion for normal ambulation without having many obvious radiographic arthritic changes. The first group of osteotomies to be discussed are used in an attempt to correct the hallux limitus before there is progression to significant arthritic changes. These procedures correct an underlying biomechanical abnormality and are best performed before significant dorsal arthritis and osteophyte formation is evident radiographically.

When a foot exhibits a congenitally tight medial band of the plantar fascia, there may be loss of the normal gliding of the proximal phalanx against the first metatarsal head. In these situations the proximal phalanx jams against the dorsal metatarsal head during dorsiflexion, and releasing the medial band of the plantar fascia theoretically will improve hallux limitus. When this condition occurs in conjunction with chronic plantar fasciitis at the origin of the plantar fascia from the calcaneus, a medial plantar fascia release may be indicated.

A Youngswick osteotomy is indicated when a foot has a first metatarsal with normal length that is believed to be elevated distally, causing the proximal phalangeal base to jam against the dorsal first metatarsal head during dorsiflexion. This procedure is similar to a distal chevron osteotomy except that a cut is made with the saw parallel to the dorsal limb, and a predetermined amount of bone is removed. The head is then impacted on the shaft and displaced plantarly. Fixation may be performed with a Kirschner wire (K-wire) (**Figure 1**). This procedure also may be performed for a concomitant, mild congruent hallux valgus deformity by displacing the capital frag-

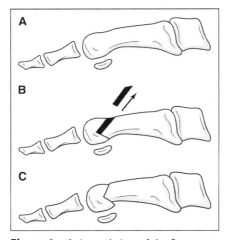

Figure 1 **A,** Lateral view of the first metatarsal. **B,** Youngswick osteotomy with bone removed from the dorsal phalanx. The initial chevron cut is made at 60°. **C,** Impaction of the head fragment with plantar displacement.

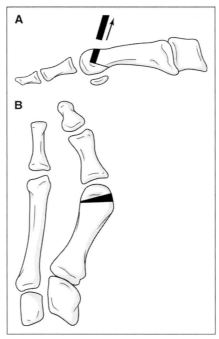

Figure 2 **A,** Lateral view of a tricorrectional osteotomy. **B,** AP view showing triangular bone removal.

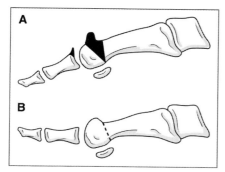

Figure 3 **A,** Watermann osteotomy cuts. **B,** Compression of the osteotomy after removal of the bone wedge.

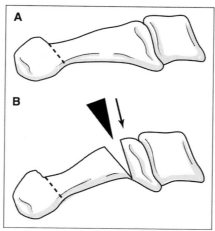

Figure 4 **A,** Watermann osteotomy. **B,** Proximal dorsal opening wedge osteotomy of the first metatarsal (sagittal Logroscino osteotomy).

ment laterally as well. As with any distal procedure, care must be taken to make the plantar limb more horizontal to avoid cutting into the metatarsosesamoid articulation. Also, the surgeon should avoid plunging the saw blade through the osteotomy sites so that damage to the lateral soft-tissue structures is avoided and the likelihood of osteonecrosis is decreased. Postoperative care is similar to that for a distal chevron osteotomy for hallux valgus deformity. A "tricorrectional" osteotomy has been described for combinations of hallux valgus and hallux limitus or rigidus in which triangular or rectangular bone wedges are resected from the dorsal limb osteotomy site (**Figure 2**).

A Watermann osteotomy is indicated when the first metatarsal is of normal length or slightly long without elevatus and there are dorsal osteophytes without articular cartilage degeneration. In this procedure a trapezoid osteotomy is made proximal to the articular cartilage of the first metatarsal head. The plantar cortex is left intact. As the osteotomy is compressed, the first metatarsal is shortened, and intact plantar cartilage rotates into the first MTP joint space (**Figure 3**). This osteotomy is most useful in younger patients in whom cartilage degeneration may be minimal. The advantage may be preservation of first MTP joint function; however, the disadvantages include

iatrogenic creation of a metatarsal elevatus and damage to the normal metatarsosesamoid articulation, forcing a difficult salvage situation. When a proximal dorsal wedge opening osteotomy is added to the Watermann osteotomy, it is referred to as a sagittal Logroscino osteotomy (**Figure 4**).

A second group of osteotomies to be considered are those performed to preserve the first MTP joint when there are more advanced degenerative changes. These osteotomies would be performed in conjunction with a dorsal cheilectomy of the first metatarsal head. The cheilectomy procedure is described in detail in the preceding chapter.

The Moberg osteotomy is indicated in hallux rigidus stages 1 and 2 when, following cheilectomy, there is insufficient dorsiflexion of the first MTP joint. However, exactly what constitutes insufficient dorsiflexion is unknown, and because intraoperative range of motion has minimal correlation with final postoperative range of motion, the quantitative indications for the Moberg osteotomy are vague. Potential complications from the phalangeal osteotomy make it prudent not to recommend it as an adjunct in every case of hallux rigidus.

The range of motion of the first MTP joint is from 30° of plantar flexion to 90° of dorsiflexion relative to the long axis of the first metatarsal. Different activities require varying degrees of dorsiflexion of the first MTP joint. It generally is desirable to obtain 60° of dorsiflexion relative to the first metatarsal long axis postoperatively. If this degree of dorsiflexion does not seem likely to occur after cheilectomy alone, then a Moberg osteotomy may be added to the procedure.

The technique involves making a dorsomedial incision over the proximal phalanx and first metatarsal head. Before surgery, range of motion must be carefully assessed to determine the amount of plantar flexion that exists relative to the floor in the first MTP joint. After performing the cheilectomy of the first metatarsal head, the proximal phalangeal base is approached. A K-wire is placed parallel and as close as possible to the articular surface without violating the concave phalangeal base. A dorsal closing wedge osteotomy is performed with the proximal cut parallel to the K-wire. The wedge can be 4 to 6 mm wide. Care must be taken to leave the center plantar cortex intact because it will act like a hinge as the osteotomy is compressed. The osteotomy can then be fixed with nonabsorbable suture, wire, crossed K-wires, or a staple. I prefer to fix the osteotomy with a malleable Hemoclip used like a staple (**Figure 5**). Postoperatively patients are asked to walk with heel-strike weight bearing for 1 week, then flat-foot in a postoperative stiff-soled shoe for 4 to 6 weeks until the osteotomy is healed. Dorsiflexion range-of-motion exercises can be begun 1 week after surgery. Plantar flexion exercises grasping the base of the hallux are begun 3 weeks after surgery. Aggressive physical therapy after the osteotomy is healed seems to increase range of motion and improve outcome.

The Regnauld procedure (enclavement) shortens the proximal

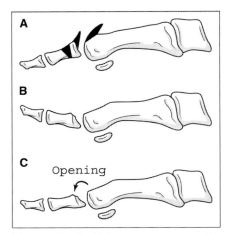

Figure 5 **A,** Moberg osteotomy with débridement of the dorsal osteophyte. **B,** Compression of the dorsal closing wedge of proximal phalanx. **C,** When the hallux touches the ground, decompression of the first MTP joint is not significant.

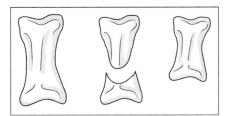

Figure 6 The Regnauld procedure shortens the proximal phalanx.

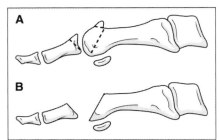

Figure 7 **A,** Valenti procedure cuts. **B,** Resection of bone decompresses the joint.

phalanx and decompresses the joint. The base of the proximal phalanx is cut, the diaphysis shortened, and the base reattached (**Figure 6**).

The third group of osteotomies are not joint-sparing procedures and are used as alternatives to resection arthroplasty, implant arthroplasty, and arthrodesis. The Valenti procedure is an ablative procedure to resect most of the first MTP joint. It preserves the plantar portion of the first metatarsal head and the first proximal phalangeal base, thereby preserving the flexor hallucis brevis insertion and sesamoid function. It is indicated for stage 3 hallux rigidus deformities (**Figure 7**).

Author's Preferred Treatment

The initial step in deciding on an appropriate treatment plan involves differentiating among hallux limitus, hallux rigidus, and global joint arthritis. Hallux limitus is best defined as limited first MTP motion with dorsal pain but no evidence of arthritis or osteophyte formation. This is an uncommon cause of pain and, in my experience, is confined mostly to adolescents and young adults. In hallux limitus, determining if the limitation is caused by a soft-tissue problem such as a tight medial plantar fascia or by a bone and joint problem, such as a pronated foot with an unstable medial column or an elevated first metatarsal, will help to determine surgical treatment. Most cases of hallux limitus can be corrected with a first metatarsal osteotomy, first tarsometatarsal arthrodesis, or selected medial column arthrodesis, such as at the naviculocuneiform joint, combined with a Moberg osteotomy without formal cheilectomy of the first metatarsal head.

I believe, as do other orthopaedic surgeons, that there is rarely a situation where metatarsus elevatus is a primary deformity. Apparent elevation of the first metatarsal off the floor is secondary to the lack of hallux dorsiflexion. Therefore, I rarely operate on the first metatarsal to perform plantar flexion osteotomies.

The diagnosis of hallux rigidus should be considered when first MTP joint dorsiflexion is limited, sesamoids are not tender, and less than 50% narrowing of the MTP joint with dorsal osteophytes is evident. In these situations, a first metatarsal head cheilectomy, with or without a Moberg osteotomy, is almost always used with good results. An appropriate cheilectomy will involve approximately 30% of the true metatarsal head exclusive of osteophytes. The Moberg osteotomy is added when the surgeon believes the patient will not achieve 60% of postoperative dorsiflexion from the first metatarsal. Global first MTP arthritis is diagnosed when there is more than 50% loss of joint space or significant sesamoid tenderness. First MTP joint arthrodesis is the procedure of choice for this diagnosis.

Management of Complications

The most common complications of these osteotomies are malunion, nonunion, stiffness, and continued pain. The main reason to consider dorsal first metatarsal cheilectomy, with or without Moberg osteotomy, is its consistency and lack of serious complications. Osteotomies of the diaphyseal portion of the proximal phalanx or proximal first metatarsal have the possibility of malunion. Shortening or dorsal angulation often results in transfer metatarsalgia. In this situation correction may require revision first metatarsal osteotomy or shortening osteotomies of the lesser metatarsals. If pain and stiffness at the MTP joint accompany the malunion, a first MTP arthrodesis may not improve the transfer metatarsalgia, and salvage may be very difficult.

References

Cavolo DJ, Davallaro DC, Arrington LE: The Watermann osteotomy for hallux limitus. *J Am Podiatry Assoc* 1979;69:52-57.

Haddad SL: The use of osteotomies in the treatment of hallux limitus and hallux rigidus. *Foot Ankle Clin* 2000;5:629-662.

Mann RA, Coughlin MJ, DuVries HL: Hallux rigidus: A review of the literature and a method of treatment. *Clin Orthop* 1979;142:57-63.

Thomas PJ, Smith RW: Proximal phalanx osteotomy for the surgical treatment of hallux rigidus. *Foot Ankle Int* 1999;20:3-11.

Coding

ICD-9 CODE

735.2   Acquired deformities of toe, hallux rigidus

CPT CODES

28289   Hallux rigidus correction with cheilectomy, débridement and capsular release of the first metatarsophalangeal joint

28310   Osteotomy, shortening, angular or rotational correction; proximal phalanx, first toe (separate procedure)

Hallux Rigidus
William G. Hamilton, MD

Definition of the Problem

Patient Presentation

Patients with hallux rigidus present with pain localized to the first metatarsophalangeal (MTP) joint and limited joint motion. The pain, caused by an associated synovitis or inflammation secondary to degenerative arthritic change, is classically evoked by activities requiring dorsiflexion of the first MTP joint. These activities include running, cross-country skiing, squatting, lunging, or walking up an inclined slope. The pain and stiffness tend to be relieved by rest. The dorsal prominence about the metatarsal head, which is typical of hallux rigidus, commonly causes pain with shoe wear. Women may report difficulty wearing high-heeled shoes because the degree of dorsiflexion required to fit in this type of shoe leads to painful impingement or jamming at the first MTP joint. Although a definite history of trauma is possible, most often the condition is idiopathic with a spontaneous onset. Symptoms of hallux rigidus can occur unilaterally or bilaterally, although both feet may not be at the same stage of disease.

Patients with hallux rigidus also may present with lateral forefoot pain, painful calluses beneath the head of the fifth metatarsal, or interdigital neuritis resulting from compensatory supination during ambulation to avoid painful pressure on the first metatarsal head during the push-off phase of gait. The compensatory supination is responsible for exacerbation of symptoms in patients with a cavus foot.

Symptoms may range from mildly uncomfortable to completely disabling. The course of the disease is progressive, ranging from a few months to a few years. In some patients pain is reduced if end-stage ankylosis develops.

Physical Examination

Inspection and palpation of the affected foot often reveal swelling around the first MTP joint and significant proliferation of dorsal osteophytes. The dorsal exostosis is often large and can be associated with an overlying bursitis, which makes palpation in this region exquisitely painful. Later-stage hallux rigidus may result in a "canoe-shaped" or plantar flexed hallux secondary to elevation of the first metatarsal head (hallux flexus). Examination of the affected foot may also reveal a callus under the proximal phalangeal head of the fifth metatarsal and, when the interphalangeal joint is stuck in flexion, an underlying plantar callus.

Assessment of range of motion of the first MTP joint should include comparison to the opposite side. Normal range of motion for the joint varies between 30° of plantar flexion and 90° of dorsiflexion. The joint should be examined by stabilizing the first ray with one hand, while the proximal phalanx is held and passively plantar flexed and dorsiflexed with the other. With hallux rigidus, dorsiflexion is limited or absent, depending on the degree of osteophyte proliferation and the degeneration of the joint's articular cartilage. Plantar flexion also is affected but to a lesser degree. Dorsiflexion of the first MTP joint classically evokes pain as the proximal phalanx is forced into apposition with the degenerated metatarsal head and dorsal osteophytic mass. Crepitus and grind often accompany sagittal motion of the joint. Application of an axial load to the affected joint typically does not evoke as much discomfort as attempted dorsiflexion, except in the most advanced stage in which the entire joint has become involved. Hyperesthesia, tingling, or a positive Tinel's sign over the digital nerves may be a result of nerve compression against the dorsolateral osteophytic mass.

The initial work-up typically includes weight-bearing AP, lateral, and oblique radiographs of the affected foot. The radiographs typically will show narrowing of the first MTP joint space, widening of the articular ends of the metatarsal head and proximal phalanx, and marginal osteophyte formation, largely on the dorsal aspect of the first metatarsal head. The radiographic studies are used in correlation with subjective observations and physical examination findings to grade the condition.

Grade I hallux rigidus is a normal or almost normal (minimally narrowed) joint space with mild to moderate osteophyte formation, typically limited to the metatarsal head without involvement of the proximal phalanx. Patients with grade I hallux rigidus have intermittent pain in the first MTP joint during ambulation. The pain is relieved by rest. Examination reveals mild restriction of MTP joint motion, with less than 35° of dorsiflexion and 20° of plantar flexion elicited. Radiographs of grade II hallux rigidus will show moderate dorsal osteophyte formation, with partial destruction of the first MTP joint indicated by joint space narrowing of the upper portion of the articular cartilage and subchondral sclerosis and/or subchondral cysts. There often is relative sparing of the plantar aspect of the MTP joint, which is best seen on the oblique view. Physical examination will demonstrate moderately restricted joint motion, with dorsiflexion and plantar flexion of less than 20°. Grade III hallux rigidus is the end stage of the disease in which there is loss of the joint space, and dorsal and plantar osteophytes are seen on the lateral radiograph. Joint motion is severely restricted in this stage, with dorsiflexion and plantar flexion of less than 10°. Patients with grades II and III hallux rigidus typically report constant pain in the affected joint, which sometimes causes severely limited ambulation and difficulty wearing shoes.

The symptoms of hallux rigidus and extent of joint damage may or may not coincide with the radiographic presentation. Some patients with radiographic evidence indicating severe disease are minimally symptomatic, and vice versa. For this reason, it is important to base treatment decisions primarily on the symptoms rather than on the radiographic results.

Differential Diagnosis
- Rheumatoid arthritis
- Muscle spasm of the great toe intrinsic muscles
- Gout
- Lyme disease

Additional Work-up

On occasion, patients may have a significant loss of motion and pain with dorsiflexion without demonstrable changes on plain radiographs. In some patients, the problem can be related to a chondral injury of the metatarsal head. MRI can be helpful in these patients, particularly if they have a history of an impaction injury involving the great toe, with prolonged pain and disability. Additional work-up to obtain a definitive diagnosis should include erythrocyte sedimentation rate and rheumatoid arthritis, antinuclear antibody, uric acid, and Lyme titers when appropriate. This work-up is important because the symptoms may be treated nonsurgically once the inflammation has been reduced.

The Solutions

Treatment Options and Rationale
NONSURGICAL TREATMENT

Treatment options should address not only the pathology in question but also the patient's needs and level of activity. Nonsurgical treatment should begin with limited activity and shoe wear modifications. The use of a steel shank and rocker-bottom sole will alleviate the discomfort that occurs with dorsiflexion of the first MTP joint during heel rise and toe-off. The use of extra-depth shoes will decrease irritation of the digital nerves on the dorsum of the great toe. As the osteophytes form and the capsule thickens, the overlying nerves can become quite irritated by compression of the shoe in this area. The avoidance of high-heeled shoes can also be quite helpful. Long-term evaluation of patients treated nonsurgically for this condition suggests that avoiding high-heeled shoes and instead wearing

shoes with an ample toe box are the most helpful. Symptoms also can be alleviated by use of orthoses with a Morton's extension to decrease motion at the MTP joint.

Nonsurgical treatment sometimes includes manipulation and injection. A retrospective study of the efficacy of manipulation and injection emphasized the importance of grading the severity of the condition before initiating treatment. The mean duration for symptomatic relief was 6 months for grade I hallux rigidus and 3 months for grade II. Surgical intervention was requested by one third of patients with grade I pathology and two thirds of patients with grade II. All patients with grade III hallux rigidus reported no relief from injections and manipulation under anesthesia and underwent surgery within 3 months. Injections and manipulation thus play a limited role in treatment.

SURGICAL TREATMENT

Several surgical options have been used to treat feet refractory to nonsurgical management. These options are directed at the degree of the involvement of the great toe, as well as the functional demands of the patient. Procedures used for grade I hallux rigidus and, therefore, a normal MTP joint, are directed at resection of the osteophyte and preservation of the joint. The most commonly used procedure, the cheilectomy, involves resection of the dorsal third of the metatarsal head to help increase range of motion and decrease the pain caused by the bony prominence. Results of cheilectomy have been favorable, and it can be used in athletes with either grade I or grade II disease.

The Moberg procedure, which consists of a closing wedge osteotomy of the proximal phalanx that, in effect, helps with dorsiflexion, also is used to treat patients with grade I disease. However, for the surgery to be successful, the patient must have adequate plantar flexion of the great toe.

This procedure is used most frequently in younger, more active people. It can be done in conjunction with a cheilectomy in patients with grade II disease. This combination is somewhat controversial, however, because the postoperative management for each is different. The cheilectomy requires immediate range of motion, and the osteotomy requires immobilization to prevent nonunion. Despite this, satisfaction rates have been 96% in patients without complications.

Patients with grade III disease are much more challenging and present a dilemma. The treatment regimen includes resection arthroplasty, fusion, and prosthetic replacement. The risks and benefits need to be carefully discussed with the patient before selecting the appropriate procedure.

The Keller procedure has been used to treat both hallux rigidus and hallux valgus, so its effectiveness could never be clearly ascertained. It eventually was abandoned because of the numerous complications that occurred postoperatively. The problems resulted from failure to lengthen the extensor hallucis longus tendon when appropriate or from removing too much of the proximal phalanx. The toe would become short and unstable, resulting in transfer lesions that further compromised patient satisfaction with the procedure. This procedure usually is reserved for older, less active individuals.

Implant procedures using Silastic became popular in the 1970s and 1980s as a means to remove the disease process while retaining function of the joint. At first these proved to be quite successful; however, the results began to deteriorate with time. Their failure resulted from fragmentation, silicone synovitis, and early loosening.

The first MTP arthrodesis is the gold standard for the treatment of hallux rigidus; it works well, and long-term postoperative problems are quite rare. A long-term review involving 100 patients followed for a minimum of 10 years nicely outlines some of the problems. Malposition (16%), interphalangeal arthritis (10%), new-onset metatarsalgia (10%), nonunion (3%), and stress fracture (2%) were complications noted in this retrospective study. The incidence of interphalangeal arthritis has been reported to be as high as 30% to 40%; however, this is rarely of clinical significance. Overall, patients are quite satisfied with the procedure and are able to bike, run, and play golf without limitations. Wearing high-heeled shoes or cowboy boots and/or participating in sports that require lunging forward (eg, tennis) are much more difficult.

An alternative procedure has been shown to be successful in treating pain without sacrificing motion or strength in patients with severe hallux rigidus. The soft-tissue arthroplasty uses the thick dorsal capsule seen in the arthritic joint, thereby avoiding the complications that occur when a foreign material is used. It attempts to preserve joint motion by resecting 25% of the proximal phalanx, as in the Keller procedure, as well as removing the dorsal third of the first metatarsal head as in cheilectomy. The dorsal capsule is interposed between the bony surfaces and sewn to the stumps of the flexor hallucis brevis tendons to prevent retraction of the sesamoids (**Figure 1**). This interposition is facilitated by tenotomy of the extensor hallucis brevis, which inserts into the capsule proximally. Before resection it is very important to release all capsular insertions from the base of the

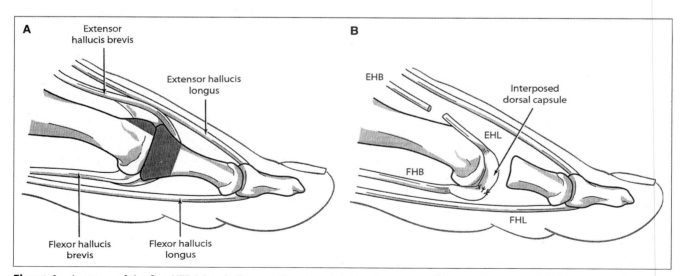

Figure 1 Anatomy of the first MTP joint. **A,** Preoperative view showing the amount of bone to be resected. **B,** Postoperative anatomy showing that the bone has been resected and the dorsal capsule has been sewn into the flexor hallucis brevis after tenotomy of the extensor hallucis brevis.

proximal phalanx, including the insertion of the flexor hallucis brevis tendons and plantar plate. The release will allow the proximal phalanx to glide rather than hinge in dorsiflexion; hinging could compromise the reconstruction by crushing the interposed capsule. Soft-tissue balancing then follows by assessing tightness of the extensor hallucis longus tendon as the foot is brought into neutral dorsiflexion. If the extensor hallucis longus is so tight that it pulls the hallux into dorsiflexion, it will require lengthening so that the great toe is in neutral position with the ankle in dorsiflexion.

When the operation was first performed in 1989, a large smooth Kirschner wire (K-wire) was placed across the MTP joint and removed 3 weeks later. Subsequently, it became apparent that recovery times and range of motion improved without the routine use of a K-wire. I currently recommend that it be used only to protect the repair when the extensor hallucis longus has been lengthened. The K-wire is left in place for 3 weeks, and then range of motion is initiated with the assistance of a physical therapist. After the procedure the stability of the toe is somewhat compromised in the early stages. Once active motion is regained this problem is alleviated because the long tendons adjust to the shortened great toe (**Figure 2**).

This procedure is intended for healthy, active patients who have symptomatic grade III hallux rigidus or failed cheilectomy that is unresponsive to nonsurgical therapy as an alternative to first MTP fusion when nonsurgical therapy has failed to control the symptoms. Absolute contraindications include poor vascular status, infection, or neuropathy. There are three relative contraindications for this procedure. First, patients whose second metatarsal is longer than the first, the so-called Morton's or Greek foot, will usually have a transfer le-sion. These patients should be advised of this possibility before undergoing the procedure. If the difference is minor, an orthotic can be used if the problem develops. If the difference is significant, I recommend concurrent plantar condylectomy of the second metatarsal head. Second, the procedure is relatively contraindicated in patients with arthritic hallux valgus because their results are unpredictable. Last, high-level athletes and professional dancers should not be considered because destruction of the windlass mechanism is associated with this procedure.

Authors' Preferred Treatment and Rationale

In my experience, patients with grade I hallux rigidus rarely seek treatment and can often be treated with shoe wear modifications alone. Patients with grade II hallux rigidus that is refractory to nonsurgical management generally undergo an extensive chei-

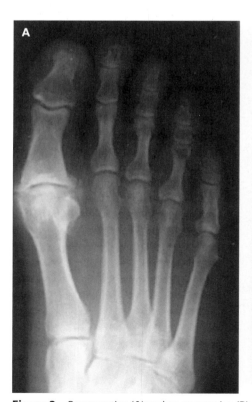
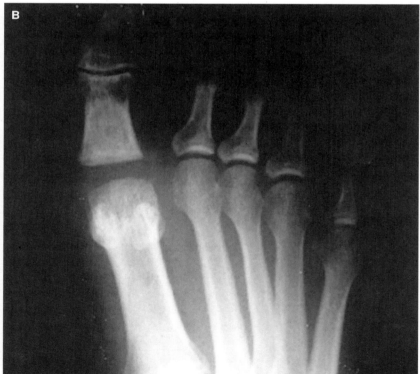

Figure 2   Preoperative (**A**) and postoperative (**B**) AP radiographs. (© Copyright William Hamilton, MD, New York, NY.)

lectomy and concurrent Moberg procedure. Patient satisfaction improved noticeably once the proximal phalangeal osteotomy (Moberg procedure) was added to the index procedure. I currently recommend capsular interposition arthroplasty for men and women in their 50s who wish to play tennis or other racquet sports and women who want to continue to wear high heels. Preliminary results show this population does exceptionally well with the procedure (women better than men). For others, I continue to encourage first MTP joint arthrodesis because of its proven effectiveness over time and high satisfaction rate.

Management of Complications

Fortunately complications of these procedures are rather limited. For cheilectomy, complications include infection, instability of the first MTP joint, recurrence of osteophytes, and hallux valgus. The infections generally are superficial and resolve with local wound care and oral antibiotics. For cases of subluxation, osteophyte recurrence, and hallux valgus, the salvage procedure is an arthrodesis.

Metatarsalgia related to this procedure can be treated with shoe wear modifications or, if necessary, metatarsal shortening procedures. For capsular interposition arthroplasty, transfer lesions have been uncommon, and complications are more often related to diminished range of motion of the great toe, which has been treated with manipulation under anesthesia or, occasionally, lengthening of the extensor hallucis longus tendon.

References

Hamilton WG, Hubbard CE: Hallux rigidus: Excisional arthroplasty. *Foot Ankle Clin* 2000;5:663-671.

Mann RA, Clanton TO: Hallux rigidus: Treatment by cheilectomy. *J Bone Joint Surg Am* 1988; 70:400-406.

Mann RA, Coughlin MJ, DuVries HL: Hallux rigidus: A review of the literature and a method of treatment. *Clin Orthop* 1979;142:57-63.

Shereff MJ, Baumhauer JF: Hallux rigidus and ostearthrosis of the first metatarsophalangeal joint. *J Bone Joint Surg Am* 1998;80:898-908.

Coding

ICD-9 CODE
735.2   Acquired deformities of toe, Hallux rigidus

CPT CODE
28293   Correction, hallux valgus (bunion), with or without sesamoidectomy; resection of joint with implant

Juvenile Hallux Valgus

Michael J. Coughlin, MD

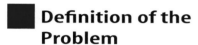

Definition of the Problem

Patient Presentation

Although a bunion may become symptomatic in later years, the onset may be observed as early as age 10 years or younger. A juvenile hallux valgus deformity differs from the typical adult deformity in several ways. Typically, the juvenile deformity has a smaller hallux valgus, intermetatarsal angle, and medial eminence; epiphyseal growth plates are frequently open; and on occasion, metatarsocuneiform hypermobility may be observed. Although the term adolescent hallux valgus is used frequently, the term juvenile hallux valgus is more appropriate because the deformity tends to occur in the preteen years. A symptomatic patient will report pain over the medial eminence with shoe wear and often will have pain with athletic endeavors. It may be difficult for the clinician to differentiate between a teenager's report of pain and his or her concern about a wide forefoot or a cosmetically unacceptable foot. It is important to identify the true complaint because pain relief is a reasonable indication for surgical repair, whereas cosmesis may be a difficult objective to obtain. Typically, the patient with juvenile hallux valgus does not have an overly wide foot and, when measured, often has a "B" width or narrower shoe size.

Metatarsus adductus occurs much more frequently in association with juvenile hallux valgus than it does in the general population. A patient with a splayfoot deformity may also report a bunionette deformity. Other forefoot problems, such as interdigital neuromas and lesser toe deformities, are very uncommon in juvenile and adolescent patients.

Physical Examination

The evaluation of a patient with a juvenile hallux valgus deformity involves both a careful physical examination and a meticulous radiographic assessment. The patient is examined in both sitting and standing positions. While the patient is sitting, attention is first directed to the ankle and Achilles tendon region. The range of motion of the ankle with the knee flexed and extended supplies important information about gastrocnemius-soleus tightness. The foot is then inspected for any deformities of the hindfoot, midfoot, or forefoot. The patient is then asked to stand, and the arch height, position of the heel (varus or valgus), presence of postural problems (pes planus or cavus), and the presence of metatarsus adductus are assessed. The hallux valgus deformity usually is accentuated while the patient is standing. The patient is then asked to walk to evaluate the gait pattern for any abnormalities, including an intoeing gait.

With the patient again in a sitting position, the forefoot is carefully assessed, and the presence of any lesser toe deformities is noted. The specific assessment of the first ray involves examination of the distal joints for position, pain, and motion. The general position of the first ray with a bunion deformity is marked by medial deviation of the first metatarsal and lateral deviation of the toe. This deviation can be accentuated by a deformity in which there is increased lateral deviation in the proximal phalanx. Hallux valgus interphalangeus occurs with greater than 10° of lateral deviation of the phalanges from their longitudinal axis. It is not uncommon to have an element of hallux valgus interphalangeus associated with a juvenile hallux valgus deformity. Most commonly, however, the principal deformity occurs at the metatarsophalangeal (MTP) joint with lateral deviation of the base of the proximal phalanx on the metatarsal head.

Although radiographic assessment is critical to determination of the correct surgical procedure, the physical examination also is helpful. Initially, the range of motion of the first MTP joint is assessed. Both active and passive plantar flexion and dorsiflexion are recorded for both feet. Then the toe is grasped between the finger and thumb of the examiner and deviated into a straight position in relationship to the first metatarsal, thus decreasing the hallux valgus deformity. The passive range of motion of the MTP joint is again assessed. With a subluxated bunion deformity, range of motion usually is not diminished. With a congruent joint associated with a hallux valgus deformity, this movement in a sagittal plane to reduce the deformity simulates what would be accomplished in surgery with an intra-articular repair (ie, sliding the base of the phalanx across the articular surface of the distal metatarsal in the correction of the deformity). With passive dorsiflexion and plantar flexion of the MTP joint in the presence of a congruent joint, motion often is observed to be diminished substantially.

Last, the mobility of the metatarsocuneiform joint is assessed. Although instability is more common in patients with collagen deficiency syndromes such as Ehlers-Danlos syndrome, instability of the metatarsocuneiform joint occasionally is associated with a juvenile hallux valgus deformity. The preferred method of physical assessment to evaluate metatarsocuneiform hypermobility requires the examiner, while sitting and facing the patient (whose ankle is in a neutral position [0° of dorsiflexion]), to grasp the lateral forefoot between the fingers and thumb of one hand and grasp the first metatarsal with the index finger and thumb of the other hand. Then with a repetitive dorsal and plantar thrust, the first ray is moved up and down in a sagittal plane to assess the mobility and/or hypermobility of the metatarsocuneiform joint. This examination is not specific for the metatarsocuneiform joint, and it may be affected by motion at the naviculocuneiform and talonavicular joints. In addition, this examination is very physician dependent because the end point of dorsal and plantar excursion is somewhat subjective. Nonetheless, with repeated examination, a sense of the degree of mobility can be gauged.

The radiographic examination is critical in the assessment of any hallux valgus deformity. The first step in this examination requires quantifying the magnitude of the deformity. The hallux valgus angle and the 1-2 intermetatarsal angle are initially used to

quantify the magnitude of the angular deformity. Marks are made in the proximal and distal metaphyses of the proximal phalanx and the first and second metatarsals. The marks are equidistant from the medial and lateral cortices of the respective bones and in the range of 1 to 2 cm from the adjacent articular surfaces. Using these reference points, longitudinal axes are drawn. The intersection of the axes of the first and second metatarsals forms the 1-2 intermetatarsal angle (**Figure 1**). The normal value is less than 9°. The intersection of the axes of the first metatarsal and proximal phalanx forms the hallux valgus

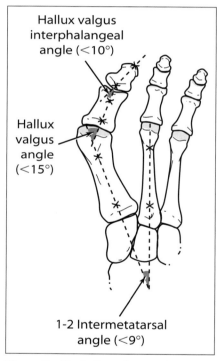

Figure 1 The hallux valgus angle and 1-2 intermetatarsal angle are formed by the intersection of the diaphyseal axes of the proximal phalanx, first metatarsal, and second metatarsal. The interphalangeal angle is formed by the axis of the distal phalanx (reference points at the tip of the phalanx and the center of the proximal articular surface) and the axis of the proximal phalanx. (Reproduced with permission from Coughlin MJ: Hallux valgus in men: Effect of the distal metatarsal articular angle on hallux valgus correction. *Foot Ankle Int* 1997;18:463-470.)

angle. The normal value is less than 15°. To quantify the magnitude of hallux valgus interphalangeus, the longitudinal axis of the distal phalanx of the hallux is created by a line drawn through reference points at the tip of the distal phalanx and at the center of the proximal articular surface at the interphalangeal joint. The intersection of this axis with the longitudinal axis of the proximal phalanx forms the interphalangeal angle of the hallux, which has a normal value of less than 10°. Attention to the orientation of the lesser metatarsal is equally important. Medial inclination of the lesser metatarsal will diminish the magnitude of the 1-2 intermetatarsal angle, giving an abnormally low value. Moreover, the presence of metatarsus adductus makes correction more difficult and may influence the selection of a particular surgical technique.

The orientation and shape of the MTP joint has a significant effect on the predisposition to a hallux valgus deformity. This joint rarely is oriented at a perpendicular angle to the long axis of the ray; rather, a slight valgus inclination of approximately 6° is considered normal. The term distal metatarsal articular angle (DMAA) is the term used to describe the magnitude of this lateral slope (**Figure 2**). Normally it is 6° or less. It is not uncommon for the DMAA to measure 10° to 15° without any MTP joint subluxation. Hallux valgus deformities that are characterized by articular surface angulation are, in general, believed to be static and rarely progress over time. However, a hallux valgus deformity with an incongruous or subluxated joint occurs when the base of the proximal phalanx deviates laterally in relationship to the articular surface of the first metatarsal head (**Figure 3**). In this type of deformity, mild subluxation may progress with time, in contrast to a hallux valgus deformity with a congruous joint that does not progress with time. Whereas many reports note the high recurrence rate of

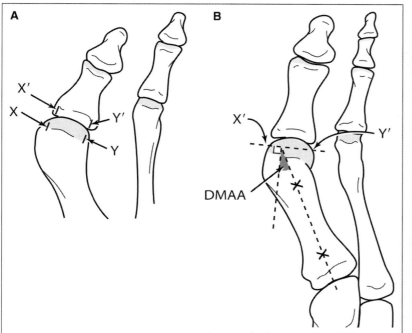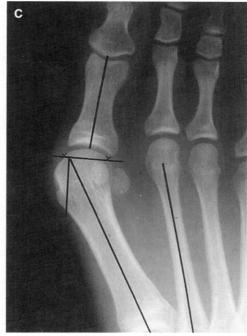

Figure 2 **A,** Congruent hallux valgus deformity. **B,** Method of determining DMAA. A line is drawn connecting points X′ and Y′, the medial and lateral extent of the distal metatarsal articular surface. A perpendicular line is drawn in relationship to X′ and Y′. The angle formed by the longitudinal axis of the first metatarsal and the perpendicular line forms the DMAA. As the DMAA increases, there is increased slope to the distal metatarsal articular surface. (Reproduced with permission from Coughlin MJ: Hallux valgus in men: Effect of the distal metatarsal articular angle on hallux valgus correction. *Foot Ankle Int* 1997;18:463-470.) **C,** AP radiograph shows increased DMAA with hallux valgus deformity (congruent deformity); lines mark the hallux valgus, intermetatarsal angles, and the DMAA.

surgery on the juvenile patient with a bunion deformity, the key may not be the age of the patient but rather the lack of recognition of a congruent MTP joint, which occurs in almost half of the patients with juvenile hallux valgus deformities. In addition, some bunion deformities treated in later years are much more difficult to treat and may have had their onset in adolescence or earlier. Surgical techniques must be tailored to the underlying anatomic abnormalities, and the differentiation of a subluxated from a congruent MTP joint is probably the most important consideration in the evaluation of the juvenile bunion.

Another consideration in the skeletally immature patient is the presence of an open epiphysis. While it has been speculated that an open epiphysis may play a role in recurrence, this concept has never been proved. More likely, recurrence re-

sults from the selection of an inappropriate procedure to correct the deformity. However, care must be taken to identify an open epiphysis in either the proximal phalanx or the proximal first metatarsal and to avoid epiphyseal injury should surgery be performed in proximity of these growth plates. Correction of a juvenile hallux valgus deformity often requires one or more osteotomies; thus, prevention of an iatrogenic epiphyseal injury is important.

Differential Diagnosis
- Neurologic or neuromuscular abnormalities
- Postural abnormalities (pes planus or pes cavus)
- Other forefoot abnormalities

Additional Work-up
While routine radiographs are typically sufficient, CT, with or without

contrast media, or MRI occasionally may be helpful in defining a congruent MTP joint. Rarely are neurologic evaluation or neurologic studies necessary in patients with routine juvenile hallux valgus deformity. Hematologic and blood chemistry studies are rarely necessary in the evaluation of a healthy adolescent.

————————————————■

■ **The Solutions**

Treatment Options and Rationale
In general the treatment options are specifically designed to treat the underlying hallux valgus deformity. The first decision in this process is made by determining the magnitude of the

angular deformity. The hallux valgus angle is less than 25° in a mild deformity, is greater than 25° but less than or equal to 40° in a moderate deformity, and is greater than 40° in a severe deformity. The next decision is based upon whether the MTP joint is characterized as subluxated or congruent. Last, the occasional presence of metatarsocuneiform hypermobility must be considered in the planning process.

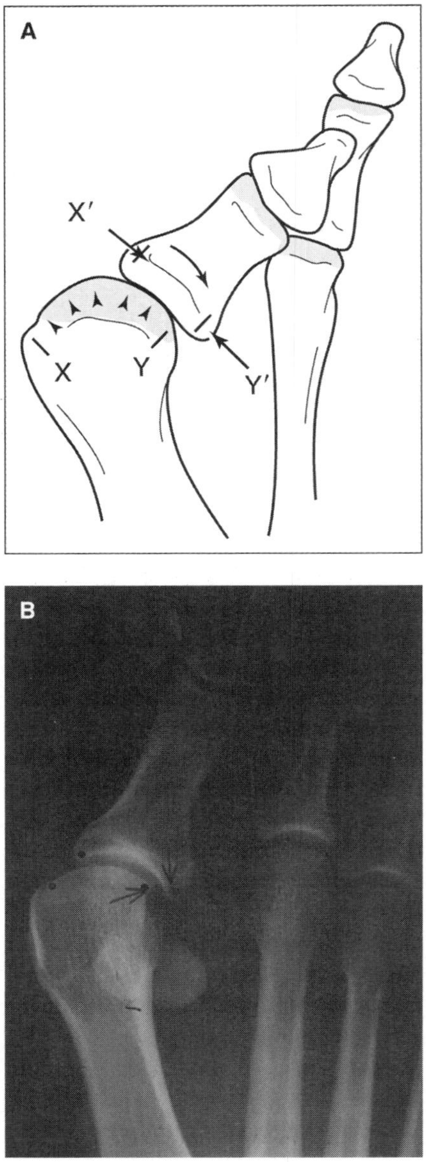

MILD DEFORMITY

For a mild deformity (hallux valgus angle less than 25°), the options are not as dramatic, and there is some overlap in the surgical considerations. For a congruent hallux valgus deformity, a distal metatarsal osteotomy is preferable. This may be a chevron osteotomy, a Mitchell osteotomy, or another type of distal metatarsal osteotomy (eg, Reverdin, Scarf, Kramer). For a subluxated deformity, a distal metatarsal osteotomy may still be the treatment of choice, but a distal soft-tissue realignment may also be considered. A distal soft-tissue realignment (ie, McBride) achieves reduction of the deformity by a lateral soft-tissue release, a medial capsulorrhaphy, and medial eminence resection. An Akin osteotomy may be combined with any of the above procedures to reduce angular deformity in the phalanx.

MODERATE DEFORMITY

For a moderate deformity (hallux valgus angle greater than 25° and less than 40°), the distinction between a congruent and incongruent (subluxated) MTP joint is again important. A distal osteotomy (eg, chevron, Mitchell) may be used with either type because reorientation of the distal metatarsal articular surface frequently can be achieved with these types of osteotomies. An Akin phalangeal osteotomy may be added to the technique to achieve increased angular realignment. For the incongruent or subluxated deformity, a distal soft-tissue realignment is often combined with a proximal first metatarsal osteotomy to reduce the intermetatarsal angle while realigning the MTP joint.

SEVERE DEFORMITY

The most challenging deformities are the severe angular deformities associated with a congruent MTP joint. The subluxated deformity can be corrected with a distal soft-tissue realignment and a proximal first metatarsal osteotomy. In the presence of metatarsocuneiform hypermobility, a Lapidus procedure (distal soft-tissue realignment with metatarsocuneiform arthrodesis) may be performed. However, in the severe angular deformity associated with a congruent MTP joint, a distal soft-tissue realignment will change a congruent joint to an incongruent joint, thereby placing the MTP joint at risk for postoperative restricted motion, later degenerative arthritis, or recurrent deformity. In this situation, a proximal osteotomy may be performed: a first cuneiform opening wedge osteotomy or a proximal first metatarsal osteotomy (crescentic, or opening or closing wedge metatarsal osteotomy). A distal first metatarsal closing wedge osteotomy and occasionally an Akin phalangeal osteotomy also may be performed. The essence of this method of treatment is the performance of periarticular osteotomies to leave the MTP joint untouched, instead achieving an extra-articular realignment.

Author's Preferred Treatment and Rationale

MILD DEFORMITY

Although many surgical options are available for the treatment of congruent and subluxated hallux valgus deformities with a mild angular deformity, a distal metatarsal osteotomy is preferable because it allows correction of either type of deformity. A Mitchell osteotomy has had substantial popularity; however, the chevron osteotomy is preferable because of its stability, its relative simplicity, and its proven reliability in treating mild and low moderate hallux valgus deformities.

Figure 3 **A,** Subluxated (incongruent) hallux valgus deformity. (Reproduced with permission from Coughlin MJ: Hallux valgus in men: Effect of the distal metatarsal articular angle on hallux valgus correction. *Foot Ankle Int* 1997;18:463-470.) **B,** AP radiograph shows subluxated hallux valgus deformity; markers are placed on medial and lateral extent of the articular surfaces.

CHEVRON PROCEDURE

The chevron procedure achieves correction by a lateral translation of the capital fragment, medial eminence resection, and medial capsulorrhaphy. A biplanar osteotomy may be performed by removing more medial bone at the osteotomy site to achieve increased reduction of the DMAA.

A 3- to 4-cm longitudinal medial incision is centered over the medial eminence and deepened to the capsule. An L-shaped capsular incision is used to expose the medial eminence, releasing the capsule along the dorsal and proximal aspects. The medial eminence is resected in line with the medial border of the foot. A transverse drill hole, oriented in a medial-lateral direction, is made in the center of the metatarsal head. This hole forms the apex of the chevron-shaped osteotomy. Two diverging osteotomy cuts are centered at the apex and diverge at a 60° angle. Care is taken to avoid deep penetration on the lateral aspect of the metatarsal head because it may injure the lateral vascular supply. After completion of the osteotomies, the capital fragment is displaced 4 to 5 mm laterally and impacted onto the metaphyses. It is then internally stabilized with a 0.062-in Kirschner wire (K-wire) that is cut so that it is covered by the overlying soft tissue. The prominent metaphysis is resected with a sagittal saw, and the capsule is repaired with interrupted absorbable sutures. The skin is approximated, and the forefoot is covered with a gauze and tape compression bandage. Ambulation is permitted in a postoperative shoe with weight bearing allowed on the lateral aspect of the foot. Dressings are discontinued 6 to 8 weeks following surgery.

DISTAL SOFT-TISSUE REALIGNMENT WITH OR WITHOUT PROXIMAL FIRST METATARSAL CRESCENTIC OSTEOTOMY

A 3- to 4-cm incision is centered over the first intermetatarsal web space and deepened to the conjoined adductor

tendon. The tendon is released from the lateral sesamoid and then from the proximal muscle leaving a 2- to 3-cm stump of tendon. The lateral capsule is released on the dorsal and proximal aspect by developing a proximally based cuff of capsule. Attention is then directed to the medial aspect of the foot.

A 3- to 4-cm longitudinal medial incision is centered over the medial eminence and deepened to the capsule. An L-shaped capsular incision is used to expose the medial eminence, releasing the capsule along the dorsal and proximal aspects. The medial eminence is resected in line with the medial border of the first metatarsal. Attention is then directed to the proximal first metatarsal. A 3- to 4-cm incision is centered over the dorsal aspect of the first metatarsal. The dissection is deepened to the metatarsal, and a crescentic osteotomy is performed 1 cm from the metatarsocuneiform joint. The concave aspect of the osteotomy is directed proximally. The osteotomy site is displaced to diminish the intermetatarsal angle, making the first and second metatarsal shafts relatively parallel. The osteotomy site is internally fixed with either smooth K-wires if the epiphysis remains open or with a K-wire and a compression screw if the epiphysis is closed. It is important to visualize the epiphysis when performing any proximal metatarsal osteotomy to minimize the chance of injury.

The medial capsule is then repaired with interrupted absorbable sutures with the toe held in a derotated realigned position. On the lateral aspect of the MTP joint, the conjoined adductor tendon and lateral capsule are repaired with interrupted absorbable sutures as well. The skin incisions are approximated and the forefoot wrapped in a gauze and tape compression dressing. Ambulation is allowed in a postoperative shoe with weight bearing on the heel and lateral aspect of the foot until radiographic healing

of the osteotomy is confirmed. Dressings are changed every 10 days for 8 weeks, holding the toes and forefoot in correct alignment.

On occasion an Akin phalangeal osteotomy is performed in conjunction with the distal soft-tissue realignment. In this case, the medial incision is extended distally approximately 1.5 cm and deepened to the phalanx with care taken to protect the distal MTP capsular attachment. A sagittal saw is used to resect a medially based wedge of bone in the proximal or distal metaphysis of the phalanx. Typically a 2- to 3-mm base is removed from the medial aspect with the cuts converging on the lateral aspect of the phalangeal cortex. The segment is removed and the osteotomy is closed and stabilized with two percutaneous 0.062-in K-wires introduced distally and driven in a proximal direction.

MODIFIED LAPIDUS PROCEDURE

A distal soft-tissue realignment is performed as described previously. A 3- to 4-cm incision is centered over the metatarsocuneiform joint and deepened to the proximal metatarsal surface. An osteotome is used to resect the articular surfaces of the first metatarsal and cuneiform. The resected surfaces are coapted with care taken to reduce the intermetatarsal angle and slightly plantar flex the first metatarsal at the time of the arthrodesis. A bone graft augmenting the arthrodesis is advantageous. Internal fixation is achieved with two or three compression screws oriented in different planes to maximize stability of the arthrodesis site. A below knee cast is applied and used until radiographic union is achieved, usually at 6 weeks after surgery. A gauze and tape compression dressing can be used if a patient is quite reliable and will refrain from weight bearing on the medial aspect of the foot.

DOUBLE AND TRIPLE FIRST RAY OSTEOTOMIES

Multiple first ray osteotomies may be necessary to correct a severe hallux valgus deformity with a congruent MTP joint. The critical osteotomy is the distal first metatarsal osteotomy. An L-shaped medial capsular release is used to expose the MTP joint and medial eminence. The medial eminence is resected in line with the medial border of the first metatarsal. With the medial capsule turned distally, a medially based closing wedge osteotomy is performed just proximal to the upper border of the sesamoids. The magnitude of this cut depends on the magnitude of the DMAA. The cuts converge on the lateral border of the first metatarsal metaphysis. The osteotomy site is closed and stabilized with two 0.062-in K-wires that are cut and left below the level of the skin (**Figure 4**).

If an Akin phalangeal osteotomy is performed, it is located at the distal end of the medial incision and is also stabilized with K-wires. The third osteotomy may be performed in the proximal metatarsal if the epiphysis is closed, and alternatively, in the first cuneiform if the proximal metatarsal epiphysis is open. If a proximal first metatarsal osteotomy is performed, a crescentic type osteotomy is preferred as it neither lengthens nor shortens the first ray. The technique described previously is used, with the osteotomy stabilized with a compression screw and K-wire. If the epiphysis remains open, the surgeon can shift the location of the crescentic osteotomy distally or consider an opening wedge cuneiform osteotomy. For a first cuneiform osteotomy, a vertical osteotomy is made at the midpoint of the cuneiform and deepened across to the lateral cortex. A lamina spreader is used to distract the osteotomy site, and an interposition iliac crest graft is placed in the interval and stabilized with two K-wires. The opening wedge cuneiform osteotomy can actually lengthen the first ray and may be considered if the ray is initially short. This osteotomy tends to decrease the intermetatarsal angle as the osteotomy site is opened (**Figure 5**).

With the combination of osteotomies, often a walking boot or cast is preferable for 6 to 8 weeks while the osteotomies heal. The position of the hallux is maintained with a gauze and tape compression dressing as well. Walking is allowed on the lateral aspect of the foot, but care must be taken to protect the multiple osteotomy sites to avoid displacement and loss of alignment.

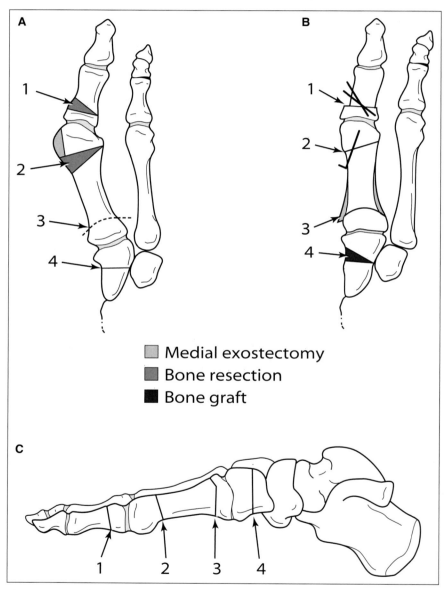

Figure 4 Triple osteotomy. **A** and **B,** AP views; **C,** lateral view. Proposed osteotomies are: (1) Phalangeal osteotomy (closing wedge); (2) Distal metatarsal osteotomy (closing wedge); (3) Crescentic proximal first metatarsal osteotomy; and (4) opening wedge cuneiform osteotomy. (Reproduced with permission from Coughlin M, Carlson R: Treatment of hallux valgus with an increased distal metatarsal articular angle: Evaluation of double and triple first ray osteotomies. *Foot Ankle Int* 1999;20:762-770.)

Management of Complications

The most common complication following surgery is recurrence. The re-evaluation of a patient following recurrence of a hallux valgus deformity is critical in defining the reasons for the previous failure. An inadequate prior correction may be a result of failure to reduce either the hallux valgus or intermetatarsal angle or to stabilize metatarsocunei- form hypermobility. The procedure may need to be redone merely to achieve adequate realignment or stabilization of the metatarsocuneiform joint. However, if an intra-articular repair with realignment of the MTP joint has been attempted in the face of a congruous joint, salvage may be achieved with periarticular osteotomies as described previously. For a patient with substantial metatarsus adductus, adequate repair of the bunion deformity may be limited by the medial inclination of the lateral lesser metatarsal. Whereas consideration may be given to multiple lesser metatarsal osteotomies, a bunion repair will often be sufficient, and the magnitude of other forefoot surgery can be avoided.

References

Coughlin MJ: Hallux valgus. *Instr Course Lect* 1997;46:357-391.

Coughlin M: Juvenile hallux valgus: Etiology and treatment. *Foot Ankle Int* 1995;16:682-697.

Coughlin MJ: Juvenile hallux valgus, in Coughlin MJ, Mann RA (eds): *Surgery of the Foot and Ankle*, ed 7. St Louis, MO, Mosby-Yearbook, 1999, pp 270-319.

Coughlin MJ, Mann RA: The pathophysiology of the juvenile bunion. *Instr Course Lect* 1987;36:123-136.

Peterson HA, Newman SR: Adolescent bunion deformity treated with double osteotomy and longitudinal pin fixation of the first ray. *J Pediatr Orthop* 1993;13:80-84.

Sangeorzan BJ, Hansen ST Jr: Modified Lapidus procedure for hallux valgus. *Foot Ankle* 1989;9:262-266.

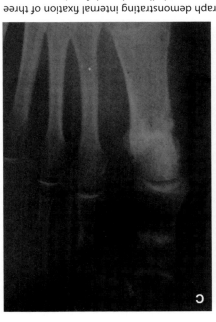
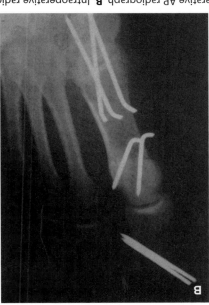
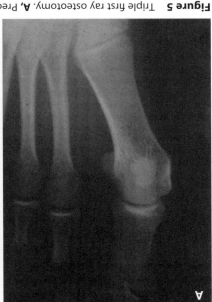

Figure 5 Triple first ray osteotomy. **A,** Preoperative AP radiograph. **B,** Intraoperative radiograph demonstrating internal fixation of three osteotomies. **C,** Follow-up 6 months after successful healing of osteotomies and correction of congruent hallux valgus deformity.

Coding

ICD-9 CODE

735.0   Acquired deformities of toe, Hallux valgus (acquired)

CPT CODES

28292   Correction, hallux valgus (bunion), with or without sesamoidectomy; Keller, McBride or Mayo type procedure

28296   Correction, hallux valgus (bunion), with or without sesamoidectomy; with metatarsal osteotomy (eg, Mitchell, Chevron, or concentric type procedures)

28297   Correction, hallux valgus (bunion), with or without sesamoidectomy; Lapidus type procedure

28298   Correction, hallux valgus (bunion), with or without sesamoidectomy; by phalanx osteotomy

28299   Correction, hallux valgus (bunion), with or without sesamoidectomy; by double osteotomy

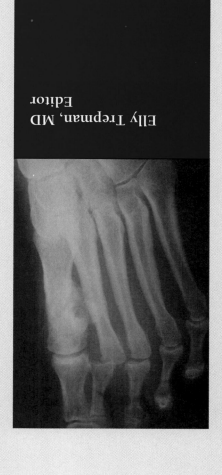

SECTION 2
Problems of the Lesser Toes

Elly Trepman, MD
Editor

Second Metatarsophalangeal Instability

William C. McGarvey, MD

Definition of the Problem

Patient Presentation

Second metatarsophalangeal (MTP) joint instability is a broad term and includes idiopathic synovitis, fixed dislocation, and crossover toe deformity. This joint is the most common chronically dislocated joint in the foot. Therefore, patients may present with a variety of symptoms.

Patients experiencing second MTP joint synovitis may report a swollen, painful area in the central forefoot. There may be swelling of the second MTP joint or the entire second toe. Pain may be diffuse, and it may be difficult to distinguish between symptoms arising directly from the joint and those from the interdigital space. Inflammatory changes within the joint may cause capsular distention and irritation of the adjacent interdigital nerve, mimicking or causing neuroma. The patient may also describe pain or calluses beneath the ball of the foot, particularly if the symptoms are associated with a long second metatarsal. Other common symptoms include difficulty with shoe wear, cramping of the second toe, or a feeling that the toes are crossing in the shoe. Pathology at the second MTP joint may arise as an alteration of the normal function of the anatomic structures. Systemic disease or chronic repetitive local trauma can cause degeneration or attrition of the plantar plate, resulting in instability and mechanical irritation. Dysfunction of the intrinsic muscles from diabetes mellitus or compartment syndrome may result in the unopposed function of the extrinsic tendons. The intrinsic minus foot has a loss of active MTP joint flexion and interphalangeal joint extension and unopposed action of the long flexors and extensors, resulting in claw toe deformity, which consists of hyperextension at the MTP joint and hyperflexion of the interphalangeal joints (**Figure 1**). Chronic malpositioning, such as the cramping imposed by a small toe box or MTP dorsiflexion in high-heeled shoes, can also lead to this deformity. In time, the deformity may become fixed. Excessive length of the second metatarsal may contribute to overload of the second MTP joint. Subluxation and dislocation of the second MTP joint also may be associated with hallux valgus deformity. The laterally deviating hallux can act as a deforming force crowding the second toe, further enhancing its buckling. Eventually the

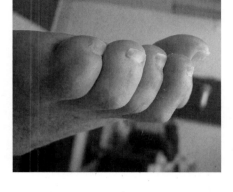

Figure 1 Typical clinical appearance of claw toe deformity. This patient had an unrecognized compartment syndrome resulting from a calcaneal fracture.

hallux valgus, if severe, may displace and elevate the second toe causing it to lie directly dorsal to the hallux as a crossover toe deformity. When second MTP instability occurs primarily, the dorsal displacement of the second toe may contribute to aggravation of the hallux valgus deformity. However, the medially subluxated or crossover second toe may present without hallux valgus deformity. Another mechanism for second MTP joint instability is idiopathic onset of inflammatory synovitis leading to attritional changes in the joint capsule. Combined with restrictive shoe wear, the third toe may be the offending agent and may impinge against the lateral second MTP joint capsule and irritate incompetent lateral tissues. This irritation may be a result of a long second metatarsal, with the second MTP joint impinging against the proximal phalanx of the third toe, aggravating the second MTP capsular erosion.

Physical Examination

The patient should be asked about vocational and recreational activity and shoe wear. Narrow or poorly fitting shoes may contribute to the problem. However, synovitis sometimes occurs as a result of overuse or chronic repetitive stress, even in properly fitting shoes, as in distance runners. The medical history may reveal comorbid conditions such as rheumatoid arthritis or gout that can lead to soft-tissue compromise and MTP joint instability.

Examination findings may be varied depending on the severity of the presentation. Toes are inspected for swelling, alignment, callosities, and deformities such as mallet toe, hammer toe, claw toe, crossover toe, hallux valgus, and swelling in other MTP joints.

Palpation may localize tender areas, identify bogginess or fullness in the area of the joint, and differentiate tenderness from intermetatarsal tenderness. If MTP joint instability is suspected, a dorsal drawer or toe translation test is performed. While grasping the proximal phalanx in one hand and the metatarsal in the other, the dorsal translation of the phalanx on the metatarsal head is assessed for pain and laxity (**Figure 2**). In some cases, the examiner may be able to completely dislocate the toe.

The degree of passive correction is assessed with the patient both sitting and standing to determine the contribution of the ankle and heel cord to the deformity. Dynamic deformation may correct with the patient in a recumbent position with the foot held in equinus. The distinction between dynamic and static deformity is crucial in implementing a treatment plan and may clarify the indications for particular surgical procedures.

Differential local anesthetic injec-

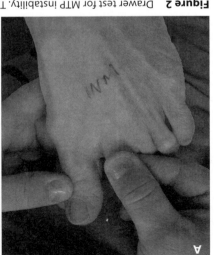
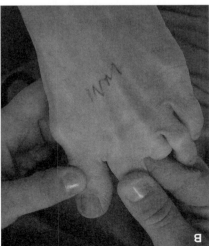

Figure 2 Drawer test for MTP instability. The foot is stabilized and the toe is manipulated, first dorsally (**A**), then plantarly (**B**). The examiner looks and feels for subluxation or dislocation of the proximal phalanx on the metatarsal head.

tion can be helpful in patients believed to have isolated MTP synovitis who may present with more vague, nonspecific symptoms. I perform the initial injection into the joint (local anesthetic only) because the nerve block from a web space injection may provide pain relief and falsely lead the examiner to believe he or she is dealing with an interdigital neuroma. Alternatively, anesthetic can

leak out of the joint, also causing a false-positive result.

Weight-bearing AP and lateral non–weight-bearing oblique radiographs are obtained to help assess anatomic anomalies, such as metatarsal length, joint incongruity, arthrosis, or Freiberg's infraction, and may reveal the degree of subluxation or dislocation (**Figure 3**). Joint distention is manifested as increased second MTP joint space compared with the adjacent MTP joint spaces.

A sesamoid view that includes the second MTP joint may be helpful in demonstrating a plantar second metatarsal head prominence, which usually is located on the fibular side.

Advanced imaging studies, such as technetium Tc 99m bone scanning or MRI, may be helpful for diagnostic dilemmas, tumors, or stress fractures.

Other studies such as serologic assays may be helpful if a systemic condition is suspected.

Differential Diagnosis
- Interdigital neuroma
- Mechanical imbalance (excessively long second metatarsal, hallux valgus)
- Poorly fitting shoes
- Inflammatory arthritides (rheumatoid arthritis, psoriasis, gout)
- Neuromuscular disorders (Charcot-Marie-Tooth disease, diabetes mellitus)
- Osteoarthritis
- Trauma or posttraumatic changes (fracture, stress fracture, osteochondral fracture)
- Freiberg's infraction

Additional Work-up
None

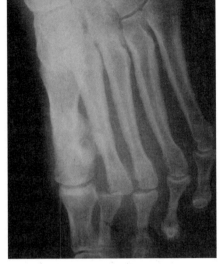
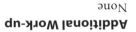

Figure 3 Complete dislocation of second toe with overlapping of the proximal phalanx on the metatarsal head.

The Solutions

Treatment Options and Rationale

Nonsurgical management of second MTP instability is increasingly unsuccessful with advancing deformity, so it is imperative that treatment be initiated as soon as the diagnosis is made. Nonsurgical treatment, which may be functional or accommodative depending on the dynamic or static nature of the deformity, meets with variable success. Synovitis is treated with nonsteroidal anti-inflammatory drugs, metatarsal support orthoses, stiff-soled accommodative and rigid rocker-bottom shoes, and judicious intra-articular steroid injections. Care must be used in the patient with impending subluxation because intra-articular steroids, although effective in alleviating symptoms, can lead to capsular attrition and precipitate subluxation or even dislocation.

Flexible deformities may be managed by taping the toe in the corrected or overcorrected position with or without metatarsal support orthoses. Careful monitoring of these patients is important because taping may restrict venous outflow and cause edema or vascular obstruction.

Fixed deformities are poorly managed nonsurgically. However, if a patient is not a candidate for surgery or does not want to undergo surgical treatment, accommodative shoe wear with a deep, wide toe box and a cushioned insole can provide reasonable relief and unload crowded toes. Factors involved in surgical decision making include the presence and degree of MTP instability, the dynamic nature of the condition, the degree of passive correction, and the magnitude and direction of the deformity.

Synovitis without deformity that has failed nonsurgical treatment may respond to surgical synovectomy. Stability must be assessed before and during surgery. Should the toe be unstable, a flexor tendon transfer into the extensor hood may prevent recurrence. The tendon transfer provides the theoretical advantage of a dynamic restraint to dorsal subluxation by restoring or reinforcing intrinsic function. In practice, however, this more likely serves as a static tenodesis that restricts dorsiflexion. In the less common instance of synovitis associated with hallux valgus that restricts space available for the second toe, the hallux deformity should be corrected concomitantly to prevent recurrence of the second toe problem and eliminate the potential deforming force from the hallux valgus.

Second MTP instability with deformity or dislocation requires more complex surgical treatment including soft-tissue release and/or reconstruction. At the very minimum, sequential release of contracted structures is required to allow for reduction of the toe into its normal anatomic position. Stepwise soft-tissue lengthening or release should begin with long and short extensor tenotomy followed by dorsal capsular tissue release and sectioning the collateral ligaments and, if necessary, the interossei. Variations exist for each of these procedures, including transverse capsulotomy, extensor Z-lengthening or tenotomy, and excision of the entire capsule, but the choice of procedure remains the surgeon's personal preference. One recommendation for collateral ligament release is to sever the distal or phalangeal attachments to maintain blood flow to the metatarsal head and avoid the theoretical complication of osteonecrosis. Maintaining blood flow is particularly important if a metatarsal osteotomy is planned because that procedure might completely devascularize the metatarsal head.

The necessity of adjunctive procedures is predicated on the reducibility and stability of the joint. Persistent instability after soft-tissue release of the MTP restraints may necessitate the addition of a flexor-to-extensor transfer. The flexor digitorum longus is removed from its insertion on the plantar surface of the distal phalanx and split evenly down its central longitudinal raphe. Each end is then brought around the proximal phalanx to attach dorsally either to itself or to the extensor expansion, thus providing a dynamic restraint to further dorsal subluxation.

Presence of a painful intractable plantar keratosis may necessitate a plantar condylectomy. Typically the fibular condyle is more prominent. Approximately 20% of the metatarsal head is resected from the plantar surface. Although this resection theoretically may increase the risk of dorsal subluxation as a result of the increased laxity of the plantar plate, in practice, however, a pin is used for 2 weeks to maintain position and allow plantar structures to scar in appropriate position, thus providing restraint against dorsal migration of the toe.

The toe that is irreducible even after complete soft-tissue release requires bony decompression. Functional shortening of the metatarsal is necessary to prevent ischemia of the small vessels under tension, to prevent overcompressing articular surfaces leading to degenerative joint disease, and to reduce the propensity of recurrence. This can be done in several ways. The most reliable ways are metatarsal shortening osteotomy and metatarsal head arthroplasty. Procedure selection is based on the specific type of deformity and the surgeon's preference.

Metatarsal shortening osteotomies in combination with the aforementioned soft-tissue releases and flexor-to-extensor transfers have gained tremendous popularity. Metatarsal shortening allows the toe to reduce into the joint and also relieves potential pressure on the metatarsal head. The distal osteotomy, though technically challenging, has been shown to have few complications, such as malunion or pseudarthrosis,

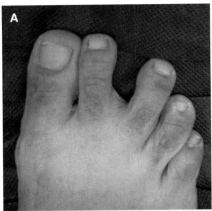
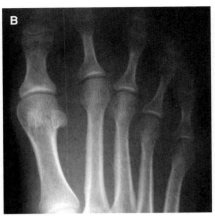
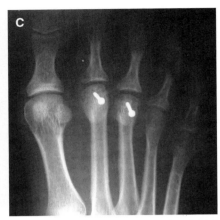

Figure 4 **A,** Splaying of second and third toes with instability. This patient underwent shortening osteotomies of both the second and third metatarsals, as well as flexor-to-extensor transfers and capsular releases. Note the relative length and incongruity on the preoperative radiograph **(B)** and the corrected length on the postoperative radiograph **(C)**.

and reliable reduction and maintenance of the joint. It also can be performed through the same incision as the soft-tissue procedure and allows 3 to 8 mm of recession of metatarsal length (**Figure 4**). Care must be taken, however, not to devascularize the metatarsal head and cause metatarsal osteonecrosis.

Metatarsal head arthroplasty (DuVries) is a reasonable alternative, but by virtue of the extensive cartilaginous débridement, it routinely leads to MTP stiffness. This procedure may be limited to low-demand patients and those with preexisting degenerative disease at the respective metatarsal head.

Patients with fixed hammer toe or claw toe deformities may require proximal interphalangeal (PIP) resection arthroplasty after unsuccessful soft-tissue release. This procedure allows for reduction of the MTP joint by extensor tenotomy and PIP capsulotomy, with or without PIP resection arthroplasty, in addition to the realignment of the PIP joint. I routinely pin these toes, and the shortening through the distal portion of the proximal phalanx reduces soft-tissue tension and relieves stress on the neurovascular bundles.

Crossover toe and a deviated toe, defined as angulation of the toe at the MTP joint not overlapping the hallux, present their own special dilemmas in determining surgical management. Concurrent hallux valgus may be corrected to allow room for the second toe to lie between the hallux and third toes (**Figure 5**). Soft tissues are then lengthened in the manner described previously, with particular attention paid to the collateral ligaments and capsule on the shortened (usually medial) side of the second toe. The first lumbrical and interosseous muscle are also released if necessary. Lateral capsular plication allows this release to be more effective by reducing the varus deviation of the second toe and providing a static lateral restraint to recurrent deformation.

In the case of long-standing deformity or systemic disease, it may be difficult to identify competent tissue, and the reliability of capsular reefing becomes suspect. More commonly, the addition of a tendon transfer for dynamic restraint or tenodesis effect is necessary.

Use of transected extensor digitorum brevis tendon has gained popularity. The distal limb of the tendon is passed inferior to the intact intermetatarsal ligament and then reattached proximally after shortening to allow for a lateral restraint to medial deviation. The tenodesis effect has been shown to be successful in maintaining toe position while preserving MTP joint motion.

Flexor-to-extensor tendon transfer may be performed to provide a restraint to medial deviation. When this procedure is done for a crossover toe deformity, the lateral limb of the split flexor tendon is preferentially tightened to correct the adduction deformity. Rotation, however, may be difficult to control. Adduction is not always completely corrected.

Direct comparison of these techniques has demonstrated excellent results in each. The advantage of the extensor digitorum brevis transfer is that it requires less soft-tissue dissection and may preserve greater MTP joint motion, but this may be at the expense of stability. Follow-up evaluation suggests that extensor digitorum brevis transfers allow slightly more laxity than properly performed flexor-to-extensor tendon transfers. Thus, it is recommended that the extensor digitorum brevis transfer preferentially be used for a lower grade medially deviated toe or flexible crossover deformity and the flexor-to-extensor tendon transfer be used for a rigid crossover toe or complete dislocation.

Toe amputation is a viable treatment alternative for the problematic second toe in limited situations. Indi-

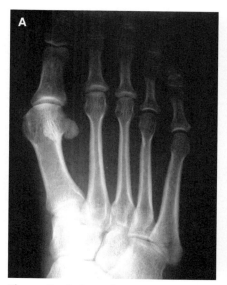 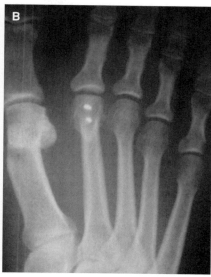 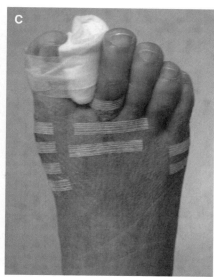

Figure 5 **A,** Second MTP instability as a result of excessive second metatarsal length and associated hallux valgus. **B,** Patient treated surgically with a metatarsal shortening osteotomy and flexor-to-extensor transfer. **C,** Hallux valgus corrected with chevron osteotomy to allow room for the corrected second toe.

cations for this procedure are the rigid claw toe, dislocated toe, or crossover second toe, which is painful or prohibits shoe wear in the elderly patient with multiple comorbidities. These patients may not tolerate extensive reconstructive forefoot surgery but may respond well and recover quickly from an amputation. Of concern are predictable progression of the hallux valgus and medial deviation of the third and fourth toes as a result of the loss of the second toe as a physical restraint. This progression may be limited with an orthotic toe filler. In addition, the stump might not heal in patients with vascular compromise.

Author's Preferred Treatment and Rationale

Second MTP instability without deformity is first managed nonsurgically. Attempts are made at taping and creating a stiffened forefoot orthosis to provide functional rest. I prefer a rigid forefoot inlay to restrict MTP motion. Nonsteroidal anti-inflammatory drugs are routinely prescribed as an adjunct. Occasional steroid injections are performed if all other treatments are unsuccessful.

Failure of nonsurgical treatment leads to surgical management. In the anatomically unaltered patient, I prefer a synovectomy combined with a flexor-to-extensor transfer. I perform a shortening metatarsal neck osteotomy if the second metatarsal is excessively long. Excessive metatarsal length is not clearly defined in the literature, but my reference is the condyle of the second metatarsal head protruding past a horizontal line drawn at the tip of the first metatarsal head. Shortening of 4 to 6 mm is routinely performed, and the osteotomy is fixed with a miniscrew. Patients may immediately bear weight on the heel in a stiff-soled shoe.

I treat instability in the face of deformity similarly. I normally perform an osteotomy first, but I position the flexor-to-extensor transfer such that the toe is in the corrected position when the limbs of the split flexor are sutured together. This position requires the release of the tight, often medial, collateral ligament and repair or reefing of the other collateral ligament. Flexor digitorum brevis transfer is used if the deformity still persists. Hallux valgus should be corrected as necessary. (If performing a distal soft-tissue procedure as part of the bunion correction, one incision in the web space may service the two procedures, if it is placed appropriately.)

Fixed, rigid deformed toes often require bony shortening to allow for correction and to avoid vascular complications. I have found PIP arthroplasty combined with complete dorsal MTP soft-tissue release and pinning to be very effective. Should the second ray be excessively long (>1 cm longer than the first), then an additional metatarsal head shortening osteotomy is added. The patient is cautioned preoperatively that the toe will be positioned properly but will remain stiff and relatively immobile. Again, hallux valgus is corrected as indicated.

Management of Complications

Complications of lesser toe procedures may be a source of patient dissatisfaction. Most lesser toe procedures will leave the toe edematous for several months after the surgery. Manual manipulation and the promotion of intrinsic strengthening exercises help reduce swelling, stiffness, scar sensitivity, or numbness that may occur after surgery.

Recurrent instability or new deformity as the result of postoperative soft-tissue contractures is a great source of patient dissatisfaction. Recurrent instability may occur despite careful attention to soft-tissue balancing to correct preoperative contractures and pin fixation to maintain correction during the healing period. Forcible reduction and pinning of the toe against moderate resistance will often result in recurrence of the deformity and a poor result. The potential for recurrence may be minimized with attention to the cause of the deformity, if known, and the soft-tissue releases or bony procedures necessary to realign the toe. Nevertheless, reappearance of chronic long-standing deformity may occur over time. Management of recurrence usually requires a more aggressive approach with bone resection adequate for neutral toe posturing and rigid fixation (pinning) for extended periods of time (at least 4 to 6 weeks).

Syndactylization is potentially helpful, using the skin as an adjunctive restraint, but it may be unreliable and cosmetically or functionally rejected by the patient.

Vascular complications are potentially the most devastating complications of lesser toe procedures. Ischemia as a result of too much tension after reduction or vasospasm can lead to complete devascularization of the toe. Ischemia that does not respond spontaneously within several minutes after deflation of the tourniquet necessitates release of the dressing, pin removal, toe manipulation, bone shortening, or all of the above to maintain viability of the toe. It is better to abort the procedure and allow for revascularization than to sustain a significant vascular insult.

The patient should also be advised of the possibility of other complications, such as neuritis, stiffness, and infection. These complications may be managed as they are with other orthopaedic procedures.

References

Deland JT, Sung I: The medial cross-over toe: A cadaveric dissection. *Foot Ankle Int* 2000;21:375-378.

Fortin PT, Myerson MS: Second metatarsophalangeal joint instability. *Foot Ankle Int* 1995;16:306-314.

Mizel MS, Yodlowski ML: Disorders of the lesser metatarsophalangeal joints. *J Am Acad Orthop Surg* 1995;3:166-174.

Richardson EG: Lesser toe deformities: An overview. *Foot Ankle Clin* 1998;3:195-213.

Trnka H, Muhlbauer M, Zettl R, Myerson MS, Ritschl P: Comparison of results of the Weil and Helal osteotomies for the treatment of metatarsalgia secondary to dislocation of the lesser metatarsophalangeal joints. *Foot Ankle Int* 1999;20:72-79.

Vandeputte G, Dereymaeker G, Steenwerckx A, Peeraer L: The Weil osteotomy of the lesser metatarsals: A clinical and pedobarographic follow-up study. *Foot Ankle Int* 2000;21:370-374.

Weinfeld SB: Evaluation and management of cross-over second toe deformity. *Foot Ankle Clin* 1998;3:215-228.

Coding

ICD-9 CODES

718.87 Other joint derangement, not elsewhere classified, ankle and foot

735.4 Acquired deformities of toe, Other hammer toe (acquired)

735.5 Acquired deformities of toe, Claw toe (acquired)

735.8 Acquired deformities of toe, Other acquired deformities of toe

735.9 Acquired deformities of toe, Unspecified acquired deformity of toe

838.09 Dislocation of toe, closed

CPT CODES

28270 Capsulotomy; metatarsophalangeal joint, with or without tenorrhaphy, each joint (separate procedure)

28285 Correction, hammertoe (eg, interphalangeal fusion, partial or total phalangectomy)

28308 Osteotomy, with or without lengthening, shortening, or angular correction, metatarsal; other than first metatarsal, each

28313 Reconstruction, angular deformity of toe, soft tissue procedures only (eg, overlapping second toe, fifth toe, curly toes)

CPT copyright © 2003 by the American Medical Association. All Rights Reserved.

Angular Deformities of the Second Toe

Jonathan T. Deland, MD

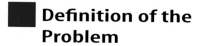 Definition of the Problem

Patient Presentation

Angular deformities of the second toe may be quite difficult to treat because patients present with a variety of symptoms and deformities. The location of each particular symptom is important. Two common symptoms stem from the change in position of the toe at the proximal interphalangeal (PIP) or metatarsophalangeal (MTP) joint. The first symptom is pain with shoe wear that is caused by pressure of a prominent PIP joint against the top of the shoe. The second is that medial or lateral deviation of the toe, most commonly medial, causes it to press against or cross over the adjacent toe. A third symptom is pain at the tip of the plantar flexed toe resulting from a flexion deformity at the interphalangeal joints. A mallet toe is a toe with plantar flexion deformity at the distal interphalangeal (DIP) joint that often is associated with callus formation at the plantar tip of the toe.

Metatarsalgia is forefoot pain in the plantar aspect of the foot. Patients may have swelling or pain about the second MTP joint from synovitis or arthritis, with dorsal and plantar tenderness. Synovitic joint pain may be difficult to distinguish from pain caused by an interdigital neuroma. Pain from an interdigital neuroma is associated with tenderness in the web space and not at the MTP joint. Meta-tarsalgia directly under the metatarsal head may occur from prominence of the head and distal migration of the underlying fat pad, with no dorsal tenderness. The orthopaedist should ascertain whether the metatarsal pain is limited to the second metatarsal or combined with one or more other metatarsal prominences.

The duration of the symptoms can indicate whether the deformity is just beginning to progress or is stable. For example, if the patient reports swelling and discomfort around the second MTP joint for only 1 to 2 months, the patient should be advised that the deformity may increase over the next several months. The synovitis can dissipate with time and with protection of a rocker-bottom shoe; the chronic deformity may not be painful so surgical treatment may not be necessary in the very earliest stages (over the first 3 to 4 months). However, if the painful deformity is allowed to become too severe, surgical correction may be more difficult.

Physical Examination

The alignment of the second toe is evaluated with the patient bearing weight. Any dorsiflexion of the MTP joint and either medial or lateral deviation of the toe should be noted. The direction of the adjacent toes is important because these toes can promote deformity if they are putting pressure on the second toe or failing to provide side-to-side support of the second toe. This would be the case for a hallux valgus with the valgus position of the great toe associated with a medial crossover toe (second toe crossing over the first) or with impingement from a third toe going under the second. If the great toe or third toe is underneath the second, deformity in those toes may need to be addressed. The hallux valgus is not necessarily part of the process that causes the medial crossover toe but can be part of that process.

Important information is gathered from the non–weight-bearing examination. First, an attempt is made to straighten the joints to assess the flexibility of deformities at the MTP, PIP, and/or DIP joints. Stability of the MTP joint can also be assessed. A dorsal drawer test is performed by holding the forefoot and second metatarsal with one hand and the proximal phalanx of the second toe with the other. The examiner attempts to subluxate the proximal phalanx dorsally at the MTP joint, and the laxity or pain can be compared with that at the other lesser MTP joints. Palpation on the dorsal aspect of the foot can determine if the joint is chronically subluxated or dislocated dorsally. Fullness of the joint may indicate the presence of synovitis. The toe is then compared with the other lesser toes. The metatarsal heads should be palpated on the plantar aspect of the foot to determine the prominence of one metatarsal head compared with the other. The metatarsal heads can be palpated individually or the index finger rolled

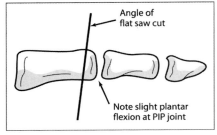

Figure 1 PIP resection.

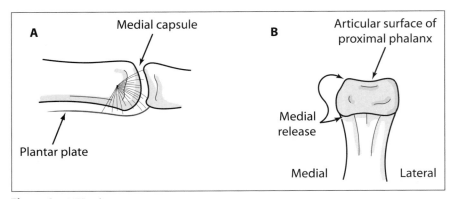

Figure 2 MTP release.

transversely across the metatarsal heads to determine prominence. The second and third metatarsal heads are the most commonly prominent. Any callus formation underneath the metatarsal heads also should be noted.

Weight-bearing AP and lateral views and a supine oblique view are standard. Because alignment of the toes and MTP joints can vary from supine to weight bearing, it is noted whether the second MTP joint on the AP view is medially or laterally deviated and whether the second metatarsal is longer than the first or third. Joint space narrowing most commonly occurs as a result of dorsal angulation of the proximal phalanx. Sclerosis with deformation of the head indicates arthritis. Full dislocation of the MTP joint will result in overlap of the proximal phalanx on the metatarsal head. MRI usually is not necessary but may be helpful for evaluation of pain around the MTP joint that cannot be explained by overload of the second MTP joint, a second web space interdigital neuroma, or findings on plain radiographs.

Differential Diagnosis
- Inflammatory arthropathies
- Freiberg's disease
- Morton's neuroma
- Metatarsal stress fracture

Additional Work-up
A rheumatoid screen should be considered if synovitis is present.

■ The Solutions

Treatment Options and Rationale
JOINT RESECTION
For fixed deformity, PIP and DIP resections are performed through a dorsal approach. Either a longitudinal or transverse skin incision can be used. After subperiosteal dissection, a retractor is placed underneath the exposed distal end of the proximal phalanx, and a small sagittal saw or bone cutter is used to resect the condyles. Optimal bone resection will reduce the joint, resolve the dorsal prominence, and give appropriate length to the toe. The cut is perpendicular to the shaft of the bone and may be angulated slightly proximal-plantar to avoid dorsiflexion at the resection site (**Figure 1**). A 0.045- or 0.062-in Kirschner wire (K-wire) is used to pin the joint in good position. At the level of the PIP joint, slight plantar flexion at the joint avoids too much elevation of the tip of the toe. This often means that the K-wire exits dorsally in the shaft or proximal metaphysis of the proximal phalanx.

MTP RELEASE
MTP release is performed through a dorsal straight, curvilinear, or zigzag incision. If severe contracture is present, a Z-lengthening of the skin is performed. The extensor digitorum brevis (EDB) tendon is released, and at the end of the procedure the extensor digitorum longus (EDL) is either released or Z-lengthened and repaired in an adequately lengthened position with the foot in neutral. The capsule is incised by taking an ellipse dorsally and releasing it halfway down on the medial and lateral sides. It is important either to tape the MTP joint in neutral during the first 6 weeks after surgery or to pin it so that it does not tend to dorsiflex. Because pins across MTP joints can bend, break, or back out with weight bearing unless a patient is in a cast or will be particularly careful, the joint is taped in neutral to slight plantar flexion, and a rigid postoperative shoe is used. If a pin is used, it is a 0.062-in and not a 0.045-in K-wire, to reduce the risk of wire breakage. However, a 0.045-in K-wire is used for the PIP and/or DIP joint pinning because the longer K-wire may exit through the proximal phalanx, which is a relatively small bone. For medial or lateral deformity (most often medial deviation) care is taken to release the collateral ligament all the way up and down the contracted side of the joint and along the plantar plate proximally. For quite significant medial deformities, the medial portion of the plantar plate may be further released from the proximal phalanx (**Figure 2**). These releases may not resolve the deformity but may discourage progression.

TENDON TRANSFER

For medial subluxation at the MTP joint that is not adequately treated by release and for which a metatarsal osteotomy is not being done, a tendon transfer to reconstruct the lateral collateral ligament can be considered. Although I do not depend on this transfer to resolve large amounts of deformity, it can be helpful to strengthen a badly torn or degenerated lateral capsule and to treat small amounts of deformity. If a metatarsal osteotomy is being performed, the EDB tendon is detached at its most distal aspect, often incorporating some of the confluence of the EDL to obtain additional length. For medial subluxation the EDB is brought back underneath the intermetatarsal ligament in the second web space and through a drill hole in the proximal phalanx at the plantar base, going to the medial dorsal distal shaft. It is tied down with the foot in neutral position and the MTP joint in slight overcorrection (**Figure 3**). Proper tensioning is important. The tendon is under moderate tension with the joint in this reduced position. The tendon lengths may need to be adjusted so the tendon end can be tied down to the drill hole in the distal aspect of the proximal phalanx. A 0.062-in K-wire can be used to hold the position of the toe; however, the wire must be carefully positioned and care must be taken to avoid driving the K-wire through the tendon transfer. This procedure also can be used in instances where a metatarsal osteotomy is being performed.

METATARSAL OR PROXIMAL PHALANX OSTEOTOMY

For treatment of large amounts of subluxation, a metatarsal or proximal phalanx osteotomy is helpful. A metatarsal osteotomy often will decompress enough of the medial or lateral deformity so a tendon transfer is not necessary. If there is metatarsalgia with prominence of the head, a metatarsal osteotomy is used. Otherwise, a proximal phalanx osteotomy can be

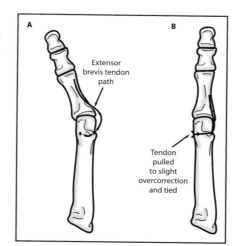

Figure 3 EDB tendon transfer.

performed for large amounts of medial or lateral deformity.

If the principal symptom is from impingement against the adjacent toe without metatarsalgia or MTP dorsiflexion, osteotomy of the proximal phalanx can be useful to manage medial or lateral deviation. A very small wedge of bone, which can be 1 to 2 mm more than the thickness of the saw cut, is resected from the base of the proximal phalanx, and the osteotomy is closed (**Figure 4**). The size of the wedge depends on the amount of deformity. Fixation can be achieved with a transosseous suture and taping of the toe toward the corrected position. A PIP resection can be performed first during the same surgical procedure as the phalanx osteotomy. However, a PIP resection is not a good treatment of considerable MTP lateral or medial deviation.

GIRDLESTONE-TAYLOR PROCEDURE

Girdlestone-Taylor flexor-to-extensor transfer can be considered for persistent dorsal subluxation at the MTP joint. It may be done with a PIP resection, and the long flexor tendon may be taken through an incision through the plantar aspect of the DIP and MTP joints, taking care to harvest as much length as possible. The long flexor is split down its raphe. With the use of a clamp, the tendon is brought from the

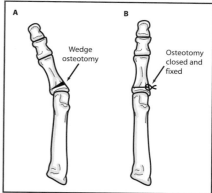

Figure 4 Wedge osteotomy.

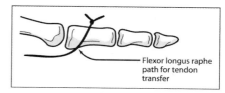

Figure 5 Girdlestone-Taylor procedure.

plantar midsection of the proximal phalanx and over the proximal phalanx dorsally, with care taken to stay adjacent to the bone (**Figure 5**). An alternative approach is to use a drill hole through the base of the proximal phalanx, but I have found that this alternative has not helped the results of the procedure. Overall, although the flexor-to-extensor tendon transfer can be helpful, the results are inconsistent. In particular, if the transfer is tied down too tightly, unwanted stiffness will result. Therefore, I use the transfer infrequently and only when I believe it is absolutely necessary and will take care not to tie the tendon transfer down too tightly. The tightness of the tendon transfer is assessed with the foot in neutral position. With one or two sutures placed, care is taken to dorsiflex the toe to confirm that the tension is approximately equal to that of the other toes and that the toe can be dorsiflexed to 40° fairly easily.

DISTAL HORIZONTAL METATARSAL OSTEOTOMY

The distal horizontal metatarsal osteotomy can be used to shorten the

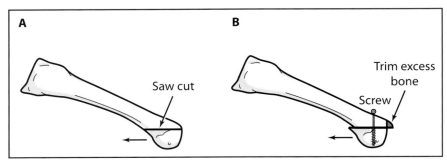

Figure 6 Distal horizontal metatarsal osteotomy.

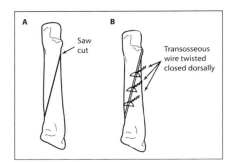

Figure 7 Proximal displacement.

second metatarsal and, with adjustment of the osteotomy, make the second metatarsal head less prominent. With the second metatarsal head exposed by plantar flexion of the MTP joint, a saw cut is made at the most dorsal aspect of its cartilaginous surface, going proximally and parallel to the plantar plane of the foot. The plantar fragment is slid proximally to the desired amount, and the osteotomy is fixed with a screw from dorsal to plantar (**Figure 6**). The remaining distal dorsal prominence of the second metatarsal head is then excised. The advantage of this osteotomy is that it heals readily and is stable. However, persistent dorsiflexion at the MTP joint and claw toe deformity can be a problem. It is therefore important to tape the toe down. Surgeons have also used this osteotomy in combination with the flexor-to-extensor transfer. If the second metatarsal head causes plantar prominence, it is important to assess the prominence after the osteotomy but before final fixation. If

the second metatarsal head still feels prominent with the osteotomy reduced, additional shaving at the osteotomy site may need to be done. Care should be taken to avoid shaving too much bone because the osteotomy cannot be adjusted back easily. If the distal horizontal metatarsal osteotomy is used to treat mild to moderate prominence of the second metatarsal head, the patient should be informed of some likely dorsal angulation or subluxation at the MTP joint and the possibility of claw toe deformity.

Osteotomies of the shaft of the metatarsal can be considered when the second metatarsal head is very prominent, and the patient reports considerable metatarsalgia. These osteotomies have the disadvantage of healing slowly; therefore, a distal horizontal osteotomy should be used when possible to avoid the slower healing time. However, for very considerable prominence of the second metatarsal head the shaft osteotomy can be used to position the head precisely. It is a technically demanding procedure. The oblique osteotomy is made dorsally from just proximal to the metatarsal neck to just distal to the base of the metatarsal (**Figure 7**). Before making this oblique saw cut, a small mark is made on the bone to allow judgment of position once the osteotomy has been mobilized. It is important to have a small Verbrugge (metatarsal) clamp (Synthes Ltd, Monument, CO) to hold the repositioned metatarsal firmly for assessment of its plantar

prominence. The prominence of the metatarsal heads can be assessed by gentle palpation of the second and other metatarsals with the foot held in neutral position. The goal is to have the second, third, and fourth metatarsals feel even on the plantar aspect. Rolling the index finger across the metatarsal heads is a good test.

With an isolated second metatarsal osteotomy, a transfer lesion to the third metatarsal head may occur. Therefore, if both the second and third metatarsals are prominent, the third metatarsal should be osteotomized and repositioned. In this situation, the third metatarsal is osteotomized to be level with the fourth metatarsal, and then the second metatarsal is osteotomized to be level with the third. Osteotomizing the second, third, and fourth metatarsals in one operation is not recommended because judgment of position is difficult with several osteotomies.

The osteotomy is temporarily fixed by placing two 0.045-in K-wires transversely across the osteotomy proximally and distally. The osteotomy is in the vertical plane so the K-wires are placed in the mediolateral plane. While the clamp is still on and after the position has been judged to be correct, the osteotomy is fixed by placing a 20-gauge wire through the K-wire holes and twisting the wire on the dorsal aspect of the bone. Careful positioning of the bone before fixation is critical. Adjustments can be made, not only in shortening of the bone but also by pushing the distal fragment slightly in the dorsal or plantar direction. It is important to achieve the desired position, apposition all along the osteotomy site, and rigid fixation. Although healing is slow, precise positioning of the metatarsals can be achieved.

Shaft osteotomies also can be done with a transverse cut and dorsal plate fixation, but for reasons of adjustability I prefer the oblique osteotomy. As with all shortening osteotomies of the metatarsals, the patient should be advised that some elevation of the toe may occur. The elevation is not as prominent as after a distal horizontal metatarsal osteotomy.

OTHER SURGICAL OPTIONS

For deformities that cannot be reduced by the above procedures, options are limited. One option is a DuVries arthroplasty, consisting of a partial metatarsal head resection. The distal and plantar portions are resected according to the amount of deformity and metatarsal head prominence. Stiffness and/or residual pain can occur. The other option is resection of the base of the proximal phalanx and syndactyly. This procedure destabilizes the MTP joint, and the proximal phalanx of the second toe remains elevated. Although it is not optimal cosmetically, the result is acceptable for pain relief and running.

If a simultaneous PIP resection is being done, excessive bone resection may result in too short a toe. The toe should be somewhat shorter than the great toe in the reduced position. This procedure does weaken the toe; therefore, a syndactyly is necessary to maintain an acceptable position. The syndactyly can be performed between the toes along the plantar aspect so that it is not too obvious cosmetically from above. On the lateral radiographic view, the proximal phalanx will not stay down at the level of the metatarsal head, but the operation does achieve two important objectives for the second toe: it provides good passive motion and usually prevents painful impingement against adjacent toes or with shoe wear.

For older patients with very severe deformities, amputation of the second toe is an alternative. This achieves the goal of quick recovery, as long as it is acceptable to the patient. Care is taken to preserve the base of the proximal phalanx in an effort to block progressive hallux valgus. The patient needs to be aware that progressive hallux valgus may occur. A plantar-based flap is used, and the nerves are resected proximally enough away

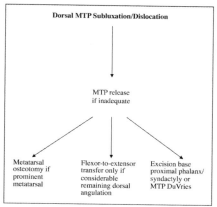

Figure 8 Algorithm for correction of dorsal MTP subluxation and dislocation.

from the skin to reduce the risk of a painful neuroma.

Author's Preferred Treatment and Rationale

For the second toe without contracture or deformity at the MTP joint and with prominence of the PIP joint resulting from its contracture, I do a PIP resection. The extensor tendon at the PIP joint need not be repaired, and the base of the middle phalanx can be roughened and trimmed at the proximal aspect, especially plantarly to discourage dorsiflexion. The base of the proximal phalanx need not be trimmed. The toe is pinned for approximately 4 weeks, after which time the toe is taped down over the proximal phalanx for an additional 4 weeks to discourage excessive MTP dorsiflexion. The patient is given plantar flexion strengthening exercises that are done with manual assistance at the MTP and PIP joints. Care is taken not to pin the PIP joint straight, but in slight plantar flexion so that the tip of the toe is not too far off the ground. This distance can be judged in the simulated plantigrade position in the operating room.

For a classic mallet toe with pain at the plantar tip, I prefer a DIP resection. If it is needed to reduce the deformity, a flexor release is performed through the same dorsal approach. Often, the second toe is long, and, therefore, a flexor release alone will risk abut-

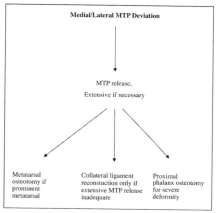

Figure 9 Algorithm for correction of medial and lateral MTP deviation.

ment of the end of the toe against the shoe. If the toe is short enough, a long flexor release through a small incision at the DIP joint can be done.

For a second toe with a PIP flexion contracture and a dorsal contracture at the MTP joint, I use a combination procedure (**Figure 8**). The PIP resection is done along with an MTP release and extensor lengthening or tenotomy. Because of the potential morbidity of pinning the second MTP joint, I usually pin only the PIP joint and tape the MTP joint in plantar flexion. Furthermore, pinning the PIP and MTP joints simultaneously can result in poor position of one of the two joints. After the PIP pin is removed at 4 weeks, plantar flexion stretching and strengthening exercises for the MTP joint can be initiated, and the MTP joint is taped down for 2 months after the procedure. This step is important to discourage MTP dorsiflexion. If there is abutment from the hallux or the third toe, the deformity at those toes must be addressed.

For the second toe with medial deviation at the second MTP joint as well as dorsal contracture and deformity at the PIP joint level, a different combination is used (**Figure 9**). The PIP resection and MTP release are performed, taking care to do an extensive release on the medial side, often releasing the medial aspect of the plantar plate. After this release, deformity can remain at the MTP joint with medial deviation. If this deformity is mild, and a metatarsal osteotomy is not being done, an EDB tendon transfer can be used. I prefer to include medial release and avoid the tendon transfer, if possible. If there is considerable deformity remaining and the metatarsal prominence is symptomatic, the tendon transfer cannot be expected to be adequate, and a metatarsal osteotomy may be performed. Shortening of the metatarsal will help lessen the medial deviation at the MTP joint. If the metatarsal head is not prominent, an osteotomy of the base of the proximal phalanx can be done. This osteotomy creates a zigzag deformity in the radiograph, but if done properly, it can restore acceptable clinical alignment. Metatarsal prominence or overload is the most common cause of deformity at the second MTP joint. If a distal horizontal metatarsal osteotomy is used, the metatarsal head can be shifted proximally and medially to resolve some of the medial deviation at the MTP joint. Another option is a DuVries MTP arthroplasty.

Whenever there is marked medial deviation, careful preoperative patient counseling is necessary. The patient should not expect that the entire toe deformity will be resolved. The toe will mold to the other toes, and some medial deviation can remain. As long as the toe is not painful and fits well in shoes, the results can be quite acceptable. Care should be taken to tape the toe in neutral to slight overcorrection to maintain correction of the dorsal subluxation and medial deviation. However, taping or pinning will not correct the deformity. Correction must be achieved via surgical release, tendon transfer, or osteotomy.

For a second toe with medial deviation, a very prominent metatarsal head, and metatarsalgia, an oblique metatarsal osteotomy is used. If the prominence is moderate to severe and I believe precise adjustment is critical, I prefer the more adjustable shaft osteotomy plus MTP release and PIP resection. I do not determine whether an extensor transfer for medial deviation is necessary until the metatarsal osteotomy. The tendon transfer usually is not necessary after the osteotomy.

If there has been complete dislocation of the second MTP joint, with proximal migration of the base of the proximal phalanx over the metatarsal neck, excision of the base of the proximal phalanx or the MTP DuVries procedure may be used as a salvage procedure. Excision of the base of the proximal phalanx does not resolve plantar metatarsal head prominence, if present. If the patient has metatarsalgia, a distal horizontal or oblique metatarsal osteotomy may precede assessment of the position of the base of the proximal phalanx. After the osteotomy, excision of the base of the proximal phalanx may not be necessary. A flexor tendon transfer can be performed with a distal horizontal metatarsal osteotomy for persistent dorsal subluxation. The toe range of motion is checked to make sure there is no impingement against the metatarsal head. If with dorsal motion of the toe, the proximal phalanx base still impinges against the second metatarsal head, then excision of the base of the proximal phalanx and syndactyly can be performed.

Although angulation resulting from abutment of the hallux against the second toe can often be managed with procedures for correction of the hallux valgus and second toe deformity, varus deformities of the lesser toes can be more difficult to treat. Commonly, the third and fourth toes can be in marked varus at the MTP joints. If these toes are asymptomatic, I avoid performing extensive procedures. Releasing the medial aspect of the MTP joints, as described for the second toe, can be considered. For severe subluxation, I release the medial attachment of the plantar plate on the proximal phalanx. If after performing the procedure on the second toe, it is clear that impingement from the third to second toe will be a problem postoperatively, I would consider the following. If the third toe curls under the second, mainly from the level of the PIP joint of the third toe, a third PIP resection along with MTP release would be appropriate. If a PIP resection at the third toe still does not resolve the prominence, a more proximal correction with a lateral closing wedge osteotomy at the base of the proximal phalanx of the third toe is performed.

Because the result can easily be less than perfect when dealing with the more severe deformities of the second toe, preoperative discussion with the patient is critical. Treatment can be both complex and controversial. The patient is counseled to expect some dorsal elevation of the tip of the toe and molding of the second toe to the adjacent toes. The patient also is informed that the most likely result is improved symptoms and reasonable rather than perfect position. It is better to achieve a pain-free or minimally uncomfortable second toe with good motion than a stiff toe in perfect position.

Management of Complications

Stiffness at the second MTP joint may occur with a flexor-to-extensor transfer or a partial distal metatarsal head resection. It can be treated with re-release or additional resection. With the excision of the base of the proximal phalanx, excessive displacement of the toe causing it to impinge on shoes is not likely to occur if the syndactyly was performed with the second toe set down enough. If excessive displacement does occur, it can be treated with readjustment of the syndactyly or plantar dermodesis. After a tight flexor-to-extensor transfer the MTP joint can be difficult to loosen at a subsequent surgical procedure, and excision of the base of the proximal phalanx may be necessary. For persistent symptomatic deformity with abutment against either the great or third toe, I assess whether there has been adequate correction at the first and third toes. If there has been adequate correction, adjustment of resection at the second PIP joint or the MTP joint can be considered.

References

Cooper P: Disorders and deformities of the lesser toes, in Myerson MS (ed): *Foot and Ankle Disorders.* Philadelphia, PA, WB Saunders, 2000, pp 308-358.

Coughlin MJ, Mann RA: Lesser toe deformities and keratotic disorders of the plantar skin, in Coughlin MJ, Mann RA (eds): *Surgery of the Foot and Ankle*, ed 7. St Louis, MO, Mosby, 1999, pp 320-436.

Deland JT, Lee K, Sobel M, Di Carlo EF: Anatomy of the plantar plate and its attachments in the lesser metatarsal phalangeal joint. *Foot Ankle Int* 1995;16:480-486.

Dockery L: Evaluation and treatment of metatarsalgia and keratotic skin disorders, in Myerson MS (ed): *Foot and Ankle Disorders.* Philadelphia, PA, WB Sanders, 2000, pp 359-377.

Myerson MS, Shereff MJ: The pathological anatomy of claw and hammer toes. *J Bone Joint Surg Am* 1989;71:45-49.

Coding

ICD-9 CODES

355.6   Lesion of plantar nerve, Morton's neuroma

726.70   Enthesopathy of ankle and tarsus, unspecified; metatarsalgia NOS

727.06   Tenosynovitis of foot and ankle

735.8   Other acquired deformities of toe

838.04   Closed dislocation, metatarsal (bone), joint unspecified

CPT CODES

28126   Resection, partial or complete, phalangeal base, each toe

28160   Hemiphalangectomy or interphalangeal joint excision, toe, proximal end of phalanx, each

28270   Capsulotomy; metatarsophalangeal joint, with or without tenorrhaphy, each joint (separate procedure)

28280   Syndactylization, toes (eg, webbing or Kelikian type procedure)

28285   Correction, hammertoe (eg, interphalangeal fusion, partial or total phalangectomy)

28308   Osteotomy, with or without lengthening, shortening or angular correction, metatarsal; other than first metatarsal, each

28312   Osteotomy, shortening, angular or rotational correction; other phalanges, any toe

28810   Amputation, metatarsal, with toe, single

28899   Unspecified

CPT copyright © 2003 by the American Medical Association. All Rights Reserved.

Failed Hammer Toe Surgery

James W. Brodsky, MD

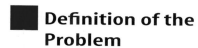 Definition of the Problem

Patient Presentation

Hammer toe is a widespread affliction, and hammer toe correction is a commonly performed surgical procedure in the shoe-wearing population. However, reported rates of patient dissatisfaction range from 14% to 17%. Although most postoperative problems will not require revision surgery, some patients may be sufficiently symptomatic to warrant an additional procedure. Scarring, swelling, and stiffness are unavoidable sequelae of all foot and ankle surgery but can be more pronounced in the toes. Despite preoperative explanations that swelling is expected and may persist, patients invariably are disturbed by it.

Corns and signs of irritation are typically caused by pressure resulting from malalignment, which is the most common cause of failed hammer toe surgery. The most common example of malalignment is a crossover second toe, which results from a metatarsophalangeal (MTP) joint that has deviated in both varus and extension.

Symptoms of pseudarthrosis are the exception rather than the rule despite the fact that in some series up to 50% of resection arthroplasties do not show evidence of fusion. Patients will frequently complain if the toe is floppy and bends back when donning a sock or stocking or if motion occurs with activity such as running or with pressure against the shoe. The lack of symptoms may be related to the fact that fibrous unions are generally stable. The original DuVries procedure for hammer toe correction was intended to produce a fibrous ankylosis because only the head of the proximal phalanx was resected, making fusion unlikely. However, it frequently produces satisfactory results.

Flexion of more than one joint usually is necessary to cause a painful corn on the distal tip of the toe. Rotation alone causes primarily a cosmetic aberration, usually with only mild pressure symptoms, unless the nail receives the pressure. However, rotation will exacerbate other deformities and may cause overlapping (**Figure 1**).

Patient factors that may influence toe deformities or hinder healing include systemic inflammatory diseases such as rheumatoid arthritis, neurologic disorders such as peripheral neuropathy or hereditary sensorimotor neuropathy (Charcot-Marie-Tooth disease), peripheral vascular disease, or a history of chemotherapy, high-dose steroids, immunosuppressive medications, or diabetes mellitus. Psychological conditions that preclude patient cooperation and compliance should not be underestimated. Unreasonable expectations (especially concerning cosmesis) are common and can devastate the outcome of the surgery.

Physical Examination

A careful history and a review of the previous medical records and surgical notes are very helpful for understanding the remaining anatomic structures and those that are damaged or absent. Obtaining information about the previous surgery is useful. For example, an attempt to correct the deformity by flexor-to-extensor tendon transfer will be frustrating if the flexor tendon has been cut and retracted. Unfortunately, the previous surgical note may not be available or sufficiently detailed, and the surgeon must rely more on physical examination. Perhaps most important to the ultimate outcome is to consider the patient's perception of the magnitude and source of the problem and the patient's expectations about treatment.

A thorough and meticulous evaluation is crucial to success in treatment of failed hammer toe surgery. During the physical examination the surgeon must assess (1) the vascular and neurologic status of the toe; (2) the condition of the skin and nail; (3) the position and function of the toe; (4) toe alignment, including its anatomic and mechanical relationship to the other toes and the influence of other toes; (5) the general alignment of the foot; and (6) cosmesis.

The anatomic effects of previous surgery to the involved or adjacent toes must be considered, including damage to nerves and the local vasculature, deep scarring, and skin contracture. The surgeon should attempt to define nerve injury as paresthesia, hyperesthesia, or hypoesthesia. Paresthesia and hyperesthesia may be asso-

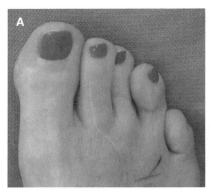
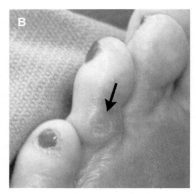
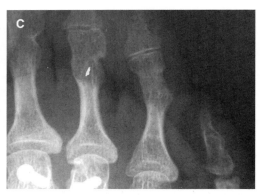

Figure 1 Combined malalignment. **A,** Dorsal view showing angulation and rotation at the PIP joint. **B,** Lateral view showing corn (*arrow*) and rotation of the fifth toe. **C,** Radiograph showing malunion. Note, however, that the rotation of the fifth toe is not visible.

ciated with local entrapment in scar tissue. Incisional neuromas should be percussed to find the area of greatest sensitivity. In unusual cases, objective vascular assessment with toe plethysmography or Doppler studies may be warranted. It may be prudent to discuss with the patient preoperatively the risk of possible vascular compromise, gangrene, or even amputation of the toe as a result of surgery. Vascular physical examination is largely limited to observation of color and capillary refill.

Damage to the nail and its surrounding structures is a major risk of distal interphalangeal (DIP) joint surgery. Preexisting irregularities, in-

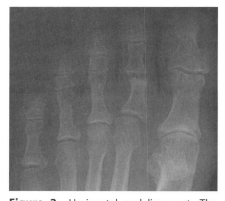

Figure 2 Horizontal malalignment. The PIP joint of the second toe is displaced in the transverse plane, with the distal end of the proximal phalanx causing pressure on the medial side and the middle phalanx causing pressure on the lateral side. (Courtesy of John Early, MD)

grown nails, paraungual corns, and onychomycosis should be noted because these may affect the cosmetic and symptomatic outcome of the secondary treatment or revision surgery. Nail irregularity or pain can be a result of damage to the matrix or of the new position of the nail in which it impinges on or is compressed by adjacent structures. In addition, the initial surgery may have brought the nail into a visible position that may be displeasing.

Evaluation includes a detailed review of alignment components. The toe may be too long, short, rigid, or floppy. It may be plantar flexed at the MTP joint, causing increased pressure against the floor, or, more commonly, elevated and suspended so that it never touches the floor.

The deformity within the toe and the ray must be analyzed into each of its components, including the sagittal plane (dorsiflexion and plantar flexion), the horizontal plane (varus and valgus), and the coronal plane (rotation in pronation or supination). It also is necessary to distinguish between angulation and translation at each of the joints. It is particularly important to discern whether the MTP or interphalangeal joints (or both) are the source of lateral and medial displacement of the toe.

Both position and alignment may cause points of increased pres-

sure in failed hammer toe surgery. These points will invariably be the focus of symptoms in most patients and may be identified on the skin by tenderness, irritation, or corns, either on the previously operated-on toe or on adjacent toes. Angulation or translation may be present in the vertical or horizontal plane, and rotation may be present in the coronal plane. Malalignment may be at the level of the MTP, proximal interphalangeal (PIP), or DIP joints, or any combination thereof. Pain resulting from pressure caused by a malaligned toe is evaluated by systematically considering each type of alignment.

Lateral angulation will cause a pressure point at the apex. Translation is a more subtle postoperative cause of pressure on the side of the toe, especially at the PIP joint. It will cause pressure at the step-off, but recognition requires scrutiny. One clue is the presence of a pressure lesion on both medial and lateral sides of the toe. For example, if the middle phalanx is translated laterally relative to the proximal phalanx, pressure will be caused by the corner of the middle phalanx on the lateral side and by the corner of the proximal phalanx on the medial side (**Figure 2**). Angulation and translation both may cause pain, with or without formation of corns, on the surgically treated and/or adjacent toes.

Vertical translation or angula-

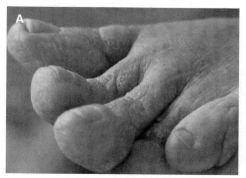
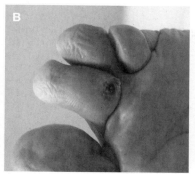

Figure 3 Vertical malalignment. **A,** Angulation deformity of the PIP joint. **B,** Pressure ulcer at the apex of the deformity.

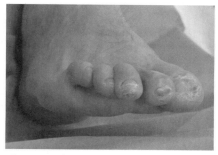

Figure 4 Varus of the second MTP joint causing pressure against the hallux, resulting in both a valgus deformity of the PIP joint and overlap.

tion may cause either dorsal or plantar pain. Dorsal prominence is more obvious and more common, but plantar prominence is more painful. Dorsal pressure may produce a hard corn as a result of shoe pressure. If the pressure is directed plantarward at the PIP joint, then the previous fusion or arthroplasty is in extension (**Figure 3**). Keratosis may be absent. This situation must be recognized both before and after surgery. Padding in the shoe is often ineffective in relieving the pain, which occurs at the toe-off stage of gait.

Coronal deformities are rotational. They are the least predictable and least reliably corrected with salvage surgery. These deformities may be caused by contracture of the soft tissues and by the forces applied by proximal malalignment. The best example is the fifth toe with a PIP resection that was treated surgically and healed in a supinated position. Derotation is unlikely to succeed. Even with more than one wire for rotational control (technically challenging in these tiny bones), the soft tissues will cause recurrence.

In the common situations in which the deformity predominantly affects one joint, usually the PIP is affected. However, there frequently are reciprocal changes at the PIP and MTP joints. For example, if the second MTP joint is deviated in varus (crossover toe) and abuts a hallux valgus,

the second toe will either overlap the hallux or develop a valgus deformity at the PIP joint (**Figure 4**).

The MTP joint may be affected alone or in combination with the PIP joint. The malalignment at the MTP level frequently is not immediately evident, and if not deliberately assessed, it may not be seen, leading to a poor result. To adequately evaluate the MTP joint, the surgeon must examine it in neutral dorsiflexion-plantar flexion of the ankle, with and without weight bearing.

The lesser MTP joints are most likely to deviate in varus, although some are deformed in valgus. Extension deformity frequently accompanies varus deviation. These MTP joint malalignments must be recognized and addressed to successfully correct deformity of failed hammer toe surgery.

A mallet toe is a flexion deformity of the DIP joint (**Figure 5**). Just as the toe that underwent surgery may influence the other toes, it also may be influenced by mechanical pressure from the hallux or one of the lesser toes (**Figure 6**). Gradual deformation of the toe after initial good postoperative alignment is often the result of molding, which is influenced both by pressure from the adjacent toes and the overall pressure from the toe box of the shoe. Molding may be desirable because it may prevent pain (from an unmolded straight toe adjacent to a bent toe). Midfoot and hindfoot defor-

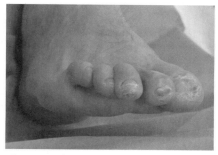

Figure 5 Mallet toe deformity of the second and third toes causing callosities at the distal edge of the toes.

mities, such as equinus or varus, may cause persistent metatarsalgia despite a good technical correction of forefoot abnormalities.

After correction of the hammer toe deformity, the structure and appearance of the toe change, both individually and relative to the other toes. Although the surgeon may see an excellent objective result, the change from normal is a frequent cause of dissatisfaction in some patients. This dissatisfaction is not entirely avoidable, but preoperative discussion that focuses on adjusting the patient's expectations to a realistic level may increase satisfaction with the surgical result. Although surgeons tend to pride themselves on their technical expertise more than they do on their powers of persuasion, the latter is often the more effective tool in revision surgery.

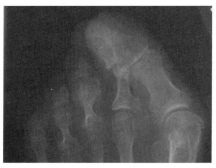

Figure 6 Pressure of the hallux on the second toe causing pressure and a valgus deformity.

Differential Diagnosis

- Infection
- Malunion
- Nonunion
- Malalignment
- Nerve Injury

Additional Work-up

No additional work-up is required.

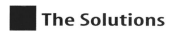

▪ The Solutions

Treatment Options and Rationale

VASCULAR PROBLEMS

If a vascular problem is recognized after deflation of the tourniquet or in the immediate postoperative period, the dressing is loosened; if ischemia persists, the Kirschner wire is promptly loosened or removed. If the problem arises insidiously, the wire is removed.

The intervention possible for an ischemic toe is limited. If amputation becomes necessary, the surgeon should always take into account the effects on the adjacent toes. Absence of a lesser toe will often cause subsequent drift of either the hallux or adjacent lesser toes into the defect. If the gangrene is limited to the distal part of the toe, partial amputation retards

these secondary deformities by providing a block to the adjacent toes. Fusion of the first MTP joint merits consideration in amputation of the second toe in some cases.

NERVE INJURY

In cases of hyperesthesia, entrapment may be present. Surgical neurolysis may be necessary. Often this is less useful than excision of the nerve, which is imbedded in scar and cannot be dissected free. A decision must be made regarding the proximal cut end of the nerve. Paresthesia is not uncommon and may or may not improve with time. If one of the complex regional pain syndromes is present, referral to a pain management consultant is appropriate.

PSEUDARTHROSIS

Salvage requires re-resection to produce fresh cancellous bone surfaces to maximize the formation of a solid ankylosis, bony or fibrous. If so much bone was resected in the first operation that there is no cancellous bone, reconstruction is much more difficult. The diaphysis of the proximal phalanx can be inserted, or impaled into the cancellous bone of the middle phalanx. Augmentation with a small bone graft may be necessary. Consideration can be given to a nonpercutaneous fixation that remains in the toe, either an absorbable or metallic pin. Overresection of bone can exacerbate the instability.

MALALIGNMENT

Initial treatment is usually nonsurgical. This step may help define the indications for surgery, the patient's expectations, and the patient's tolerance for frustration, all of which are important in decision making. Shoe wear modification consists primarily of pressure reduction with wider, softer, or more open-toed shoes. Various toe pads, caps, and spacers are commercially available. Taping is satisfactory

to some patients. After a previous poor surgical result, patients may be more willing to try these methods.

POSTOPERATIVE MANAGEMENT

The patient is kept in a rigid-soled postoperative shoe for at least 6 weeks. Some patients are uncomfortable in the surgical shoe either because it has no heel or because the foot slides in the shoe. In this situation, the use of an ankle-high boot is recommended. Thereafter, shoe wear is advanced slowly, with the patient using sandals or a very wide shoe for at least 2 more months. Taping may be necessary after removal of the Kirschner wires.

Author's Preferred Treatment and Rationale

NERVE INJURY

We favor placing the nerve end in bones such as the metatarsal or midtarsal bones. A tunnel is drilled in the bone and a looped suture or pull-out suture is placed around the nerve end. It is then drawn through the tunnel with a straight needle, which can be brought through the plantar surface of the foot.

MALALIGNMENT

After correction of malalignment at the PIP joint, we leave the percutaneous pins in for approximately 4 weeks, although the duration can be extended. Our preferred treatment of floppy, short toes is nonsurgical.

Surgical salvage is aimed to correct malalignment. For malalignment at the PIP joint level, it is usually sufficient to resect, realign, and re-fuse the joint in correct position. Resecting the bony corners resulting from translational malalignment in the horizontal or vertical planes has the limitation that the remaining small surface area may be unstable, but this may be very useful in decreasing bony prominence. Caution must be exercised to remain in the metaphysis of the proximal phalanx, if at all possible, and not to resect down to the diaphysis because the metaphysis is cancellous bone and has a wider surface area, promoting fusion, whereas the diaphysis has a smaller diameter and is cortical bone (**Figure 7**). Furthermore, excessive bony resection may increase the risk of instability.

Malalignment at the MTP joint may be addressed by soft-tissue procedures, bone procedures, or a combination of both. Soft-tissue realignments usually require MTP joint capsulotomy. Although the role of extensor tendon lengthening and flexor-to-extensor tendon transfer (modified Girdlestone-Taylor procedure) has been emphasized in the literature, there is a strong role for capsulorrhaphy. A reefing reconstruction is done with the proximal and distal flaps of the MTP joint capsule using No. 2-0 or No. 0-0 Vicryl (Ethicon, Somerville, NJ) suture. Metatarsal shortening osteotomy, especially with resection of a section or wedge of bone, can be performed with or without correction of rotation.

A variant of the Akin procedure can be used in the lesser toes. Either a medial or a lateral closing wedge osteotomy at the base of the proximal phalanx can realign the toe when complete correction through the MTP joint cannot be achieved. However,

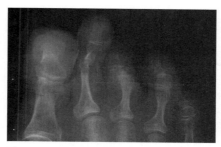

Figure 7 The proximal phalanx of the second toe with atrophic, narrow bone surfaces.

this procedure is less successful distally in the toe because the compensatory deformity makes a zig-zag shape in the toe that may be uncomfortable. If the MTP joints are severely dislocated dorsally, resection of the metatarsal heads (Hoffman procedure) may be beneficial. Resection of two metatarsal heads is likely to lead to transfer metatarsalgia under the two remaining lesser metatarsal heads. DuVries condylectomy of the metatarsal head is likely to lead to MTP joint arthritis, especially in the presence of a flexor-to-extensor tendon transfer.

Malalignment at the DIP joint, causing mallet toe, is corrected as primary mallet toe. The flexor digitorum longus tendon is fully divided because retention of the flexor fibers has been demonstrated to be a risk factor in recurrence of this deformity.

Floppy, short toes are disturbing when present but cause symptoms variably. When they cause catching or there is intense dissatisfaction with the cosmesis, a soft-tissue procedure such as a V- to Y- or Z-plasty may be performed with or without partial metatarsal head resection. Syndactylization has been recommended for this problem. Unfortunately, the floppy, extended toe may deform the adjacent toe after syndactylization. Bone grafting may be attempted to lengthen and stabilize the toe. These are the least rewarding and least predictable salvage cases in the lesser toes.

If all else fails, amputation of the offending toe can be a reasonable salvage procedure but is associated with the potential for secondary deformity of the adjacent toes described previously.

Management of Complications

Any of the complications mentioned for primary surgery on hammer toes may occur after revision surgery. Detailed evaluation, painstaking planning, attention to detail, and meticulous surgical technique may improve the potential for patient satisfaction. The most common risk in salvage surgery is poor soft-tissue healing.

The author wishes to acknowledge the contribution of Efrain D. Leibner, MD, PhD, in the creation of this chapter.

References

Coughlin M: Lesser toe abnormalities. *Instr Course Lect* 2003;52:421-444.

Coughlin M, Dorris J, Polk E: Operative repair of the fixed hammertoe deformity. *Foot Ankle Int* 2000;21:94-104.

Coughlin M, Mann R: Lesser toe deformities, in Coughlin M, Mann R (eds): *Surgery of the Foot and Ankle*, ed 7. St. Louis, MO, Mosby, 1999.

Dhukaram V, Hossain S, Sampath J, Barrie JL: Correction of hammer toe with an extended release of the metatarsophalangeal joint. *J Bone Joint Surg Br* 2002;84:986-990.

Lehman D, Smith R: Treatment of symptomatic hammertoe with a proximal interphalangeal joint arthrodesis. *Foot Ankle Int* 1995;16:535-541.

Coding

ICD-9 CODES

718.27   Pathological dislocation of joint, foot and ankle

718.47   Contracture of joint, foot and ankle

735.4   Other hammer toe (acquired)

736.79   Other acquired deformities of ankle and foot

905.8   Late effect of tendon injury

CPT CODES

28124   Partial excision (craterization, saucerization, sequestrectomy, or diaphysectomy) bone (eg, osteomyelitis or bossing); phalanx of toe

28234   Tenotomy, open, extensor, foot or toe, each tendon

28270   Capsulotomy; metatarsophalangeal joint, with or without tenorrhaphy, each joint (separate procedure)

28285   Correction, hammertoe (eg, interphalangeal fusion, partial or total phalangectomy)

28308   Osteotomy, with or without lengthening, shortening or angular correction, metatarsal; other than first metatarsal, each

Fifth Toe Deformity

Lowell D. Lutter, MD

◼ Definition of the Problem

Patient Presentation

Fifth toe positional problems usually cause difficulties with footwear. The position of the toe leads to skin irritation and callus formation. Three varieties of deformities, a cock-up deformity, a plantar flexion deformity, and an overlapping deformity, occur at the metatarsophalangeal (MTP) joint of the fifth toe. Although each deformity produces symptoms related to footwear, they have different physical examination findings, etiology, and treatment. Surgical repair may be unsuccessful if the underlying cause of the deformity is not understood.

In general, a cock-up deformity is a progressive deformity that often is associated with a hammer toe. It is seen most frequently in older age groups. The usual presentation is a dorsiflexed and adducted fifth toe. The onset is often insidious, and the patient does not seek treatment until he or she has difficulties fitting shoes, pain, or callus.

The plantar flexion deformity and overlapping deformities tend to occur in younger age groups and often are congenital. Generally signs and symptoms of a plantar flexion deformity are similar to those of a cock-up deformity. The patient has difficulty with shoes fitting correctly. The underlapping fifth toe produces difficulties at the edge of the fifth nail bed and may cause a painful ingrown toenail. The dorsal skin of the toe may become painful. An overlapping deformity is characterized by dorsal overlapping of the fifth toe on the fourth toe. Symptoms generally are associated with difficulties with footwear and problems from skin contact of the fifth onto the fourth toe.

A corn is an accumulation of the keratotic layer of the epidermis in re-

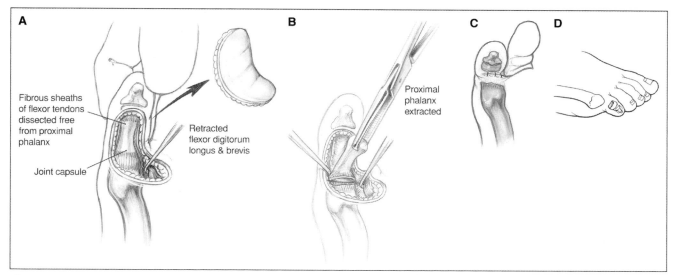

Figure 1   Ruiz-Mora procedure. **A,** The fibrous sheaths of the flexor tendons are dissected free from the proximal phalanx. The retracted flexor digitorum longus and brevis are held by the instrument. The excised ellipse of skin is shown. **B,** The extracted proximal phalanx is held by the instrument. **C,** The skin is closed transversely in the area where the previous ellipse of skin had been removed. **D,** The appearance of the toe after bone removal and skin closure. (Reproduced with permission from Lutter LD: Toe deformities, in *Atlas of Adult Foot and Ankle Surgery*. St. Louis, MO, Mosby-Yearbook, 1997, pp 91-111.)

sponse to pressure or friction. Footwear often has been cited as a cause, with compression of the toes producing the accumulation of the keratosis. The patient usually has pain between the fourth and fifth toes that is associated particularly with wearing shoes. When the corn develops in the web space, maceration, which produces a very painful "soft corn" that usually cannot be treated with pads and may become infected, may be caused by the moisture in this area. Corns distal to the web space often are on the fourth toe and are across from a bony prominence on the fifth toe.

A bunionette is a prominent distal fifth metatarsal head with secondary lateral bursa. This occurs frequently in a patient with a relaxed, splayed forefoot. Symptoms generally include pain along the lateral aspect of the foot, particularly in association with tight footwear. There may also be an intractable keratosis below the fifth metatarsal head.

Physical Examination

The MTP joint usually is dorsiflexed in a cock-up deformity. Generally a rotational component with axial rotation of the toe is present. Early in the process, the joint is flexible and easily can be plantar flexed. With time, the capsule and extensor mechanism become contracted and the MTP joint cannot be plantar flexed. Frequently, there is a callus on the dorsum of the toe over the interphalangeal (IP) joint. In a plantar flexion deformity, the toe is in a plantar flexed position, often with pronation of the distal phalanx. Generally, there is a flexion contracture of the soft tissues and the flexor digitorum longus tendon. This contracture prevents bringing the toe to a neutral position; when stretched upward, the toe will snap back into a flexed position.

An overlapping deformity may be either congenital or developmental. The fifth toe rests on the dorsal base of the fourth toe. There may be a

fixed contracture and a rotational component of the distal portion of the fifth toe. In the congenital form, the deformity is fixed and cannot be brought into the corrected position with taping or splints. Early in the developmental form, the toe can be brought into the neutral position. With time, it progresses to a fixed deformity.

Radiographs of a foot with a cock-up deformity usually show subluxation of the proximal phalanx on the metatarsal head, occasionally as-

sociated with rotation of the toe. The metatarsal articular surface is often at a 90° angle to the phalanx. A radiograph of the area with a corn may show a bony prominence of the fifth toe, or in the case of a deep web corn, a bony prominence of the base of the fifth toe.

The radiographic appearance of the foot with a bunionette deformity is characteristic. It may involve an abnormality of the fifth metatarsal, consisting of prominence of the distal lateral portion, or there may be an ab-

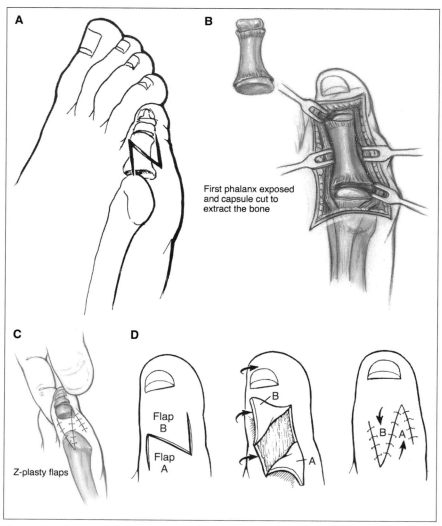

Figure 2 Thompson procedure. **A,** Z-plasty is performed with the incision beginning laterally. **B,** The proximal phalanx is excised. **C,** The toe is rotated from the plantar position and dorsiflexed. **D,** The Z-plasty is then closed to derotate and dorsiflex the toe. (Reproduced with permission from Lutter LD: Toe deformities, in *Atlas of Adult Foot and Ankle Surgery*. St. Louis, MO, Mosby-Yearbook, 1997, pp 91-111.)

normally increased angulation between the fourth and fifth metatarsal shafts.

Differential Diagnosis
• Mycotic infection

Additional Work-up
If there is suspicion of a mycotic infection in the area with a corn, a culture should be obtained.

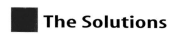

The Solutions

Treatment Options and Rationale
NONSURGICAL TREATMENT
Taping and padding generally are not successful for a cock-up deformity because the soft-tissue contractures cause the deformity to recur after removal of the tape and padding. Wide shoes with a deep toe box can temporize the deformity and may be all that is needed in the elderly or in patients with low physical demands. The toe box may be stretched or a bubble patch may be applied to the shoe to remove pressure of the toe box from the toe.

Taping or pads can temporarily control symptoms of a plantar flexion deformity, but the flexion contracture prevents permanent solution of the problem. Adequate length of footwear is also helpful.

The presence of an overlapping deformity does not categorically mean that it requires repair. With the congenital form, it is customary to delay repair until the child is old enough (usually age 4 to 5 years) where the soft-tissue aspects of the repair can be done easily. This problem persists in many adults in a mild form without difficulties. The indications for treatment include a marked rotational component that produces difficulty wearing shoes and a painful callus.

The use of lamb's wool or other absorbent material placed into the interdigital area helps reduce the maceration and provides padding for an interdigital corn. If the corn is more distal, soft padding may be all that is necessary.

Specific treatment of a keratosis, such as padding directly on the area or a metatarsal bar, may provide some relief for a bunionette deformity. A wide toe box used with a semirigid insert may also provide relief.

SURGICAL TREATMENT
Minimal cock-up deformity generally is characterized by the presence of a hammer toe, and a resection arthroplasty of the proximal IP joint is necessary. The standard hammer toe procedure can be performed. In association with this procedure, an extensor tendon lengthening or tenotomy and MTP dorsal capsule release are necessary.

Surgical treatment of a severe hammer toe deformity should be performed in a sequential manner. If the soft-tissue release used for the minimal deformity does not provide correction, then a more extensive procedure should be performed. Options include a partial proximal phalangectomy with syndactylization to the fourth toe or a complete proximal phalangectomy with soft-tissue repair (Ruiz-Mora procedure) (**Figure 1**).

Syndactylization of the fourth and fifth toes is an option for surgical treatment of a plantar flexion deformity. A second option is the Thompson procedure (**Figure 2**) in which a dorsal Z-plasty is performed in conjunction with a proximal phalangectomy.

The selection of a specific procedure is related to the severity of the

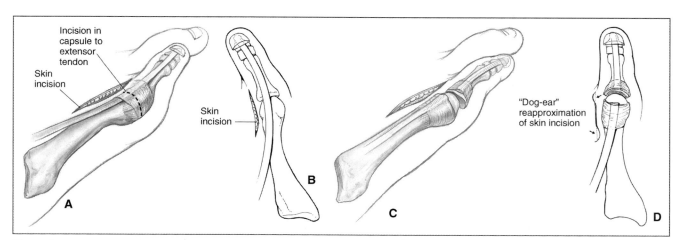

Figure 3 DuVries procedure. **A** and **B,** The incision begins at the space between the metatarsal heads and extends proximally. **C,** A complete soft-tissue release is performed. **D,** The skin is closed to remove "dog ears" and release any tension. (Reproduced with permission from Lutter LD: Toe deformities, in *Atlas of Adult Foot and Ankle Surgery*. St. Louis, MO, Mosby-Yearbook, 1997, pp 91-111.)

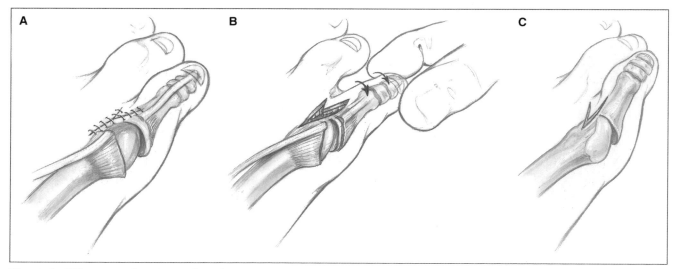

Figure 4   Wilson procedure. **A,** A V-shaped incision is made over the MTP joint. **B,** A complete soft-tissue release is performed as in the DuVries procedure. **C,** Closure is performed changing a V to a Y. There is some asymmetry of the limbs of the Y to accommodate any persistent deformity. (Reproduced with permission from Lutter LD: Toe deformities, in *Atlas of Adult Foot and Ankle Surgery*. St. Louis, MO, Mosby-Yearbook, 1997, pp 91-111.)

overlapping deformity in terms of its contracture and rotation. Three surgical procedures can be used for this problem. The DuVries procedure (**Figure 3**) uses a dorsal incision between the fourth and fifth toes with a complete release of the extensor tendons and dorsal capsule. A soft-tissue dressing is held in place for 6 weeks. The Wilson procedure (**Figure 4**) is similar to the DuVries procedure with the exception that a V-shaped incision is made over the MTP joint. At closure, the V is converted to a Y. The Lapidus procedure uses a curved incision on the dorsum of the MTP joint (**Figure 5**). The extensor digitorum longus tendon is cut at the joint, passed plantarward, and attached to the abductor digiti tendon. Rotation and adduction can be controlled by tensioning the repair. Correction is then maintained with a smooth pin for 3 weeks and a soft dressing for an additional 3 weeks.

The DuVries and Wilson procedures are less extensive but do not correct the rotational component. The Lapidus procedure should be used when there is a large amount of mal-

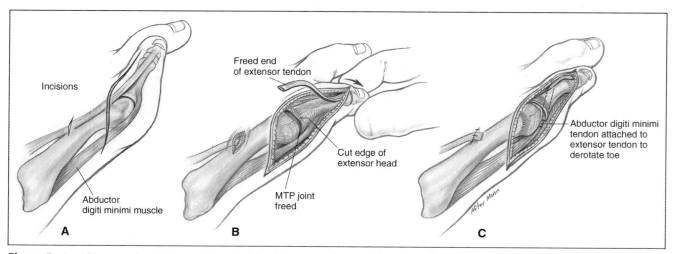

Figure 5   Lapidus procedure. **A,** A curvilinear incision is begun at the medial portion of the proximal phalanx. **B,** The extensor tendon is divided proximally. It is then brought into the wound and mobilized. The MTP joint capsule is divided to allow the proximal phalanx to be derotated. **C,** The distal tendon segment is passed medial to lateral under the proximal phalanx and sutured to the abductor and short flexor of the fifth toe. (Reproduced with permission from Lutter LD: Toe deformities, in *Atlas of Adult Foot and Ankle Surgery*. St. Louis, MO, Mosby-Yearbook, 1997, pp 91-111.)

rotation of the proximal phalanx on the metatarsal.

A distal corn can be treated with a partial condylectomy of the area below the corn or a complete condylectomy similar to that used for hammer toe correction. For a proximal corn deep within the web space, simultaneous procedures on the medial condyle of the proximal phalanx of the fifth toe and the lateral condyle of the proximal phalanx of the fourth toe, respectively, should be performed. It is important to confirm the identity of the bony prominence with a lead marker on radiographs. Syndactylization can be performed as an isolated procedure or in conjunction with a condylectomy.

The selection of a specific surgical procedure for bunionette defor-

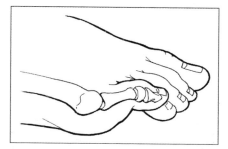

Figure 6 Type I bunionette deformity. Simple excision of the lateral eminence and capsular plication will alleviate pain.

mity is based on the type of deformity present. Difficulties from a bunionette can be the result of an enlarged fifth metatarsal head (type I deformity) (**Figure 6**), fifth metatarsal shaft bowing (type II deformity), or an increased angle between the fourth and fifth metatarsals (type III deformity).

Procedures available for correction of bunionette deformity include lateral metatarsal head condylectomy, plantar metatarsal head arthroplasty, distal shaft osteotomy, diaphyseal (midshaft) osteotomy, and metatarsal head resection. A specific diagnosis of the type of deformity should be made before selection of a surgical procedure.

For a type I deformity, a lateral metatarsal head condylectomy will decompress the area and provide relief. In elderly or inactive patients, excision of the lateral eminence and capsule plication should provide satisfactory results. In the presence of a prominent plantar callus, a metatarsal head arthroplasty can be performed by removing the plantar surface of the metatarsal head. However, removing the plantar surface as an isolated pro-

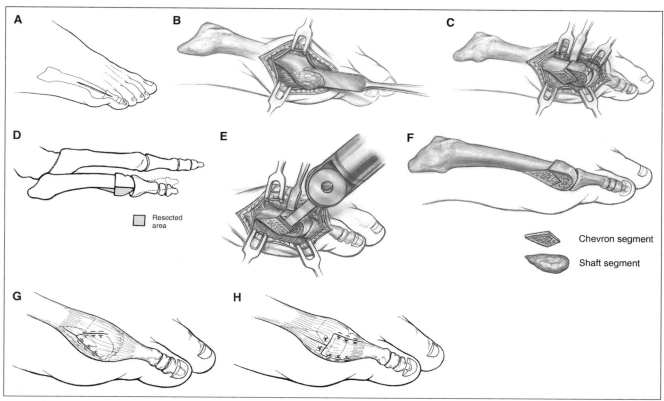

Figure 7 Distal chevron osteotomy. **A,** An incision, approximately 2 cm, at the lateral portion of the joint extends over the metatarsal head. **B,** A simple lateral eminence excision is performed, followed by a chevron cut (**C**) in which the dorsal limb is longer than the plantar. **D,** The metatarsal head is shifted medially approximately one third of the width of the shaft. **E,** The remaining overhanging bone can be excised. **F,** The final construct can be stabilized with a smooth in. Soft-tissue closure can be either a V-Y closure (**G**) or a distally shifted tongue-type cut (**H**). (Reproduced with permission from Lutter LD: Toe deformities, in *Atlas of Adult Foot and Ankle Surgery*. St. Louis, MO, Mosby-Yearbook, 1997, pp 91-111.)

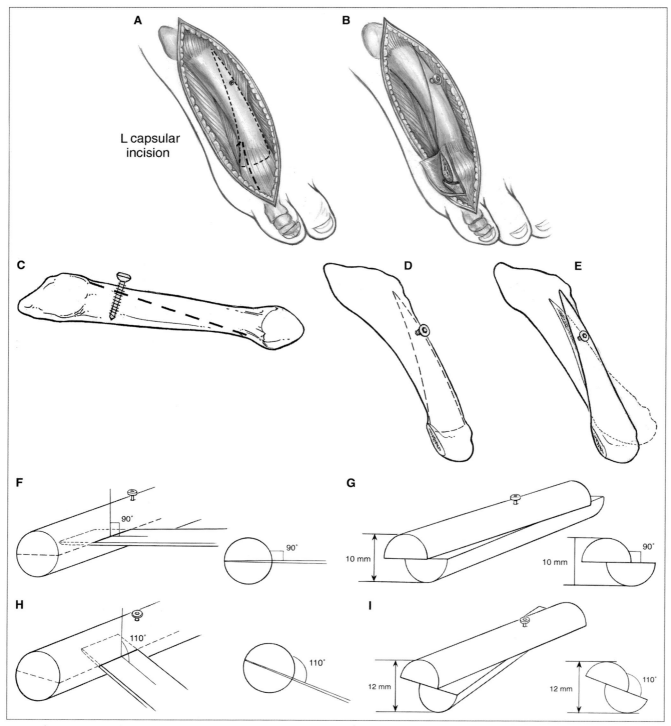

Figure 8 Diaphyseal osteotomy (oblique shaft osteotomy). **A** and **B,** The skin incision does not need to expose the metatarsal head. The osteotomy is 45° when viewed from the lateral cortex. The proximal cut should be made first to both cortices and the distal cut only through the lateral cortex. **C,** A screw is placed proximally but not tightened. **D,** The screw contacts both cortices. **E,** The osteotomy is completed to the medial cortex and the entire head is moved medially and upward out of the plantar surface. **F,** This shows position of the hand and the cut when no elevation is desired. **G,** When the osteotomy is shifted, the metatarsal head will be neither elevated nor depressed. **H,** This shows diagrammatically what will occur if the hand is dropped cutting the metatarsal. **I,** When the metatarsal head then is shifted, it is elevated. (Reproduced with permission from Lutter LD: Toe deformities, in *Atlas of Adult Foot and Ankle Surgery*. St. Louis, MO, Mosby-Yearbook, 1997, pp 91-111.)

cedure is associated with a high rate of recurrence of symptoms.

A distal shaft osteotomy is effective with this type of deformity. A chevron cut, step cut, or oblique osteotomy can be used. The goal of each of these procedures is to produce a medial shift of the distal metatarsal fragment.

A distal chevron metatarsal osteotomy (**Figure 7**) will correct problems caused by a type II deformity. A simple lateral condyle excision will not correct the angular deformity, and recurrence is high if this is done as an isolated procedure. If the 4-5 intermetatarsal angle is greater than 12°, then a diaphyseal osteotomy may be performed.

Type III deformities are large deformities associated with painful calluses. The diaphyseal osteotomy is a more complex procedure but may correct a large deformity (**Figure 8**). With this procedure, the metatarsal head may be elevated and moved medially. A metatarsal head resection is a salvage procedure. It is effective as part of a multiple metatarsal head resection for the treatment of rheumatoid arthritis.

Author's Preferred Treatment and Rationale

The Ruiz-Mora procedure entails excising a longitudinal ellipse from the plantar surface skin and removing the entire proximal phalanx. The skin is closed by converting the longitudinal ellipse into a transverse incision, bringing the distal most edge to the proximal edge (**Figure 1**). One helpful modification entails leaving the base of the proximal phalanx; this provides better stability to the toe postoperatively. Postoperative care should include a dressing for approximately 6 to 8 weeks that maintains the alignment of the toe and helps prevent floppiness. Dressings are changed weekly. A longitudinal Kirschner wire (K-wire) may assist in controlling the toe and is left in place for 3 to 4 weeks.

Even with all of these measures, the toe may remain floppy or unstable when healed.

The Thompson procedure for correction of a plantar flexion deformity allows for the rotation and dorsiflexion of the toe. Because there is a tendency for an unstable toe following this procedure, a longitudinal pin should be placed for 3 weeks. After removal of the pin, the position should be maintained for an additional 6 to 8 weeks with taping or a soft dressing. If instability is still present, buddy taping to the fourth toe for an additional 6 weeks is recommended.

For a deep web corn, I prefer the excision of both medial and lateral condyles of the fifth and fourth toes, respectively, combined with a proximal syndactylization. The syndactylization should go only to the midpoint of the proximal phalanx of the fifth toe.

I prefer to use a distal oblique or chevron osteotomy for a type I bunionette deformity. The major difficulties have been with fixation. If the patient is small, an oblique distal shaft osteotomy provides more secure fixation than a distal chevron osteotomy, using a small K-wire.

Management of Complications

Bunionette may form at the fifth toe after treatment of a cock-up deformity. Prolonged taping to the fourth toe (buddy taping) is a satisfactory method to treat a bunionette deformity when it is first recognized. After a deformity is established, management is the same as a primary bunionette. A hammer toe of the fourth toe also may occur, and continuous taping for approximately 12 weeks or use of a soft dressing to maintain flexion of the fourth toe will help prevent this problem. If a painful hammer toe of the fourth toe develops, surgical repair may be necessary. Shortening of the fifth toe is always associated with some instability and may manifest as a floppy toe. Usually there is no functional problem except catching on socks.

Recurrence of the overlapping deformity may occur if the toe is undercorrected. At the time of surgery, the toe should lie in the corrected position before placement of the pin. Placement of a pin for 3 weeks will not correct a soft-tissue deformity that has not been corrected at surgery.

Neurovascular structures should be protected because the working space is small and the potential for injury is present. The patient should be counseled that the toe will not have full function after surgery because there has been shortening of the toe and disruption of the extensor mechanism. Numbness occasionally is related to irritation of a digital nerve during surgical treatment of an interdigital corn. Before surgery, the patient should be informed that there may be a sense of stiffness after a complete condylectomy. Instability of the proximal IP joint may occur if a large partial condylectomy is performed or if there is inadequate closure of the capsule and soft tissue over the area. Pin fixation at the time of surgery may lessen the sense of instability.

Loss of correction of a bunionette deformity can occur if adequate fixation is not used. The distal osteotomy can be difficult if the fragment is small and unstable. The use of threaded pins or small screws has been helpful for this problem.

If undercorrected, the deformity can recur. Nonunion or delayed union of both distal and diaphyseal shaft osteotomies can occur frequently. If a nonunion or fibrous union is asymptomatic, the decision to perform revision with addition of bone graft should be based on symptoms and not the radiographic appearance.

The skin incision for all bunionette procedures should be placed either midline or slightly dorsal to that because placement of a plantar lateral skin incision can result in a painful callosity. Fifth toe varus is unlikely because the fourth toe holds it in place.

References

Coughlin MJ: Etiology and treatment of bunionette deformity. *Instr Course Lect* 1990;39:37-48.

Coughlin MJ: Lesser toe abnormalities. *Instr Course Lect* 2003;52:421-444.

Lutter LD: *Atlas of Adult Foot and Ankle Surgery*. St. Louis, MO, Mosby-Year Book, 1997, pp 102-111.

Myerson MS: *Foot and Ankle Disorders*. Philadelphia, PA, WB Saunders, 2000, pp 335-341.

Coding

ICD-9 CODES

700   Corns and callosities; callus, clavus

727.1   Other disorders of synovium, tendon, and bursa, bunion

735.8   Acquired deformities of toe, other acquired deformities of toe

CPT CODES

28110   Ostectomy, partial excision, fifth metatarsal head (bunionette) (separate procedure)

28150   Phalangectomy, toe, each toe

28270   Capsulotomy; metatarsophalangeal joint, with or without tenorrhaphy, each joint (separate procedure)

28280   Syndactylization, toes (eg, webbing or Kelikian-type procedure)

28285   Correction, hammertoe (eg, interphalangeal fusion, partial or total phalangectomy)

28286   Correction, cock-up fifth toe, with plastic skin closure (eg, Ruiz-Mora-type procedure)

28288   Ostectomy, partial, exostectomy or condylectomy, metatarsal head, each metatarsal head

28306   Ostectomy, with or without lengthening, shortening or angular correction, metatarsal; first metatarsal

28313   Reconstruction, angular deformity of toe, soft-tissue procedures only (overlapping second toe, fifth toe, curly toes)

Recurrent Metatarsalgia After Distal Horizontal Metatarsal Osteotomies

Pascal F. Rippstein, MD

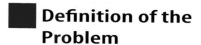 ## Definition of the Problem

Patient Presentation
Metatarsalgia may recur after a distal horizontal metatarsal osteotomy as a result of metatarsophalangeal (MTP) joint instability, postoperative MTP joint stiffness, an oblique osteotomy that is not in the horizontal plane of the foot (**Figure 1**, *A*), and excessive shortening. The patient describes symptoms typical of metatarsalgia—pain under one or more metatarsal heads that occurs when walking or standing and increases with walking distance. If the metatarsalgia is the result of excessive metatarsal shortening, then during push-off the patient might have pain underneath the adjacent metatarsal head that became relatively too long in relation to the shortened one. Walking barefoot may aggravate the pain, but wearing good shoes with stable soles and soft insoles may reduce it. No pain is present when the patient is sitting or lying. Callosities that occur under the metatarsal heads have to be removed frequently to diminish the pain. If there is dorsal MTP subluxation, the patient may have pain over the elevated proximal interphalangeal joint caused by friction with the shoe and pain with swelling about the MTP joint.

Physical Examination
The classic clinical finding is a painful callus underneath the involved metatarsal head. After the removal of this callus with a sharp blade, the metatarsal head is palpated and found to be too prominent plantarly when compared with the other metatarsal heads. The toe might not touch the floor when the patient is standing if the MTP joint is subluxated, and recurrence of a hammer toe is common. Depending on the degree of stiffness, the toe might or might not be reducible passively at the MTP joint.

Depending on the underlying problem, AP, oblique, and lateral radiographs may show subluxation at the MTP joints, with or without discontinuity in the metatarsal break curve. A metatarsal head that is in an excessively plantar position as a result of excess obliquity of the osteotomy is very difficult to assess radiographically, and the diagnosis is based on clinical examination. Very rarely, there may be radiographic findings of necrosis or nonunion of a metatarsal head that may be associated with diffuse MTP joint pain.

Differential Diagnosis
- Morton neuralgia
- Functional insufficiency of the first ray (hallux valgus, failed hallux valgus surgery, true first ray instability, short first metatarsal, Keller arthroplasty, transfer lesion)
- Gastrocnemius contracture
- Bursitis
- Rheumatoid arthritis and rheumatoid nodule
- Plantar fat pad atrophy
- Systemic connective tissue disorder
- Freiberg's infraction

Additional Work-up
None

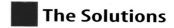

The Solutions

Treatment Options and Rationale
UNSTABLE MTP JOINT ASSOCIATED WITH RECURRENT DORSAL SUBLUXATION
Dorsal MTP subluxation is caused primarily by a rupture of the plantar plate. After reduction of the subluxation with an extensive soft-tissue release and a distal horizontal metatarsal osteotomy, scar formation around the MTP joint, especially on the plantar side, should build a stabilizing structure that prevents recurrence of the subluxation. If this fails to happen, then the MTP joint will remain unstable and the toe will subluxate again. This subluxation increases plantarward pressure on the metatarsal head and leads to recurrent metatarsalgia. Such conditions may be treated non-

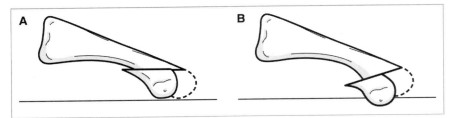

Figure 1 **A,** On the second and the third metatarsals, the distal horizontal metatarsal osteotomy should be performed strictly horizontally to leave the metatarsal head on the same horizontal plane when moving it proximally for shortening. **B,** An oblique osteotomy brings the metatarsal head more plantar while pushing it proximally for shortening.

surgically with a toe-strap orthosis, which holds the toe reduced in its MTP joint. Surgical treatment options include dynamic stabilization with the transfer of the flexor digitorum longus tendon to the dorsum of the proximal phalanx (Girdlestone-Taylor procedure).

DORSAL MTP SUBLUXATION ASSOCIATED WITH STIFFNESS

If recurrent metatarsalgia after distal horizontal metatarsal osteotomy results from MTP stiffness and dorsal subluxation of the toe within approximately 4 to 6 months after surgery, then a closed toe manipulation may be attempted because retracted scar tissues may be stretched only during this short period of time. Initial nonsurgical treatment limited to insoles and shoe modifications is not recommended at such an early stage because the potential to improve the problem

with a simple closed reduction could be missed. This closed toe mobilization can be performed in the orthopaedist's office with the foot under an ankle block. If the closed reduction succeeds, then it is essential for the patient to stretch the involved toe intensively several times a day. In addition to this stretching, a splint that holds the toe in plantar flexion (Darco toe alignment splint [Darco International, Huntington, WV], for example; **Figure 2**) is worn at night for approximately 1 to 2 months.

If closed reduction fails, then an open dorsal soft-tissue release is considered. The same approach as for the initial surgery is applied. Extensor tendons are tenotomized or lengthened in a "Z" fashion without reapproximating. The soft tissues all around the MTP joint are carefully released (**Figure 3**). Soft tissues must be released until the toe is spontaneously reduced during the intraoperative "push-up" maneuver, in which the surgeon puts a hand under the metatarsals and pushes dorsally until the

foot is in a neutral position. The foot is otherwise in plantar flexion on the operating table, and the extensor tendons are pulling the toes dorsally. To secure the reduction, a Kirschner wire (K-wire) is introduced from the tip of the toe through the MTP joint into the corresponding metatarsal, with slight plantar flexion at the MTP joint. This K-wire will be removed in about 4 to 6 weeks. After the K-wire has been removed, the patient stretches the toe frequently and wears a toe splint at night.

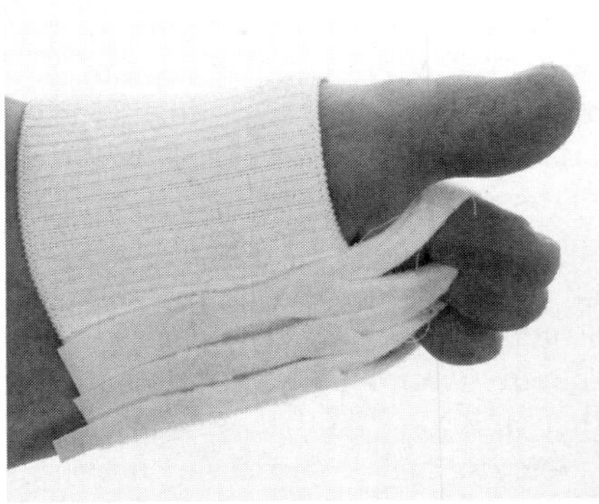

EXCESSIVELY PLANTAR POSITIONED METATARSAL HEAD

If a distal horizontal metatarsal osteotomy is oblique from distal-dorsal to proximal-plantar, then the metatarsal head will move plantar while it is pushed proximally to achieve metatarsal shortening (**Figure 1**, *B*). A more plantar position of one metatarsal head in relation to the other metatarsal heads is responsible for excessive pressure under the involved head and leads to an intractable plantar keratosis and metatarsalgia.

Because the fourth and the fifth metatarsals are less oblique than the second and the third metatarsals, a strict horizontal fourth or fifth metatarsal osteotomy is not possible (**Figure 4**, *A*). Therefore, the cut has to be slightly oblique from distal-dorsal to proximal-plantar, but this will displace the metatarsal head plantarward while it is moved proximally for the shortening. Because the fourth and fifth metatarsals are much more mobile in their proximal joints (Lisfranc joints) than the second and third metatarsals, they usually can compensate a more plantar position of the metatarsal head with increased dorsiflexion at the tarsometatarsal joint. If this compensation mechanism is insufficient, or if the osteotomy has been performed much too obliquely, then the patient may have metatarsalgia. Therefore, the distal horizontal metatarsal osteotomy on the fourth and

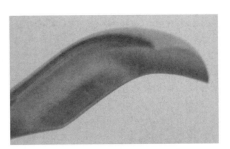

Figure 2 A splint stretches the toes in plantar flexion and may be worn at night for 1 to 2 months to prevent dorsal contractures and recurrent subluxation at the MTP joints.

Figure 3 The curved elevator is very efficient in releasing the soft tissues around the MTP joint, especially on the plantar aspect.

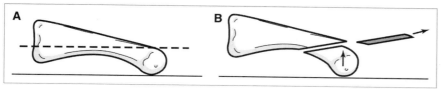

Figure 4   **A,** A strictly horizontal distal horizontal metatarsal osteotomy on the fourth and fifth metatarsals would end proximally into the tarsometatarsal joint. Therefore, the cut has to be slightly oblique. **B,** To compensate for the plantar displacement of the metatarsal head, a small bony slice is removed at the level of the osteotomy and allows a more dorsal position of the head. (Reproduced with permission from Rippstein P: Rheumatoid forefoot deformities. *Surg Tech Orthop Traumatol* 2001;10:55-68.)

fifth metatarsals should be made with a double cut, removing a 2-mm thick slice of bone. This procedure will displace the metatarsal head dorsally and compensate the effect of the oblique osteotomy (**Figure 4**, *B*).

If nonsurgical treatment fails or is not acceptable for the patient, then three surgical options may be helpful. The easiest way to relieve the plantar pressure is to perform a horizontal condylectomy on the plantar aspect of the metatarsal head. However, this is possible only when the excessive plantar position of the head does not exceed 3 to 4 mm; otherwise, too much of the head would have to be removed, and MTP joint dysfunction could result. An alternative is to remove a horizontal slice of bone at the level of the previous distal horizontal metatarsal osteotomy to bring the metatarsal head back dorsally at a corrected level in relation to the other metatarsal heads.

Another alternative is a proximal closing wedge osteotomy of the involved metatarsals to bring the meta-

tarsal head back dorsally to a corrected position. A very long, almost horizontal, closing wedge osteotomy in the proximal metatarsal metaphysis may be very efficient in the correction of such problems (**Figure 5**). When performing this osteotomy, care is taken not to cut the plantar cortical bone, which acts as a hinge. If the resected wedge provides the exact amount for the correction, then a compression screw (2.0-mm screw) will stabilize the osteotomy. If the wedge is too large, then the orthopaedic surgeon pushes the metatarsal head until it reaches the correct level and holds it while the assistant places a screw without compression, with the osteotomy slightly open. This screw can be replaced if needed until the metatarsal head is at the correct position. Bone graft (eg, calcaneal graft) is then placed into the open gap left by this osteotomy.

METATARSAL OVERLENGTH

The length of each metatarsal is very crucial and has a strong interaction with the length of the other metatar-

sals (metatarsal curve). Each metatarsal has to be shorter than the adjacent metatarsal on its medial side, except for the third metatarsal which might be equally long as the second metatarsal. If one metatarsal is longer than the next medial metatarsal, this relative overlength will produce increased plantar pressure under the metatarsal head, especially during the push-off phase, and the patient will have metatarsalgia from heel-rise to toe-off.

This metatarsalgia usually is not improved sufficiently with insoles alone. Because the painful overpressure occurs mainly during push-off, a shoe with a rigid rocker-bottom sole may be helpful. Surgical options include restoration of a correct metatarsal length with a second distal horizontal metatarsal osteotomy at the same level. The new position of the metatarsal head may be verified with a C-arm to ensure adequate correction. The length of the lateral metatarsals is also checked for any overlength. Additional shortening of the metatarsals will be indicated to achieve a correct metatarsal curve and avoid other secondary metatarsalgia.

Author's Preferred Treatment and Rationale

I prefer nonsurgical treatment of mild metatarsalgia without significant deformities. For all other conditions, I prefer early and aggressive surgical management because such conditions do not improve over time and may be more difficult to salvage later on.

I perform closed mobilization of dorsally retracted scar tissues with or without dorsal MTP subluxation if intensive stretching therapy does not sufficiently improve the condition within 1 month. This decision is not difficult to make because this therapy is efficient, easy to perform, and not necessarily invasive.

If a metatarsal head has been placed in too plantar a position and surgical correction is performed, I usually prefer a second osteotomy in-

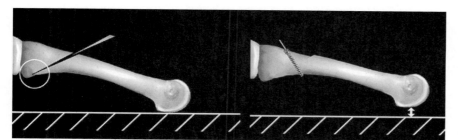

Figure 5   The proximal (extra-articular) closing wedge metatarsal osteotomy may elevate metatarsal heads that have been displaced too much toward plantar with a distal horizontal metatarsal osteotomy. (Reproduced with permission from Barouk LS: *Forefoot Reconstruction.* New York, NY, Springer-Verlag, 2003.)

stead of condylectomy. Condylectomy may lead to new bone formation underneath the resected area and to recurrent metatarsalgia. In addition to this, it is not always easy to predict if such a condylectomy will be sufficient to bring the metatarsal head to a correct level.

Of the two osteotomies that have been described, I prefer the proximal osteotomy. The distal osteotomy with removal of a bony slice has a limited ability to move the metatarsal head more dorsally, and with a larger slice removed, there is a smaller surface area for fixation. Although metatarsal head necrosis or nonunion is rare, such complications are more likely to occur after a second distal horizontal metatarsal osteotomy. Finally, if too much bone has been resected, and the metatarsal head has been moved too dorsally, it is difficult to bring it back to a more plantar position. The advantages of this technique are that the procedure is quite fast and release of the contracted soft tissues can be performed through the same approach.

The proximal metatarsal osteotomy allows correction even with metatarsal heads that are severely too plantar. Because of its long and almost horizontal cut, this osteotomy usually heals. The position of the metatarsal head is adjusted by opening or closing the osteotomy until the exact position is reached. MTP joint stiffness is not expected because this osteotomy is purely extra-articular. The osteotomy also can be used as a pure open wedge osteotomy in the rare instance where a metatarsal head has been displaced too dorsally, such as when an excessively large bony slice has been removed.

Management of Complications

After revision surgery, the vascular condition of the skin and the toe can be severely impaired. The tourniquet should be released under sterile conditions and the local perfusion observed until it has returned to a satisfactory condition. If after 15 minutes there are still areas of white skin, the K-wire may be removed, leaving the MTP subluxated if necessary.

A common postoperative complication is a recurrent dorsal contracture at the MTP joint. Therefore, it is very important to immobilize the reduced MTP joint in slight plantar flexion for 4 to 6 weeks with a K-wire.

Metatarsal head necrosis and nonunion after a second distal horizontal metatarsal osteotomy are severe complications that are not easy to salvage. Resection of the lesser metatarsal head is a reliable and safe procedure for such a difficult condition, even if toe function is going to be diminished.

———————————■

References

Barouk LS: *Forefoot Reconstruction.* New York, NY, Springer-Verlag, 2003.

Rippstein P: Rheumatoid forefoot deformities. *Surg Tech Orthop Traumatol* 2001;10:55-68.

Trnka HJ, Nyska M, Parks BG, Myerson MS: Dorsiflexion contracture after the Weil osteotomy: Results of cadaver study and three-dimensional analysis. *Foot Ankle Int* 2001;22:47-50.

Coding

ICD-9 CODES

715.17 Osteoarthrosis, localized, primary, ankle and foot

718.27 Pathological dislocation, ankle and foot

718.37 Recurrent dislocation of joint, ankle and foot

718.47 Contracture of joint, ankle and foot

719.07 Effusion of joint, ankle and foot

719.47 Pain in joint, ankle and foot

719.77 Difficulty in walking, ankle and foot

735.4 Other hammer toe (acquired)

CPT CODES

28270 Capsulotomy; metatarsophalangeal joint, with or without tenorrhaphy, each joint (separate procedure)

28308 Osteotomy, with or without lengthening, shortening or angular correction, metatarsal ; other than first metatarsal, each

28309 Osteotomy, with or without lengthening, shortening or angular correction, metatarsal; multiple (eg, Swanson type cavus foot procedure)

SECTION 3
Flatfoot

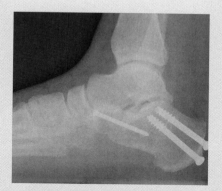

Glenn B. Pfeffer, MD
Editor

Stage II Adult Acquired Flatfoot Deformity: Treatment Options and Indications

David B. Thordarson, MD

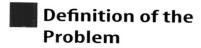

Definition of the Problem

Patient Presentation

Most patients who present with an adult acquired flatfoot deformity initially have posteromedial ankle pain. Approximately half of all patients will recall some type of trauma, often minor, to the involved ankle. Frequently, patients are misdiagnosed by their primary care physician as having an "ankle sprain," which leads to a delay in diagnosis. Many patients presenting to an orthopaedic surgeon's office have had pain for 3 or more months because of failed treatment of a presumed ankle sprain. The predominant presenting symptom is pain with secondary weakness or easy fatigue with walking. In most patients, a variable flatfoot deformity will develop over time. As the deformity progresses, many patients begin to notice lateral hindfoot pain as a result of subtalar inflammation, and in more extreme cases, calcaneofibular abutment or even peroneal tendinitis. In some patients with severe deformities, a fibular stress fracture may develop that will lead to a sudden increase in pain.

Most patients are 30 to 50 years of age. Women are more commonly affected than men. The condition is also more common in obese patients and patients with chronic flatfoot deformities.

Physical Examination

The physical examination should include evaluations while the patient is in both standing and seated positions. In a standing position, a unilateral flatfoot deformity will be noted. In addition to the loss of the longitudinal arch (**Figure 1**), the patient will have an abduction deformity of the forefoot. When the patient is viewed from behind, increased hindfoot valgus can be observed. Forefoot abduction is demonstrated by a patient having a "too many toes" sign (**Figure 2**).

The most sensitive diagnostic clinical test for posterior tibial tendon insufficiency is a single heel rise test. In the first part of this test, the patient should be standing on the tip toes of the unaffected side. As the patient stands on tip toes, movement of the heel into an inverted position can be observed. The test is then repeated on the involved side. An insufficient posterior tibial tendon is demonstrated by either of the following: (1) an inability to perform the test because of weak-

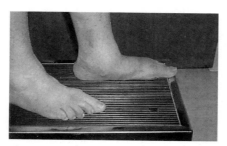

Figure 1 Patient demonstrating loss of longitudinal arch of the left foot.

ness or pain or (2) weak plantar flexion with no evidence of inversion of the hindfoot as the patient rises on the ball of the foot.

While the patient is seated, tenderness and edema localized in the distal portion of the posterior tibial tendon can be noted. In more long-standing cases, patients may also have tenderness over the sinus tarsi or the tip of the fibula because of inflammation caused by impingement in that area. The inversion of the involved side should be symmetric to that of the uninvolved side in a stage II flexible deformity. The degree of flexibility is important because a fixed deformity cannot be addressed with soft-tissue, nonfusion methods of treatment.

The tightness of the gastrocnemius-soleus complex should be assessed in all patients with an adult acquired flatfoot deformity. This test should be performed when the patient is in a seated position with the knee both extended and flexed. While checking for tightness, the hindfoot must be held in a subtalar neutral position with the navicular reduced onto the head of the talus, which usually involves mildly inverting the foot. With the foot held in subtalar neutral and the knee flexed and extended, ankle dorsiflexion is assessed (**Figure 3**). Knee flexion relaxes any tightness of the gastrocnemius. An inability to dorsiflex past 0° in either of the two positions indicates tightness of either the gastrocnemius alone (with the

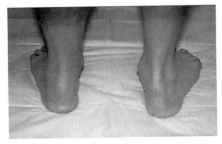

Figure 2 Normal hindfoot alignment on the left side with increased hindfoot valgus and a "too many toes" sign on the right side.

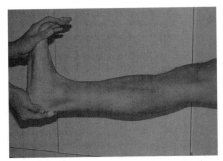

Figure 3 Examining the gastrocnemius for tightness with the knee fully extended and subtalar joint held in neutral position with hand on the posterior aspect of the heel and the other hand maximally dorsiflexing the ankle.

knee fully extended) or both the gastrocnemius and soleus (if also present with the knee flexed).

Weight-bearing AP and lateral radiographs of the foot should be obtained to determine the site and degree of the deformity. On the lateral radiograph, the talo-first metatarsal angle is a good measure of the degree of deformity (**Figure 4**). The sag is usually present at the talonavicular joint, but instability or sag at the naviculocuneiform joint and tarsometatarsal joint can also be present. The degree of lateral peritalar subluxation of the navicular on the head of the talus can be observed on the AP radiograph (**Figure 5**). Occasionally, deltoid ligament laxity will develop, leading to a valgus tilt of the talus in the mortise, which is classified as a stage IV flatfoot deformity.

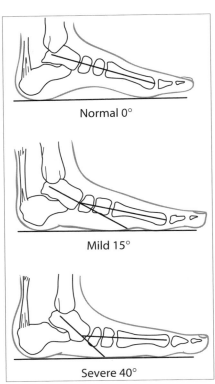

Figure 4 Normal, mild, and severe deformities of the longitudinal arch with increased talo-first metatarsal angle with progressing deformity.

Differential Diagnosis
- Unilateral inflammatory arthropathy or degenerative arthritis of the hindfoot
- Tarsal coalition
- Soft-tissue injuries to the plantar fascia or ligaments
- Malaligned Lisfranc arthritis

Additional Work-up
Although MRI can demonstrate the integrity of the posterior tibial tendon, it is generally unnecessary in the management of this condition because treatment is predicated on the response to conservative treatment and the presence of flexible versus fixed deformity.

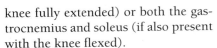

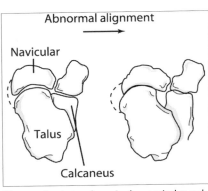

Figure 5 Lateral navicular peritalar subluxation with increasing deformity.

■ The Solutions

Treatment Options and Rationale
NONSURGICAL TREATMENT
A trial of nonsurgical treatment should be attempted in all patients with adult acquired flatfoot deformity before surgical interventions are considered. Younger patients and those with more severe deformities, however, are less likely to have a successful outcome from nonsurgical interventions. The goal of nonsurgical treatment is to protect the inflamed structure (ie, the posterior tibial tendon) and to prevent further deformity. Off-the-shelf and custom-made longitudinal arch supports can be helpful in the management of this condition. These orthotic devices can either be posted medially to approximately 1/8-in, or a 1/8-in or 1/4-in wedge can be added to the heel of the shoe medially (**Figure 6**). Patients with a tight gastrocnemius-soleus complex should stretch these muscles. Although physical therapy can provide transient relief, it generally does not result in any lasting benefit. Examples of ankle support include soft supports, lace-up ankle braces, walking boots, and articulated or nonarticulated ankle-foot orthotics. The use of walking casts may also be considered. In general, if an arch support with or without an in-shoe ankle brace is un-

successful, surgery is generally indicated.

SURGICAL TREATMENT

In general, approximately 75% of patients will have a contracture, with approximately three fourths of these being isolated gastrocnemius contractures. Treatment options include either a gastrocnemius recession (Strayer procedure) or percutaneous Achilles tendon lengthening.

The gastocnemius recession has the advantage of weakening only the tight muscle (ie, the medial and lateral heads of the gastrocnemius) while entirely preserving the soleus. However, many patients, especially women, find a midline longitudinal scar objectionable (**Figure 7**). Frequently in thinner patients, there is dimpling of the subcutaneous tissue as a result of the diastasis of the fascia following this release.

Another treatment option for a tight gastrocnemius is a percutaneous triple hemisection Achilles tendon lengthening (TAL). The advantage of this procedure is that is it easy to perform. A TAL can be completed in approximately 30 seconds by hemisecting the tendon distally and laterally, proximally and medially, and again proximally and laterally. With the correction usually necessary with this condition, these incisions can usually be made 3 cm apart (**Figure 8**). The disadvantage of this procedure is that it weakens both the gastrocnemius and the soleus. However, if the patient has contractures of both the gastrocnemius and soleus, making them unable to dorsiflex to neutral with the knee both flexed and extended, then a TAL is necessary.

POSTERIOR TIBIAL TENDON RECONSTRUCTION

The damaged posterior tibial tendon is generally reconstructed with adjacent normal tendon. Most orthopaedic surgeons transfer the flexor digitorum longus (FDL) tendon to the

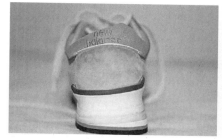

Figure 6 Athletic shoe with a 1/4-in medial heel wedge added.

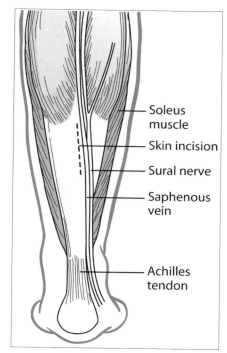

Figure 7 Standard midline incision for gastrocnemius recession.

navicular. This is an established procedure that has been shown to provide good pain relief. By dividing the FDL tendon in the midplantar arch, it should be possible to transfer the tendon from plantar to dorsal through the navicular and suture the tendon to itself (**Figure 9**). As part of this procedure, most orthopaedic surgeons resect the diseased portion of the tendon and perform a side-to-side tenodesis between the posterior tibialis and FDL tendon proximal to the flexor retinaculum. Simply débriding the damaged posterior tibial tendon and per-

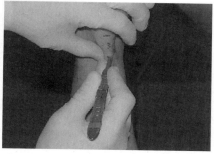

Figure 8 Inraoperative photograph showing midmedial hemisection of the Achilles tendon 3 cm proximal to the distal lateral release.

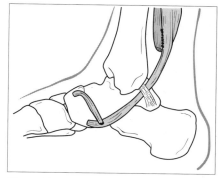

Figure 9 FDL transfer placed from plantar to dorsal and sutured to itself through the navicular. Note the retained portion of the flexed retinaculum at the posterior aspect of the medial malleolus and side-to-side tenodesis with the posterior tibialis proximally.

forming a side-to-side tenodesis to the FDL has also been described. Theoretically, this procedure could be associated with persistent symptoms because the diseased portion of the posterior tibial tendon is retained. Other orthopaedic surgeons have advocated transferring the FDL tendon to the medial cuneiform to prevent progression or the development of a naviculocuneiform sag. Although attractive in theory, it is often difficult to obtain FDL tendon of sufficient length to perform this transfer.

Another type of tendon reconstruction is the transfer of the flexor hallucis longus (FHL) muscle to the navicular. The FHL is stronger than the FDL and thus provides a stronger tendon transfer. However, this is a

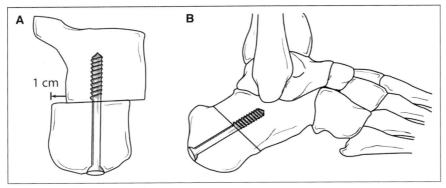

Figure 10 Medial calcaneal sliding osteotomy. **A,** Axial view of 1-cm medial shift of the posterior tuberosity with single screw fixation. **B,** Lateral view showing oblique osteotomy of the posterior tuberosity with single cancellous screw fixation.

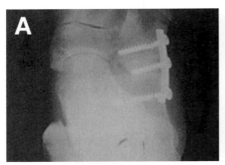
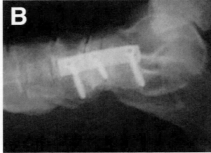

Figure 11 AP (**A**) and lateral (**B**) postoperative radiographs following calcaneocuboid distraction arthrodesis with allograft femoral head and three-hole 1/3 tubular plate fixation.

technically difficult operation and has the potential disadvantage of weakening the great toe. Some recent work has also evaluated transferring the peroneus brevis to the FDL tendon reconstruction to increase the strength and decrease the deforming force of the peroneus brevis.

FLATFOOT DEFORMITY

Acquired flatfoot deformity is generally the result of a damaged posterior tibial tendon; however, reconstruction of the posterior tibial tendon alone does not reconstruct the arch. Deformity develops because of attenuation of the ligamentous soft-tissue supporting structures, particularly structures in the arch, including the plantar calcaneonavicular ligament (spring ligament). Although there are some encouraging reports of reconstruction of the spring ligament, in my

experience, tightening of this poorly vascularized tissue does not lead to a durable correction. Other soft-tissue reconstructions have been described, including the use of allograft Achilles tendon, peroneus longus tendon run through a drill hole, and tibialis anterior tendon. Although these procedures can lead to improvement in the arch configuration, with appropriate bony work, they are generally unnecessary.

Various bony procedures have been described to correct the flatfoot deformity. Perhaps the most commonly performed procedure is the medial calcaneal sliding osteotomy. In this procedure, an oblique osteotomy of the posterior tuberosity of the calcaneus is performed, and the posterior tuberosity is translated 1 cm medially (**Figure 10**). In general, a single cancellous screw provides adequate fixa-

tion of this osteotomy. Care should be taken, especially in thin patients, to bevel the bone edge laterally so that the patient will not have a bony prominence in this subcutaneous region of the hindfoot. The calcaneal osteotomy works by statically correcting the hindfoot valgus, dynamically shifting the pull of the Achilles insertion medially, and statically increasing the longitudinal arch of the foot.

Another option for correcting the flatfoot deformity is to lengthen the lateral column of the foot. For calcaneocuboid distraction arthrodesis, the lengthening procedure is performed through the fusion site of the calcaneocuboid joint. In general, a 1- to 1.5-cm wedge of bone is placed in the calcaneocuboid joint, which pushes the forefoot out of abduction and increases the longitudinal arch sagittally. This procedure has been performed with autogenous tricortical iliac crest bone graft and, more recently, with allograft bone (**Figure 11**). Theoretically, a drawback to the use of allograft bone is the risk of collapse and nonunion. Although these grafts have been used without internal fixation, there is a risk of nonunion. Thus, I recommend using some type of internal fixation, either an H-plate, low profile cervical plate, or 1/3 tubular plate, with bone grafts.

Another option for lengthening the lateral column is to avoid the calcaneocuboid joint and to lengthen the anterior portion of the calcaneus with an Evans lengthening procedure. This procedure is generally performed approximately 1 to 1.5 cm posterior to the calcanecuboid joint. Internal fixation is recommended to minimize the risk of collapse of the bone graft. Allograft or autograft bone can be used in this lengthening procedure. This procedure has the theoretical advantage of preserving the motion of the calcaneocuboid joint. A disadvantage is the risk of calcaneocuboid degenerative arthritis developing because of increased joint pressures and a risk of calcaneocuboid subluxation.

Other bony procedures that can correct flatfoot deformity include selected midfoot fusions. Although most patients have a talonavicular sag that will correct passively with either a calcaneocuboid distraction arthrodesis or calcaneal osteotomy, some patients will have a naviculocuneiform or tarsometatarsal sag. These deformities are not corrected by a calcaneal osteotomy or lateral column lengthening. Thus, either a single joint fusion or extensive fusions of the midfoot may be treatment options. The advantage of these procedures is the correction of the sites of the deformity. The disadvantage is the risk of nonunion associated with each of the multiple joint fusions used.

Recently, hindfoot fusion with tendon reconstruction has gained some attention. A subtalar fusion to correct the hindfoot valgus combined with an FDL tendon reconstruction of the posterior tibial tendon to correct forefoot abduction has been described with good results. In addition, triple arthrodesis should remain a therapeutic option, particularly for morbidly obese patients.

Author's Preferred Treatment and Rationale

I prefer to begin with nonsurgical treatment in all patients. If nonsurgical treatment fails, then surgical intervention is indicated. For the gastrocnemius-soleus contracture, I usually perform a percutaneous TAL because of its decreased morbidity and improved cosmesis. For a patient who wants to be active in sports and who is not opposed to its potentially less than desirable cosmesis, I would perform a gastrocnemius recession. With regard to the tendon reconstruction, I prefer an FDL transfer to the navicular because it is a predictable operation. In patients with mild to moderate deformity, I prefer a medial sliding calcaneal osteotomy because of its predictable, rapid healing. In cases of more severe deformity, such as a greater than 15° talo-first metatarsal angle on a lateral radiograph or greater than 25% uncovering of the talar head on an AP radiograph, especially in patients who are overweight, the lateral column lengthening through a calcaneocuboid distraction arthrodesis is a much more powerful correction. In general, I have found midfoot fusion to be unnecessary unless there is demonstrable instability of these joints instead of simply a sag on a standard lateral radiograph. If there is any question regarding the stability of these joints, stress radiographs can be obtained in both plantar flexion and dorsiflexion. If a naviculocuneiform sag corrects to neutral on plantar flexion stress, I would fuse the joint. Visible plantar gapping at the first tarsometatarsal joint indicates instability that should be treated with a fusion.

In general, the only soft-tissue procedure performed medially is the FDL reconstruction because spring ligament reconstruction and other procedures have not been proved to be necessary and are not as durable. Finally in morbidly obese patients, especially those with lower functional demand, or in elderly patients, a triple arthrodesis or other hindfoot fusion is far more predictable in achieving a correction even in the presence of a flexible deformity.

Management of Complications

The most common postoperative complication is persistent pain, with or without persistence and recurrence of deformity. Initially, all patients with persistent pain deserve a course of nonsurgical treatment following the principles described previously. If a 6-month course of nonsurgical treatment including the modalities listed above fails, a fusion procedure is likely to be required. For these patients, it is generally best to proceed to a true salvage operation, a triple arthrodesis, as it provides excellent deformity correction and will eliminate all three of the hindfoot joints as potential sources of persistent pain.

Wound complications and occasionally infection are not infrequent after surgical interventions. These complications generally can be successfully treated with local wound care. Nonunion of the calcaneocuboid distraction arthrodesis or other hindfoot fusions is possible and should be treated with additional fusion procedures and bone grafting as indicated. The most common complication of a medial sliding osteotomy is residual deformity. Medial sliding osteotomy is rarely complicated with nonunion.

———————■

References

Guyton GP, Jeng C, Krieger LE, Mann RA: Flexor digitorum longus transfer and medial displacement calcaneal osteotomy for posterior tibial tendon dysfunction: A middle-term clinical follow-up. *Foot Ankle Int* 2001;22:627-632.

Johnson JE, Cohen BE, DiGiovanni BF, Lamdan R: Subtalar arthrodesis with flexor digitorum longus transfer and spring ligament repair for treatment of posterior tibial tendon insufficiency. *Foot Ankle Int* 2000;21:722-729.

Mosier-LaClair S, Pomeroy G, Manoli A II: Intermediate follow-up on the double osteotomy and tendon transfer procedure for stage II posterior tibial tendon insufficiency. *Foot Ankle Int* 2001;22:283-291.

Myerson MS, Corrigan J, Thompson F, Schon LC: Tendon transfer combined with calcaneal osteotomy for treatment of posterior tibial tendon insufficiency: A radiological investigation. *Foot Ankle Int* 1995;16:712-718.

Wacker JT, Henessy MS, Saxby TS: Calcaneal osteotomy and transfer of the tendon of flexor digitorum longus for stage-II dysfunction of tibialis posterior: Three- to five-year results. *J Bone Joint Surg Br* 2002;84:54-58.

Coding

ICD-9 CODE
726.72   Tibialis tendinitis

CPT CODES

27606   Tenotomy, percutaneous, Achilles tendon (separate procedure); general anesthesia

27687   Gastrocnemius recession (eg, Strayer procedure)

27691   Transfer or transplant of single tendon (with muscle redirection of rerouting); deep (eg, flexor digitorum longus to midfoot or hindfoot)

28300   Osteotomy; calcaneus (eg, Dwyer or Chambers type procedure), with or without internal fixation

28740   Arthrodesis, midtarsal or tarsometatarsal, single joint

Stage III Acquired Flatfoot Deformity

Jeffrey E. Johnson, MD

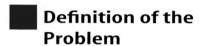

Definition of the Problem

Patient Presentation

The adult acquired flatfoot deformity most often is associated with either elongation or attritional rupture of the posterior tibial tendon. Less often, a flexible physiologic pes planovalgus deformity may begin to progress to a more severe deformity secondary to degenerative changes in the hindfoot joints and/or capsuloligamentous insufficiency. A stage III acquired flatfoot deformity is characterized by a stiff, fixed deformity of the subtalar or transverse tarsal joints that often is associated with osteoarthritis of all or one of these joints. Usually a middle-aged or elderly patient presents with a flexible acquired flatfoot deformity (stage II) that he or she has had for several years and that has become progressively worse and more painful. In the initial stages of the deformity, the pain may be located in the medial arch area; however, as the foot stiffens and the hindfoot progresses into greater degrees of valgus, the calcaneus comes into contact with the distal fibula, causing lateral impingement pain. This pain is often the most predominant presenting symptom. The pain and swelling over the distal portion of the posterior tibial tendon, which are common in stages I and II of posterior tendon insufficiency, often are not seen in stage III.

Physical Examination

Examination of a standing patient will reveal a pes planovalgus deformity characterized by varying degrees of hindfoot valgus and forefoot abduction with loss of the longitudinal arch. There often is a painful callosity on the plantar medial aspect of the navicular tuberosity or the medial cuneiform. In the presence of calcaneofibular abutment, tenderness to palpation is common in the sinus tarsi and at the tip of the distal fibula. Tenderness around the joint line of the talonavicular and calcaneocuboid joints is also common.

When the patient is seated, the orthopaedist cannot completely correct the hindfoot. The forefoot often will remain in a fixed varus position after the heel is corrected to neutral, and the orthopaedist cannot rotate the forefoot back into a plantigrade position while holding the heel in neutral. With the hindfoot held in as corrected a position as possible and the knee in extension, a significant equinus contracture secondary to gastrocnemius muscle tightness is seen in the ankle. Long-standing pes planovalgus deformity often will result in osteoarthritis or instability at the first metatarsocuneiform joint. During the physical examination, this joint should be palpated to determine the amount of hypermobility of the medial column midtarsal joints.

Differential Diagnosis

- Neuropathic arthropathy
- Rheumatoid arthritis
- Osteoarthritis with deformity at the tarsometatarsal joints (primary or posttraumatic)

Additional Work-up

Work-up should include weight-bearing AP, lateral, and medial-oblique radiographs of the foot (**Figure 1**). In addition, a weight-bearing AP view of the ankle is needed to identify any evidence of valgus tilt of the talus within the mortise, which may occur from chronic attrition of the deltoid ligament with long-standing pes planovalgus deformity (ie, stage IV disease). It is important to identify valgus malalignment of the tibiotalar joint preoperatively because it may alter the choice of procedures required to correct the deformity. Correction of the foot deformity alone would not be expected to correct all of the valgus deformity of the hindfoot if the ankle joint has a valgus talar tilt.

CT in two planes (semicoronal and axial) through the hindfoot and ankle joints is helpful to determine the severity of osteoarthritis of the hindfoot joints. If the physical examination is equivocal, differential diagnostic injections sometimes are used to identify which joints are causing pain and need to be fused. These injections are best performed under fluoroscopy with the use of an arthrogram to confirm needle placement before injection of a long-acting local anesthetic.

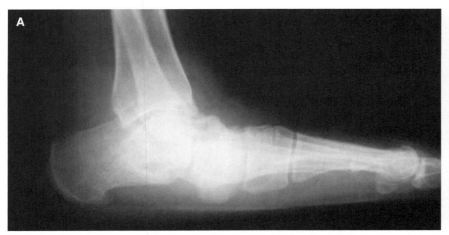
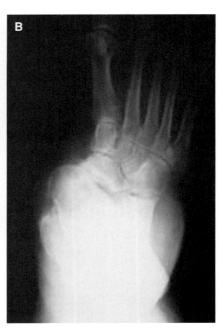

Figure 1   Stage III posterior tendon dysfunction in a 49-year-old woman treated with a triple arthrodesis with a tricortical iliac crest distraction bone graft placed into the calcaneocuboid joint. A medial displacement calcaneal osteotomy helped provide additional correction of the hindfoot valgus. The gastrocnemius also was lengthened. **A,** Preoperative lateral radiograph shows significant lateral subluxation of the calcaneus in relation to the talus, with marked angulation of the talo-first metatarsal line. **B,** Preoperative AP radiograph shows significant lateral perialar subluxation of the foot with degenerative changes of the transverse tarsal joint.

■ The Solutions

Treatment Options and Rationale

Nonsurgical treatment is aimed at accommodating a fixed pes planovalgus deformity that is not passively correctable. Appropriate extra-depth shoes that are wide enough through the midfoot area are necessary. Some manufacturers of specialty footwear make a shoe with a wide-shank last to accommodate these types of deformities. In addition, the last, or shape, of these shoes can be changed by a certified pedorthist, and the shoes can be fit with custom total-contact inserts. Occasionally a severe deformity will require a custom molded shoe. Severe deformities, especially those with tibiotalar valgus alignment, will require use of an ankle-foot orthosis (AFO). The traditional full-length short leg molded polypropylene AFO or metal double uprights can be used; however, the trend has been to use shorter style braces. A plastic reinforced leather ankle gauntlet-style AFO is less bulky and cumbersome than the other types of braces and, with the leather padded

lining, provides a level of comfort not found with metal or plastic braces.

Surgical treatment options include an isolated subtalar joint arthrodesis, double (talonavicular and calcaneocuboid joint) arthrodesis, or a triple arthrodesis. Other procedures may be added to any of the above procedures to fully correct the tripod of the foot. A medial displacement calcaneal osteotomy is added when there is residual hindfoot valgus despite reduction and stabilization of the subtalar joint. An opening wedge plantar flexion osteotomy of the first cuneiform could be performed to help plantar flex the medial column if it is still elevated, despite rotational correction of the foot at the transverse tarsal joint. Alternatively, arthrodesis of the first tarsometatarsal joint can be performed if there is painful arthritis at that joint or dorsal subluxation through the joint. A gastrocnemius or Achilles lengthening is almost always required in conjunction with a triple arthrodesis for a pes planovalgus deformity.

An isolated subtalar joint fusion is performed when the degenerative

changes are isolated to the subtalar joint and the transverse tarsal joint is passively correctable to neutral when the heel is reduced into neutral. However, if there is any stiffness in the tarsal joint that will not allow the forefoot to be passively corrected to neutral, an isolated subtalar joint fusion would result in a fixed residual forefoot varus that would cause both pain and excessive weight bearing on the lateral border of the foot.

Some authors advocate a double arthrodesis for the transverse tarsal joint deformity that cannot be corrected passively, leaving the subtalar joint unfused. However, this procedure creates the same amount of hindfoot stiffness as a triple arthrodesis and may have a slightly higher rate of nonunion than a triple arthrodesis. Double arthrodesis is better suited for isolated arthritis of the transverse tarsal joint associated with minimal valgus deformity.

Author's Preferred Treatment and Rationale

After initial evaluation of a patient who has not tried bracing, I often recommend the short molded plastic re-inforced leather ankle gauntlet that laces anteriorly and fits nicely into an extra-depth shoe. The surgical treatment of stage III acquired flatfoot deformity is a major operation, and bracing, especially in the elderly patient, is often satisfactory. If the patient has not improved after 2 to 3 months of bracing, then surgical treatment is recommended. Failure of brace therapy not only helps determine which patients truly require surgical treatment but also helps simplify the decision-making process because the patient has fully evaluated and experienced the results of nonsurgical treatment.

If the pes planovalgus deformity is not correctable at the transverse tarsal joint, a triple arthrodesis is performed. If there is a significant amount of forefoot abduction, a tricortical iliac crest bone block may be placed into the calcaneocuboid joint at the time of the triple arthrodesis to help lengthen the lateral column and correct the foot abduction. A medial displacement osteotomy often is required for patients who had a physiologic pes planovalgus deformity before the acquired flatfoot deformity developed. In these patients, anatomic repositioning of the subtalar joint will only return the joint to its premorbid state, which is a valgus deformity. Therefore, the medial displacement osteotomy will help fully correct the hindfoot valgus. Full correction of the hindfoot to neutral is particularly important in the patient with mild to moderate valgus talar tilt at the ankle.

Placement of the incisions is critical to prevent wound complications if a medial displacement calcaneal osteotomy and subtalar joint fusion are to be performed at the same time. An oblique longitudinal incision along the lateral aspect of the calcaneal tuberosity is made for the osteotomy, and a parallel incision is made from the tip of the distal fibula to the base of the fourth metatarsal for completion of the subtalar and calca-

neocuboid joint portions of the triple arthrodesis. Care is taken to avoid undermining the skin or subcutaneous tissue as the exposure is made. Additional care is taken in handling the skin during the procedure, and no self-retaining retractors are used (**Figure 2**).

Gastrocnemius lengthening almost always is required before any hindfoot osteotomy or fixation. Lengthening usually is done near the myotendinous junction on the posterior aspect of the calf.

Proper preparation of the joints is critical if a high percentage of solid arthrodeses is to be obtained. It is important to remove all the cartilage and to expose the subchondral bone of all joints to be fused. The next step is to expose the underlying cancellous bone by using a small osteotome to "feather" the surface or by using a 2.5-mm drill bit to make multiple holes through the subchondral bone. The ligaments on the medial side of the subtalar joint must be lax enough to allow reduction of the valgus deformity or must be débrided so that the hindfoot can be returned manually to its normal position beneath the talus during the reduction maneuver. Lamina spreaders, both with and without teeth at the end of the blades, are very useful for distracting the hindfoot joints to allow proper exposure, preparation, and reduction of the joint fusion surfaces. Distraction of the subtalar joint allows visualization across the joint to the medial capsule. Under direct vision a pituitary rongeur can be used to remove the medial capsule to loosen and aid in joint reduction. Care is taken to avoid injury to the flexor hallucis longus tendon or the flexor digitorum longus tendon, which reside along the medial aspect of the subtalar joint.

The talonavicular joint is exposed through a dorsomedial incision along the lateral border of the anterior tibialis tendon. Dissection is carried through the interval between the an-

terior tibialis tendon and the extensor hallucis longus tendon down to the dorsal capsule of the talonavicular joint. Further dissection, medial and lateral to this area, is subperiosteal.

Once all the joints have been prepared for fusion, and the ligaments of the talonavicular joint, the calcaneocuboid joint, and the medial side of the subtalar joint have been adequately released, the foot is corrected in segments from proximal to distal. The subtalar joint is repositioned first. The surgeon places the thumb of one hand on the medial side of the talar neck and the thumb of the other hand along the lateral side of the calcaneus. The calcaneus is pushed medially and internally rotated back under the talus by pushing the thumbs toward one another. This maneuver also decreases any lateral translation of the calcaneus in relation to the talus. The subtalar joint is held in this repositioned location while a Steinmann pin is placed from the neck of the talus across the subtalar joint. A lateral C-arm image is then obtained to ensure the proper relationship of the talus to the calcaneus. The posterior facet of the subtalar joint should appear congruent. The inferior portion of the talar head and neck should be slightly overlapped by the anterior tuberosity of the calcaneus, and the posterior border of the body of the talus should be even with the posterior edge of the posterior facet of the calcaneus (**Figure 3**).

Once proper reduction has been confirmed, one or two 6.5-mm cannulated screws are placed from the posterior inferior tuberosity of the calcaneus across the subtalar joint and into the talus. The thread length of the screws should be chosen such that the threads do not cross the subtalar joint, and each screw will act as a lag screw.

Next, the transverse tarsal joint is reduced by simultaneously pushing the forefoot into adduction and pronating it to reduce the talonavicular joint. In severe deformities, a lamina

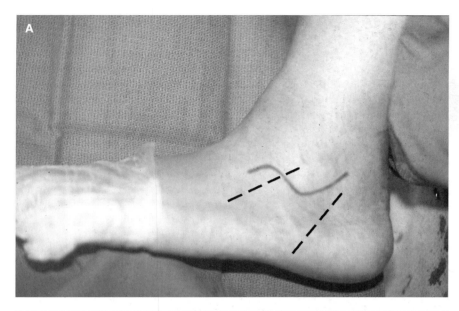

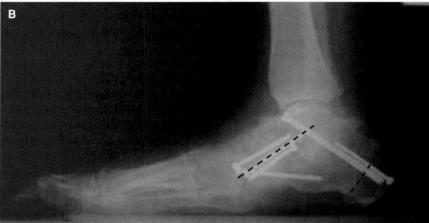

Figure 2 Clinical photograph (**A**) and lateral radiograph (**B**) showing incision placement for triple arthrodesis with medial displacement calcaneal osteotomy. Two parallel incisions are used. The subtalar joint and calcaneocuboid joint are exposed through an incision from the tip of the distal fibula to the base of the fourth metatarsal. The medial displacement calcaneal osteotomy is performed through an oblique parallel incision over the posterior tuberosity. An attempt to perform both of these procedures through the same extensile lateral incision is more difficult and may create wound healing problems from necrosis of the skin flaps.

reduced, two 4.5-mm cannulated screws are placed from the navicular tuberosity into the talar head and neck. Finally, the calcaneocuboid joint is fixed with crisscrossing 4.5-mm cannulated screws. One screw is placed percutaneously from the cuboid into the anterior calcaneus, and the head is countersunk. The second screw is placed from the antero-superior process of the calcaneus inferiorly and distally into the plantar medial portion of the cuboid. Staples may be used at the calcaneocuboid joint if a tricortical bone block has not been inserted.

Given the significant deformity in the stage III flatfoot, bone grafting material is usually needed to fill the voids created by anatomic reduction of the joints. It is my preference to place autogenous bone graft into the joints after reduction and before fixation to fill any small voids that occur at the joint surfaces. Allograft or autograft tricortical iliac crest can be used for distraction of the calcaneocuboid joint or cuneiform osteotomy. Morcellized allograft or some type of bone graft substitute can also be used for filling the voids in these joints or to augment autograft.

Postoperative management includes 10 to 14 days in a short leg compression splint with the ankle in neutral. This is followed by suture removal and 4 weeks in a short leg non–weight-bearing cast. Radiographs are obtained, then a short leg walking cast is applied for an additional 4 weeks until the patient is fully weight bearing and all the joints are consolidated. Physical therapy for ankle range of motion and calf muscle strengthening is then begun. A knee-high support stocking and a removable walker boot are helpful during the transition from a cast to an in-depth shoe.

This is an extensive surgical procedure, and the patient often will require 9 to 12 months to achieve maximal improvement. The postoperative use of an AFO sometimes will be nec-

spreader placed into the calcaneocuboid joint will help push the foot out of abduction. In these deformities, a tricortical iliac crest bone graft placed into the calcaneocuboid joint will help maintain the length of the lateral column and the reduction of the forefoot. Anatomic reduction of the hindfoot joint may not be possible due to a severe deformity and limitations imposed by tight ligaments and

skin. In these cases, the medial column of the foot is shortened by removing some of the talar head. This may also avoid the need for a distraction graft in the calcaneocuboid joint. However, my preference is to maintain the conformity of the joints and perform reduction of the hindfoot bones to restore the most anatomically shaped foot possible.

Once the talonavicular joint is

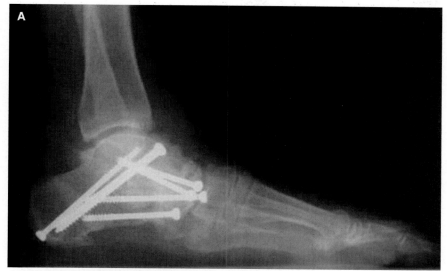

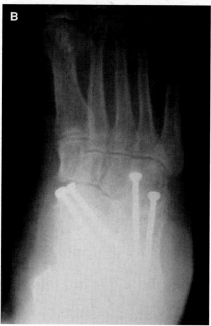

Figure 3 Postoperative radiographs of the patient described in Figure 1. **A**, Lateral radiograph shows restoration of the talocalcaneal relationship and the lateral talo-first metatarsal line. **B**, AP radiograph shows a tricortical iliac crest bone block placed in the calcaneocuboid joint to lengthen the lateral column and help achieve reduction of the talonavicular joint.

essary for the patient with a residual valgus talar tilt at the tibiotalar joint.

Two additional procedures can be done to ensure correction of the flatfoot. If the talonavicular joint is reduced, but the medial column of the foot remains elevated relative to the lateral column, a plantar flexion opening wedge medial cuneiform osteotomy or an arthrodesis of the first tarsometatarsal joint with plantar flexion at the joint can be performed. For both of these procedures, the tal-

onavicular joint incision is extended distally over the cuneiform and base of the first metatarsal. For the opening wedge cuneiform osteotomy, a small microsagittal saw is used to make an osteotomy cut from dorsal to plantar while care is taken to protect the articular surface of the second cuneiform. The plantar cortex of the cuneiform can be kept intact and hinged open. A small osteotome is used to pry open the bone, then a 5- to 7-mm dorsally based wedge of tricortical iliac

crest bone graft is harvested and tapped into the cuneiform to create a snug fit. A percutaneous 0.062-in Kirschner wire or a 4.0-mm cannulated screw across the osteotomy site is used for fixation.

If at the time of subtalar joint reduction the heel remains in valgus relative to the long axis of the tibia, a medial displacement calcaneal osteotomy will help to restore the mechanical alignment of the hindfoot. This osteotomy is made before definitive fixation of the subtalar joint. An incision is made over the lateral aspect of the calcaneal tuberosity just posterior to the sural nerve and parallel to the subtalar joint incision. Dissection is carried down to the subcutaneus border of the calcaneus without undermining the adjacent soft-tissue planes. A microsagittal saw is used to make a transverse osteotomy that then is distracted with a lamina spreader to stretch the periosteum on the medial side. The tuberosity is shifted laterally along the line of the osteotomy about 1 cm (or whatever is needed) to correct the hindfoot alignment and fixed with a 0.062-in Kirschner wire. A 4.5-mm or 6.5-mm cannulated screw is then placed from the tuberosity of the calcaneus into the anterior calcaneus. A second (6.5-mm) screw is placed from the tuberosity into the talar body or from the anterior neck of the talus across the subtalar joint and into the tuberosity of the calcaneus. The talar neck screw is inserted through and a 2-cm incision is made along the medial edge of the anterior tibial tendon. Care is taken to avoid overcorrecting the heel into varus with this osteotomy. (See chapter 33, Malunited Triple Arthrodesis.)

Management of Complications

Early complications of a triple arthrodesis for a severe valgus hindfoot include lateral wound breakdown resulting from excessive tightness of the closure, wound infection, and sural nerve injury. A superficial skin breakdown or superficial infection is treated with local wound care and antibiotics. Deep infection requires return to the operating room for débridement as necessary and antibiotics. An attempt is made to leave the hardware in place unless it is directly exposed in the open wound after débridement. Sural nerve injury is often a transient neurapraxia, and reassuring the patient that sensation should return is helpful.

Late complications include non-union resulting from inadequate fixation or preparation of the joint surfaces. Smoking also has an adverse effect on union rate. Because this is an elective procedure, I prefer to postpone surgery until the patient has been able to stop smoking for least 1 month.

Failure to adequately reduce the hindfoot valgus deformity often places additional stresses on the ankle joint and may accelerate a valgus tilting of the tibiotalar joint. A valgus hindfoot that has been fused in situ can be salvaged with a medial displacement calcaneal osteotomy and a transverse osteotomy across the calcaneocuboid and talonavicular joints to rotate the forefoot and midfoot back into neutral position.

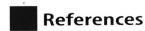

References

Fortin PT, Walling AK: Triple arthrodesis. *Clin Orthop* 1999;365:91-99.

Graves SC, Mann RA, Graves KO: Triple arthrodesis in older adults: Results after long-term follow-up. *J Bone Joint Surg Am* 1993;75:355-362.

Pell RF IV, Myerson MS, Schon LC: Clinical outcome after primary triple arthrodesis. *J Bone Joint Surg Am* 2000;82:47-57.

Saltzman CL, Fehrle MJ, Cooper RR, Spencer EC, Ponseti IV: Triple arthrodesis: Twenty-five and forty-four-year average follow-up of the same patients. *J Bone Joint Surg Am* 1999;81:1391-1402.

Coding

ICD-9 CODES

715.97   Osteoarthritis

719.47   Pain, foot/ankle

727.81   Contracture gastrocnemius-soleus muscle

734   Acquired flatfoot deformity

754.61   Congenital flatfoot deformity

905.8   Late effects of tendon injury

CPT CODES

20902   Bone graft, any donor area; major or large

27685   Lengthening or shortening of tendon, leg or ankle; single tendon (separate procedure)

28300   Osteotomy; calcaneus (eg, Dwyer or Chambers type procedure), with or without internal fixation

28304   Osteotomy, tarsal bones, other than calcaneus or talus

28715   Arthrodesis; triple

28740   Arthrodesis, midtarsal or tarsometatarsal, single joint

(The – 59 modifier will need to be added to the codes for the adjunctive procedures to denote that they were made through a separate location and not part of the triple arthrodesis itself.)

Stage IV Flatfoot: Alternatives to Tibiocalcaneal or Pantalar Procedures

Arthur K. Walling, MD

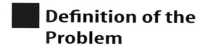

Definition of the Problem

Patient Presentation

Patients presenting with stage IV flatfoot tend to be middle-aged to older women who are overweight. However, stage IV flatfoot can occur in anyone and has additional causes such as inflammatory arthritis. Although the pathomechanics of the deformities are different, the clinical presentation of patients with inflammatory arthritis is similar enough to that of other patients that both groups can be discussed as a single entity.

By definition, patients with stage IV flatfoot usually present with long-standing symptoms and deformity. These patients have very limited inversion through the subtalar joint and minimal adduction of the transverse tarsal joints, or they may have a totally fixed deformity. They also will have a fixed forefoot varus greater than 15°. In addition to the fixed hindfoot deformity, these patients have medial ankle laxity and lateral tibiotalar arthritis, with loss of articular cartilage in the lateral portion of the ankle joint (**Figure 1**). This loss leads to even more valgus malpositioning of the hindfoot and to pain in both the hindfoot and the ankle.

Patients with stage IV disease will report significant limitations in their ability to perform the normal activities of daily living, including walking. They are uncomfortable wearing any type of shoe, and most attempts at shoe modification or bracing have failed.

Physical Examination

The deformity of these patients is obvious. They have marked valgus of both the ankle and hindfoot when viewed from behind. They have no arch and often have a rocker-bottom deformity, as well as a plantar prominence of the talar head. These patients are unable to raise a heel off the ground when asked to perform a single stance heel rise. Essentially all inversion and eversion occur through the ankle joint. It often is difficult for patients to determine whether most of their pain emanates from the ankle or the hindfoot. The valgus position of the hindfoot in some patients is so great that their pain is a result of fibular impingement by the calcaneus or of an unrecognized fibular fracture secondary to the impingement (**Figure 2**).

Weight-bearing radiographs of the foot and ankle are necessary to evaluate the degree of deformity.

Differential Diagnosis
- Posterior tibial dysfunction
- Fracture malunion
- Inflammatory arthritis
- Deltoid insufficiency

Additional Work-up

Because the amount of pain attributed to the deformity at the ankle can vary widely, I recommend a 5-mL intra-articular injection of lidocaine to attempt to determine whether the ankle is actually symptomatic in patients who do not have significant valgus tilt or arthrosis of the ankle.

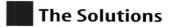

The Solutions

Treatment Options and Rationale

Nonsurgical management of stage IV flatfoot deformity is very difficult because of the fixed position of the hindfoot and the bony prominences caused by the deformity. The prominence of the talar head medially cannot tolerate much pressure, and, because of the fixed valgus of the hindfoot and ankle, any attempt to correct the malposition results in painful pressure. In fact, any attempt to correct the fixed deformity will cause pain and result in skin breakdown. In patients who are not candidates for surgical repair or who refuse to consider surgery, I have had better success with either ankle stirrups (such as those used for ankle sprains) or immobilizer-type boots. I have not been particularly impressed with patient acceptance of solid or articulated ankle-foot orthoses. The goal of bracing is to provide symptomatic relief; it probably is impossible

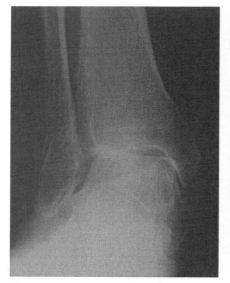

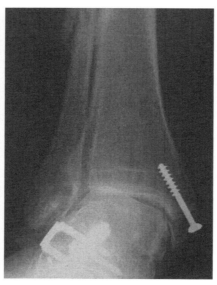

Figure 1 AP radiograph of the ankle shows valgus positioning with lateral articular loss secondary to the fixed valgus position of the hindfoot, typical in stage IV flatfoot.

Figure 2 AP radiograph shows incomplete correction of hindfoot valgus following triple arthrodesis. In this patient, the fibular impingement increased to the point that fracture eventually occurred.

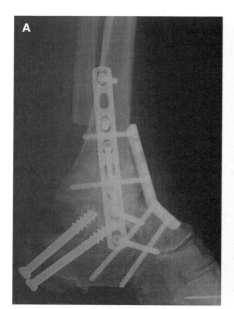

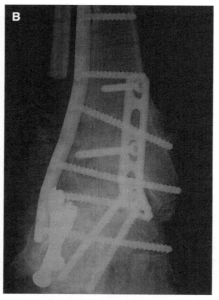

Figure 3 Radiographs of arthrodeses of the ankle and subtalar joints for stage IV deformity. **A,** Lateral view shows that a medial sliding calcaneal osteotomy was also used to obtain physiologic positioning. **B,** AP view shows that fusion was initially attempted through a transfibular approach with resection of the fibula. These patients often drift into valgus. A lateral plate was used to counteract the loss of the fibula.

to arrest progression and prevent further arthrosis with bracing. Successful nonsurgical treatment remains the exception rather than the rule.

The greatest difficulty in surgical treatment of patients with stage IV flatfoot deformity is the fact that they have two levels of involvement, and

that treatment of one will influence the other. To assess overall treatment, the hindfoot deformity and the ankle deformity need to be assessed individually and together. Two clinical situations can occur. In the first, less common, situation, the patient has stage IV disease with a fixed hindfoot deformity, talar tilt (with or without deltoid insufficiency), and no symptomatic ankle arthritis. In the second, more common, situation, the patient has fixed hindfoot deformity (with or without deltoid insufficiency) and symptomatic ankle arthritis. I will discuss treatment of the second situation.

Author's Preferred Treatment and Rationale

The two main surgical options for patients with stage IV deformity and symptomatic ankle arthritis involve tibiotalocalcaneal or pantalar arthrodesis (**Figure 3**). Although these two procedures may produce satisfactory pain relief and provide an alternative to amputation, they both have substantial functional consequences and complications and are considered salvage procedures.

In patients who have minimal ankle arthritis and whose primary symptoms are related to the fixed hindfoot deformity, the option of performing a triple arthrodesis without initially addressing the ankle should be seriously considered. The preservation of ankle motion significantly benefits function. However, these patients need to be informed preoperatively that their ankle arthritis or valgus tilt may progress with time and that they may require a second procedure to address either situation. The key to this approach is complete correction of the hindfoot deformity at the time of the triple arthrodesis. Any residual hindfoot malalignment will be poorly tolerated and lead to increased talar tilt, arthritis, or both. The severity of symptoms or the progression of arthritic changes in the ankle may be surprisingly minimal (**Figure 4**).

For patients in whom both the hindfoot and ankle deformities have to be addressed, the option of hindfoot fusion and ankle joint arthroplasty should be considered. However, this approach remains largely untested and undocumented. Encouraging early results have been reported for the newer generation of ankle replacements that rely on porous ingrowth fixation. However, it is recognized that any hindfoot or ankle malalignment represents a much more challenging surgical correction and can result in higher patient dissatisfaction and earlier component loosening if the malalignment is not addressed.

The success of hindfoot arthrodesis plus ankle replacement depends on complete correction of the hindfoot malalignment and the amount of deltoid insufficiency. I believe it is much better to approach this as a two-stage procedure than to attempt simultaneous hindfoot arthrodesis and ankle replacement. Because it is imperative to achieve full hindfoot correction at the time of triple arthrodesis, stress radiographs of the ankle mortise should be taken during this procedure. These radiographs confirm that the hindfoot is corrected when the talus is in a parallel position relative to the tibia. In addition, they will help the surgeon determine whether most of the ankle valgus is secondary to arthritic narrowing of the lateral ankle joint or secondary to deltoid ligament incompetence.

Total ankle replacement is reasonable when the valgus malposition of the ankle is primarily a result of articular narrowing secondary to arthritic changes, and the ankle is symptomatic. This procedure may be timed so that its immobilization period coincides with that for the hindfoot arthrodesis (**Figure 5**).

The choice of procedures becomes much more difficult if there is significant incompetency of the deltoid ligament. Although sizing of the prosthetic components can bring about some tensioning of the ligaments, significant laxity cannot be overcome in this manner. Procedures for correcting deltoid ligament insufficiency (deltoid ligament advancement, plication, and tendon substitutions) have been described, but their efficacy, especially in conjunction with ankle replacement, has not been tested adequately. I recommend that total ankle replacement be abandoned if the deltoid is so incompetent that it needs reconstruction.

Another contraindication to total ankle replacement is progression to stage IV disease after triple arthrodesis. This progression usually is a consequence of inadequate correction of the hindfoot deformity, with secondary changes occurring in the ankle. The malunion of the hindfoot must be corrected before consider-

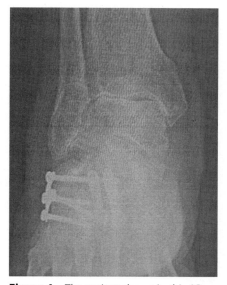

Figure 4 The patient shown in this AP radiograph, despite having a significant flatfoot deformity and secondary ankle changes, had a passively correctable hindfoot without significant arthritis. Following an attempt at correction with a lateral column lengthening and calcaneal medial slide, he remains asymptomatic.

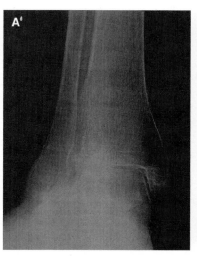
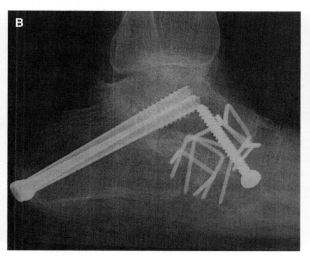
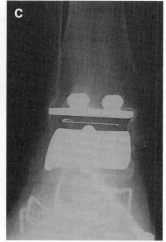

Figure 5 **A,** Preoperative AP radiograph of a patient with rheumatoid arthritis and stage IV flatfoot. **B,** Lateral view following correction of the hindfoot deformity with triple arthrodesis. **C,** AP view of the ankle following staged total ankle replacement.

ation of total ankle replacement. Medial displacement calcaneal osteotomy, complete revision of the arthrodesis, or a combination of both may be necessary to achieve correction. If satisfactory correction is not obtained, or if deltoid insufficiency remains significant, total ankle replacement should not be considered. No clinical results of these scenarios have been published, and they should be considered untested at this time.

Management of Complications
The usual postoperative complications of wound healing and infection probably are compounded because of the multiplicity of procedures concentrated in a relatively small area. However, they certainly are manageable and require the same diligence as any arthrodesis or joint arthroplasty. The greater concern is residual malalignment or deltoid insufficiency because either of these may be a catastrophic consequence for which there are few recognized solutions. When encountered, these complications usually will require resorting to a salvage extended arthrodesis or amputation.

──────■

References

Walling AK: Symposium: Adult acquired flatfoot. *Clin Orthop* 1999;365:2-99.

Pomeroy GC, Pike RH, Beals TC, Manoli A II: Acquired flatfoot in adults due to dysfunction of the posterior tibial tendon. *J Bone Joint Surg Am* 1999;81:1173-1182.

Kelly IP, Nunley JA: Treatment of stage 4 adult acquired flatfoot. *Foot Ankle Clin* 2001;6:167-178.

Coding

ICD-9 CODES
715.97   Osteoarthrosis, unspecified whether generalized or localized, ankle and foot

736.72   Other acquired deformities of limbs, Other acquired deformities of ankle and foot, Equinus deformity of foot, acquired

CPT CODES
27698   Repair, secondary disrupted ligament, ankle, collateral (eg, Watson-Jones procedure)

27702   Arthroplasty, ankle; with implant ("total ankle")

28300   Osteotomy; calcaneus (eg, Dwyer or Chambers type procedure), with or without internal fixation

28715   Arthrodesis; triple

Painful Congenital Pes Planus in the Adult

Andrew K. Sands, MD

Definition of the Problem

Patient Presentation

Patients with congenital pes planus or, more accurately, pes plano abducto valgus (PPAV) usually present with a history of always having had flatfeet. They often required shoe modifications and bracing as children (molded insert, navicular "cookie," or boots and bars). They often are seen again during their adolescence or as young adults. Some patients may be accompanied by a concerned parent, and the main complaint may be cosmetic, although the deformity may have become painful. Young adults may seek medical attention when they move from a locale where they get around by car to one where walking is more popular, especially to areas where there are hard concrete sidewalks. Long-standing PPAV may become a problem in patients who have gained a lot of weight. PPAV may also result from overcorrected clubfoot surgery. In general, all of these presentations are characterized by new onset of pain in previously asymptomatic patients with long-standing deformity.

Physical Examination

The patient should have bare feet during this examination. The weight-bearing part of the examination will reveal PPAV or flatfoot. There is loss of medial arch height, the calcaneal tuber is in valgus, and the forefoot may be abducted

and pronated. There may be an associated hallux valgus, especially if there is concomitant hypermobility of the medial column, which makes the PPAV deformity worse.

Single-leg heel rise should be tested. Patients with posterior tibialis insufficiency or failure are unable to raise their heels off the ground. Patients with long-standing deformity (congenital) may have an intact single-leg heel rise, despite the deformity. Usually, an equinus contracture, which adds to the stress on the foot and contributes to the progression, is also present.

The hindfoot should be examined for inversion and eversion. If the subtalar joint is supple, motion-sparing reconstruction should be considered.

AP, oblique, and lateral radiographs of the weight-bearing foot show the site of the deformity. Often the radiographs show peritalar subluxation with dorsal and lateral subluxation of the navicular through the coxa pedis-talonavicular joint. The deformity can also be through the midfoot tarsometatarsal area. A talocalcaneal or calcaneonavicular coalition is less common. Examination in the presence of a coalition reveals decreased range of motion through the hindfoot and should raise suspicion. Further imaging studies are helpful.

Differential Diagnosis
- Posterior tibialis insufficiency or failure
- Hindfoot coalition (talocalcaneal or naviculocalcaneal)

- Posttraumatic deformity (hindfoot or midfoot)
- Overcorrection of previous congenital deformity (clubfoot)

Additional Work-up

Although MRI might show a cartilaginous or fibrous coalition, CT with reconstruction is less expensive and yields a more detailed image with better resolution. CT with sagittal and coronal reformatting is the imaging study of choice.

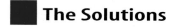

The Solutions

Treatment Options and Rationale
NONSURGICAL

The advent of new high-tech materials and footwear designs makes the use of cushioned footwear a good choice for treatment of these foot deformities. The footwear should have medial support but not be too rigid. The material should be a closed-cell viscoelastic material that should not be irreversibly compressible like some of the older open-cell materials. Hard plastics should be avoided. Custom orthotics have not been shown to be any more efficacious than off-the-shelf cushioned inserts; however, they can be harmful and increase pain. Forced dorsiflexion (ie, an improperly made custom orthotic), especially in the presence of an equinus contracture, often causes more pain. Physical therapy, in the form of aggressive calf (and hamstring) stretching can be tried. Stretching maintains or may even improve subtalar and complex hindfoot motion. Strengthening of the posterior tibialis will help to support the medial arch and possibly prevent further loss of medial arch height. Although bracing has been described as a treatment of congenital PPAV, it is not corrective and may hasten hindfoot rigidity. Bracing is not recommended except in patients who are low demand or who are medically contraindicated for surgical intervention.

SURGICAL

Fusion, with resultant loss of complex hindfoot motion, used to be the standard of care; it now is known that this treatment should be avoided whenever possible. The long-term results of fusion are now well known. The adjacent joints begin to wear because of the increased stress of the fused joints, and within a few years, these joints show symptomatic arthritic changes. Wear on the adjacent joints of patients who underwent fusion as children shows by their late 20s or early 30s (or sooner). This wear leads to a treatment dilemma because further fusion in an active young patient only accelerates the degeneration. Therefore, motion-sparing procedures are preferable, especially in younger patients. Fusion should be reserved for those patients who are much older and sedentary and whose activity level involves nothing more strenuous than "mall walking." Hindfoot fusion impairs the two important functions of the hindfoot: accommodation and adaptation to uneven terrain and shock absorption, which prevents transmission of forces to the ankle. This fusion can be used in older, more sedentary, heavier patients or in patients whose

hindfoot deformity has become rigidly fixed.

SURGICAL APPROACHES

Medial Utility Incision Start 1 cm below the medial malleolus and extend the incision distally over the medial navicular prominence, along the medial midaxial line. The incision can extend all the way down to the hallux if a long flexor hallucis longus (FHL) transfer is needed. This incision allows access to the talonavicular joint and the anterior and middle facets of the subtalar joint. For flexor digitorum longus (FDL) transfer, the tendon is found just posterior and inferior to the posterior tibialis at the medial malleolus. Follow the FDL distally to the master Knot of Henry. Differentiate the FDL from the FHL by wiggling the lesser toes. Cut the FDL and remove the paratenon. The FDL distal stump can be whipstitched to the FHL, but this is not required if the master knot fibers have not been completely dissected.

For FDL transfer, a bony trough under the naviculocuneiform area is made with a curet and/or rongeur. It is not necessary to transfer the FDL tendon through bone because the point of maximum healing is the periosteum. Drill down from the top, pass a suture, whipstitch the free FDL tendon end, then drill another hole and pass the suture up from below. Secure by pulling upward and completing a horizontal mattress stitch.

Lateral Incision The two most commonly used lateral incisions are the Ollier and axial. The axial is preferred because there is less chance of cutting sensory nerves along the anterior lateral ankle. It can also be extended distally if needed for better visualization of the calcaneocuboid (CC) joint. For lateral column lengthening (LCL), the Ollier incision can gap open, and closure may therefore cause tension across the wound. An axial incision is not under pressure after LCL. After the skin is opened, take

care to maintain the extensor digitorum brevis muscle belly because its blood supply helps in healing the incision and the osteotomy. The peroneal tendons are retracted plantarly, and the extensor digitorum brevis muscle belly is retracted dorsally. This procedure allows access to the sinus tarsi, the CC joint, and the posterior facet. Progress from lateral to medial through the lateral incision to expose the lateral half of the talonavicular joint and the anterior and middle facets.

Dorsomedial Incision This incision is useful for tarsometatarsal/intertarsal fusion, often along with smaller medial incisions along the medial utility line.

PROCEDURES

No single procedure can be used for correction because this deformity really is not a single deformity but rather a constellation of deformities throughout the foot and ankle. A thorough understanding of hindfoot mechanics, as well as static and dynamic correction, is required before surgical treatment of this deformity is considered.

Lateral Column Lengthening Two techniques for LCL have been described: (1) through the CC joint with resection of the joint and CC fusion, or (2) as an Evans-type procedure through the distal calcaneus with an intact CC joint. When LCL was first used to treat PPAV, it was thought that LCL through the calcaneus would lead to increased forces and subsequent arthritis of the CC joint, but this turned out not to be the case. A large series of LCLs performed through the distal calcaneus has shown that subsequent need for CC fusion was rare. Medial column FHL transfer and Achilles tendon lengthening usually are done in conjunction with LCL. Residual hypermobility of the medial column was believed to be a problem, but it has been shown that the retensioning of the peroneus longus by the LCL helps to stabilize the medial column, often obviating the need for medial column stabilization or fusion (**Figure 1**).

LCL is performed using a small external fixator-distractor or cervical spine distractor. The correction is slowly applied as the surgeon looks at the hindfoot and forefoot. When good correction has been achieved, the defect is measured and the graft is harvested from the anterosuperior iliac crest. The distractor is then used to overdistract the LCL gap, the graft is impacted in place, and the tension is removed (**Figure 1**, *B*). A static, fully threaded solid 4.0-mm screw is placed through the distal calcaneus, through the graft, and into the calcaneal body (**Figure 1**, *C*).

Examine the foot after completion of the LCL. If further correction is needed or if the heel is still in valgus, a tuber medial slide osteotomy of the calcaneus can be added to the degree needed. If a calcaneal tuber medial slide osteotomy is needed and performed, the screws are aimed superiorly so they do not hit the LCL screw (**Figure 2**). Care should be taken to avoid damaging the post facet with the screws holding the tuber medial slide osteotomy.

Hindfoot Fusion Selective fusions such as double fusion (CC and talonavicular) and isolated talonavicular fusion have been described in surgical treatment of PPAV. Triple arthrodesis (**Figure 3**) is the treatment of choice because other fusions can be difficult to obtain. Isolated talonavicular fusion, especially with a single approach, has a high nonunion rate. Double fusion has been shown to provide good correction of the deformity but leaves the subtalar joint in place, but the joint can become painful. The addition of subtalar fusion does not significantly add to morbidity or duration of the procedure. It adds stability, pain relief, and deformity correction.

Medial Column Stabilization Medial column stabilization is often performed in conjunction with tar-

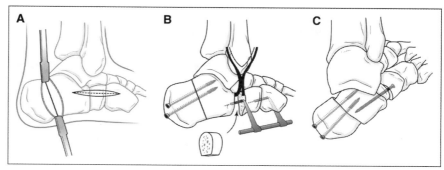

Figure 1 **A,** Approaches for LCL and tuber osteotomy. **B,** Double osteotomy. Tuber medializing slide osteotomy completed; LCL in progress using distractor, lamina spreader, and iliac crest bone graft. **C,** Double osteotomy. Tuber medializing slide osteotomy and LCL.

sometatarsal-intertarsal corrective osteotomy and fusion, calcaneal medial slide osteotomy, and FDL transfer to the underside of the naviculocuneiform area; it occasionally requires naviculocuneiform fusion. This grouping of procedures can provide good symptom relief, especially in older, more sedentary patients, but it does not work as well for younger, more active patients.

Coalition In the case of PPAV secondary to hindfoot coalition, the quandary is whether to resect the coalition and reconstruct the PPAV as a later secondary procedure or to do both at one sitting. Previously, the coalition was resected first because the postoperative care included aggressive hindfoot range-of-motion exercises, whereas PPAV reconstruction requires immobilization to facilitate healing. However, with the advent of better internal fixation, the possibility of doing the reconstruction immediately after resection of the coalition is more likely.

Achilles Tendon Lengthening All patients with PPAV require Achilles tendon lengthening in the presence of equinus contracture. PPAV without calf tightness is exceedingly rare. The lengthening is performed either distally or at the gastrocnemius musculotendinous junction (Strayer).

If the ankle is tight with the knee extended but releases with the knee flexed, the contracture is in the gas-

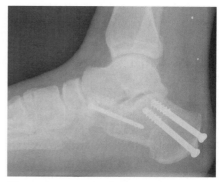

Figure 2 Lateral radiograph showing LCL. The apparent elevation of the distal talus does not represent overreduction. Slight overcorrection may be desirable because the foot tends to settle back a bit over time.

trocnemius complex and the lengthening can be done higher in the calf. The advantage of doing a Strayer-type lengthening is that it heals faster with less scarring. If, however, ankle dorsiflexion does not improve with knee flexion, a contracture of the triceps surae complex more distally is indicated, and a distal lengthening is required. Distal lengthening often is done via a percutaneous step-cut technique.

Closure Undyed, bioabsorbable braided No. 0 and No. 00 suture is used on the deep layers with No. 000 absorbable suture used on the skin. Tension-relieving nonabsorbable suture can be used as needed. A nonadherent dressing with antibiotic ointment is used. This moist type of

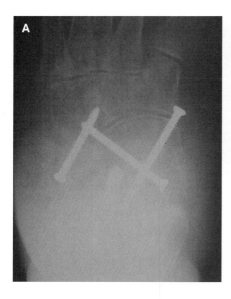

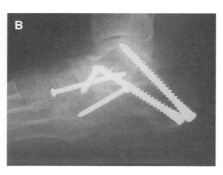

Figure 3 Triple arthrodesis. AP **(A)** and lateral **(B)** views showing rigid internal fixation of all joints.

dressing seals the wound area and prevents the dressing from adhering to the wound or surrounding skin. Sterile dressings and cast padding are placed under sterile conditions in the operating room. A three-sided splint or short leg cast (with a swelling strip removed) is then used. The plaster and dressings are left in place for 2 weeks. Sterile conditions are rarely maintained at the bedside or in the office; therefore, leaving the dressing and cast intact until the patient is seen back in the office in 2 weeks can decrease wound problems and infection rates.

Author's Preferred Treatment and Rationale

When treating congenital PPAV, we try to stretch the indications to avoid motion-sacrificing fusions. A properly informed patient understands the long-term problems of fusion. Every attempt should be made to perform a motion-sparing procedure. If the mechanical issues are discussed and properly explained, the patient usually will consent to the attempt at a motion-sparing procedure. Failure of the motion-sparing procedure usually does not burn any bridges; it can be converted to a fusion if it fails.

In any fusion, several factors can help ensure success. Proper joint surface preparation is necessary. All articular cartilage of each joint surface should be denuded without damaging the subchondral bone. When performing a triple arthrodesis, it is important to ensure that the dissection is carried all the way through the sinus tarsi to allow access to the lateral half of the talonavicular joint and anterior and middle facets of the subtalar joint. Proper dissection and joint surface preparation should be performed in a deliberate, meticulous fashion; this is not the time to move quickly. Before internal fixation is placed, a burr can be used to create a small (5-mm) pocket in the center of the joint. This spot weld helps prevent shear across the joint and hastens proper fusion. Shear strain relief grafting is also performed around the periphery of all joints after the internal fixation is placed.

If assistance is needed in aiming the drill, an anterior cruciate ligament aiming guide can be helpful. We would not recommend cannulated screws if possible. If the aiming guide is used to place a guide wire, the cannulated drill can then be used, but placement of a solid, fully threaded screw is preferable. Remove all soft tissue from the sinus tarsi and fill with bone graft before closing.

One of the best places to obtain autologous bone graft when performing foot surgery is the proximal tibia. This site is easily prepared into the surgical field, unlike a pelvic donor site. Harvest of up to 30 mL of good quality cancellous bone has been reported. The donor site cortical window is closed over Surgicell (Ethicon, Somerville, NJ) and bioabsorbable gelatin sponge. The small incision is then covered with a dressing and a breathable but water-impervious membrane. New biologic solutions are exciting, but their success in foot surgery has not yet been proved.

Management of Complications

Complications in reconstruction of PPAV can be avoided if sound surgical and mechanical principles are followed. Surgery should be avoided in any patient who is currently using any tobacco product. These procedures are purely elective; therefore, cessation of tobacco use should be a prerequisite for reconstructive surgery. The time between cessation and surgery has been debated, with reports suggesting from 6 weeks to 3 months. It is well known that tobacco use causes wound breakdown, failure of soft-tissue healing such as tendon transfers, and most importantly, failure of fusion and incorporation of structural bone grafts.

LATERAL COLUMN LENGTHENING

Although rarer when done through the calcaneus, nonunion or delayed union of as high as 25% has been reported in LCL done through CC joint resection. Loss of position and graft resorption have also been reported, but these complications are less likely with autograft (structural iliac crest is the preferred material) and better and stronger internal fixation. Treatment includes repeat bone grafting of the LCL site and fixation with an

H plate instead of a screw. H plates have also been used primarily, but problems with these occurred because of prominence under the peroneal tendons. However, if there is any concern at time of surgery, plate fixation should be used instead of screw fixation.

TRIPLE ARTHRODESIS

Nonunion and delayed union are less common now with bone graft (autograft or biologic graft) and stronger internal fixation. Loss of position in a triple arthrodesis usually is the result of improper choice of hardware. Partially threaded, cannulated screws do not give as secure rigid internal fixation as fully threaded solid screws, especially in overweight patients. Fully threaded, solid screws are less likely to break or allow the bone to lose position while the bone graft heals and fu-

sion occurs. Often the calcaneus tries to slide out laterally from under the talus (recurrence of the original deformity). This problem is less likely to occur with fully threaded, solid screws.

Bone stimulators (usually external) can help facilitate healing of the osteotomy and fusion sites. The screw heads may become symptomatic in the plantar tuber area. Removal of the prominent (tuber) screws should be delayed until after the osteotomy has healed.

A rare problem after LCL is unexplained sinus tarsi pain. The pain is relieved by injection into the sinus tarsi of local anesthetic (although usually temporarily). Removal of the LCL screw and débridement of all soft tissue from sinus tarsi has yielded good pain relief.

Finally, an unrecognized concomitant condition can lead to recur-

rent deformity. Unrecognized or early neuropathy, as in patients with diabetes mellitus, can result in loss of correction at a different site. In one patient, LCL provided correction of the original PPAV. Over the following 2 years, however, the foot collapsed through the Chopart-midfoot area. The patient has good sensation, intact skin, and good overall alignment and is still happy with the result, despite the radiographic appearance. The patient is aware that an extended triple arthrodesis is the salvage/revision procedure should skin breakdown problems or further deformity develop.

The author wishes to acknowledge the contribution of Jessica Gallina, MD, in the creation of this chapter.

References

Chao W, Wapner KL, Lee TH, Adams J, Hecht PJ: Nonoperative management of posterior tibial tendon dysfunction. *Foot Ankle Int* 1996;17:736-741.

Cooper PS, Nowak MD, Shaer J: Calcaneocuboid joint pressures with lateral column lengthening (Evans) procedure. *Foot Ankle Int* 1997;18:199-205.

Evans D: Calcaneo-valgus deformity. *J Bone Joint Surg Br* 1975;57:270-278.

Mosier-LaClair S, Pomeroy G, Manoli A: Operative treatment of the difficult stage 2 adult acquired flatfoot deformity. *Foot Ankle Clin* 2001;6:95-119.

Neufeld S, Myerson M: Complications of surgical treatment for adult flatfoot deformities. *Foot Ankle Clin* 2001;6:179-191.

Weinfeld S: Medial slide calcaneal osteotomy. *Foot Ankle Clinics* 6:89-90.

Coding

ICD-9 CODES

718.87 Other joint derangement, not elsewhere classified, ankle and foot

728.4 Laxity of ligament

728.9 Unspecified disorder of muscle, ligament, and fascia

735.0 Hallux valgus, acquired

736.70 Other acquired deformities of ankle and foot

754.61 Congenital pes planus

754.70 Other congenital deformities of feet, talipes, unspecified

755.67 Anomalies of foot not elsewhere classified, tarsal coalitions

755.8 Other specified anomalies of unspecified limb

CPT CODES

20902 Bone graft, any donor area; major or large

27606 Tenotomy percutaneous, Achilles tendon (separate procedure); general anesthesia

27687 Gastrocnemius recession (eg, Strayer procedure)

27691 Transfer or transplant of single tendon (with muscle redirection or rerouting); deep (eg, anterior tibial or posterior tibial through interosseous space, flexor digitorum longus, flexor hallucis longus, or peroneal tendon to midfoot or hindfoot)

27692 Transfer or transplant of single tendon (with muscle redirection or rerouting); each additional tendon (List in addition to code for primary procedure)

28116 Ostectomy, excision of tarsal coalition

28300 Osteotomy; calcaneus (eg, Dwyer or Chambers type procedure), with or without internal fixation

28715 Arthrodesis; triple

28725 Arthrodesis; subtalar

28730 Arthrodesis, midtarsal or tarsometatarsal, multiple or transverse

28735 Arthrodesis; with osteotomy (eg, flatfoot correction)

28737 Arthrodesis, with tendon lengthening and advancement, midtarsal, tarsal navicular-cuneiform (eg, Miller type procedure)

28740 Arthrodesis, midtarsal or tarsometatarsal, single joint

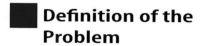

Tarsal Coalition

W. Hodges Davis, MD

Definition of the Problem

Patient Presentation

Symptomatic tarsal coalition is an uncommon condition that affects less than 2% of the population. Tarsal coalition is a failure of differentiation and segmentation of the primitive mesenchyme during intrauterine development. Association with autosomal dominant heredity has been described in the literature. Tarsal coalitions also have been associated with other congenital syndromes; however, these coalitions are typically more extensive and rarely symptomatic. Calcaneonavicular and talocalcaneal coalitions account for more than 90% of coalitions and occur in equal frequency. Talonavicular, naviculocuneiform, and calcaneocuboid coalitions are also seen. Occurrence is bilateral in approximately 50% of patients. There is also a slight predominance of female patients.

Coalitions may present as fibrous, cartilaginous, or osseous. They also are described as complete or incomplete. Coalitions may develop between two or more bones in the midfoot, hindfoot, or a combination thereof. These coalitions compromise the complex synchronized motions of the midtarsal, subtalar, and tibiotalar joints during the gait cycle. Although these coalitions can be complete and osseous in nature, they typically continue to allow decreased but limited motion in the adjacent midtarsal or subtalar joint.

Calcaneonavicular coalitions form between the anterior process of the calcaneus and the posterior inferior margin of the navicular. The calcaneus and navicular do not share a true joint. Talocalcaneal coalitions develop between the anterior, middle, or posterior facet; the most common presentation is a middle facet coalition with or without anterior facet involvement.

Adult and adolescent patients typically present with gradually increasing pain resulting in altered function. The pain is typically vague, is associated with weight bearing and activity, and may have a variety of causes. Advancing arthritic changes, arthrofibrosis of adjacent joints, and stress fractures of the coalition all are believed to contribute to tarsal coalition pain.

Patients may report a history of foot problems or frequent sprains after minor trauma as well as a family history of similar symptoms. The classic presentation has been described as spastic peroneal flatfoot or rigid flatfoot, but this presentation may have been overemphasized in the literature. However most patients do present with planovalgus feet. Although coalition is the most common cause of peroneal spastic flatfoot, any pathology that involves the subtalar joint may irritate the peroneal tendon. However, this situation does not preclude a patient with normal hindfoot position or even a cavovarus foot from having a coalition.

Adolescents present predictably depending on the type of coalition and the expected timing of ossification of their tarsal bones. As the coalition consolidates, patients often will have increased pain and decreased function. Calcaneonavicular coalitions mature in patients between the ages of 8 and 12 years, whereas talocalcaneal coalitions mature in patients between the ages of 12 and 16 years. In adults, a separate traumatic event often precedes the discovery of a coalition. The degree and timing of symptoms and limitation of motion can be altered by the nature (fibrous, cartilaginous, and osseous) and the degree (complete and incomplete) of coalition present.

Physical Examination

Patients should be examined thoroughly while in the sitting, standing, and supine positions. Visual inspection often reveals atrophy of the calf on the involved side. In addition, asymmetric involvement often results in an altered dependent sitting position. The forefoot is abducted; there may be flattening of the medial longitudinal arch, as well as a prominence

One or more of the authors or the departments with which they are affiliated have received something of value from a commercial or other party related directly or indirectly to the subject of this chapter.

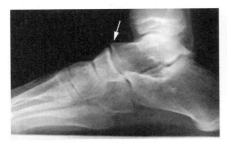

Figure 1 Tarsal beak (arrow) on lateral radiograph of the foot.

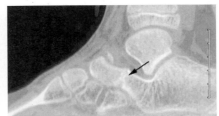

Figure 3 Sagittal CT scan showing calcaneonavicular coalition (arrow).

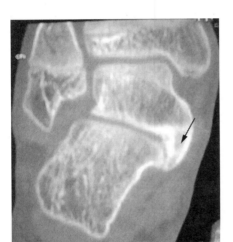

Figure 2 Coronal CT scan of a talocalcaneal coalition shows the plantar slope of the sustentaculum tali (arrow).

along the posteromedial hindfoot. Physical inspection reveals a near rigid hindfoot and midfoot complex.

Patients with calcaneonavicular coalitions typically lose midtarsal motion but may retain limited subtalar motion. Those with talocalcaneal coalitions lose almost all of their subtalar motion but retain a greater degree of midtarsal motion. These alterations in midtarsal and subtalar motion also contribute to a loss of terminal ankle dorsiflexion and plantar flexion moments. The hindfoot may present in a valgus position that does not correct with passive, active, or dynamic testing. Dynamic testing consists of inspection of the hindfoot position during toe raise. There may be tenderness in the medial sustentaculum tali or sinus tarsi region in talocalcaneal coali-

tion and directly over the coalition in the anterolateral foot in calcaneonavicular coalition. Peroneal tenderness also may be present. Occasionally patients may present with symptoms classic for tarsal tunnel that are related to a middle facet coalition. The examiner needs to be reminded that because 50% of coalitions are bilateral, side-to-side comparisons can be misleading.

AP, lateral, and oblique radiographs of the foot should be obtained in all patients suspected of having a tarsal coalition. Calcaneonavicular coalitions most often are seen on medial oblique views. An axial view may delineate a talocalcaneal coalition. The observation of talar beaking on the anterior aspect of the talus has been considered pathognomonic of a coalition (**Figure 1**).

Most osseous talocalcaneal coalitions can be found definitively on coronal CT. The middle facet will often have an altered sustentaculum tali that is more cephalad than the lateral margin and has a plantar slope with hypertrophy of the adjacent joint space (**Figure 2**). CT will also identify calcaneonavicular coalitions in the axial and sagittal views (**Figure 3**). We routinely obtain CT scans for preoperative planning to assess the size of the coalition and to identify any sclerosis or degenerative changes. MRI is also useful to identify purely fibrous or cartilaginous coalitions and show marrow elements extending across the joint in osseous coalitions.

Differential Diagnosis

- Trauma (talus fracture, anterior process of calcaneus fracture, subtalar dislocation)
- Fracture
- Subtalar arthritis
- Transverse tarsal arthritis
- Osteoid osteoma
- Fibrosarcoma

Additional Work-up

A triple-phase bone scan will show increased uptake in the region of the coalition; however, it lacks specificity, and we rarely order these when the diagnosis is established.

---◼

◼ The Solutions

Treatment Options and Rationale

Patients who present in adolescence or early childhood with gradual onset of pain or symptoms following minor trauma require a short course of immobilization followed by a weight-bearing short leg cast for 4 to 6 weeks. Pain relief should be almost immediate with the cast applied. After cast removal, the use of nonsteroidal anti-inflammatory drugs, ice, and a longitudinal arch support or medial wedge orthotic can be attempted. If the basic orthotic fails, a hindfoot controlling brace (ankle-foot orthotic or University of California, Berkeley orthotic) can be tried. The judicious use of differential injection into the region of a fibrous coalition may also help guide treatment options. Patients with an incomplete or fibrous coalition tend to have less deformity as well as more normal motion and, therefore, tend to respond more favorably to a period of immobilization and bracing. Patients with a more rigid and excessive deformity such as a talocalcaneal middle facet coalition are less likely to improve after immobilization and probably will require surgical intervention.

Surgical treatment consists of excision of the coalition, subtalar fusion, or triple arthrodesis. The main diagnostic tools to determine the degree of surgical intervention needed are the physical examination and CT. The latter helps to identify the size of the lesion and to evaluate for arthritic changes in the adjacent joints.

With a minimal amount of deformity on physical examination and normal appearance of adjacent joint spaces on the CT scan, a simple excision of the coalition can be undertaken. However, this recommendation should be tempered by the size of the lesion.

CALCANEONAVICULAR COALITIONS

Calcaneonavicular coalitions historically have responded favorably to resection as long as degenerative changes were not seen in the adjacent joints. Complete resection should be attempted initially whether the coalition is fibrous, cartilaginous, or osseous. Adolescents have been shown to have better results than adults. Adults typically respond more favorably to resection of fibrous coalitions than to osseous coalitions. Moreover, talar beaking does not appear to contraindicate a simple resection. Patients with significant degenerative changes or deformity that does not appear to be conducive to simple resection should have a subtalar arthrodesis. The talar beak also should be removed. We believe that this is a critical step to allow increased motion and eliminate a potential source of pain.

TALOCALCANEAL COALITIONS

Talocalcaneal coalitions typically involve the middle facet with fewer incidences of anterior and posterior facet involvement. Many talocalcaneal coalitions appear to be asymptomatic; however, pain in a previously asymp-

tomatic patient may respond to a selective injection into the subtalar joint. CT is critical for identification of the amount of degenerative change in the joints as well as the size of the coalition. The size of the lesion can be estimated by viewing consecutive cuts on the CT scan. It has been suggested that excision of the coalition should not be attempted if the lesion occupies more than 50% of the joint. We attempt excision in adolescents with less than 50% involvement of the middle facet. Adolescents with a marked planovalgus deformity and less than 50% involvement of the facet should be treated with an excision of the coalition and a calcaneal osteotomy to correct the malalignment of the hindfoot. However, a subtalar arthrodesis is performed in adolescents with more than 50% involvement or any adult with middle facet involvement. Good results have been reported with isolated subtalar arthrodesis in patients without arthritic involvement in the Chopart joints, and we strive to preserve adjacent joints if possible. The talar beak is excised through a separate incision.

Author's Preferred Treatment and Rationale
CALCANEONAVICULAR COALITIONS
SURGICAL TECHNIQUE

A lateral incision as described by Ollier is used. The extensor digitorum

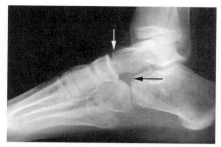

Figure 4   The patient shown in Figure 1 after resection of calcaneonavicular coalition (black arrow). Note excision of talar beak (white arrow).

brevis muscle is dissected and reflected distally. The coalition is then identified between the calcaneus and navicular. An aggressive resection is then required. All cartilage must be removed to prevent possible recurrence. The defect created should be at least 1 cm in length, and care must be taken not to create a convergence in the depths of the wound. The piece removed should be rectangular, not triangular or trapezoidal. Care also must be taken not to violate the talonavicular joint and ligaments. Damage to the ligaments may allow the navicular to subluxate over the talus. The bone edges are covered with bone wax, and Gelfoam sterile sponge (Pharmacia and Upjohn, Kalamazoo, MI) can be inserted into the defect. The extensor digitorum brevis is repaired to the sinus tarsi. A separate incision is also used to resect the talar beak (**Figure**

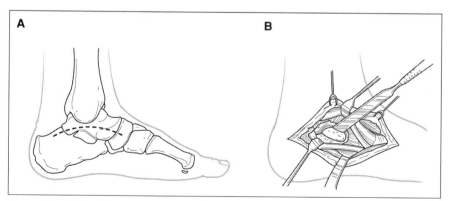

Figure 5   **A,** Curvilinear incision based medially over the sustentatculum tali. **B,** Interval between the flexor digitorum longus and neurovascular bundle superiorly and the flexor hallucis longus tendon inferiorly.

4). The foot is placed in a non–weight-bearing short leg splint in a neutral position of the hindfoot and ankle. The patient's splint and sutures are removed at the first postoperative visit at 2 weeks, and a removable boot is applied. The patient is encouraged to begin active range-of-motion exercises and progressive weight bearing. The boot is discontinued at 6 weeks, and physical therapy is instituted if the patient is not progressing with motion. The patient is allowed to resume normal activity when he or she is pain-free and normal motion and strength are regained. An arch support or orthotic can also be prescribed for long-term use.

TALOCALCANEAL COALITIONS
SURGICAL TECHNIQUE

A medial talocalcaneal coalition is excised through a medial incision over the sustentaculum tali (**Figure 5**). The flexor retinaculum is divided, and the flexor digitorum longus tendon and neurovascular bundle are identified and protected. The flexor hallucis longus tendon is identified under the sustentaculum tali. The coalition is iden-tified in the interval between the flexor digitorum longus superiorly and the neurovascular bundle and the flexor hallucis longus inferiorly. The extent of the coalition is exposed with subperiosteal dissection. Adequate re-traction is required to visualize the posterior facet, the inferior surface of the sustentaculum tali, and the distal extent of the coalition. A combination of osteotome, rongeur, and burr is used to resect the coalition. The coali-tion should be resected back to nor-mal articular cartilage or to where there is space between the two bones that allows increased subtalar motion. Bone wax is applied to the bone sur-faces and Gelfoam is placed into the defect. The retinaculum and skin are closed, and a non–weight-bearing short leg splint is applied. The staples and splint are removed at the first postoperative visit at 2 weeks. The pa-tient is then placed into a removable boot and allowed to begin range-of-motion exercises without weight bear-ing. Progressive weight bearing is al-lowed at 6 weeks. The patient is allowed to resume normal activities when he or she is pain free and has regained strength. This is typically in 4 to 6 months.

Management of Complications

Wound healing problems resulting from the extent of the dissection con-stitute the most common surgically related complication. Late complica-tions most commonly are related to continued pain and arthrofibrosis, typically resulting from a progression of arthritic changes. The progression of deformity is also a potential compli-cation stemming from a destabilizing simple resection of the coalition. The removal of a segment that caused a rigid foot may now result in a flexible hindfoot that may collapse. Contin-ued pain or deformity in a talocalca-neal resection can be salvaged with an isolated subtalar arthrodesis, with or without a calcaneal osteotomy, if there is no significant deformity. The salvage surgery is a triple arthrodesis.

The author wishes to acknowledge the contribution of Simon Lee, MD, in the creation of this chapter.

References

Cohen BE, Davis WH, Anderson RB: Success of calcaneonavicular resection in the adult population. *Foot Ankle Int* 1996;17:569-572.

Harris RI: Follow-up notes on articles previously published in the journal: Retrospect-peroneal spastic flatfoot (rigid valgus foot). *J Bone Joint Surg Am* 1965;47:1657-1667.

Scranton PE: Treatment of symptomatic talocalcaneal coalition. *J Bone Joint Surg Am* 1987;69:533-539.

Swiontkowski ME, Scranton PE, Hansen S: Tarsal coalition: Long-term results of surgical treatment. *J Pediatr Orthop* 1983;3:287-292.

Varner KE, Michelson JD: Tarsal coalition in adults. *Foot Ankle Int* 2000;21:669-672.

Coding

ICD-9 CODE
755.67   Anomalies of foot not elsewhere classified

CPT CODE
28116   Ostectomy, excision of tarsal coalition

Glenn B. Pfeffer, MD
Editor

Acute Peroneal Tendon Dislocation

Paul T. Fortin, MD

◼ Definition of the Problem

Patient Presentation

Acute peroneal tendon dislocation mimics lateral ankle sprain and may occur at the same time as lateral ankle ligament injury, making diagnosis in the acute period difficult. Although associated commonly with downhill skiing, traumatic dislocation of the peroneal tendons has been reported with numerous activities and sports. Patients often relate a history of an acute snapping sensation and intense pain in the posterolateral aspect of the ankle after a rapid deceleration such as when a skier digs the ski tip into the snow. The patient typically is unable to continue activities and often is unable to walk. Usually the tendons subluxate transiently over the fibula and spontaneously reduce. A violent contraction of the peroneal musculature is required to overcome the soft-tissue restraints. The position of the foot at the time of injury is variable. With the ankle dorsiflexed and everted, maximal peroneal contraction can create an anterolateral force against the superior peroneal retinaculum that is sufficient to cause anterior subluxation of the tendons (**Figure 1**). Conversely, dorsiflexion and inversion tightens the calcaneofibular ligament, thereby elevating the floor of the peroneal tunnel, forcing the tendons up against the retinaculum and over the posterior ridge of the fibula.

Physical Examination

Spontaneous reduction of the peroneal tendons and swelling may obscure the diagnosis of acute dislocation. In contrast to a typical lateral ankle sprain, maximal tenderness and swelling are along the posterior sulcus of the distal fibula rather than over the anterior talofibular ligament. Eversion against resistance elicits pain and apprehension. Overt dislocation, however, may not be tolerated in the acute setting. Lateral ankle ligament injury and instability may occur concomitant with peroneal tendon dislocation, further obscuring the diagnosis in the acute setting. In these circumstances, peroneal tendon dislocation may not become evident until swelling and discomfort have subsided and, therefore, necessitates reevaluation when a more valid examination can be performed.

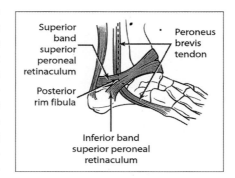

Figure 1 Lateral view of the ankle showing the most common orientation of the superior peroneal retinaculum, the superior band attaching to the Achilles tendon, and the inferior band that parallels the calcaneofibular ligament and attaches to the lateral wall of the calcaneus.

It is important to evaluate the opposite side for any evidence of congenital or developmental peroneal tendon dislocation. Hindfoot alignment should be assessed. It has been suggested that hindfoot valgus may predispose to tendon dislocation.

Differential Diagnosis
- Lateral ankle ligament sprain
- Congenital/developmental peroneal tendon dislocation
- Lateral/posterior talar process fracture
- Peroneal tendon tear
- Achilles tendon rupture

Additional Work-up

Diagnosis of peroneal tendon dislocation is based primarily on clinical examination. Imaging studies can be helpful to guide preoperative planning. Plain radiographs may show avulsion of the posterolateral edge of the fibula. This "rim fracture" typically is seen as a small linear fragment. It is best visualized on the mortise view of the ankle. When the posterior rim is fractured, the peroneal tendons are believed to pass through the fracture. Abrasion of the tendons against the fractured surface may lead to tearing, especially of the peroneus brevis tendon. The two basic types of injury leading to incompetence of the superior peroneal retinaculum are detachment of the retinaculum from the fibula and avulsion of the posterolateral fibular rim. Midsubstance tearing of the retinaculum itself is very rare.

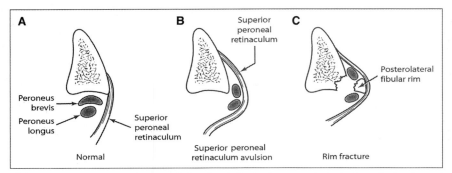

Figure 2 Cross-sectional view of the distal fibula. **A,** Normal. **B,** Retinacular/periosteal sleeve stripped from the fibula. **C,** Posterolateral fibular rim fracture.

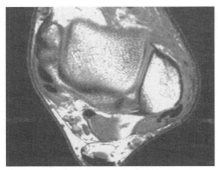

Figure 3 Axial MRI scan following acute peroneal tendon dislocation showing the peroneal tendons displaced anterior to the posterolateral rim of the fibula.

The superior peroneal retinaculum is contiguous with the fibular periosteum and commonly has two distinct bands. The superior band extends transversely to insert at the level of the Achilles tendon. The inferior band parallels the calcaneofibular ligament and inserts on the lateral wall of the calcaneus. This parallel relationship suggests that inversion stress to the ankle potentially challenges both structures (**Figures 1** and **2**).

CT can be used to define the anatomic relationships among the distal fibula, peroneal tendons, and superior peroneal retinaculum. It will also identify other bony injury. The shape of the fibular sulcus has been implicated as a predisposing factor for tendon dislocation, and CT helps to define anatomic variations such as a shallow or convex posterior fibular surface. A flat or convex posterior fibular sulcus has been reported to occur in 18% to 28% of patients. This information may influence the type of surgical reconstruction chosen. It is also useful when occult bony injury is suspected. MRI is usually more informative and is the study of choice. It clearly defines the detachment of the superior peroneal retinaculum from the posterior border of the fibula, any peroneal tendon or ligamentous pathology, and fibular anatomy (**Figure 3**). It also identifies anomalies such as a peroneus quartus muscle and low-lying peroneus

brevis musculature. Stress radiographs of the ankle can be useful if concomitant lateral ankle instability is suspected.

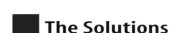

The Solutions

Treatment Options and Rationale

NONSURGICAL TREATMENT
There are isolated reports of successful nonsurgical treatment of acute peroneal tendon dislocation. The small sample sizes and wide variety of treatment methods in these series preclude identifying a reproducible nonsurgical regimen. Casting in 20° of plantar flexion and heel inversion for 6 to 8 weeks can be considered if the injury is diagnosed within 7 to 10 days, and MRI demonstrates that the tendons are anatomically reduced. In most circumstances, surgical management probably should be considered.

SURGICAL TREATMENT
The rationale for surgical treatment of acute peroneal dislocation is a result of the following three observations. (1) Attrition and longitudinal splitting of the peroneus brevis are common findings in chronic peroneal dislocation. (2) Displaced tendons may

lead to an aberrant line of pull and adaptive shortening with loss of power of the peroneal musculature. (3) A high incidence of recurrence has been reported with nonsurgical treatment.

Several surgical procedures have been described to stabilize dislocated peroneal tendons. They can be divided into three categories: soft-tissue repair or reconstruction of the superior peroneal retinaculum; bone procedures to deepen or reorient the peroneal groove; and rerouting of the peroneal tendons.

When the retinaculum is intact but stripped from the fibula and there is an adequate fibular sulcus, it is repaired directly by incision and advancement of the anterior margin through drill holes to the posterolateral corner of the fibula. This scenario is the most common with acute retinacular injury, and this relatively simple surgical procedure has led to consistently good results, with most patients returning to their previous level of activity. In the rare circumstance of midsubstance tearing of the retinaculum, the tear is plicated in a vest over pants fashion. Rim fractures should be reduced and fixed. The size of the fragment usually dictates the method of fixation. Larger fragments may be amenable to screw, suture anchor, or pin fixation. Small fragments can be reduced and secured with nonabsorbable suture.

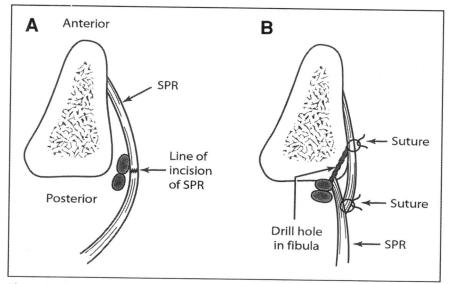

Figure 4 Reconstruction of superior peroneal retinaculum (SPR). **A,** The retinaculum is incised and advanced to the posterolateral rim of the fibula. **B,** Sutures are passed through drill holes. The anterior limb is plicated over the reattached retinaculum.

Fibular osteotomy, groove deepening, and tendon rerouting have been described for acute peroneal dislocation. Results are comparable to those for direct retinacular repair. It is therefore difficult to justify their routine use for acute injuries. In the rare circumstance in which the retinaculum is insufficient or irreparable, consideration should be given to these supplementary procedures to ensure that the tendons are sufficiently stabilized. Various types of osteotomies and groove deepening procedures have been described, but no one is clearly superior to the others. The most popular fibular groove deepening procedure involves creating an osseous flap of the posterior fibula and removing a portion of the cancellous bone, thereby recessing the posterior cortex (**Figure 4**). Fibular osteotomies are intended to reorient the fibula so that it acts as a bony block to tendon displacement. The tendons deep to the calcaneofibular ligament have been rerouted by sectioning the ligament or the tendons, or by raising the ligament in a bone-block fashion and routing the peroneal tendons medial to the ligament.

Author's Preferred Treatment and Rationale

For most acute peroneal tendon dislocations without rim fracture, the retinacular/periosteal sleeve can be reattached and plicated. Fibular osteotomy, groove deepening, or tendon rerouting procedures should not be necessary in the acute setting. An incision is made over the posterolateral edge of the fibula. Care is taken to avoid the sural nerve in this region. The redundant retinacular/periosteal sleeve is identified and then divided in its midsubstance such that the leading edge of the retinaculum can be advanced to the anatomic point of insertion on the posterolateral corner of the fibula. Sectioning the retinaculum too far posteriorly will prevent the leading edge from being advanced all the way to the posterior rim of the fibula. Sectioning it too far anteriorly will leave it redundant after it is advanced and may leave the tendons unstable (Figure 4). The desired point of attachment on the posterolateral corner of the fibula is roughened with a small burr or rongeur. Drill holes are made from the posterolateral corner to the lateral face of the fibula. Heavy, nonabsorbable sutures are woven in the posterior limb of the retinaculum. Suture anchors also may be used. The foot is held everted, and the sutures are tied. The anterior limb of the retinacular/periosteal sleeve is oversewn with absorbable sutures. A short leg cast is worn for 6 weeks, and ankle rehabilitation is then initiated.

When a posterolateral fibular rim fracture is present, reduction and fixation of the fracture typically stabilizes the tendons. Small avulsed fragments are advanced and fixed with nonabsorbable sutures. Larger fragments may be amenable to screw, suture anchor, or pin fixation.

On rare occasion the retinacular tissues are insufficient or irreparable. A reinforcement of the retinaculum can be created using a 1-cm posteriorly based flap of fibular periosteum that is folded and attached to the calcaneus with a suture anchor. If the tendons are not stable within the peroneal groove, débridement of a tear or excursion of the peroneus quartus tendon may be sufficient. A relatively simple groove deepening procedure may also be required and is usually my preferred method. After surgical exposure and division of the retinaculum, the peroneal tendons are retracted anteriorly. A cortical window is made on the posterior surface of the fibula using an oscillating saw that is 3- to 4-cm long and approximately 1-cm wide. The posteromedial border of the window is left intact and acts as a hinge. The cortical osteoperiosteal window is hinged posteromedially, and sufficient cancellous bone is removed to facilitate deepening the groove several millimeters. The flap is then tamped back into place. If there is any available retinacular tissue, it is advanced to the posterolateral corner of the fibula. If the retinacular tissue is insufficient, a periosteal flap from the lateral face of the fibula can be used (**Figure 5**).

If there has been significant injury to the lateral ankle ligaments, consideration should be given to their concomitant repair. Intraoperative assessment of lateral ankle stability is important with all peroneal tendon reconstructions. Intraoperative stress radiographs of both ankles may be helpful in determining the extent of ligamentous injury. A primary repair of the ligaments is usually all that is necessary. The inferior extensor retinaculum can be advanced to the fibula in a manner similar to the modified Broström technique to augment the repair.

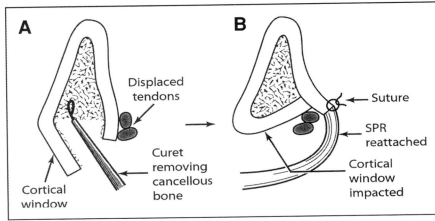

Figure 5   Fibular groove deepening procedure. **A,** A medially based cortical window is made on the posterior aspect of the fibula. **B,** Cancellous bone is removed, and the window is impacted. The superior peroneal retinaculum (SPR) is advanced to the posterolateral rim of the fibula.

Management of Complications

Fortunately, surgical management of acute peroneal dislocation is successful in most patients. Recurrence of tendon dislocation after surgical treatment, the most commonly reported complication, is rare. Recurrent dislocation after retinacular repair alone should be treated with a supplemental stabilization procedure, débridement of a peroneal tear if present, excision of the peroneus quartus, and a possible groove deepening procedure.

Persistent pain despite a stable repair can be from a tear of a peroneal tendon, which will require treatment. Peroneal tenosynovitis may also be a source of pain. This pain is more common following supplemental stabilization procedures such as osteotomy, groove deepening, and rerouting of the tendons; it typically is not functionally limiting and does not require further surgical intervention. Other reported complications include sural nerve injury and fracture following fibular osteotomy.

References

Das De S, Balasubramaniam P: A repair operation for recurrent dislocation of peroneal tendons. *J Bone Joint Surg Br* 1985;67:585-587.

Eckert WR, Davis EA Jr: Acute rupture of the peroneal retinaculum. *J Bone Joint Surg Am* 1976;58:670-672.

Mason RB, Henderson JP: Traumatic peroneal tendon instability. *Am J Sports Med* 1996;24:652-658.

Zoellner G, Clancy W Jr: Recurrent dislocation of the peroneal tendon. *J Bone Joint Surg Am* 1979;61:292-294.

Coding

ICD-9 CODES

727.06 Other disorders of synovium, tendon, and bursa, Synovitis and tenosynovitis, Tenosynovitis of foot and ankle

727.9 Other disorders of synovium, tendon, and bursa, Unspecified disorder of synovium, tendon, and bursa

824.2 Fracture of ankle, Lateral malleolus closed

845.02 Sprains and strains of ankle and foot, Ankle, Calcaneofibular (ligament)

905.7 Late effects of musculoskeletal and connective tissue injuries, Late effect of sprain and strain without mention of tendon injury

905.8 Late effects of musculoskeletal and connective tissue injuries, Late effect of tendon injury

CPT CODES

27675 Repair, dislocating peroneal tendons; without fibular osteotomy

27676 Repair, dislocating peroneal tendons; with fibular osteotomy

27695 Repair, primary, disrupted ligament, ankle; collateral

27696 Repair, primary, disrupted ligament, ankle; both collateral ligaments

27792 Open treatment of distal fibular fracture (lateral malleolus), with or without internal or external fixation

CPT copyright © 2003 by the American Medical Association. All Rights Reserved.

Peroneal Tendon Injury

Glenn B. Pfeffer, MD

■ Definition of the Problem

Patient Presentation

The symptoms of peroneal tendinopathy are usually insidious in onset, with a patient reporting chronic, dull, achy pain on the posterolateral aspect of the ankle. A patient may relate the onset of the symptoms to a period of increased activity, a direct blow to the lateral ankle, or an ankle sprain that occurred months in the past. Symptoms are usually worsened by activity and improved with rest. Specific reports of intermittent snapping may relate to recurrent subluxation or dislocation of the tendons.

The presentation of peroneal tendinopathy is highly variable because of the frequent occurrence of associated problems. For example, a patient report of lateral pain and weakness may be secondary to peroneal tendinosis and associated laxity of the lateral ankle ligaments. A prior calcaneal fracture or progressive flattening of the arch may be the cause of lateral symptoms from peroneal impingement. In the initial evaluation of peroneal injury, the extensive differential diagnosis of lateral ankle pain should always be considered. Occult fracture, subtalar pathology, and systemic disorders, such as gout or rheumatoid arthritis, are often overlooked.

Severe, acute peroneal pain usually results from traumatic rupture or dislocation of the tendons. Complete rupture is a rare problem. The mechanism of injury and presentation of a patient with an acute rupture are similar to those of a patient with a severe lateral ankle sprain. The diagnosis is easily missed. Focal tenderness and ecchymosis directly over the peroneal sheath without significant anterolateral tenderness should alert the examiner to this diagnosis. A similar diagnostic problem occurs with acute dislocation of the peroneals, although in this case the patient often relates a history of the tendons "popping" out. MRI is usually diagnostic for both conditions.

Chronic tendinopathy of one or both peroneals is a relatively common problem. The tendons are susceptible to injury where they experience high mechanical stress. There are two common zones of injury. Peroneus brevis injury usually occurs proximally at the level of the distal fibula. The tear probably occurs when the tendon is forced against the posterior ridge of the fibula during an inversion injury (**Figure 1**). Over time or with repeated inversion injuries, the tear propagates, local inflammation develops, and progressive degeneration of the tendon occurs. Peroneus longus injury usually occurs more distally in one of two places: (1) along the lateral wall of the calcaneus inferior to the trochlear process, or (2) in the cuboid tunnel where the tendon changes from vertical to horizontal as it passes into the plantar aspect of the foot.

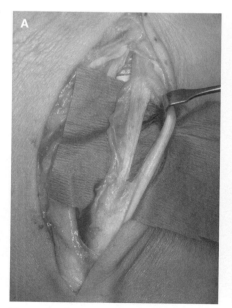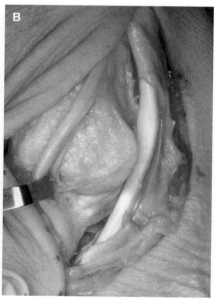

Figure 1 **A,** Complex tear of the peroneus brevis. **B,** Peroneus brevis tear at the distal fibula.

Physical Examination

The key component of the physical examination is localization of maximal tenderness. Peroneal tendinopathy causes focal tenderness over the injured portion of the tendon, the peroneus brevis usually just distal to the tip of the fibula, and the peroneus longus at the trochlear process or just proximal to the calcaneocuboid joint. In a patient with peroneus brevis tendinopathy, focal pressure over the tendon will cause pain, especially when accompanied by resisted active dorsiflexion of the ankle and eversion of the hindfoot (**Figure 2**). In a patient with peroneus longus tendinopathy, focal pressure over the injured tendon causes pain, especially when accompanied by resisted plantar flexion of the first ray.

The orthopaedist should look for swelling over the peroneals or palpable thickening of their sheath. A large trochlear process may be present and cause irritation when the patient is wearing shoes. Ankle and subtalar stability always should be assessed. Varus laxity of the ankle often occurs in conjunction with peroneal pathology. Focal bone and joint tenderness should be evaluated.

Active circumduction of the hindfoot may reproduce a patient's symptoms. Recurrent dislocation of the tendons, if present, can often be reproduced with this maneuver. Range of motion of the ankle and subtalar joints should be measured bilat-erally. Because it is easy to miss loss of subtalar motion in a patient with significant valgus laxity of the ankle, both sides always should be compared. Subtalar arthritis, tarsal coalition, or a fracture of the lateral process of the talus can cause a decrease in subtalar motion and tenderness over the posterior facet. Guarding from painful excursion of the peroneal tendons can also cause a decrease in subtalar motion.

The orthopaedist should percuss over the superficial peroneal and sural nerves, first plantar flexing the ankle and inverting the heel to place tension on the nerves. Dysesthesias in the nerve distribution may indicate a local entrapment from a fibrous band, ganglion, or underlying prominence of bone.

The orthopaedist should note whether the patient has a cavus foot. Patients with a cavus foot have a high incidence of peroneal injury. A varus heel increases stress on the lateral hindfoot and predisposes a patient to ankle sprains, instability, and peroneal tendon injury. The position of the heel should be evaluated from behind. Heel varus often has to be corrected surgically at the same time as the peroneals. The position of the forefoot should be noted with the hindfoot in neutral (talus and navicuar in alignment). A fixed forefoot valgus of 10° or more predisposes a patient to peroneal injury and may require correction.

Differential Diagnosis

ACUTE

Rupture or dislocation of peroneal tendon

Fracture (avulsion or stress fracture of the distal fibula, lateral process of the talus, osteochondral lesion of the lateral talus, anterior process of the calcaneus, os trigonum, os peroneum, base of the fifth metatarsal)

Acute peroneal tenosynovitis

Syndesmotic sprain of the ankle

CHRONIC

Occult bone injury or nonunion

Prominent trochlear process

Subtalar arthritis

Subtalar synovitis

Tarsal coalition

Calcaneocuboid arthritis

Lateral gutter of the ankle (synovitis, loose body, osteochondral lesion)

Posterior ankle impingement (os trigonum, etc)

Ankle or subtalar laxity (intermittent symptoms related to episodes of giving way)

Retrocalcaneal bursitis (posterior to peroneals, with bilateral tenderness)

Sural neuralgia (postoperative neuroma, rare neurapraxia)

Superficial peroneal nerve entrapment

Chronic subluxation and/or dislocation

Peroneal tenosynovitis

Peroneal tendinosis

Painful os peroneum

Impingement of peroneals (secondary to severe pes planus or malunion of a calcaneal fracture)

Tendinopathy of anomalous tendon (peroneus quartus)

Additional Work-up

Radiographs should include three views of the ankle and three views of the foot, including a weight-bearing AP and both obliques. It is often difficult to differentiate a chronic peroneal injury from an underlying bone or joint injury. Fractures, nonunion, and arthritic changes in the ankle, subtalar, or calcaneocuboid joints should be excluded. Often overlooked fractures include the posterior and lateral processes of the talus, the lateral talar dome, and the anterior process of the calcaneus. It should be noted whether an os peroneum is present and if it is fractured or deformed. Arthritic changes in the posterior facet of the subtalar joint should be carefully evaluated. Stress radiographs may be

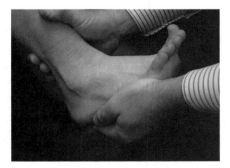

Figure 2 Examination of the peroneals with resisted dorsiflexion and eversion.

required to evaluate laxity of the ankle and subtalar joints.

Occult bone injury of the hindfoot may be difficulty to detect by routine radiographs. A technetium Tc 99 bone scan is very helpful in both detecting occult bone injury and confirming that radiographic bone or joint changes are abnormal. The scan should be limited to the feet and ankle, bilaterally, with AP, posteroanterior, medial, and lateral views. After radiographs, a bone scan is my study of choice for sorting out a confusing clinical presentation in a patient with more than 3 to 4 months of chronic lateral ankle pain.

In an acute injury, MRI is helpful in excluding acute peroneal rupture and confirming reduction of the peroneals after traumatic dislocation. In a patient with chronic injury, MRI is most helpful for detecting the degree of peroneal tendinopathy. Occult fracture and arthritic changes can also be detected. When requesting the study, the specific diagnosis and exact location of suspected injury should be conveyed to the radiologist. Ultrasound evaluation of the peroneals is a cost-effective technique that will probably have an increasing role in the future. Peroneal tenogram is of historic interest only.

A small number of patients with peroneal tendinopathy will have an MRI scan that is read as normal, with pathology not detected by the scanning sequence. In these patients, a differential injection of 3 mL of lidocaine into the peroneal sheath will help make the correct diagnosis. A 23-gauge needle should be used to inject the lidocaine directly into the peroneal sheath where the patient has maximum tenderness. If the patient's symptoms are cured, the diagnosis of peroneal tendinopathy is likely. This approach is less helpful distal to the trochlear process, where the peroneus brevis and longus have separate sheaths. A small amount of radiopaque dye may be used with the

lidocaine to confirm by radiograph that the solution is within the sheath and does not extravasate into the surrounding tissue. In 15% of patients there is a communication between the peroneal sheath and the ankle or subtalar joint that can confuse the interpretation of a positive response to the injection.

■ The Solutions

Treatment Options and Rationale
ACUTE INJURY
Acute peroneal rupture is rare and usually involves the peroneus longus. The mechanism of injury is invariably a severe inversion injury that occurs during sports activity in a young athlete. A correct diagnosis requires a high index of suspicion. The patient will usually hold the hindfoot in an inverted position and is unable to perform active eversion. Surgical repair of the tendon is appropriate once the acute swelling has resolved. The rupture usually occurs at the level of the trochlear process. Rupture can also occur at the musculotendinous junction. Fracture through an os peroneum with separation of the fracture fragments has also been reported. Retraction of the ruptured tendon usually is not a problem, and it is easily repaired at 10 to 14 days postinjury. At the time of surgery, the peroneal sheath should be carefully palpated for any bone spurs or sharp ridges on the trochlear process that may have contributed to the rupture. The tendon ends are repaired with a nonabsorbable No. 3-0 suture. If a fracture of the os peroneum is present, excision of the bone segments will probably be required.

CHRONIC PERONEAL DYSFUNCTION
Tenosynovitis without tendinosis can occur. Nonsurgical care should in-

clude a walking cast for 4 to 6 weeks. One corticosteroid injection may be appropriate. Persistent symptoms will usually respond to a surgical tenosynovectomy. Under loupe magnification the thickened tenosynovium is easily stripped off the tendons. Involvement of both the peroneus brevis and peroneus longus requires a wide exposure. An effort should be made to preserve a 1-cm portion of the extensor retinaculum at the level of the fibula. This preservation, along with a strong vest-over-pants repair of the remaining extensor retinaculum, will allow early range of motion of the tendons. After the tenosynovectomy is complete, all sides of each tendon should be inspected to detect a tear that can be hidden on the deep surface of the tendon. If a partial-thickness longitudinal tear is present, it can be repaired with a running No. 4-0 nonabsorbable suture with the knot buried.

PROMINENT TROCHLEAR PROCESS
On rare occasions, a prominent trochlear process may be the source of symptoms in the absence of peroneal pathology. The giant process causes irritation of the skin in shoe wear. A local bursitis can develop along with compression of the sural nerve or one of its branches. If shoe modification fails, the treatment is excision. A 2-cm incision is made over the trochlear process, with care taken to protect branches of the sural nerve. Loupe magnification is helpful. The trochlear process is exposed using an end-cutting blade. The peroneus brevis and longus are carefully protected. The bone is excised with a rongeur and smoothed down with a power rasp. A small amount of bone wax is applied, and the inferior extensor retinaculum is repaired directly over the exposed bone.

PERONEUS BREVIS TENDINOPATHY
A longitudinal tear of the peroneus brevis is the most common peroneal injury. An isolated full-thickness tear

of the peroneus brevis is amenable to repair using a No. 4-0 nonabsorbable suture. Interrupted sutures with buried knots or a running suture can be used. Several authors have recommended tabularization of the remaining tendon. If multiple longitudinal tears of the tendon are present, each can be repaired in a similar fashion. Irreparable areas should be excised longitudinally before repair. To facilitate a tight repair of the extensor retinaculum, the distal centimeter of the peroneus brevis muscle can be excised to make more room within the peroneal tunnel and decrease pressure on the sheath. If a peroneus quartus is present, it can be excised without disability (**Figure 3**). In my experience, a bone-deepening procedure is almost never required. More extensive degeneration of the tendon may necessitate complete excision of several centimeters followed by a reconstructive procedure that uses an intercalary graft, tenodesis, or tendon transfer.

PERONEUS LONGUS TENDINOPATHY

As the peroneus longus passes beneath the trochlear process, it is sus-

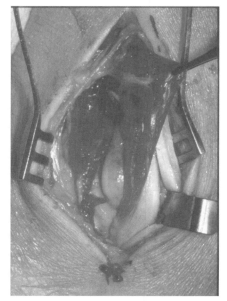

Figure 3 The peroneus quartus sits within the peroneal tunnel.

ceptible to high stress, especially in a patient with a cavus foot. The trochlear process is an attachment for the inferior extensor retinaculum and a division between the sheaths of the peroneus longus and brevis. It can develop a knife-like edge, which literally cuts into the peroneus longus. Multiple tears can develop, which are treated with a similar approach to tears of the peroneus brevis. Both tendons should be removed from their individual sheaths and carefully examined because simultaneous tears of both tendons, although unusual, can occur. An end-cutting blade can be used to expose the trochlear process, which can be smoothed down or excised. In the presence of any heel varus, a corrective ostoetomy should be performed. On rare occasions, extreme forefoot valgus may also require correction.

PAINFUL OS PERONEUM

Another area of high stress on the peroneus longus is within the cuboid tunnel, where the tendon turns from vertical to horizontal around the lateral border of the foot. A fibrocarilaginous sesamoid with the substance of the tendon is always present to protect the tendon from stress. The sesamoid (os peroneum) is ossified in about 20% of patients. As with any sesamoid in the body, the os peroneum can fracture, degenerate, or develop chondromalacia on its articular surface. Each of these conditions can lead to pain and local tenderness. A bone scan can demonstrate increased uptake over the os peroneum, and MRI can demonstrate local inflammatory changes and edema within the bone. There is, however, a high false-negative rate. Surgical treatment consists of exploration of the peroneus longus distally and excision of the os peroneum, which can easily be shelled out of the tendon with an end-cutting blade. The defect is repaired with a No. 4-0 nonabsorbable suture.

ADVANCED TENDON DEGENERATION

Simple dèbridement or repair of a tendon may not always be possible. End-stage degeneration of either the peroneus brevis or longus necessitates a more extensive reconstruction. The degenerated segment of the tendon requires excision. Several options exist for restoration of function. An intercalary autograft or allograft restores excellent function if the proximal and distal segments of the tendon are healthy, and there is good muscle excursion. Another option is a tenodesis of the tendon ends to the adjacent tendon. With degeneration of both tendons, a flexor digitorum longus transfer to the insertion of the peroneus brevis at the base of the fifth metatarsal will restore some eversion strength. A subtalar fusion will also restore adequate function if both tendons are unsalvageable.

Author's Preferred Approach and Rationale

Acute tendon rupture should be repaired. The surgical approach is common to all peroneal surgery. With the patient under anesthesia, the ankle and subtalar joints are examined for laxity, which should be corrected if present. A thigh tourniquet is used with the patient in a lateral decubitus position. Loupe magnification is often helpful. A curvilinear incision is begun just inferior to the base of the fifth metatarsal and extended to the tip of the fibula. The incision can be extended proximally if further exposure of the tendons is required. Care should be taken to protect the sural nerve and its branches, especially in the distal third of the incision. The superior peroneal retinaculum is divided longitudinally 5 mm posterior to the fibula. It is important to leave this cuff of tissue attached to the posterior fibula for the final meticulous repair of the sheath. If possible, a 1-cm portion of the sheath at the distal end of the fibula is left intact to facilitate early postoperative range of motion of the tendons.

When the retinaculum has avulsed off the fibula because of tendon dislocation, it can be tacked down with several bioabsorbable suture anchors. A tight vest-over-pants repair of the retinacular sheath is performed at the end of the procedure. If there is too much pressure on the repair, the contents of the tunnel should be decompressed by cutting back the distal 1 cm of the peroneus brevis muscle belly and excising any accessory tendons. A bone-deepening procedure is almost never required. Distally, both the peroneus brevis and longus sheaths are opened to facilitate careful inspection of the tendons. I have often found it difficult to repair these distal sheaths and now often leave them open.

The peroneus brevis and longus are both examined on all surfaces. There is always a fibrous thickening of the tendons where they are exposed to increased stress: at the tip of the fibula, beneath the trochlear process, and within the cuboid tunnel. This thickening is normal and should not be mistaken for degeneration of the tendon. An acute rupture can usually be repaired directly. Gentle tension for 30 seconds should be placed on the proximal portion to bring the tendon out to length. The tendon should be trimmed slightly using a sharp blade on a wet tongue depressor. A No. 3-0 nonabsorbable modified Kessler suture is used to repair the ends. The foot is held in 20° of plantar flexion and eversion to take tension off of the repair. A running No. 6-0 nylon suture can be used to reinforce the repair circumferentially. The fragments of a fractured os peroneum should be shelled out of the tendon using an end-cutting blade. A postoperative splint is used for 12 days followed by a short leg cast with the hindfoot in sufficient equinus and valgus to take tension off the repair. Protected range-of-motion exercise is started at 2 to

4 weeks, depending on the strength of the repair. The patient is allowed to start bearing weight at 4 weeks with a cast boot, which is discontinued 2 weeks later. An air splint is used for an additional 2 weeks.

Chronic tendinopathy is the most common reason for surgery. If there is any question, always check for anterior and varus instability of the ankle once the patient is under anesthesia. Significant laxity should be corrected. Once the tendons are exposed, they are carefully palpated with a moist glove to detect areas of tendinosis. Longitudinal tears in the tendon are identified. In general, I have had better results with longitudinal excision of the torn or fibrotic portions of the tendon rather than repair (**Figure 4**). Repair adds a foreign body to an already compromised and hypovascular tendon. Invariably, at least one third of the tendon can be preserved, which is sufficient for normal function and strength. Postoperative rupture does not occur, even with longitudinal excision of 65% of the tendon; if the remaining tendon is healthy, I no longer tabularize it. A similar approach can be used when there is simultaneous injury to both tendons.

On occasion, one of the tendons has extensive tears or fibrosis that requires complete excision of a portion

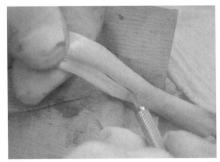

Figure 4 Longitudinal débridement of the peroneus brevis tendon.

of the tendon. Usually 4 to 5 cm of the tendon must be excised. The proximal and distal ends can be attached to the adjacent tendon. This approach is usually most applicable to degeneration of the peroneus brevis just distal to the tip of the fibula (**Figure 5**). A Pulver-Taft weave using No. 4-0 nonabsorbable suture provides a very strong repair that allows range-of-motion exercise within 2 to 3 weeks. To preserve the appropriate muscle tension, mark the position of the tenodeses proximally and distally before excising the degenerated portion of the peroneus brevis. The foot and ankle should be held in a neutral position to gauge the final tension.

Distal degeneration of the peroneus longus may not be amenable to the same technique because a distal healthy end of the tendon cannot eas-

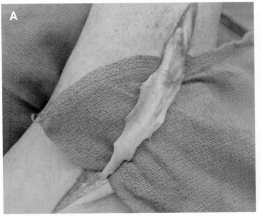
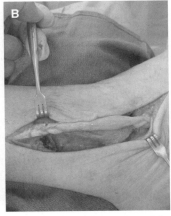

Figure 5 **A,** Advanced degeneration and fibrosis of the peroneus brevis. **B,** Tenodesis of the proximal and distal peroneus brevis to the peroneus longus.

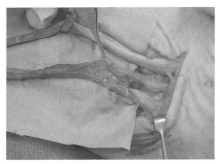

Figure 6 Advanced degeneration of the peroneus longus tendon.

ily be reached (**Figure 6**). In this situation, only the proximal portion of the peroneus longus is sutured into the intact peroneus brevis to provide increased eversion strength. Because many of the patients with distal peroneus longus degeneration have cavus feet, the loss of peroneus longus function may not be significant, and a tenodesis does not necessarily have to be performed. This is especially the case if there is any decreased function in the peroneus longus muscle belly. It always is important to ensure that there is normal excursion in the muscle of an injured tendon; tenodesis of a tendon that has a fibrotic, dysfunctional muscle is contraindicated.

Another alternative to tenodesis, especially in a young or athletic individual, is the use of an intercalary graft. The tendon has degenerated but not ruptured; therefore, the muscle has been kept to length and should

function well. A toe extensor, plantaris, or slip of the Achilles tendon can be used. I prefer a semitendinosis allograft. In the rare instance in which both tendons are degenerated, a flexor digitorum longus transfer woven into the insertion of the peroneus brevis will usually provide adequate eversion strength. The ultimate salvage for failure of this repair is a subtalar fusion.

Peroneal tendinopathy, particularly of the peroneus longus, occurs in patients with a cavus heel. These patients place increased stress on their peroneal tendons and have a high incidence of repeated ankle sprains and varus laxity of the ankle. A corrective osteotomy of a varus heel should be performed at the same time as the peroneal surgery. The tendon repair and calcaneal osteotomy can be performed through one extensile incision. If a simultaneous Broström repair is performed, however, I prefer two incisions with one anterior for the tendons and ligaments and the other posterior for the osteotomy over the calcaneal tuberosity. An oblique biplanar closing wedge Dwyer-type osteotomy can be held with staples or a screw placed across the osteotomy from posterior to anterior. The osteotomy is cut with a sagittal saw. The medial wall of the calcaneus should be left intact to act as a hinge and for added stability. If a fixed forefoot varus of more than 10° is present, a closing wedge osteotomy of the first

ray, performed dorsally through the base of the fist metatarsal, may be added. An osteotomy of the heel usually is sufficient. After surgery a splint is kept in place for 12 days. A short leg non–weight-bearing cast is then used until 4 to 6 weeks after surgery, depending on the stability of the osteotomy. The patient may then start bearing weight in a removable cast for an additional 4 weeks. Range-of-motion exercises can be started as early as 3 weeks if the fixation of the osteotomy and tendon repair are good.

Management of Complications
The most common problem with peroneal tendinopathy is persistent symptoms postoperatively. Although most patients are improved, it is not uncommon for a patient to describe continued discomfort, weakness, and difficulty walking for prolonged periods on uneven ground. The use of a soft lateral ankle brace may be helpful. A molded ankle-foot orthosis can be used for refractory symptoms. Skin slough is the most serious complication and can be minimized by the cessation of smoking preoperatively and the use of two incisions in those patients who need both a calcaneal osteotomy and a Broström reconstruction of the ankle ligaments.

References

Brandes CB, Smith RW: Characterization of patients with primary peroneus longus tendinopathy: A review of twenty-two cases. *Foot Ankle Int* 2000;21:462-468.

Krause JO, Brodsky JW: Peroneus brevis tendon tears: Pathophysiology, surgical reconstruction, and clinical results. *Foot Ankle Int* 1998;19:271-279.

Sammarco GJ: Peroneal tendon injuries. *Orthop Clin North Am* 1994;25:135-145.

Sobel M, Bohne WH, Levy ME: Longitudinal attrition of the peroneus brevis tendon in the fibular groove: An anatomic study. *Foot Ankle* 1990;11:124-128.

Coding

ICD-9 CODES

727.06   Other disorders of synovium, tendon, and bursa, Synovitis and tenosynovitis, Tenosynovitis of foot and ankle

727.68   Other disorders of synovium, tendon, and bursa, Rupture of tendon, nontraumatic, Other tendons of foot and ankle

CPT CODES

27659   Repair, flexor tendon, leg; secondary, with or without graft, each tendon

27680   Tenolysis, flexor or extensor tendon, leg and/or ankle; single, each tendon

27691   Transfer or transplant of single tendon (with muscle redirection or rerouting); deep (eg, anterior tibial or posterior tibial through interosseus space, flexor digitorum longus, flexor hallucis longus, or peroneal tendon to midfoot or hindfoot)

Achilles Tendinopathy

Richard M. Marks, MD

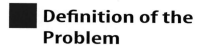

Definition of the Problem

Patient Presentation

The acute presentation of Achilles tendinopathy includes warmth and swelling of the paratenon and/or tendon. Patients often present with symptoms of discomfort on arising for physical activities. This discomfort tends to improve after an initial period of activity as the patient continues with a session of exercise. Typically, symptoms are relieved with rest. Once the tendinopathy becomes chronic, symptoms are often unremitting.

Men are more commonly affected than women. Individuals with seronegative spondyloarthropathies, gout, hypercholesterolemia, sarcoidosis, and those who have had a renal transplant have an increased incidence of Achilles tendinopathy. Age-dependent changes in collagen quality and diminished circulation within the Achilles tendon may also contribute to the development of disorders of the Achilles tendon.

Individuals who have tight hamstrings and diminished Achilles flexibility or those who excessively pronate as a result of excessive subtalar motion, tibiovarum, or calcaneovalgus have a predisposition to Achilles tendinopathy. Participation in repetitive, high-impact activities, particularly running and jumping, may increase the risk of Achilles tendinopathy. Changes in training regimens such as increases in frequency, duration, and/or intensity of running have also been implicated. The use of improper shoes that allow excessive pronation of the foot exacerbates Achilles tendinopathy. Use of intratendinous steroid injections or the use of systemic steroids are other contributing factors. The use of fluoroquinolone antibiotics may increase the risk of Achilles tendinopathy; however, this effect is usually self-limited and improves with the cessation of the drug.

Physical Examination

All areas of tendon degeneration and concomitant bony deformity must be identified so that appropriate interventions can be initiated. Examination of Achilles tendinopathy frequently reveals warmth and swelling about the tendon and paratenon, with variable fullness and/or nodularity. Patients with acute inflammation may exhibit crepitus with palpation and range of motion of the Achilles tendon. This indicates inflammation within the peritendinous space. It is often difficult to differentiate between inflammation of the tendon and inflammation of the paratenon. The painful arc sign allows for this differentiation. With primary tendon inflammation, the point of maximal tenderness will migrate with ankle dorsiflexion and plantar flexion because of the mobility of the tendon. The paratenon, which remains in a constant position during ankle plantar flexion and dorsiflexion, will exhibit a constant point of maximal tenderness (**Figure 1**). Distinct nodularity may be encountered, and in chronic Achilles tendinopathy, may not be tender to palpation. The orthopaedic surgeon should differentiate noninsertional from insertional tendinopathy, although these conditions may coexist. Insertional disorders may be limited to inflammation secondary to Haglund's deformity or may encompass posterior insertional degeneration. Combinations of noninsertional and insertional disorders must also be recognized.

The medial and lateral aspects of the calcaneal tuberosity should be palpated, as should the posterior-central insertion of the Achilles tendon. In addition, the retrocalcaneal space is palpated for tenderness. A Haglund's deformity is typically most tender along the lateral aspect of the calcaneal tuberosity, with concomitant lateral bony prominence. Patients with insertional tendinopathy exhibit tenderness directly posterior to the insertion of the Achilles tendon. This tenderness may occur in association with calcification of the tendon insertion. Not infrequently, patients may also have pre- or retrocalcaneal bursitis.

The physical examination should include evaluation of both ankle and subtalar range of motion. Ankle dorsiflexion should be tested with the foot in a neutral position and the knee in both extended and flexed positions; this allows for proper assessment of a gastrocnemius contracture. A contracture that exists solely with the

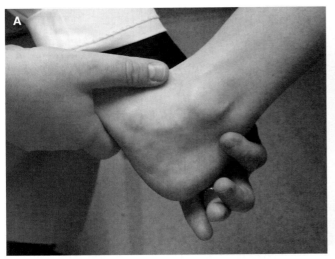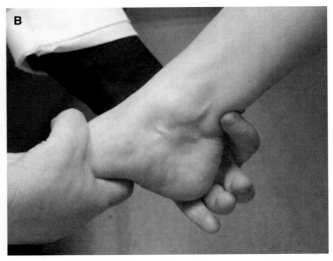

Figure 1 The painful arc sign allows for differentiation of primary tendon inflammation and inflammation of the paratenon. With inflammation of the tendon, the point of maximal tenderness will migrate with ankle dorsiflexion (**A**) and plantar flexion (**B**) because of the mobility of the tendon. The paratenon, which remains in a constant position during ankle plantar flexion and dorsiflexion, will exhibit a constant point of maximal tenderness.

knee extended is caused by a proximal gastrocnemius contracture about the knee. A contracture noted with the knee flexed denotes a distal gastrocnemius-soleus contracture. In addition, subtalar motion should be evaluated to test for excessive rigidity or laxity.

The physical examination includes tests performed with the patient standing. Cavus or pes planovalgus deformities should be noted. Gait should also be evaluated for stride length and the presence or absence of limp; the presence or absence of functional pronation should also be noted. Poor push-off strength and increased ankle dorsiflexion in terminal stride may indicate a functionally incompetent tendon or chronic elongated rupture.

The work-up of a patient with Achilles tendinopathy should include a lateral radiograph of the heel to evaluate for intrasubstance calcification, insertional calcification, and the presence of a Haglund's deformity. The presence or absence of an os trigonum should be noted. If present, an os trigonum may contribute to retrocalcaneal symptoms.

Differential Diagnosis
- Achilles tendinosis
- Peritendinitis
- Insertional tendinopathy
- Haglund's deformity
- Retrocalcaneal bursitis
- Seronegative spondyloarthropathy (Reiter's)
- Sever's apophysitis
- Os trigonum

Additional Work-up
Axial MRI scans allow assessment of the percentage of tendon involved and sagittal MRI scans help determine the length of the tendon abnormality. Intrasubstance longitudinal splits with intrasubstance edema and evidence of mucoid degeneration indicate chronic tendinopathy. The axial images will reveal loss of the ovoid, coffee-bean shape of normal tendon, which becomes more rounded and thickened with chronic degeneration. MRI also facilitates evaluation of peritendinitis. In patients with peritendinitis, the tendon will have a normal appearance with increased fluid within the peritendinous space.

Ultrasonography may also be used in the evaluation of the Achilles tendon. This allows for rapid, real-time evaluation as well as the possibility of evaluation under dynamic conditions. This technique, however, is operator-dependent, and substantial skills are required to use ultrasonography to accurately evaluate the Achilles tendon. In addition, ultrasonography has less specificity than MRI for the evaluation of insertional disorders because of distortion at the tendon-bone interface.

The Solutions

Treatment Options and Rationale
Treatments of Achilles tendinopathy may be categorized as either acute or chronic interventions. Acute Achilles tendinopathy is defined by symptoms of less than 3 months' duration. Chronic tendinopathy is defined by the presence of symptoms for more than 3 months and the failure to respond to acute intervention. Unfortunately, the

point at which acute inflammation leads to irreparable changes that only respond to surgical intervention has not been fully elucidated. Therefore, these definitions of acute and chronic phases are only considered general guidelines.

ACHILLES TENDINOPATHY

Treatment goals for acute Achilles tendinopathy include pain relief and reduction of inflammation so that a rehabilitation program may be instituted. An estimated 90% to 95% of patients with acute tendinopathy can be successfully treated with the interventions described below. The initial treatments of noninsertional and insertional disorders are identical.

Activities are restricted, and the stretch of the Achilles tendon is adjusted either with the use of a 3/8-in heel lift placed in a shoe or the application of a removable boot brace in 10° of equinus with a 3/8-in heel lift. Nonsteroidal anti-inflammatory drugs are recommended, and an organized physical therapy program is started. In severe cases, physical therapy is withheld until inflammation has diminished. Modalities such as ice massage, contrast baths, ultrasound, phonophoresis, and/or iontophoresis are implemented. Corticosteroid injections are contraindicated because of the danger of intratendinous injection and subsequent tendon rupture.

Once the acute inflammation has diminished, stretching of the Achilles tendon and eccentric strengthening exercises are instituted. Physical therapy should also attempt to increase the flexibility of the hamstrings. Based on the evaluations of structural abnormalities, corrective heel wedges or functional orthoses are used as indicated. Training regimens are reviewed and modified as necessary. In runners, hill training is avoided during the initial rehabilitation phase.

CHRONIC ACHILLES TENDINOPATHY

Chronic noninsertional disorders may be characterized as peritendinopathy, which principally involves the paratenon; tendinopathy, which principally involves the tendon; or pantendinopathy, which involves both the paratenon and the tendon. For patients with tendinopathy, the surgeon must identify the extent of tendon involvement. Involvement of less than 50% of the cross-sectional diameter of the tendon is usually amenable to débridement and repair of the degenerated tendon. If, however, the degenerative condition is greater than 50% of the cross-sectional diameter, or greater than 6 cm in length, resection of the degenerated tendon with either proximal tendon lengthening and repair or treatment with tendon transfer should be considered.

Chronic insertional tendinopathy requires tendon débridement and frequently requires partial or full detachment of the insertional portion of the Achilles tendon. Reattachment with the use of suture anchors is necessary. This reattachment is typically performed through a posterior tendon-splitting approach. If the chronic degeneration is secondary to a prominent Haglund's deformity, this procedure can be performed through a lateral peritendinous approach. Retrocalcaneal bursitis can be addressed through either the posterior or lateral approaches. More extensive insertional degeneration will require a posteromedial approach to allow for harvesting of the flexor hallucis longus (FHL) tendon distally for a graft.

Author's Preferred Treatment and Rationale

NONSURGICAL TREATMENT

Nonsurgical treatment of acute noninsertional or insertional Achilles tendinopathy requires rest, immobilization, and rehabilitation. Structural abnormalities are addressed with either heel wedges or a functional

orthosis, and training regimens are modified as necessary. Running shoes are also evaluated for excessive medial or lateral wear and for support provided.

Chronic tendinopathy and pantendinopathy, if not extensive, may be treated nonsurgically with heavy-load eccentric strengthening exercises. This physical therapy protocol has been quite effective in the treatment of chronic Achilles tendinopathy and has been found to be superior to conventional treatment regimens and comparable to open débridement of the tendon.

SURGICAL INTERVENTION

Surgical intervention is required for chronic disorders that have failed to respond after 3 months of acute treatment. Peripheral circulation should be evaluated preoperatively. A history of smoking and diabetes mellitus are relative contraindications to surgery. Good to excellent results are achieved with surgical treatment of chronic peritendinopathy in approximately 80% of patients. Better results are observed in patients who undergo early mobilization and in those with inflammation limited to the peritendinous tissue. The interpretation of some studies of surgical interventions, however, can be difficult because some trials failed to adequately describe the patient populations, procedures used, and the extent of tendon degeneration evaluated.

TREATMENT OF CHRONIC PERITENDINOPATHY WITH BRISEMENT OR LIMITED OPEN DÉBRIDEMENT

Chronic peritendinopathy, verified by a constant point of maximal tenderness that does not change with ankle motion and MRI revealing no tendon abnormality but fluid in the peritendinous space, may be treated with brisement or limited open débridement. Brisement, which is the mechanical lysis of adhesions, is performed by the rapid infusion of 5 to 15 mL of local

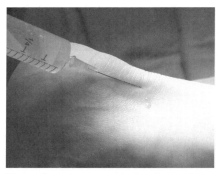

Figure 2 Brisement, which is the mechanical lysis of adhesions, is performed by rapid infusion of local anesthetic into the peritendinous space.

anesthetic into the peritendinous space (**Figure 2**). This allows for an immediate, aggressive rehabilitation program with range-of-motion exercises. The advantage of this treatment is that it obviates the need for formal surgical intervention. Patients who present with peritendinopathy alone tend to have the best outcomes.

OPEN SURGICAL DÉBRIDEMENT OF THE PARATENON

Open surgical débridement of the paratenon allows for direct visualization of both the paratenon and the underlying tendon. This technique is preferred when there is concern about concomitant tendon abnormality. Supine positioning may be used for a medial approach, which avoids the sural nerve laterally. I prefer the use of a thigh tourniquet and surgery performed under a regional or general anesthetic. The incision is made down through the superficial crural fascia directly to the paratenon, taking care to avoid undermining of the subcutaneous tissue. The length of the incision is determined by the extent of the paratenon pathology. This helps to avoid wound healing complications and postoperative scarring. The paratenon is sharply entered, and inflammatory and fibrous tissues are excised. Care is taken to avoid extensive anterior dissection to protect the mesotenal blood supply, which is the

main blood supply source of the Achilles tendon. The remaining healthy paratenon is repaired with No. 4-0 absorbable sutures, and No. 4-0 nylon is used for the skin. Initially, the leg is maintained in a resting equinus position. To minimize postoperative adhesions, range-of-motion exercises are started as soon as wound healing allows.

TREATMENT OF BOTH CHRONIC TENDINOPATHY AND PANTENDINOPATHY

The surgical treatment of patients with both chronic tendinopathy and pantendinopathy follows the same guidelines. Under tourniquet control and with the patient in a prone position, which allows for proximal extension of the incision and greater ease of visualization, a medially based incision is made and continued down to the level of the paratenon. No subcutaneous undermining is performed. The paratenon is entered and débrided accordingly. Longitudinal incisions are made within the substance of the tendon, and intrasubstance degeneration is thoroughly débrided. If less than 50% of the cross-sectional area of the tendon is involved, intrasubstance repair of the viable tendon is performed, followed by a running superficial suture. If more than 50% of the cross-sectional diameter is involved, or tendon degeneration stands for greater than 6 cm, then the diseased portion of tendon needs to be removed in its entirety. For defects less than 6 cm in length, a V-Y proximal tendon advancement or central third turndown can be performed to achieve primary anastomosis.

FHL TENDON TRANSFER

If the extent of degeneration is greater than 6 cm, an FHL tendon transfer is necessary. A V-Y advancement can be performed in conjunction with the tendon transfer to decrease the length of the bridging repair with the FHL tendon. Closure and immobilization

are similar to those described previously. Early mobilization of the tendon is performed when intrasubstance repair is possible. If V-Y advancement, central third turndown, or tendon transfer is necessary, then equinus cast immobilization is performed for the first 4 weeks, followed by controlled range-of-motion activities thereafter.

PERCUTANEOUS LONGITUDINAL TENOTOMY

Tendinopathy and pantendinopathy that involve a discrete portion of tendon, typically less than 4 cm in length, are amenable to percutaneous longitudinal tenotomy (PLT). This newer technique uses five incisions performed in line with the tendon fibers. With the patient under a local or regional anesthetic, the area of tendon degeneration is either palpated or located using ultrasound for guidance. The initial percutaneous incision is performed centrally, and the ankle is put through a full range of motion to maximize the excursion of the No. 11 scalpel blade. Two incisions are made proximal to this spot along the medial and lateral aspects, and the ankle is taken through a similar range of motion. Two distal incisions are made medially and laterally in a similar manner. In theory, this technique allows increased local circulation that in turn facilitates a controlled inflammatory process and, ultimately, results in a reparative response. Early range of motion and weight bearing is instituted immediately. In one study of this technique, 77% of patients (37 of 48) had good to excellent results. Ten of 11 patients who had a failed intervention had coexisting peritendinitis. Therefore, I recommend performing a brisement procedure in conjunction with the PLT in patients with coexisting peritendinitis.

TREATMENT OF ISOLATED CHRONIC TUBEROSITY IMPINGEMENT

Chronic insertional disorders with isolated tuberosity impingement (Haglund's deformity) must be distinguished from those that occur in conjunction with insertional tendinopathy. Isolated chronic tuberosity impingement is treated by resection of the prominent tuberosity and the retrocalcaneal bursa through a lateral paratendinous approach with the patient in a lateral decubitus position. Care must be taken to adequately decompress the area of impingement and avoid leaving a prominent ridge of bone at the insertion site. Early range-of-motion exercises are started once adequate soft-tissue healing has occurred. In some cases, a second medial incision may be necessary to adequately decompress the posterior heel; however, it is rarely used because of concerns about an adequate skin bridge.

TREATMENT OF TRUE INSERTIONAL TENDINOPATHY

Patients with true insertional tendinopathy, with or without concomitant Haglund's deformity, require a posterior tendon-splitting approach. With the patient in a prone position, the surgeon makes a longitudinal incision directly over the insertion of the Achilles tendon. This incision is carried directly through the paratenon and the Achilles tendon is split longitudinally. The medial and lateral attachments are reflected in their respective directions. The prominent calcaneal tuberosity is resected, and the insertional portion of tendon is débrided. Care must be taken to fully débride the tendon at its insertion, removing all calcifications and degenerated tendon. If extensive detachment of the insertion is required, then suture anchors are used to reattach the tendon. A V-Y advancement or central third tendon turndown may be necessary if a defect is created as a result of débridement. For defects greater than 6 cm in length, or if more than 50% of the cross-sectional area of the tendon is débrided, an FHL tendon transfer is indicated.

The rehabilitation program is determined by the extent of tendon débridement. Early range-of-motion plantar flexion is performed, but dorsiflexion that may disrupt the tendon repair should be avoided. If more extensive débridement and tendon transfer are required, a 4-week course of cast immobilization may be necessary. Rates of good to excellent results for this treatment range from 75% to 91%.

Management of Complications

Postoperative complications include continued symptoms following surgical intervention, wound healing problems, and scarring. Not infrequently, the extent of tendon degeneration is underestimated by the surgeon intraoperatively or inadequate tendon débridement is undertaken because of concern that the tendon will be weakened. Intraoperatively, all degenerated tendon must be removed. If the surgeon is unsure of additional areas of degeneration, longitudinal cuts can be made within the tendon to allow for direct visualization. If

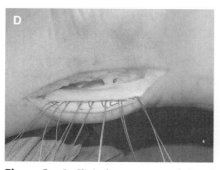
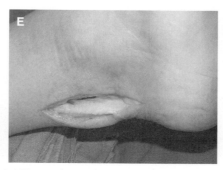
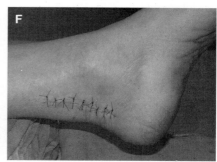

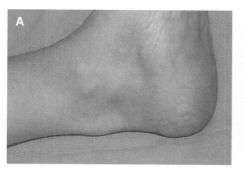
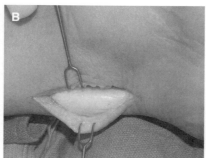
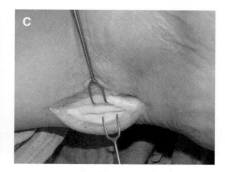

Figure 3 **A,** Clinical appearance of chronic Achilles tendinopathy. **B,** Medial incision performed through scleral fascia, exposing tendon and peritenon. **C,** Tendon exposed with intrasubstance degeneration. **D,** Intrasubstance repair with No. 2-0 nonabsorbable suture. **E,** Final repair with No. 4-0 running bioabsorbable suture. **F,** Closure with No. 4-0 nylon suture.

extensive degeneration of the tendon is encountered, the surgeon should perform either a V-Y advancement, central third tendon turndown, or FHL tendon transfer after adequate débridement (**Figure 3**). Wound healing problems frequently occur as a result of excessive undermining of the subcutaneous tissues or inadequate repair of the paratenon after tendon débridement. Inadequate paratenon repair can result in scarring of the tendon and the subcutaneous tissues. Postoperative adhesions can prevent proper glide of the tendon and may lead to wound breakdown.

————————■

■ References

Alfredson H, Pietila T, Jonsson P, Lorentzon P: Heavy-load eccentric calf muscle training for the treatment of chronic Achilles tendinosis. *Am J Sports Med* 1998;26:360-366.

Johnston E, Scranton P Jr, Pfeffer GB: Chronic disorders of the Achilles tendon: Results of conservative and surgical treatments. *Foot Ankle Int* 1997;18:570-574.

Maffulli N, Testa V, Capasso G, Bifulco G, Binfield PM: Results of percutaneous longitudinal tenotomy for Achilles tendinopathy in middle- and long-distance runners. *Am J Sports Med* 1997;25:835-840.

McCrory JL, Martin DF, Lowery RB, et al: Etiologic factors associated with Achilles tendinitis in runners. *Med Sci Sports Exerc* 1999;31:1374-1381.

Paavola M, Kannus P, Paakkala T, Pasanen M, Jarvinen M: Long-term prognosis of patients with Achilles tendinopathy: An observational 8-year follow-up study. *Am J Sports Med* 2000;28:634-642.

Coding

ICD-9 CODES

726.71   Achilles bursitis or tendinitis

726.91   Exostosis of unspecified site

CPT CODES

27630   Excision of lesion of tendon sheath or capsule (eg, cyst or ganglion), leg and/or ankle

27654   Repair, secondary, Achilles tendon, with or without graft

27680   Tenolysis, flexor or extensor tendon, leg and/or ankle; single, each tendon

27685   Lengthening or shortening of tendon, leg or ankle; single tendon (separate procedure)

28118   Ostectomy, calcaneus.

CPT copyright © 2003 by the American Medical Association. All Rights Reserved.

Chronic Achilles Tendon Rupture

Keith L. Wapner, MD

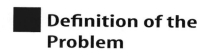 Definition of the Problem

Patient Presentation

Patients with an old or missed Achilles tendon rupture will present with plantar flexion weakness of the ankle during walking, climbing, carrying objects, and other activities of daily living that require push-off power in gait. With chronic ruptures, patients report gradual onset of progressive aching pain in the Achilles tendon that worsens over time, accompanied by a gradual thickening of the Achilles tendon associated with their symptoms, without any distinct history of a traumatic rupture. Reports of start-up pain in the morning when getting out of bed or arising after sitting for a prolonged period of time are common. These symptoms may develop over weeks or months with increasing severity.

Patients with missed ruptures recall an episode of trauma and pain followed by an initial decrease in symptoms. Some have ruptures that were misdiagnosed as ankle sprains, and others fail to seek initial medical attention. As time progresses, patients with partial ruptures notice symptoms similar to those of patients with chronic ruptures. Patients with complete ruptures report resolution of pain followed by increased weakness and a palpable defect in the tendon.

Physical Examination

Misdiagnosis at the time of the rupture has been reported in up to 20% of patients. Initially, there may not be an obvious defect but with time the ends of the rupture separate, and the overlying skin shrinks to conform with the back of the ankle, presenting as a hatchet-type defect. This defect may look like an overgrowth of the posterior calcaneus. The Thompson, or calf squeeze, test will be positive but will not cause much pain in an old injury.

Tendon rupture from progressive degenerative tendinosis presents with an insidious course. On examination, active but weakened plantar flexion is maintained by the extrinsic toe flexors and the posterior tibial and peroneal tendons. There is progressive thickening of the tendon and lengthening with loss of function and increased pain. In these patients, a defect will not be present unless an acute-on-chronic traumatic rupture occurs. In general, the tendon will be markedly thickened and tender to palpation.

Differential Diagnosis

- Soft-tissue tumor
- Chronic infection
- Inflammatory nodule

Additional Work-up

Radiographs should be obtained to rule out avulsion of the posterior tuberosity of the calcaneus, bony deformities, and calcification of the tendon. MRI may be helpful in the uncertain diagnosis of an Achilles tendon rupture and chronic tendinosis (**Figure 1**). It is most helpful in a sagittal plane to determine the length of tendon injured and to anticipate the type of surgical procedure needed.

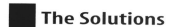

The Solutions

Treatment Options and Rationale

Nonsurgical management with shoe modifications including heel lifts will alleviate pain but will not improve function. Lace-up high-top shoes, boots, or braces, such as a molded ankle-foot orthosis, may improve gait in addition to controlling pain. Work or activity modifications may also be tried to decrease the need to plantar flex the foot. However, these modalities cannot restore push-off power.

The rupture usually occurs 2 to 6 cm from the calcaneal insertion, which is the most avascular region of the tendon. If the defect, by clinical examination or MRI, is less than approximately 3 cm, and the injury occurred within the past 3 months, then direct end-to-end repair is often possible. If the gap is greater than 3 cm after scar tissue débridement and the remaining tendon tissue is healthy, then a V-Y lengthening to close the gap may be considered. If the remaining tendon tissue has chronic tendinosis, then augmentation with transfer of the flexor hallucis longus (FHL) can be used.

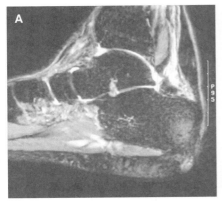
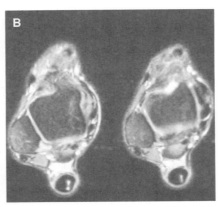

Figure 1 Axial (**A**) and sagittal (**B**) MRI scans demonstrating chronic tendinosis of the Achilles tendon with marked fusiform swelling of the tendon.

Surgery is indicated to restore normal push-off power. The surgical procedure is selected by analyzing the mechanism of injury, the time from the initial injury, and the quality of the tissues. The longer the time from the initial injury, the less likely a primary end-to-end repair can be performed. In my experience, primary end-to-end repair can be done up to 3 months postinjury. Connective tissue diseases such as rheumatoid arthritis, diabetes mellitus, obesity, autoimmune disorders, and malnutrition may inhibit the ability to perform end-to-end repair and necessitate augmentation. Local factors that make the repair weaker or cause postoperative wound problems include ischemia resulting from peripheral vascular disease, scars, and infections about the foot.

Author's Preferred Treatment and Rationale

My preferred procedure for chronic tendinosis and missed ruptures is FHL transfer. The patient is placed in a supine position with the foot externally rotated. This position allows easy access to the midfoot if tendon augmentation with graft is indicated. An incision is made over the medial side of the distal leg along the anterior border of the Achilles tendon (**Figure 2**). This site avoids irritation of the scar with shoe wear postoperatively and avoids the sural nerve. The dissection is carried down full thickness to the level of the paratenon. The paratenon

is opened and all dissection performed for exposure deep to the paratenon to avoid compromise of the skin flaps. The tendon is inspected, and any adhesions proximally and distally are freed up. In patients with a missed complete rupture, the size of the gap present is determined.

It often is possible to free up proximal adhesions within the tendon sheath up to the level of the muscles of the gastrocnemius-soleus complex. By placing a tag suture on the proximal stump of the Achilles tendon and sustaining a pulling force distally for about 5 to 10 minutes, the size of the gap between the tendon ends often can be significantly narrowed. If the gap can be closed and the tendons ends have viable tissue, direct end-to-end repair can be done. The repair is performed using No. 2-0 nonabsorbable braided suture. If inspection of the tendon reveals mucinous degeneration and thickening of the tendon fibers indicating chronic tendinosis, then augmentation should be considered.

If the tendon ends are viable and the gap is less than 3 cm, a V-Y slide can be used to close the gap and lengthen the Achilles tendon for end-to-end repair. The paratenon of the gastrocnemius is exposed and opened to the proximal end of the myotendinous junction. An inverted V incision is made, leaving the underlying muscle attached to the anterior paratenon. The flap is then advanced distally and the rupture repaired as described above for an end-to-end repair. The proximal portion is repaired by closing the inverted V to a Y. This V-Y technique is most helpful when a defect of more than 3 cm is present after the Achilles tendon is débrided to healthy tissue. If the gap is large, then a very long V with an acute angle is necessary to provide the proper length of tendon advancement. In my experience, the V cut can be advanced one half of its length without the need for augmentation. Up to about 5 cm

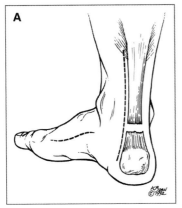
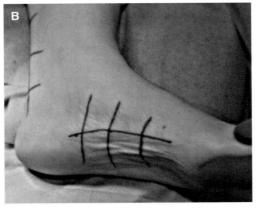

Figure 2 **A,** Diagram of incisions used for FHL reconstruction of Achilles tendon. **B,** Clinical demonstration of incisions.

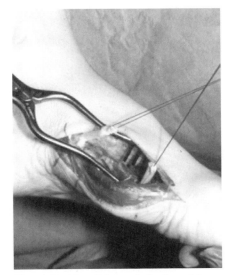

Figure 3 The abductor hallucis and flexor hallucis brevis are reflected in a plantar direction, and the FHL tendon is identified. The FHL has been tagged and divided at the level of the proximal third of the first metatarsal.

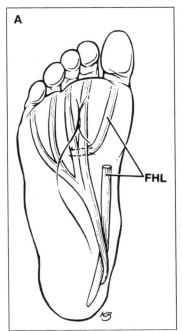
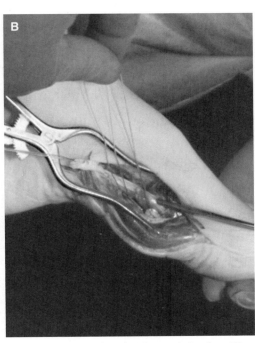

Figure 4 **A,** Diagram of FHL and FDL anastamosis. (Reproduced with permission from Wapner KL, Pavlock GS, Hecht PJ, Naselli F, Walther R: Repair of Chronic Achilles tendon rupture with flexor hallucis longus tendon transfer. *Foot Ankle* 1993;14:443-449.) **B,** The FDL is identified and tagged, and the distal FHL is sewn into the FDL with all the toes held in neutral.

can be spanned in some instances, but the diameter of the remaining tendon tissue will be compromised and its tensile strength diminished. Augmentation should be considered in these instances.

Most frequently, the tendon ends are not viable in chronic missed tears, and significant débridement is necessary to get to the level of healthy tissue. The remaining gap is then too large to close, or the remaining tissue too tenuous to withstand the tensile loads necessary to preclude rerupture. Augmentation with tendon tranfer facilitates repair in this instance. Augmentation is also useful when there is chronic tendinosis and the degenerative part of the Achilles tendon must be débrided. I prefer to add augmentation if more than one quarter of the tendon is débrided.

The FHL tendon is harvested from an incision along the medial border of the midfoot, just above the level of the abductor muscle from the navicular to the head of the first metatarsal (**Figure 2**). The skin and subcutaneous tissues are sharply divided down to the level of the abductor hal-

lucis fascia. The abductor is reflected in a plantar direction and a small Weitlander retractor is placed in the wound. The flexor hallucis brevis is then reflected in a plantar direction, and the origin is released exposing the deep midfoot anatomy.

The FHL and flexor digitorum longus (FDL) tendons are identified within the midfoot. They usually are covered by a layer of adipose tissue. Identification of the tendons is assisted by placing a finger over the lateral wall of the short flexor and manually plantar flexing and dorsiflexing the first toe proximal interphalangeal joint. The motion of the tendon can be felt, and dissection can be carried down to identify the tendons of the FHL medially and the FDL laterally. The FHL is divided as far distally as possible, generally at the level of the midshaft of the first metatarsal, but the surgeon must allow an adequate distal stump to be transferred to the FDL (**Figure 3**). The proximal portion is tagged with a suture. The distal limb

of the FHL is sewn side to side into the FDL with all five toes in a neutral position, providing flexion to all five toes via the FDL (**Figure 4**). Exposure of the FHL and FDL tendons can be aided by release of the origin of the flexor hallucis brevis to gain access to the Knot of Henry and the more proximal portion of the tendons.

In the posteromedial incision, the fascia overlying the posterior compartment of the leg is incised longitudinally directly over the muscle belly of the FHL. Pulling on the distal tag suture in the midfoot allows the surgeon to identify the level of the muscle belly, indicating where to open the fascia. The tendon is then retracted into the posterior incision from the midfoot (**Figure 5**).

A transverse drill hole is made just distal to the insertion of the Achilles tendon (generally 2 cm below the dorsal surface of the calcaneus) halfway through the bone from medial to lateral. A second vertical drill hole is made (1 cm anterior) just anterior to

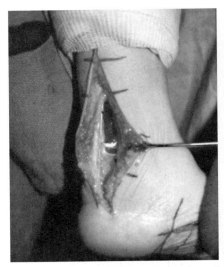

Figure 5 A posterior incision is made, and the posterior fascia of the leg is opened to allow transfer of the FHL into the wound.

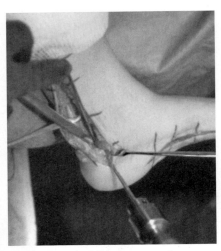

Figure 6 Two drill holes are made, one superior and the other medial, to intersect in the posterior body of the calcaneus to create a tunnel for tendon transfer.

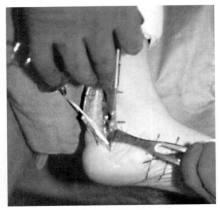

Figure 7 The FHL tendon is passed through the superior hole and out the medial side of the tunnel.

the attachment of the Achilles tendon to meet the first hole (**Figure 6**). A large towel clip is used to augment the tunnel created. A suture passer is placed through the tunnel from distal medial to proximal. The suture is pulled through the tunnel, drawing the FHL tendon through the drill hole (**Figure 7**).

A tendon weaver is used to weave the FHL from distal to proximal through the Achilles tendon (**Figure 8**). The tendon weaver is passed through the Achilles tendon creating a tunnel in the tendon. The tag suture on the FHL is then grasped and pulled back through the tunnel, bringing the flexor tendon through the Achilles tendon. The FHL is woven through the Achilles and then the sutures are put across both tendons using a figure-of-eight configuration. This process is repeated to use the full length of tendon harvested. The tendon is secured with multiple sutures of No. 1-0 nonabsorbable braided suture. After completion of the reconstruction, the paratenon is repaired. The subcutaneous tissue and skin are closed. Compressive dressings and plaster splints are applied to maintain 15° of ankle plantar flexion.

I believe that in instances where there is substantial tendinosis, there is added value to bringing the FHL tendon as a weave through the remaining Achilles tissue. My experience with this technique continues to be positive, and there have not been any reruptures. Other authors report good results for cutting the FHL at the level of the posterior ankle joint and inserting it into the calcaneus with suture anchors. No studies comparing the techniques have been conducted. In either technique, there is little morbidity with harvesting of the tendon, and I believe the added value of FHL augmentation of the Achilles tendon is beneficial.

Postoperatively the patient is placed in a short leg non–weight-bearing cast at 15° of equinus for 4 weeks. Sutures are removed at 2 weeks. When the patient returns at 4 weeks the cast is removed, and with the patient seated on an examining table with the hip flexed, the forefoot is placed on a foot rest and allowed to stay in this position until the foot reaches neutral. The foot is then placed into a short leg

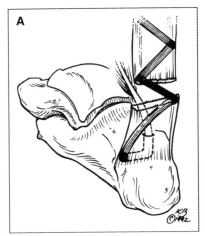
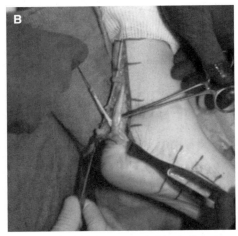

Figure 8 **A,** Diagram of completed weaving of the FHL through the Achilles tendon demonstrating the orientation of the tunnel through the posterior calcaneus. (Reproduced with permission from Wapner KL, Pavlock GS, Hecht PJ, Naselli F, Walther R: Repair of chronic Achilles tendon rupture with flexor hallucis longus tendon transfer. *Foot Ankle* 1993;14:443-449.) **B,** The FHL is woven through the Achilles tendon using a tendon weaver.

walking cast or removable cast walker with the ankle at neutral for an additional 4 weeks, and weight bearing is begun. A rehabilitation program for strengthening and range of motion is begun 8 weeks postoperatively. The patient is maintained in a removable cast walker for community ambulation until 10° of dorsiflexion is obtained and grade 4/5 strength is demonstrated. In-home ambulation is allowed with a 7/16-in heel lift during this time. The patient is then advanced to regular shoe wear and continued on a home strengthening program with stretch cords. Athletic activity is restricted for 6 months after surgery.

Management of Complications

The main complications are wound necrosis, infection, rerupture, ankle stiffness, and sural neuroma formation. Wound edge necrosis is pre-vented by keeping the posterior flap as thick as possible and performing all dissection deep to the paratenon, avoiding excessive flap retraction. Very careful wound closure and an adequate postoperative period of wound compression and immobilization are also important. If skin necrosis occurs, débridement, soaks, and antibiotics should allow healing by secondary intention. In instances of large sloughs, skin grafting may be necessary once the wound granulates. If the defect is too large and a large portion of tendon is exposed, a free flap may be required. Patients are encouraged to stop smoking before surgery and are informed of the potential detrimental effect on healing if they do not stop.

Infection is closely related to wound necrosis. If an infection occurs deep to a wound that was closed by pri-mary intention, treatment consists of débridement and drainage and parenteral antibiotics. Primary closure may be possible, or the wound may be left open to heal by secondary intention.

Rerupture is unusual if the rehabilitation is gradual and allows hypertrophy of the repaired tendon. It is important that healthy tissue be used to span the site of repair. Rerupture has not been reported after augmentation with FHL transfer.

Sural nerve neuroma formation is possible if a lateral approach is used. Leaving the adipose tissue around the nerve after identification is important. If the nerve is injured inadvertently, then a more proximal nerve transection in a relatively undisturbed subcutaneous site will decrease the sensitivity of the resulting end-bulb neuroma.

References

Schweitzer ME, Karasick D: MR imaging of disorders of the Achilles tendon. *AJR Am J Roentgenol* 2000;175:613-625.

Wapner KL, Hecht PJ, Mills RH Jr: Reconstruction of neglected Achilles tendon injury. *Orthop Clin North Am* 1995;26:249-263.

Wapner KL, Pavlock GS, Hecht PJ, Naselli F, Walther R: Repair of chronic Achilles tendon rupture with flexor hallucis longus tendon transfer. *Foot Ankle* 1993;14:443-449.

Coding

ICD-9 CODE
727.67   Other disorders of synovium, tendon, and bursa, Rupture of tendon, nontraumatic, Achilles tendon

CPT CODE
27654   Repair, secondary, Achilles tendon, with or without graft

CPT copyright © 2003 by the American Medical Association. All Rights Reserved.

Problems of the Flexor Hallucis Longus Tendon

G. James Sammarco, MD

◼ Definition of the Problem

Patient Presentation

Acute laceration of the flexor hallucis longus (FHL) tendon from a penetrating wound or inadvertent surgical cut is uncommon. The location of the wound, often in the forefoot or midfoot, is similar to that of tendon disruption. The hallux interphalangeal (IP) joint lies in extension, and active flexion at that joint is lost, whereas active flexion of the metatarsophalangeal (MTP) joint is present but weak.

In the athlete, symptoms of tendinitis occur after running, climbing, or rapid side-to-side movements. Those participating in contact sports, such as football, basketball, and soccer, have vague posteromedial ankle pain. Because they dance in a strictly controlled low to medium impact environment, ballet and modern dancers tend to have symptoms that are insidious in onset. Characteristically, an ache occurs at the posteromedial aspect of the ankle. Symptoms occur as the dancer raises to half pointe (ie, on the ball of the foot), and the pain increases when the dancer rises sur les pointes (ie, to her toes).

In acute tendinitis, swelling may occur at the posteromedial aspect of the ankle. Its presence suggests a mass (a pseudocyst) surrounding the tendon. The mass is soft and movable and can be collapsed by gentle pressure. Symptoms may occur at the beginning of dance class, decrease during activity, and then return within an hour after the end of class. The patient may feel a grinding sensation posteriorly as the ankle is flexed and extended. These symptoms of "dancer's tendinitis" may occur suddenly when changing a dance step, changing technique, or performing a new dance without appropriate warm-up or preparation.

If the muscle is hypertrophied at the distal end of the musculotendinous junction, the enlarged muscle mass or nodule may prevent the tendon from sliding distally into its fibro-osseous tunnel and, thereby, prevent the hallux from dorsiflexing. This is the "stopper-in-bottle" phenomenon, wherein the hallux passively flexes as ankle dorsiflexion is attempted.

In patients with chronic tendinitis, pain and crepitus increase over time. As longitudinal tears within the tendon occur, fusiform thickening develops at the proximal or distal end of the tear, preventing the tendon from sliding smoothly through its fibro-osseous tunnel and creating the classic "trigger toe." As the thickening in the tendon enlarges, triggering becomes more pronounced until the nodule restricts sliding altogether, and the hallux remains either in a flexed position with the nodule locked proximal to the fibro-osseous tunnel or in an extended position with the nodule locked distal to the tunnel.

Pain is not always the predominant symptom; the dancer may present reporting difficulty performing tendu (ie, the ankle in a plantar flexed position and the toe pointing while stretching the leg in a straight line), relevé (ie, slowly rising up on the ball of the foot), or plié (ie, bending of the knees before beginning or landing from a jump). All these activities are part of the barre exercises. Symptoms are aggravated by dance techniques that require increased use of deep compartment muscles as foot and ankle stabilizers rather than use of the gastrocnemius-soleus complex muscle to stabilize the foot and ankle.

Physical Examination

Trauma to the FHL tendon or muscle, such as a laceration or compartment syndrome following fractures, dramatically affects its function. Primary disease involving the tendon alone occurs commonly in athletes, laborers, and dancers. Unfortunately the location of the tendon, deep in the soft tissues behind the ankle, often makes tendon pathology difficult to diagnose and can delay treatment.

Physical examination includes observing ankle dorsiflexion and plantar flexion with the patient sitting. This motion may elicit a sudden snapping of the hallux and indicates the presence of trigger toe. The test for identifying pathology in the tendon is as follows: The patient sits with the knee flexed to relax the gastrocnemius-soleus muscle complex and allow full dorsiflexion of the ankle. The ankle and hallux MTP and IP joints are all brought passively into full extension, anterior to the Achilles tendon at the level of the ankle joint. The patient is asked to extend the knee while at the same time plantar flexing the ankle and hallux. The motion is then reversed.

With tendinitis, tenderness is elicited and crepitus (ie, "leather bottle" sensation) is palpable at the fingertip throughout the maneuver. In trigger toe, the hallux snaps or "triggers" if the toe hangs up in extension and then snaps into flexion with a palpable pop beneath the fingertip at the ankle. This occurs during flexion and/or extension. If the tendon is locked proximally or there is muscle hypertrophy, dorsiflexion of the hallux is prevented when the ankle is dorsiflexed. The hallux cannot be dorsiflexed actively or passively because the nodule or hypertrophic muscle prevents the tendon from sliding distally into its tunnel. This is the so-called "stopper-in-bottle" phenomenon. If the tendon is locked distally, the hallux cannot be flexed with active plantar flexion of the ankle and hallux because the nodule on the tendon is prevented from sliding proximally.

These findings can be subtle; however, only palpation of a "pop" or crepitus at the ankle with pain is necessary to indicate that there is significant disease within the tendon. Although uncommon, tenderness beneath the first metatarsal head and snapping at the MTP joint with active motion suggest tendinitis at the level of that joint. Also, the presence of a pseudocyst and tears, which may be several centimeters in length, can produce tenderness in the arch distal to the sustentaculum tali. Although complete rupture rarely occurs, it prevents active flexion, allowing the hallux to remain fully extended during active and passive motion at the ankle.

The test to differentiate between tendinitis and posterior impingement at the ankle is as follows. The patient rises on the ball of the foot. If pain occurs at the posterior ankle, the pa-

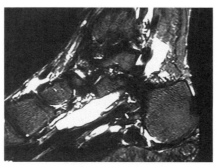

Figure 1   Sagittal T2-weighted MRI scan of the foot and ankle shows dumbbell appearance of a pseudocyst of the FHL tendon. Note that one portion of the fluid-filled cyst is posterior to the ankle and the other is anterior to the sustentaculum tali. The cyst surrounds the tendon and represents an inflammatory response with or without a tear of the tendon.

tient then sits and the ankle is passively plantar flexed to its limit. If the same pain occurs posteriorly with passive plantar flexion, it is more likely to be caused by posterior impingement or os trigonum syndrome than by tendinitis.

Differential Diagnosis

• Synovitis of the ankle
• Posterior impingement or os trigonum syndrome
• Insertional Achilles tendinitis
• Achilles tendinitis
• Tarsal tunnel syndrome
• Posterior tibial tendon insufficiency (early stages)

Additional Work-up

Radiographs of the ankle rule out the presence of an os trigonum. MRI of the foot and ankle is helpful in differentiating posterior impingement from FHL tendinitis. The MRI scan may show degeneration within the tendon and fluid surrounding the tendon. A pseudocyst is best visualized on T2-weighted images in sagittal and axial views (**Figure 1**). A "dumbbell" appearance of the pseudocyst is seen best on sagittal sections. A collection of fluid is present proximal and distal to the sustentaculum tali with fluid

connecting the two parts along the FHL tendon. The fibro-osseous tunnel causes narrowing of the cyst beneath the sustentaculum tali. Electrodiagnostic testing is indicated if tarsal tunnel syndrome is suspected.

——————————■

■ The Solutions

Treatment Options and Rationale

It is important to establish goals for the patient. Because this condition occurs in laborers, athletes, and dancers, goals for each group must be clarified. In the laborer, stability with endurance and functional range of motion of the foot and ankle is reasonable. In the athlete, particularly those involved in contact sports such as running and jumping, full painless range of motion with maximum strength and agility is necessary. In the dancer, the goals are similar to those required of a concert pianist's hand: flexibility, strength, full symmetric range of motion, and coordination.

Nonsurgical treatment is directed toward reducing swelling and triggering with anti-inflammatory medication and physical therapy. Corticosteroid injections are not recommended because of the risk of inadvertent intratendinous injection. Deposition of steroid within the tendon tends to contribute to further degeneration and may increase symptoms. If symptoms are chronic, a full insole, semirigid functional orthotic is helpful to aid in supporting the longitudinal arch and to allow the patient to stand for long periods of time, increasing endurance and decreasing fatigue. For acute symptoms in the athlete involved in contact sports, nonsteroidal anti-inflammatory medication and physical therapy including ultrasound and taping should be tried.

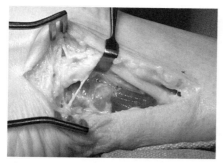

Figure 2 Surgical photograph of the pseudocyst herniating into the wound as the FHL tendon is exposed.

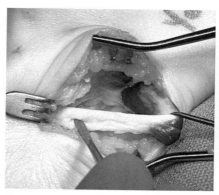

Figure 3 Surgical photograph showing longitudinal rent in the tendon, which may be accompanied by a nodule in the tendon that can cause triggering of the hallux.

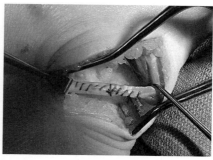

Figure 4 After the cyst is excised and the tendon débrided, the fibro-osseous tunnel is released and the tendon tear is repaired. The tendon should slide through its tunnel smoothly.

Full insole, semirigid functional orthotics are prescribed if symptoms persist. These orthotics allow movement while supporting the longitudinal arch and slowly increasing muscle strength in the leg. Dancers are advised to increase their warm-up and cool-down periods before and after class, respectively. The use of a water barre (ie, barre exercises performed in a pool with the dancer submerged to the chest to eliminate gravity) is recommended. If these modalities fail to alleviate symptoms over time, the patient may be offered surgical intervention.

Author's Preferred Treatment and Rationale

The surgical approach begins with a 5-cm incision along the posteromedial aspect of the ankle 2 cm anterior to the Achilles tendon at the level of the ankle joint. The deep fascia and flexor retinaculum are divided, the neurocirculatory bundle is retracted medially, and the muscle belly of the FHL is identified. A pseudocyst, if present, may herniate into the wound (**Figure 2**). Careful dissection of the cyst is necessary to free it from soft tissue near the neurocirculatory bundle. Plantar flexing the ankle and applying traction on the tendon with a tendon hook deliver into the wound any remaining portion of the cyst and tendinitis to be excised. A longitudinal tear and nodule may be present on the

tendon (**Figure 3**). The nodule is thinned by sharply skiving off the broad portion of its fusiform shape so that the tendon is uniform in diameter throughout its length. The longitudinal tear is repaired with running No. 2-0 Ethibond suture (Ethincon, New Brunswick, NJ) (**Figure 4**). The fibro-osseous tunnel begins just below the level of the ankle and subtalar joints. The proximal portion of the fibrous tunnel is released with a Metzenbaum scissors. If the muscle belly is hypertrophied, the muscle is debulked by removing enough muscle to allow the tendon full excursion.

Flexing the ankle and hallux and applying traction on the tendon can move 5-cm long tendon tears into the wound. A tear extending distal to the sustentaculum tali requires a second incision along the medial longitudinal arch. The tendon is exposed by dissection beneath the anterior calcaneus, retracting the abductor hallucis and neurocirculatory bundle plantarward. The distal portion is repaired in the manner described above. When the repair is complete, the tendon should slide easily throughout its full excursion.

Closure is with No. 3-0 subcutaneous suture and No. 4-0 absorbable subcuticular suture. The ankle is immobilized for 2 weeks with active and passive gentle range of motion in a

range of motion walking boot. At 3 weeks after surgery the boot is removed, and a full physical therapy program, including power building and flexibility, is begun.

Management of Complications

Complications stemming from treatment of FHL tendon disease are related to the tendon itself or to surrounding structures. For complete rerupture of a repaired tendon as in the young athlete, direct repair using No. 2-0 Ethibond suture is recommended. Although uncommon, complete rupture at the level of the MTP joint or at its insertion is repaired with No. 2-0 Ethibond suture using a Krackow or crisscross stitch end-to-end or securing the tendon to the distal phalanx with a transosseous suture. The medial or plantar surgical approach may be used. Progressive degeneration of the tendon following surgical intervention produces symptoms related to painful scar formation and recurrent triggering, which limit function. Reexploration of the tendon, lysis of adhesions, and excision of the scar with retubularization of the tendon using a running nonabsorbable No. 4-0 braided suture with buried knots are recommended. Early motion beginning 3 weeks postoperatively is recommended. If the tendon is so damaged that it cannot be repaired directly, a tendon graft using a regional donor tendon such as the plantaris is recommended. Extensile exposure on the medial aspect of the foot provides access to the FHL tendon in the distal tarsal tunnel and midfoot.

Because of the position of the tarsal tunnel and its proximity to the neurovascular structures at the posteromedial aspect of the ankle, postoperative neuritis associated with neurapraxia can occur as a result of pressure on the nerves from retraction or from postoperative edema. Scarring in and about the repair can also produce symptoms. Burning and pain in the foot along the distribution of the plantar nerves can be present for up to 1 year. In the great majority of cases, symptoms subside. Treatment with nonsteroidal anti-inflammatory drugs or gabapentin controls these symptoms. In my experience, exploration of the nerve and the contents of the tarsal tunnel has not been required. Careful retraction of the tibial nerve at the time of surgery reduces the risk of compression. The fibrous sheath surrounding the FHL tendon at the posterior ankle should be released with care, mindful that the neurocirculatory bundle lies close to the tendon as it passes beneath the sustentaculum tali. Releasing the fibrous tunnel using blunt dissection avoids injury to the medial plantar nerve. Inadvertent sectioning of the medial plantar nerve will cause numbness in the forefoot and weakness of the medial intrinsic muscles of the foot, primarily the hallux. Exploration of the nerve is indicated if symptoms warrant. Complete transsection of the nerve results in significant symptoms, and excision of the medial plantar nerve and neuroma to an area of reduced pressure is recommended. A full insole semirigid accommodative orthosis with relief beneath the area of nerve sensitivity helps to reduce symptoms.

Physical therapy, including range-of-motion exercises, power building, and proprioceptive treatment modalities is helpful in treating postoperative problems that result from scar formation. Ultrasound is often helpful in the midfoot and hindfoot; however, the use of ultrasound over the incision at the posteromedial ankle may irritate the posterior tibial nerve and should be discontinued if nerve irritation occurs.

References

Hamilton WG: Stenosing tenosynovitis of the flexor hallucis longus tendon and posterior impingement upon the os trigonum in ballet dancers. *Foot Ankle* 1982;3:74-80.

Sammarco GJ, Cooper PS: Flexor hallucis longus tendon injury in dancers and non-dancers. *Foot Ankle Int* 1998;9:356-362.

Coding

ICD-9 CODE
727.68   Other disorders of synovium, tendon, and bursa, Rupture of tendon, nontraumatic, Other tendons of foot and ankle

CPT CODE
27659   Repair, flexor tendon, leg; secondary, with or without graft, each tendon

Anterior Tibial Tendon Disorders

Andrea Cracchiolo, III, MD

Definition of the Problem

Patient Presentation

The patient with paratenonitis usually presents with swelling and tenderness about the tendon and may have some weakness in dorsiflexion as a result of pain. The patient may not know that he or she has injured the tendon and may modify his or her gait to accommodate the dorsiflexion weakness. If the tendon has ruptured, symptoms may be mild, with some swelling and tenderness that promptly resolve. At times, however, a spontaneous rupture is insidious, and the patient may present many weeks or months after the rupture occurs with weakness or fatigue with walking, aching over the lower leg, and a sensation of dragging the foot.

Physical Examination

Disorders involving the anterior tibial tendon are rare and, therefore, may not be readily recognized. The tendon can be surrounded by an inflammation (paratenonitis), can develop an intratendinous degeneration (tendinosis), can rupture spontaneously or as a result of a traumatic force, and can be lacerated.

The anterior tibialis is a powerful dorsiflexor of the foot (**Table 1**). The anterior tibial tendon courses just beneath the deep subcutaneous tissues and can be easily seen and palpated along the anteromedial side of the ankle and hindfoot (**Figure 1**). Because the tendon rests just under the skin, synovial hypertrophy around the tendon can easily be seen.

PARATENONITIS WITH OR WITHOUT TENDINOSIS

The anterior tibial tendon is enveloped by a synovial sheath that is approximately 8 cm long. An inflammation can be caused by a systemic arthritis such as rheumatoid arthritis (**Figure 2**) or Reiter's syndrome. It also can occur secondary to athletic activities such as running and hiking, particularly on slopes, and irritation can be produced by boots worn for activities such as skiing and ice hockey. The condition usually is diagnosed by the history and physical examination. Tendinosis involving the anterior tibial tendon is very rare. The condition is degeneration within the tendon and may be associated with reduced intratendinous blood supply. This reduction may occur in an older patient or as a result of overuse. On examination, the area of tendinosis will feel like a nodule and will usually be tender. Swelling, if any, will be mild, and symptoms are usually chronic. If the tendinosis is associated with a paratenonitis, there can be an increased incidence of tendon rupture.

RUPTURE OF THE ANTERIOR TIBIAL TENDON

This condition usually occurs in men older than age 60 years who usually report some history of tripping or a missed step, a stumble, or even a short fall. The mechanism producing the rupture is a contraction of the anterior tibial tendon against a plantar flexed ankle. Physical examination will demonstrate weakness of dorsiflexion, loss of a palpable tendon, and palpability of the bulbous end at the proximal part of the rupture.

Because dorsiflexion will be performed by the extensor tendons of the foot, especially the extensor hallucis longus; there will be hyperextension of the hallux and the lateral toes (**Figure 3**). These tendons

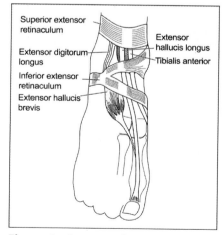

Figure 1 Anatomy of the anterior tibial tendon as it courses under the superior and inferior extensor retinaculum.

Table 1 Anatomy of the Anterior Tibialis Muscle and Tendon

Origin of the muscle	Lateral tibial condyle, proximal lateral anterior tibia, interosseous membrane, intermuscular septum.
Origin of the tendon	Begins at the junction of the middle and distal one third of the anterolateral tibia; 1 cm wide.
Course of the tendon (Proximal to distal)	Under superior extensor retinaculum, passes between deep and superficial portions of the superomedial bands of the inferior extensor retinaculum (potential site of compression and paratenonitis), and under the inferomedial band of the inferior extensor retinaculum.
Tendon rotation	Gradual 90° rotation from the musculotendinous junction.
Tendon insertion	Medial side of the medial cuneiform and the inferomedial side base of the first metatarsal.
Tendon sheath	From proximal to superior extensor retinaculum to the proximal portion of the inferior extensor retinaculum; approximately 8 cm long, contains a complete mesotendon and vincular apparatus giving a large portion of blood supply to the tendon.
Areas of hypovascularity	None
Function	Controls deceleration of the foot to the floor after heel strike; assists in ankle and foot dorsiflexion after toe-off; provides 80% of dorsiflexion strength; and has a maximum excursion of 2.9 cm.

also produce an eversion of the foot in dorsiflexion. A progressive flatfoot deformity has been reported in older patients. Drop foot can be distinguished from a peroneal nerve palsy because the extensor hallucis longus, extensor digitorum longus, and the peroneal tendons are intact, and there is an absence of paresthesias. A rupture occurring at the musculotendinous junction usually is associated with a systemic disease such as gout, rheumatoid arthritis, or diabetes mellitus.

Differential Diagnosis
- Paratenonitis
- Tendinosis
- Inflammatory arthritis
- Tendon laceration
- Tendon rupture
- Common peroneal nerve palsy, compression, or laceration
- Peripheral neuropathy
- Drop foot due to lumbar nerve root compression (ruptured intervertebral disk)

Additional Work-up
Patients with a paratenonitis should be evaluated by a rheumatologist for an underlying inflammatory arthritis. Neurologic evaluation is indicated if a peripheral neuropathy is suspected. Careful clinical evaluation of the peripheral circulation is necessary in older patients about to undergo surgical reconstruction. Although the diagnosis of a tendon rupture can be made clinically, MRI can be useful to confirm any pathology involving the anterior tibial tendon. It would be most useful in identifying a complete tendon rupture, a paratenonitis, or a tendinosis

and could aid in making treatment decisions.

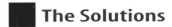

The Solutions

Treatment Options and Rationale
Surgical repair of a ruptured anterior tibial tendon has been shown to be a very effective procedure with low complications. Thus, it should be considered and offered to most patients, particularly to young, active patients. Age alone should not be a consideration, however, because many older patients are very active (eg, playing golf, tennis, walking). Even patients who initially were functional following their rupture and have subsequently experienced symptoms should be considered for surgical repair.

Nonsurgical treatment probably should be considered if the condition is chronic or if the patient is older and has a sedentary lifestyle, has other orthopaedic pathology that restricts activities, or a disease such as diabetes mellitus or a peripheral vascular disease that poses substantial risk to a surgical procedure. A custom orthotic device such as an ankle-foot orthosis made of polypropylene that may provide a few degrees of dorsiflexion or a double upright metal drop-foot brace attached to the patient's shoe can be helpful. Patients frequently discard braces; therefore, brace treatment should be ordered only if the patient truly understands the type of device and is willing to use it. If the patient has adapted to the lack of dorsiflexion strength, then a brace probably will be unnecessary. However, an orthotic device should be worn because a progressive flatfoot deformity has been reported in older patients.

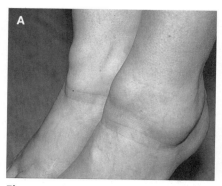
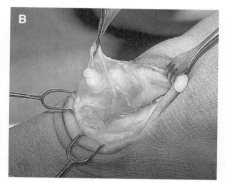
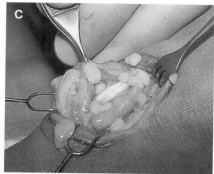

Figure 2   Preoperative views of a patient with rheumatoid arthritis. **A,** Swelling over the anterior tibial tendons (right and left). **B,** Extensive synovitis about the anterior tibial tendon. **C,** Synovial hypertrophy and rice bodies surrounding the anterior tibial tendon. Tendon decompression should be done promptly to avoid tendon rupture in these patients.

Author's Preferred Treatment and Rationale

DIRECT REPAIR OF RUPTURED ANTERIOR TIBIAL TENDON

Traumatic ruptures usually occur about 1 to 1.5 inches from the tendon's insertion. The tendon proximal to the rupture can retract to the level of the inferior extensor retinaculum where it is held by the superomedial and inferomedial bands through which the tendon normally passes. Direct repair is ideal and is usually possible in younger patients who have had a traumatic rupture less than 3 months before surgery. The tendon rupture is usually quite distal. If the distal stump is viable then a direct suture technique, such as the Bunnell, Kessler, or Krackow technique, can be performed using a No. 1 nonabsorbable suture. The tendon is exposed through a dorsal longitudinal incision that usually is placed between the anterior tibial and extensor hallucis longus tendons. Exposure is from the tendon insertion distally to the inferior extensor retinaculum. After minimal débridement, the tendon is sutured holding the foot in about 10° of dorsiflexion. The synovial sheath can be repaired. The portion of the extensor retinaculum that is or may be over the suture line should not be repaired to prevent development of subsequent adhesions. Care must be taken to care-

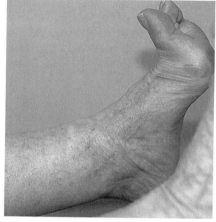

Figure 3   Overactivity of the extensor hallucis longus in a patient with a ruptured anterior tibial tendon who is attempting to dorsiflex his left foot.

fully close the skin because there is very little subcutaneous tissue, and any impairment of wound healing would result in failure.

TENDON TRANSFER

Although the ideal repair of a ruptured anterior tibial tendon may be anatomic repair, delay in diagnosis appears to be a factor that makes the procedure difficult to perform. The proximal tendon stump retracts, and even with extensive mobilization there is insufficient anterior tibial tendon to bridge the rupture gap.

Extensor hallucis longus trans-

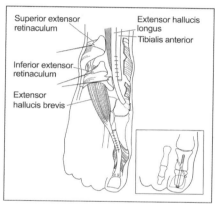

Figure 4   Transfer of the extensor hallucis longus to bridge a defect in the anterior tibial tendon. The distal portion is sutured to the extensor hallucis brevis. If the entire length of the extensor hallucis longus is required (especially if the distal portion of the anterior tibial tendon is abnormal or deficient and the surgeon needs or wishes to suture the tendon transfer into bone), then an arthrodesis of the hallux interphalangeal joint is required (inset).

fer appears to be the most commonly used reconstruction procedure for patients with this problem (**Figure 4**). The exposure is similar to that for a direct tendon repair. The surgeon can then measure the length of extensor hallucis longus necessary to bridge the gap. If the distal part of the ruptured tendon appears viable it may be necessary only to divide the extensor hallucis longus distally so that it can be sutured both distally and proximally to the anterior tibial tendon. The remaining distal portion of the extensor hallucis longus is then sutured to the extensor hallucis brevis. However, if the distal part of the ruptured anterior tibial tendon is of poor quality or if the surgeon wants to secure the distal transfer through a bony tunnel in the medial cuneiform, it will be necessary to mobilize the entire length of the extensor hallucis longus, which would then require an arthrodesis of the hallux interphalangeal joint. However, it usually is not necessary to perform the transfer in this manner.

Several other options are possible when considering the surgical treatment of a ruptured anterior tibial tendon. (1) If the rupture has occurred near the insertion of the tendon, it may be possible to reattach the tendon directly to the navicular using at least two bone anchors and a No.1 nonabsorbable suture. The tendon is not long enough to be reattached through a drill hole in the bone. (2) Transfer of the extensor digitorum longus from the second and third toes has been described. These tendons are sutured to the distal stump of the anterior tibial tendon. The distal portions of the transected extensor digitorum longus of the second and third toes are sutured to the extensor digitorum brevis of each toe. (3) For a sliding graft of the proximal stump, the anterior tibial tendon is exposed both proximal and distal to the rupture. The inferior extensor retinaculum must then be divided. If the gap is between 2 and 4 cm wide and the proximal tendon appears healthy, it is possible to slide half of the proximal tendon distally. The tendon is then sutured proximally and distally. The retinaculum is not repaired to avoid forming adhesions to the lesion. (4) Free tendon grafts, usually using the long exterior tendon to the second and third toes, have also been performed.

Postoperative care is similar regardless of the type of repair used. After surgery a short leg cast is placed with the foot in neutral or about 10° of dorsiflexion. Weight bearing can begin at about 3 weeks, and the cast can be removed after 6 weeks. Depending on the patient, a walking boot that restricts plantar flexion can be used for about 2 weeks. Physical therapy is usually helpful. Athletic activities can be started gradually about 12 weeks postoperatively.

Management of Complications

Although no large series have been reported because this is a very uncommon tendon rupture, almost all reports note that the few patients who underwent surgery had good results no matter which surgical technique was used. It is difficult to find many complications to these operations. Care must be taken in the dissection to avoid creating postoperative adhesions and to avoid injury to the deep peroneal nerve and dorsalis pedis artery, which are just lateral to the extensor hallucis longus. Wound closure must be meticulous to avoid wound breakdown and infection.

It is noteworthy that the existing literature does not mention an equinus contracture in a patient with a ruptured anterior tibialis tendon. The remaining extensors, although much weaker than the triceps surae, may provide sufficient strength that an equinus contracture will not occur. However, the basic principles of tendon transfer would be violated if a surgeon attempted a tendon transfer or even a direct repair in patients with an equinus contracture. It is important that the foot be brought, at least, to a neutral position when doing these repairs. I prefer holding the foot in about 10° of dorsiflexion during the first 3 to 4 weeks after surgery while the foot and leg are in a short leg cast. This position reduces tension on the suture sites and the dorsal skin incision. Thus, in a patient with a tight Achilles tendon, the surgeon should consider either (1) a gastrocnemius-soleus recession or (2) a three-step percutaneous lengthening of the Achilles tendon, which would preclude a more proximal and somewhat longer skin incision.

───────────▶

■ References

Coughlin MJ: Disorders of tendons, in Coughlin MJ, Mann RA (eds): *Surgery of the Foot and Ankle*, ed 7. St Louis, MO, Mosby, 1999, pp 790-795.

Markarian GG, Kelikian AS, Brage M, Trainor T, Dias L: Anterior tibialis tendon ruptures: An outcome analysis of operative versus nonoperative treatment. *Foot Ankle Int* 1998;19:792-802.

Coding

ICD-9 CODE

727.68   Other disorders of synovium, tendon, and bursa, Rupture of tendon, nontraumatic, Other tendons of foot and ankle

CPT CODES

27664   Repair, extensor tendon, leg; primary, without graft, each tendon

27665   Repair, extensor tendon, leg; secondary, with or without graft, each tendon

27690   Transfer or transplant of single tendon (with muscle redirection or rerouting); superficial (eg, anterior tibial extensors into midfoot)

CPT copyright © 2003 by the American Medical Association. All Rights Reserved.

SECTION 5
Arthritis

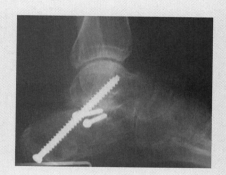

Roy W. Sanders, MD
Editor

Ankle Arthrodesis

Keith A. Heier, MD

■ Definition of the Problem

Patient Presentation

Patients report arthritic pain in the ankle on presentation. A careful history should help determine whether the patient has primary osteoarthritis or posttraumatic, infectious, inflammatory, or congenital arthritis. It is also vital to ensure that the patient's discomfort emanates from the ankle joint (not an adjacent joint) and to determine whether the pain is activity related (mechanical) or present at rest or night (possible infection or tumor). If the patient has already had an ankle arthrodesis, the previous postoperative course must be investigated with special attention to any wound problems and to the postoperative period of immobilization and patient compliance.

A history of diabetes mellitus, inflammatory arthritis, neuropathy, or psychiatric problems is an indication of potential postoperative problems. Social factors such as tobacco and alcohol use also should be evaluated.

Physical Examination

The physical examination is an important part of the preoperative work-up. The most important step is to identify the location and source of the patient's pain. In a patient with ankle arthritis, pain should be caused by dorsiflexion and plantar flexion. Pain with eversion and inversion may indicate that the discomfort is related to the subtalar or talonavicular joint. With the patient bearing weight, the presence of a flatfoot or a cavovarus foot should be checked. The forefoot and especially the first ray should be examined to determine whether a corrective osteotomy is needed to realign the foot. Fixed and dynamic deformities of the lower extremity should be noted, including hip and knee motion and limb-length discrepancy. The overall appearance of the leg must be assessed, and in the case of a revision fusion or previous ankle surgery, the location of previous incisions and traumatic wounds should be noted (**Figure 1**). Soft-tissue coverage, including previous skin grafts or flaps and the pliability of the skin around the sites of future incisions, must be inspected closely. Any signs and symptoms of infection (eg, swelling, erythema, previous draining wounds, or sinuses) should be noted. All leg pulses should be documented to prevent future healing problems. Sensation should be checked globally (light touch and Semmes-Weinstein filaments) and locally because the patient may have a neuroma or a vascular injury from previous trauma or surgery.

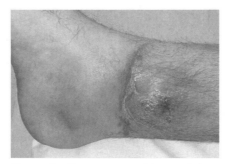

Figure 1 Transverse medial wound from previous open fracture.

Differential Diagnosis

Primary arthrodesis
- Infection
- Charcot arthropathy
- Adjacent joint arthritis (subtalar, talonavicular, calcaneocuboid, midfoot, knee)
- Deformity above or below the ankle (tibia, hindfoot, forefoot)

Revision arthrodesis
- Nonunion
- Malunion
- Infection (soft tissue or osteomyelitis)
- Complex regional pain syndrome (CRPS) or reflex sympathetic dystrophy (RSD)
- Symptomatic hardware
- Malleolar impingement
- Subtalar arthritis
- Tendon disorders
- Stress fracture
- Lymphedema

Additional Work-up

Ankle fusion is an elective operation, and a well-considered preoperative work-up can help prevent any potential problems. Radiographic studies and laboratory tests can be done to correctly diagnose the problem and plan any future surgical interventions. Standard weight-bearing and non–weight-bearing radiographs to determine static and dynamic deformity will help evaluate for varus or valgus tilt in the ankle or in the subtalar complex. CT is an excellent tool to visualize degenerative changes in the adjacent joints (**Figure 2**) and, in the case of a suspected nonunion, to verify union (**Figure 3**). MRI provides information that is not available on CT and is the best way to visualize soft tissues in and around the ankle. MRI can help diagnose a bony or soft-tissue infection and will help rule out less common causes of pain such as stress fractures, tendon problems, or tumor. Degenerative joint changes will appear as increased signal intensity on T2-weighted images as a result of

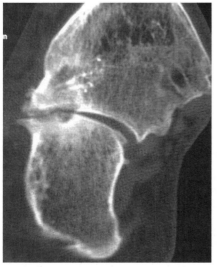

Figure 2 CT scan demonstrating severe subtalar arthritis after an ankle arthrodesis.

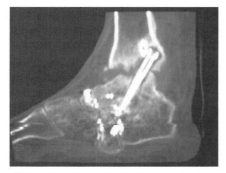

Figure 3 CT scan demonstrating nonunion of the tibiotalar joint.

edema. Although MRI shows infection in the bone and especially the soft tissues, a bone scan or Indium In 111 scan is more specific in diagnosing osteomyelitis and is the best option when the patient has preexisting hardware, which limits the effectiveness of CT and MRI. Once CT and/or MRI detects other possible arthritic joints, selective steroid and anesthetic blocks can be administered in an attempt to eliminate the patient's pain. The other joints may be the sole source of discomfort or an additional source of pain that may need to be addressed in the definitive surgery.

In addition to radiographic and nuclear medicine studies, laboratory studies may be necessary. Erythrocyte sedimentation rate, C-reactive protein, and white blood cell count are needed to determine whether there is an infection. Slightly elevated values usually are not diagnostic of osteomyelitis, but elevated values should at least raise the index of suspicion and necessitate an MRI or Indium In 111 scan. Serum glucose levels should be evaluated to rule out diabetes mellitus. In the presence of diabetes or severe open fractures, vascular studies (Doppler, arteriography) and electromyography and nerve conduction velocity studies can help plan incisions and prevent postoperative complications.

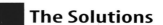

■ The Solutions

Treatment Options and Rationale
APPROACHES
Multiple surgical approaches are available to the skilled surgeon performing an ankle arthrodesis. The location of the incision depends on the surgeon's preference and training, the patient's previous incisions, the de-

gree of deformity, and the fixation technique. The surgeon must be comfortable with all of the exposures to successfully perform revision surgery. Previous incisions, especially if they are well placed and adequately healed, often should be used to prevent potential wound problems. Additionally, all or part of previous incisions will be needed to remove retained hardware. If previous incisions were slow to heal or had drainage and/or infection, other distant incisions should be used. An adequate skin bridge is needed to prevent a wound slough. This bridge is usually between 5 and 7 cm but depends on location, the age of the incision, and the patient's blood supply.

ARTHROSCOPIC
This approach is excellent for patients with minimal deformity and soft-tissue concerns. To minimize complications, arthroscopy should be performed with two or three portals and without skeletal traction. This technique is learning curve dependent and typically should not be used on a revision arthrodesis unless a clear technical error is noted on the primary fusion.

MINIARTHROTOMY
This is one of the most common techniques because it requires minimal soft-tissue dissection, affords good joint visualization, and is less technically demanding than the arthroscopic technique. This exposure comprises two small incisions: one medial to the anterior tibial tendon and one lateral to the peroneus tertius tendon. This technique is best suited for primary arthrodeses but not for revision cases or patients with bone loss or deformity.

ANTERIOR
This is the most common exposure used in ankle arthroplasty. It uses the interval between the anterior tibial tendon medially and the extensor ten-

dons and neurovascular bundle laterally. This approach provides an excellent exposure of the ankle joint but is commonly associated with neuromas of the deep and superficial peroneal nerves and with wound healing problems because of the subcutaneous nature of the joint. This incision is one of the workhorse incisions for complicated fusions, especially after a total ankle arthroplasty.

LATERAL TRANSFIBULAR INCISION

The other workhorse incision for complicated and revision arthrodeses provides excellent visualization of the ankle and subtalar joints via a lateral incision and the subsequent removal of the distal fibula. The removed fibula can be used for bulk bone graft, or it can be used as a lateral vascularized strut graft for added stability and healing. The drawbacks of this approach are the limited medial exposure of the joint and the destruction of the normal ankle anatomy.

POSTERIOR

This uncommon incision uses a trans-Achilles interval to reach the back of the ankle. It is useful in double hindfoot fusions, especially those with previous infections and anterior soft-tissue concerns from previous incisions or open fractures.

FIXATION TECHNIQUES

Many types of fixation are available to perform an ankle fusion, and the well-prepared surgeon must be skilled in their use.

CANNULATED SCREWS

These screws are the most common source of fixation in primary fusions and are reportedly more biomechanically stable than external fixators. Excellent compression across the fusion site can be obtained, and multiple screws can be precisely and safely placed with the use of fluoroscopy. Most authors recommend using at

least three large screws (6.5 to 8.0 mm) placed from the tibia to the talus in the following pattern: medial tibia to medial talus, posterolateral tibia to anteromedial talus, and lateral tibia to lateral talus. In the lateral approach, additional screws can be placed from the lateral talus into the tibia. The use of cannulated screws is limited in patients with bone loss in whom there is insufficient bone to obtain a good purchase distally or when compression across the fusion is not desired, such as in an attempt to maintain height.

PLATES AND SCREWS

These are often needed in complex fusions, especially in patients with bone loss and deformity. Anterior tension plates can be used in conjunction with cannulated screws to reinforce a fusion. A laterally placed blade plate is commonly used in revision surgery, particularly when the fusion is extended to include the subtalar joint. The main drawback associated with the use of plates is the extensive dissection needed to implant the hardware.

ORTHOPAEDIC STAPLES, KIRSCHNER WIRES, AND CERCLAGE WIRES

These implants have no significant place in modern ankle fusions. They offer less stability and compression relative to the other options and should be used only in rare situations in combination with other implants.

INTRAMEDULLARY NAIL

This nail is used only for salvage in ankle fusions because the subtalar joint must also be sacrificed; it is ideal for patients with severe deformity and significant bone loss, especially in the talus. An intramedullary nail is relatively easy to insert but can cause plantar foot pain and may offer limited compression across the fusion sites in patients with poor bone quality.

EXTERNAL FIXATORS

External fixators, specifically ring fixators (ie, Ilizarov), are useful for complex ankle fusions and are ideal for patients with previous infection, bone loss, or deformity. An Ilizarov fixator can simultaneously correct deformity, compress across a fusion site, and lengthen the tibia to correct a limb-length discrepancy caused by bone loss from a failed total ankle arthroplasty. However, the use of fixators has a steep learning curve associated with many complications, and fixators often are poorly tolerated.

FUSION TECHNIQUES

Nonunions, delayed unions, and malunions can be minimized by close attention to detail while preparing the joint surface and in placing the appropriate hardware. The preferred position of the foot in an ankle arthrodesis is as follows: neutral flexion, 5° to 10° external rotation, 5° valgus, and posterior displacement of the foot relative to the tibia. Many proven techniques are used to prepare the fusion site, but they all adhere to the same principles. Unless there is a severe deformity that only can be corrected with straight cuts, I recommend anatomic preparation of the joint surface with curets and osteotomes. This technique will minimize bone loss and prevent thermal necrosis of the bone, which may limit healing.

Whenever possible, it is important to minimize soft-tissue stripping of the joint to maintain the blood supply. All of the cartilage and fibrous tissue must be removed to expose healthy, underlying vascularized bone. Eburnated bone should be improved by fish scaling with an osteotome or drilling with a 2.0- or 2.5-mm drill bit to create vascular access channels.

Fluoroscopy should be used to ensure the appropriate placement of the selected implants. The hardware should be placed meticulously; the near cortex may be notched with a burr to prevent a fracture when inserting sharply angled screws, and the screw threads should be completely across the fusion site to prevent distraction of the joint.

BONE GRAFTING

Many published articles report adequate ankle fusion rates with the use of allograft or no bone graft at all; however, this practice should apply only to the patient who has no nonunion risk factors and is undergoing a primary fusion. Nonunion risk factors include smoking, previous infection, previous open injury, neuropathy, spasticity, pilon fracture, talus osteonecrosis, noncompliance, and major medical problems.

The major sources of autograft are the proximal tibia, the iliac crest, and the ankle (the medial malleolus or distal fibula). Autograft should be used for any revision fusion or any patient with nonunion risk factors. Bone graft can easily be harvested from the proximal tibia with no additional site preparation and with minimal morbidity to the patient. Cancellous bone can be harvested through a small bone window in the proximal lateral tibia; however, the amount of adequate bone is limited, and no structural bone can be obtained. The proximal tibia is best suited for the basic fusion with no significant bone loss or deformity or in addition to allograft.

Whenever there is a large bony defect, the iliac crest should be used because of the large amount of available cancellous and cortical bone. The downside of the iliac crest is the associated morbidity, especially when structural graft is obtained. The last option for bone graft is to sacrifice one or both malleoli. This is not recommended for a primary fusion but can enhance the exposure and give valuable bone for a primary or revision with bone loss and deformity. Additionally, allograft such as cancellous chips or demineralized bone matrix and systems that combine fibrin and the patient's own platelet-rich plasma

can be added to the autograft to extend its use.

Occasionally, large bulk allograft (femoral head, strut grafts) can be used in conjunction with autograft to fill large bone defects. Unfortunately, this technique is associated with an increased nonunion and malunion rate, and the amount of structural allograft used should be limited. Furthermore, the use of allografts is associated with lower fusion rates in patients with previous infection. Options for very large defects include vascularized grafts such as the fibula or the use of an Ilizarov fixator to slowly regenerate the required amount of bone.

BONE STIMULATORS

Implantable electric stimulators may be beneficial in enhancing fusion rates in patients with previous nonunion or in unfavorable healing environments. Previous studies have shown a relationship between electric current and new bone growth. Although no controlled studies prove the efficacy of implantable stimulators, multiple anecdotal reports show that they do appear to be helpful and safe in obtaining fusions in difficult situations. External electric bone stimulators may also be beneficial for complicated fusions; however, their success rates are lower because of the extended periods of time that they are required to be worn and the subsequent patient noncompliance.

Another option to enhance bone healing is ultrasound (Exogen, Smith and Nephew, Andover, MA). Multiple studies have shown accelerated fracture healing with the use of low-intensity pulsed ultrasound. The use of ultrasound in ankle fusions is only anecdotal at this time, but this treatment option is well tolerated by patients because it is used for only 20 minutes once or twice per day. Fusion rates may also be improved by pharmacologic means. Medicines typically used to treat osteoporosis (calcium, alendr-

onate sodium, calcitonin-salmon) may be able to enhance fusion rates in select patient populations. None of the specific bone stimulating options are statistically proven to increase fusion times and rates, but their use should be strongly considered in patients with complicated fusions and nonunion risk factors.

ADDITIONAL PROCEDURES

Normal overall limb alignment is important in obtaining a functional and pain-free ankle arthrodesis. Malalignment increases point contact forces, which can lead to chronic overload arthritis and instability. The basic tenet is that proximal deformities should be corrected first. Moreover, correction should be obtained at the level of the deformity and not by compensatory cuts at distal sites. For dynamic problems, soft-tissue procedures such as an Achilles tendon lengthening, gastrocnemius recession, or tendon transfers can be done. For fixed deformity, osteotomies are usually required. For deformity above the ankle, which affects the alignment of the leg, a supramalleolar osteotomy is indicated to restore the normal axis. For patients with smaller deformities, opening or closing wedge osteotomies can be performed at the medial tibia with plates and screws. For larger deformities, an external fixator may be used to help generate new bone and prevent additional shortening.

When deformity exists at the ankle joint, but does not affect overall limb axis, such as in a fracture malunion, a simple malleolar osteotomy can be performed to prevent impingement and improve the cosmetic appearance of the joint.

Deformities distal to the ankle joint also should be addressed to provide the patient with a plantigrade foot. In patients with a varus or valgus hindfoot, a calcaneal osteotomy is indicated. With a varus ankle, a Dwyer calcaneal osteotomy can be done at the same time as the ankle fusion. Similarly, a medializing calcaneal slide can be done for a valgus hindfoot. Attention also should be paid to the forefoot. In a cavovarus or planovalgus foot, the first metatarsal may need to be realigned with a dorsiflexing or plantar flexing osteotomy.

Author's Preferred Treatment and Rationale

All of the previously discussed treatment options must be considered when approaching the surgical decision-making process. Although the overall principles and goals for fusions remain the same, there are many acceptable plans for each specific case, as described below.

BASIC FUSION

For a simple fusion with minimal deformity and bone loss, I recommend miniarthrotomy with anatomic bony cuts and the placement of three large cannulated screws (**Figure 4**). I usually use proximal tibial autograft; however, if a patient has minimal nonunion risk factors, demineralized bone matrix can be used. For surgeons skilled in arthroscopic techniques, this approach can be used in basic or revision arthrodeses with no deformity.

ANKLE WITH DEFORMITY

The deformity must be located and addressed before the ankle fusion. In patients with milder deformities, the anterior approach is used to spare the malleoli. However, the lateral approach often is used in more severe deformity. Additional procedures (supramalleolar, calcaneal, or metatarsal osteotomies) may be needed to restore the normal axis of the leg. Deformity localized to the ankle can be corrected with bony cuts or soft-tissue balancing. Straight cuts can be used to realign the joint with previous varus or valgus deformity. Bone-sparing cuts should be used to prevent significant shortening of the leg. If flat bony surfaces can be obtained, cannulated screws can be used. To further stabilize the fusion site, I often place a small plate (one third tubular or 3.5 dynamic compression plate) anteriorly over the ankle joint in addition to the cannulated screws (**Figure 5**).

On occasion, structural bone graft must be added to correct the deformity and prevent shortening of the leg. Whenever possible, autograft (iliac crest) should be used when structural bone is needed. Plates and screws are commonly used to secure the structural bone graft and to stabilize the fusion site by holding it in position until the graft is incorporated. The plate should be placed near the graft site to contain the graft and give added stability. Cannulated screws are not recommended for this purpose because their compression may recreate the deformity or they may fracture the structural bone graft.

NONUNION

Before operating on a patient with a nonunion, the cause of the nonunion must be determined. Three major causes are technical error (the surgeon), noncompliance (the patient), and local or systemic problems. In the case of a technical error, the hardware should be removed and the fusion approached like a primary fusion, with the addition of autograft and cannulated screws and the possible use of a postoperative bone stimulator.

Noncompliant patients should be cautioned about the risk of nonunion with cigarette smoking and re-educated about the postoperative weight-

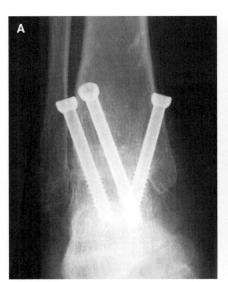
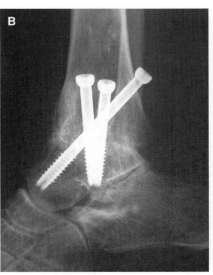

Figure 4 AP **(A)** and lateral **(B)** radiographs of the ankle showing cannulated screw technique. The lateral view shows possible screw penetration of the subtalar joint. Intraoperative Broden views can help in the safe and proper placement of the screws.

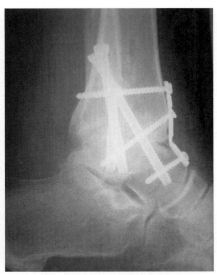

Figure 5 Lateral radiograph of the ankle showing fusion with cannulated screws and an anterior tension plate.

bearing expectations. They may require cannulated screws and plates for extra stability. Furthermore, the noncompliant patient may benefit from an implantable bone stimulator (**Figure 6**).

Local and systemic problems refer to previous or present infections, soft-tissue problems, or medical problems (ie, diabetes mellitus, neuropathy). Each of these specific problems must be addressed in the new treatment plan. Soft-tissue problems may require a plastic surgery or vascular surgery consult to prevent further problems. General medical problems are associated with lower fusion rates; therefore, these patients should have limited soft-tissue dissections, autograft, stable constructs, and consideration for a bone stimulator.

INFECTION

In most patients, any previous or present infection must be eradicated before obtaining a solid fusion. Infection should be treated in a staged fashion; the first step is to débride the infected bone and soft tissues and place antibiotic-impregnated beads. The patient then usually needs to be treated with 6 weeks of intravenous antibiotics. Laboratory tests can be monitored

to check if the infection has been adequately treated. Once the infection has been addressed, the beads can be removed and a fusion performed. I usually use an external fixator to minimize the amount of hardware in the ankle. Additionally, the fixator can be used to correct any deformity resulting from the surgical débridement.

TALAR OSTEONECROSIS

MRI and/or CT may be used to determine the extent of talar osteonecrosis and the involvement of the subtalar joint. If there is no bone loss and no subtalar joint involvement, a simple fusion can be performed with cannulated screws and a proximal tibial bone graft. In the case of talar bone loss but no subtalar joint disease, an ankle fusion can be performed with autograft and an external fixator or plates and screws, depending on the amount of talus available for fixation. When there is subtalar joint destruction, a tibiotalocalcaneal fusion is recommended. This fusion is performed by a lateral approach, harvesting the fibula for bone graft and fixing the ankle with a lateral plate or an intramedullary nail (**Figure 7**). Finally, when there is severe talar destruction, a tibiocalcaneal fusion is preferred over a Blair procedure (sliding tibial bone graft). The tibiocalcaneal fusion should be done with a laterally placed

blade plate to maximize the limited purchase in the calcaneus.

FUSION AFTER A FAILED TOTAL ANKLE ARTHROPLASTY

The difficulty in performing a fusion after a total ankle arthroplasty depends on three main factors: the amount of bone loss present once the implant is removed, the remaining talus and subtalar involvement, and the presence of infection. The other factor to consider is how the patient wants to treat a possible limb-length discrepancy. A defect less than 2 cm warrants primarily bone grafting and then using shoe modifications to make up the deficit. A defect greater than 2 cm will result in a noticeable limb-length discrepancy unless either a bulk structural autograft (iliac crest) or an Ilizarov-type device is used to lengthen the leg. It is important to discuss the limb-length discrepancy with the patient before surgery because the patient's choice to accept or correct this problem dictates the rest of the care.

If the bone defect is less than 2 cm, a fusion can be attempted in the typical fashion. The entire defect does not have to be made up to ensure a good result but, if the patient consents, structural autograft from the pelvis and/or the fibula can be used to fill the defect and enhance the fusion.

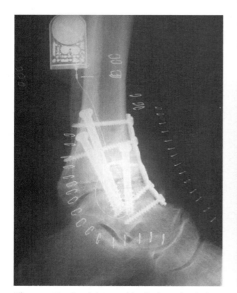

Figure 6 Revision ankle fusion depicting implantable bone stimulator.

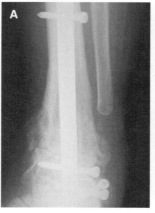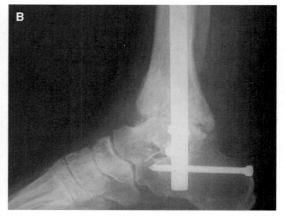

Figure 7 AP (**A**) and lateral (**B**) radiographs of the ankle and subtalar fusion with an intramedullary nail.

I prefer a plate and screws for fixation because there usually is not enough remaining bone to use cannulated screws alone. Depending on the previous incisions and any deformity, a large spoon plate can be placed anteriorly or a cannulated blade plate can be placed laterally.

If there is a major bony defect, but the patient is not committed to the required procedures to restore the previous length, I recommend packing as much autograft as possible with additional nonstructural allograft and performing the fusion as previously discussed. The medial and/or lateral malleoli may need to be resected to prevent malleolar impingement if there is significant shortening of the tibia on the talus. Large bulk allograft, such as a femoral head, can be used to fill the bony defect, but many authors have reported decreased fusion rates with structural allograft in the ankle. Even if the patient elects to fuse the ankle in the shortened position, the leg can be lengthened at a later time if the patient is unhappy with the outcome.

If the patient is committed to correcting a large defect, I recommend using an Ilizarov or ring fixator to perform a bone transport and lengthening with a simultaneous ankle fusion in a staged fashion. In the first stage, the ankle implant is removed and the joint is débrided. An Ilizarov frame is placed on the tibia and ankle, and a proximal tibial corticotomy is performed. For the ankle, pins are placed in the distal tibia and wires and pins are placed in the calcaneus. The tibia is lengthened proximally, and the tibial segment is transported distally. Any deformities resulting from the implant can be corrected at this time. Prior to docking of the tibia on the talus, the patient is brought back to the operating room and the ankle joint is débrided and bone grafted with iliac crest, distal fibula, or allograft putty.

At this time, a pin or wire is placed in the talus for extra stability. It is placed in this delayed fashion to prevent early loosening associated with placement at the time of the original corticotomy. Once the ankle is grafted, the Ilizarov is used to obtain circumferential compression across the ankle and to allow early weight bearing.

In patients whose ankle implant has failed and caused destruction of the talus, a tibiotalocalcaneal fusion is indicated. I recommend using the distal fibula for bulk autograft to regain some of the lost length. If leg length is not a major concern, the intramedullary nail is an excellent way to perform the fusion and stabilize the hindfoot. The other option is to use a cannulated blade plate placed laterally into the calcaneus. Again, if there is a large bony defect, an Ilizarov can be used to assist with the fusions and/or correct the leg lengths.

Infection is the final problem concerning fusion after a total ankle arthroplasty. The ankle implant must be removed, and then the joint should be thoroughly débrided and antibiotic-impregnated beads placed. The patient should receive 6 weeks of intravenous antibiotics and then a course of oral antibiotics. In patients with previous infections, bulk bone grafting with internal fixation is less likely to succeed because of the risks of nonunion and recurrent infection. I recommend the use of an external fixator to obtain an ankle fusion in this select group of patients. Additionally, a bone transport can be used to enhance the blood supply to the fusion and correct any limb-length discrepancy.

Management of Complications

Not only is it important to know how to perform the fusion, but it is also necessary to know how to diagnose and treat potential postoperative complications. Wound problems should be actively managed with local wound care, dressing changes, and immobilization. Larger wounds should be surgically débrided and evaluated by a plastic surgeon. Clean wounds can be treated with becaplermin or suction therapy if plastic surgery coverage is not necessary.

Oral and/or intravenous antibiotics should be used for cellulitis. Drainage or persistent swelling and redness in the legs should be further evaluated for deep infection via laboratory tests and MRI and/or Indium In 111 scan.

Deep venous thrombosis and/or pulmonary embolus should be considered in any patient with persistent leg swelling, palpable cords in the leg, or unexplained shortness of breath. Venous doppler, nuclear medicine studies, or spiral lung CT should be ordered to rule out these potentially fatal complications. Patients at risk for deep venous thrombosis should be taking pharmacologic prophylaxis during the initial postoperative period.

Incisional neuroma can be treated with scar desensitization and steroid and marcaine injections. Persistent pain can be treated with excision of the neuroma and burying the nerve in bone or muscle.

Adjacent joint pain is treated initially with orthotics and shoe wear modifications; however, it may require a fusion for persistent pain. Use compression stockings and aggressive physiotherapy for lymphedema. The key to treatment of chronic regional pain syndrome is the early diagnosis. In these instances, the patient should be referred to a pain specialist for therapy, medication, and possible injections.

Delayed union can be diagnosed with CT. Consider an indolent infection in patients with previous drainage. If there are no signs of infection, the patient may benefit from a bone stimulator.

References

Buck P, Morrey BF, Chao EYS: The optimum position of arthrodesis of the ankle. *J Bone Joint Surg Am* 1987;69:1052-1062.

Carlsson AS, Montgomery F, Besjakov J: Arthrodesis of the ankle secondary to replacement. *Foot Ankle* 1998;19:240-245.

Mann RA, Rongstad KM: Arthrodesis of the ankle: A critical analysis. *Foot Ankle* 1998;19:3-9.

Manoli A, Beals TC, Hansen ST: Technical factors in hindfoot arthrodesis. *Instr Course Lect* 1999;48:347-356.

Midis N, Conti SF: Revision ankle arthrodesis. *Foot Ankle Int* 2002;23:243-247.

Coding

ICD-9 CODES

250.02	Diabetes mellitus without mention of complication; type II (non-insulin dependent type) (NIDDM type) (adult-onset type) or unspecified type, uncontrolled
711.97	Arthropathy associated with infections, arthroplasty associated with other bacterial diseases, ankle and foot
714.0	Rheumatoid arthritis and other inflammatory polyarthropathies, rheumatoid arthritis
716.97	Other and unspecified arthropathies, arthropathy, unspecified, ankle and foot
718.4	Other derangement of joint, contracture of joint
719.27	Villonodular synovitis, ankle and foot
726.91	Exostosis of unspecified site
727.81	Other disorders of synovium, tendon, and bursa, contracture of tendon (sheath)
730.07	Acute osteomyelitis, ankle and foot
730.17	Chronic osteomyelitis, ankle and foot
733.81	Other disorders of bone and cartilage, malunion and nonunion of fracture, malunion of fracture
733.82	Malunion and nonunion of fracture, nonunion of fracture
736.74	Other acquired deformities of ankle and foot, claw foot, acquired
736.81	Other acquired deformities of limbs, acquired deformities of other parts of limbs, unequal leg length (acquired)
892.1	Open wound of foot except toe(s) alone, complicated
905.4	Late effects of musculoskeletal and connective tissue injuries, late effect of fracture of lower extremities
905.7	Late effect of sprain and strain without mention of tendon injury
996.4	Complications peculiar to certain specified procedures, mechanical complication of internal orthopaedic device, implant and graft

Coding

CPT CODES

20680 Removal of implant; deep (eg, buried wire, pin, screw, metal band, nail, rod or plate)

20692 Application of a multiplane (pins or wires in more than one plane), unilateral, external fixation system (eg, Ilizarov, Monticelli type)

20900 Bone graft, any donor area; minor or small (eg, dowel or button)

27606 Tenotomy, percutaneous, Achilles tendon (separate procedure); general anesthesia

27640 Partial excision (craterization, saucerization, or diaphysectomy) bone (eg, osteomyelitis or exostosis); tibia

27641 Partial excision (craterization, saucerization, or diaphysectomy) bone (eg, osteomyelitis or exostosis); fibula

27687 Gastrocnemius recession (eg, Strayer procedure)

27704 Removal of ankle implant

27705 Osteotomy; tibia

27707 Osteotomy; fibula

27715 Osteoplasty, tibia and fibula, lengthening or shortening

27720 Repair of nonunion or malunion, tibia; without graft (eg, leg compression technique)

27870 Arthrodesis, ankle, open

28300 Osteotomy; calcaneus (eg, Dwyer or Chambers type procedure), with or without internal fixation

28306 Osteotomy, with or without lengthening, shortening, or angular correction, metatarsal; first metatarsal

28725 Arthrodesis; subtalar

CPT copyright © 2003 by the American Medical Association. All Rights Reserved.

fixation for distraction. The Agility

sure is applied. Almost all loose talar components are associated with some degree of settling. Unless the talus is split, the component will collapse until it reaches the subchondral bone of the posterior facet of the talus, at which point it will stop. It will then move in a "windshield wiper" pattern, creating a wider fin slot in the medial to lateral direction. If difficulty is encountered in removal, the external fixator is placed on the previously inserted pins, and distraction is applied. Care must be taken to avoid prying against a stable tibial component and loosening it. If the polyethylene component is in the way, it is removed. The newer polyethylene inserts have short side pillars for easy extraction, but older inserts have long pillars that may make them difficult to remove. In these instances, an osteotome is used to split the insert. Although a saw can be used, its use is avoided to minimize polyethylene debris.

Once the polytheylene insert and the talar component are removed, the tibial tray is tested for stability. If it is stable, attention turns to the talus, which is cleaned of bone debris, osteophytes, and fibrous tissue. The external fixator is then used to reposition the talus so that it is parallel to the tibial tray. The cut surface of the talus may have to be recut to be parallel, and this step may require a freehand cut using a sagittal saw. In my experience, replacing the jig is exceedingly difficult and not worth the tourniquet time it expends. The fin slot should be very carefully prepared, with great care taken to minimize bone removal because at the present time, no wide fin revision components exist. In my experience, no additional bone graft can be added to the talus. Graft can neither be secured nor develop ingrowth at the bone-bone and bone-metal interface quickly enough to guarantee component stabilization. As a result, no graft is used on the talar side.

Trial components are then placed, using a 2-mm polyethylene insert and

usually a 2-mm tibial trial component. This will add 4 mm to the arthroplasty and usually suffices in restoring the loss of height due to the settling of the talar component. Rotation of the talar component is critical, and the alignment handle often is inserted into the tibial tray to confirm position of the talus relative to the tibia and the foot. Gutters are carefully evaluated after distraction is released from the external fixator because once the patient begins weight bearing, excess talar bone will impinge on the long metal pillars of the tibial tray. This bone is removed, using a reciprocating saw, after the trial components are removed. If the talar trial component is grossly unstable and cannot be secured, revision is aborted and the ankle is fused.

Once height and gutters are deemed acceptable, trial components are removed, and the ankle is washed and dried until it is clean, dry, and absent of bone debris. The ankle is gently distracted using the external fixator. The tibial polyethylene component is then placed in the tibial tray.

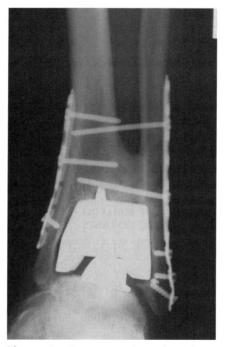

Figure 4 Custom prosthesis for a large erosion defect of the tibia.

The talar component fin and under-surface are covered with PRP to assist in healing, and the component is inserted. The external fixator may have to be removed to allow maximum plantar flexion to insert the talar component. Once the talus is seated, it is evaluated for stability, and it should be fairly stable. Occasionally, manual compression applied in a open-handed striking motion to the heel is required. If the component is deemed stable, standard closure and splinting are performed. Total tourniquet time should not exceed 150 minutes.

Aftercare requires that the patient be placed in a short leg weight-bearing cast. The patient is instructed to remain in non–weight-bearing status for at least 6 weeks, except for 10 minutes each morning and evening. During this time, the patient stands with his or her weight evenly distributed on both legs. Rocking, single leg stance, and ambulation are strictly avoided. Sutures are removed at 6 weeks, the patient is placed in a pre-fabricated removable boot at this time, and partial weight bearing is begun in the boot with either crutches or a walker. The patient should be able to begin unsupported weight bearing by 12 weeks based on fluoroscopically controlled radiographic evidence of healing across the bone-implant interface.

TIBIAL COMPONENT

If the tibial component is loose, and the syndesmosis is healed, there is no way at the present time to remove the prosthesis without removing the talar component, even if it is stable. This is a limitation of the current design, which hopefully will be corrected in the future. If the tibial component is loose without erosion of the tibia, both components are removed, and a new, larger size total ankle prosthesis is inserted using standard methods. If erosion of the tibia is evident, then structural iliac crest bone graft is obtained to allow repositioning of the implant. Allograft is not advised because no ingrowth into a dead piece of

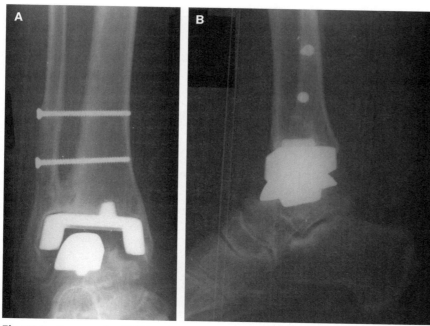

Figure 5 Preoperative AP (**A**) and lateral (**B**) views of failed total ankle arthroplasty secondary to recurrent synovitis and foreign body reaction.

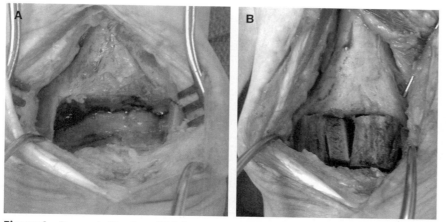

Figure 6 Removal of implants (**A**) followed by interposition of tricortical iliac crest graft (**B**). Allograft may be used instead.

bone will occur, and this lack of ingrowth may ultimately cause loosening of the prosthesis again. If excessive erosion is evident on preoperative radiographs, a custom prosthesis is considered (**Figure 4**).

REVISION TO AN ANKLE ARTHRODESIS
Although anecdotal evidence suggests that a double hindfoot fusion is required to salvage failure of an Agility Total Ankle Replacement, this has not been my experience with the six conversions to ankle fusion that I have performed (**Figure 5**). The technique described below allows for sparing of the subtalar joint and will restore the length and alignment to the affected limb.

Once the prosthesis has been removed and the decision to fuse the ankle has been made, all bone surfaces are curetd back to healthy bleeding bone (**Figure 6**). A laminar spreader can be inserted into the defect, and correct tension can be seen with use of lateral fluoroscopic control. The gap is then measured with a ruler, and a fresh-frozen femoral head allograft is obtained. Once the allograft has soaked in a water bath, it is shaped until it fits perfectly into the defect. The bone that was removed from the allograft during shaping is morcellized and mixed with demineralized bone matrix and PRP. Similarly, the femoral head allograft is soaked in PRP until it has percolated through the entire allograft.

The slurry of bone graft is then applied to all the raw bone surfaces and the ankle joint, and PPR is injected into this area again. The femoral head interpositional allograft is then inserted, and position and alignment are verified using intraoperative fluoroscopy. A large fragment (4.5-mm) spoon plate (Synthes, Paoli, PA) is then placed across the ankle (**Figure 7**). The plate may require slight bending distally to fit but should be almost acceptable without much manipulation. It is secured to the tibia with a bicortical screw in the middle of the slot hole to permit sliding of the plate if needed. With the C-arm in the lateral position, three 6.5-mm fully threaded (noncannulated) screws are inserted through the three horizontal holes at the distal end of the plate into the talar body, avoiding the subtalar joint. Except in the most severe situations, ample bone exists to secure these screws. Once the screws are inserted, the articulating tension device (ATD) is applied to the proximal end of the plate, the screw in the slot hole is loosened slightly, and gentle compression is applied. When compression is obtained, the screw is retightened, and the remaining screws are applied in the plate. The ATD and the screw in the slot hole are removed, and position and alignment are verified. Additional lag screws may be placed if needed, but care should be

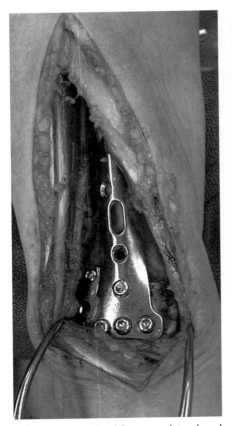

Figure 7 Anterior AO spoon plate placed anteriorly across the ankle.

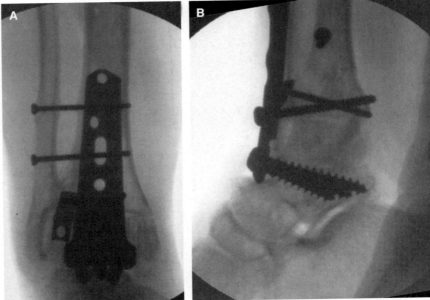

Figure 8 AP (**A**) and lateral (**B**) views of a completed fusion sparing the subtalar joint.

taken not to split the graft. A final lag screw may be placed from the fibula into the talar body if needed. The remainder of the graft and PRP are applied, and the wound is closed in a standard manner. To prevent loss of the PRP, no drain is used. The tourniquet is removed, and a splint is applied.

Aftercare includes casting and non–weight-bearing status for 12 weeks until evidence of fusion is observed (**Figure 8**). Sutures are usually removed at 6 weeks. Physical therapy and progressive weight bearing in a prefabricated boot may be begun at 12 weeks. The patient should be back to activities of daily living by 14 weeks after surgery.

Management of Complications
When a superficial infection is evident, suppressive antibiotics coupled with rest may prevent a deep infection; however, once a deep infection exists failure ultimately will occur. There are rare instances in which an acute deep infection can be eradicated with aggressive open débridement and intravenous antibiotics. Most patients will present with signs and symptoms of a deep-seated infection months after successful implantation of the prosthesis. Treatment is similar to that of other total joint arthroplasties.

The patient is brought to the operating room for removal of the prosthesis. Cultures are obtained, and obviously dead bone is removed using a high-speed burr. Antibiotic-impreg-nated beads or an antibiotic-impregnated cement spacer (made of 1 g tobramycin per packet of bone cement) is inserted and the wound closed. Culture-specific antibiotics are begun intravenously, with the patient typically followed-up by an infectious disease specialist for management of the antibiotic course and duration. After several surgical washouts, the patient is discharged to home. After appropriate antibiotic treatment, usually 6 to 8 weeks, the patient is brought back to the operating room for débridement and cultures. If the cultures are postive, the above sequence is repeated; if they are negative, a fusion as described in the previous section can be performed. However, tricortical iliac crest graft should be used. Aftercare is similar to that for fusion without infection.

References

None

Coding

ICD CODE

733.8   Nonunion and malunion of fracture

CPT CODES

20680   Removal of implant; deep (eg, buried wire, pin, screw, metal band, nail, rod, or plate)

20902   Bone graft, any donor area; major or large

27620   Arthrotomy, ankle, with joint exploration, with or without biopsy, with or without removal of loose or foreign body

27640   Partial excision (craterization, saucerization, or diaphysectomy) bone (eg, osteomyelitis or exostosis); tibia

27641   Partial excision (craterization, saucerization, or diaphysectomy) bone (eg, osteomyelitis or exostosis); fibula

27687   Gastrocnemius recession (eg, Strayer procedure)

27703   Arthroplasty, ankle; revision, total ankle

27704   Removal of ankle implant

27871   Arthrodesis, tibiofibular joint, proximal or distal

28120   Partial excision (craterization, saucerization, sequestrectomy, or diaphysectomy) bone (eg, osteomyelitis or bossing); talus or calcaneus

29894   Arthroscopy, ankle (tibiotalar and fibulotalar joints), surgical; with removal of loose body or foreign body

No code Insertion antibiotic beads/spacer

CPT copyright © 2003 by the American Medical Association. All Rights Reserved.

Pantalar Arthritis
George E. Quill, Jr, MD

Definition of the Problem

Patient Presentation

Patients with pantalar arthritis present with symptoms at the ankle (tibiotalar), subtalar (talocalcaneal), and/or transverse tarsal (talonavicular and calcaneocuboid) joints. Most patients do not have arthritic involvement in all these sites.

The history, physical examination, and radiographs are usually sufficient for establishing which joint or joints are affected. Additional imaging studies such as tomography, CT, MRI, or arthrography, as well as differential injection of local anesthetic, can further elucidate the diagnosis in more complicated cases.

Pantalar arthritis may occur in adolescents, adults, or the elderly. Pain, swelling, and limited range of motion (usually a loss of dorsiflexion associated with anterior tibiotalar osteophytes) are common. Patients occasionally describe locking resulting from intra-articular loose bodies or incongruities. Patients with ankle arthritis do not necessarily have worse symptoms when walking on uneven ground than when walking on level surfaces, but they often have difficulty ascending and descending stairs. Those with tibiotalar arthritis may give a history of prior trauma or frequent, repetitive ankle sprains. Patients with subtalar pathology almost always have more difficulty ambulating on uneven ground than on level

surfaces. Locking is less common than stiffness in these patients. Patients with arthritis of the transverse tarsal joints will often have a fallen arch or a stiff, painful foot. These patients may have deformity in any plane or a normal biomechanical axis while bearing weight.

Physical Examination

A thorough physical examination is necessary to evaluate the relative position of the hip and knee, calf atrophy, peroneal spasm, joint range of motion, trophic changes, callus formation, abnormal gait pattern, or shoe wear abnormalities. Thorough sensory, vascular, motor, and reflex examinations are necessary as well.

Patients with advanced ankle arthritis have a warm joint with synovial hyperplasia manifested by circumferential thickness. Anterior drawer and varus-valgus tilt testing may confirm or rule out pathologic instability.

With subtalar arthritis there is more tenderness at the sinus tarsi than medially. Because the sinus tarsi is more voluminous than the superficial ankle and transverse tarsal joints, swelling may not always be obvious in patients with mild to moderate ankle arthritis. The fat pad at the anterior process of the calcaneus and origin of the intrinsic toe extensors may be more prominent with subtalar involvement.

The transverse tarsal joints are more superficial, and swelling in this region is more easily seen. With ad-

vanced involvement, there may be subluxation of the talonavicular complex, loss of the normal longitudinal medial arch, and prominence of the talar head plantar medially. A valgus hindfoot, an abducted and varus forefoot, and loss of the longitudinal arch may be associated with subfibular impingement and lateral abutment that may occur with peroneal tenosynovitis.

Pantalar arthritis may accompany pes cavovarus deformity and a plantar flexed first ray with abnormal wear on the lateral border of the foot and a rigid varus hindfoot. There may be associated tibiotalar instability. The peroneal tendons may be subluxated from the fibula, crepitant, and thickened.

Radiographic evaluation includes weight-bearing AP and lateral views of the foot, a weight-bearing AP view of the ankle, and a 30° internal oblique view of the foot. The standard AP, mortise, and lateral views of the ankle can be obtained if needed. Broden views may be obtained by positioning the supine lower extremity with 10° to 15° of internal rotation and angling the x-ray beam 10° to 30° cephalad from vertical. These views may be helpful in evaluating the posterior facet of the subtalar joint after trauma or open reduction of a calcaneal fracture.

Joint space narrowing, osteophyte formation, and subchondral sclerosis or cysts are characteristic of osteoarthritis. Posttraumatic fracture deformity and hardware from prior fixation may be present. Rheumatoid arthritis and other inflammatory arthritides may be associated with periarticular erosions, soft-tissue swelling, and osteopenia.

Neuropathic arthrosis or Charcot neuroarthropathy is characterized by numerous fractures or microfractures in various stages of healing, hypertrophic new bone formation, and loss of normal weight-bearing architecture. Bone resorption may be seen along with vascular calcification and joint subluxation or dislocation.

Plain tomography may be helpful in evaluating union of fractures or arthrodesis and the integrity of existing hardware. CT in the axial and coronal planes (section width, 1.5 mm) may be helpful, but three-dimensional reconstructions are not helpful in the routine setting. MRI may complement CT by evaluating for fluid in and around the joints, bone marrow edema, infection, talar vascularity, and periarticular tendon and ligament pathology.

Technetium Tc 99m bone scans may be useful in the evaluation of osteonecrosis after talus fracture, arthritic involvement of one or several joints, stress fracture, or neoplasm. Indium-labeled white blood cell scans can be helpful in the diagnosis of osteomyelitis or septic arthritis.

Differential Diagnosis

- Primary and secondary osteoarthrosis, including posttraumatic osteoarthritis

- Rheumatoid arthritis and other inflammatory arthritides (gout, pseudogout, pigmented villonodular synovitis, septic arthritis, psoriatic arthritis, spondyloarthropathy, Reiter's syndrome)

- Neuropathic (Charcot) arthropathy (diabetes mellitus, spinal cord injury, hereditary sensory motor neuropathy, syringomyelia, congenital indifference to pain, alcoholism, peripheral nerve disease, tabes dorsalis, and leprosy)

- Infectious arthritis (sepsis, open trauma, or previous surgical procedures for fixation of fractures)

- Arthritis and joint subluxation resulting from generalized ligamentous laxity, mixed connective tissue disease, posterior tibial tendinopathy, spring ligament insufficiency

Additional Work-up

The selective injection of local anesthetic may help locate the exact anatomic source of the patient's pain. It is not uncommon for a patient being evaluated for the possibility of pantalar arthritis to have a painful, stiff joint that appears normal on radiographs. The injection of 5 to 10 mL of 1% lidocaine into the subtalar joint or of even lesser quantities into one of the transverse tarsal joints can clarify whether the joint in question is contributing to the patient's pain. Alternatively, the injection may be carefully placed in the tenosynovial sheath of the peroneal tendons when evaluating a patient who may have tendon pathology but a more normal- appearing ankle or hindfoot joint.

The Solutions

Treatment Options and Rationale

The goals of management are to alleviate pain, correct deformity, and improve function. Nonsurgical treatment options include bracing and shoe wear modifications. However, bracing alone without surgery will not alleviate symptoms while the patient is barefoot, halt the progression of the arthritis, or correct any fixed deformity.

The goals of managing pantalar arthritis can usually be attained by adhering to the following principles: (1) fuse painful joints; (2) fuse as few joints as possible; (3) correct the deformity and maintain the normal biomechanical axis in three planes; (4) consider the patient's age, height, and desired activity level before recommending a treatment plan; (5) consider ankle arthroplasty, which is controversial but may be helpful; (6) provide rigid fixation for arthrodesis; (7) use bone grafts and cast immobilization where indicated; (8) consider external or implantable electrical bone stimulation for revision or neuroarthropathy; and (9) provide frequent postoperative follow-up, including rehabilitation, shoe wear selection, and restoration of the patient to the highest possible level of function.

There are several options for treatment of the patient with pantalar arthritis. A nonarticulated polypropylene ankle-foot orthosis (AFO) is often helpful after ankle or tibiotalocalcaneal arthrodesis in the patient with continued transverse tarsal disease. The patient with late ankle problems after triple arthrodesis may benefit from a nonarticulated or articulated AFO.

Steroid injection is justified infrequently and only of temporary benefit for the patient with pantalar arthritis. There are no published long-term data to confirm significant benefit with injected viscosupplementation of the ankle or hindfoot joints.

Ankle or even subtalar arthroscopy is reserved for patients with monarticular mechanical problems such as intra-articular loose bodies, abutting osteophytes, or talar dome osteochondral defects. Open or arthroscopic synovectomy may be helpful for patients with rheumatoid arthritis. Abrasion chondroplasty has not been proved to be of long-term benefit. Arthroscopic or open anterior tibiotalar cheilectomy can improve ankle dorsiflexion by removing abutting osteophytes if joint architecture posterior to the osteophytes is normal.

Osteotomy of the distal tibia, distal fibula, or calcaneus is rarely helpful in the patient with mild osteoarthritis associated with angular deformity. There is no proven benefit from osteotomy in patients with inflammatory arthritis because of involvement of the entire joint.

The primary procedure for the orthopaedist managing pantalar arthritis is arthrodesis. Total ankle replacement is controversial but is gaining wider acceptance, and short-term data are favorable for appropriately selected patients.

Author's Preferred Treatment and Rationale

In practice, the orthopaedic surgeon treating pantalar arthritis relies on the following five procedures: ankle (tibiotalar), subtalar (talocalcaneal), tibiotalocalcaneal, triple (subtalar and transverse tarsal), and pantalar (fusion of the talus to all the bones with which it articulates: tibia, calcaneus, navicular, and cuboid) arthrodesis. Arthroplasty options include total ankle arthroplasty as an isolated procedure or combined with subtalar or triple arthrodesis. The arthroplasty can be performed simultaneously with the arthrodesis or secondarily as a staged procedure after the arthrodesis. The indications for these procedures are best illustrated by example.

Isolated tibiotalar arthritis usually is treated with ankle arthrodesis, which can be done using a transfibular approach with cannulated screw fixation. Isolated subtalar arthritis, such as that observed after displaced intra-articular calcaneus fracture, is managed with in situ subtalar arthrodesis. If there is major diminution of the talar declination angle, bone-block distraction subtalar arthrodesis is indicated. Cannulated screw fixation and

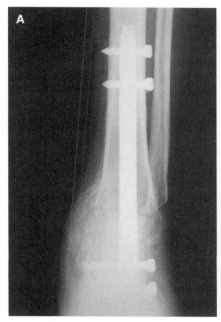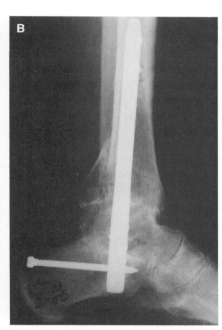

Figure 1 AP **(A)** and lateral **(B)** radiographs of a 55-year-old woman with diabetes mellitus who has profound neuropathic arthropathy 3 months after undergoing tibiotalocalcaneal arthrodesis. She had a trimalleolar fracture-dislocation that was initially treated with open reduction and internal fixation, but it progressed to nonunion. It was successfully salvaged with removal of the initial hardware and tibiotalocalcaneal arthrodesis with intramedullary nail fixation.

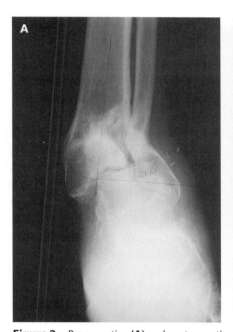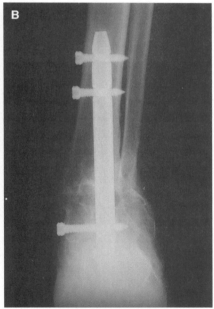

Figure 2 Preoperative **(A)** and postoperative **(B)** radiographs of a 60-year-old woman with oxygen-dependent emphysema who had an open ankle fracture-dislocation with resultant osteomyelitis and persistent deformity. She underwent numerous prior attempts at salvage and was referred for consideration of below-knee amputation. The ankle was salvaged successfully with distal tibiotalar realignment osteotomy and tibiotalocalcaneal arthrodesis with intramedullary nail fixation. She currently is ambulatory with a plantigrade foot and has no sign of infection.

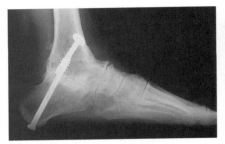

Figure 3 Weight-bearing lateral radiograph of a 51-year-old woman 10 years after undergoing successful tibiotalocalcaneal fusion using cannulated screw fixation. Note the presence of osteophytes and joint space narrowing at the transverse tarsal joints.

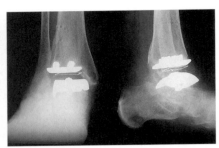

Figure 4 Radiograph of a 68-year-old woman with pantalar rheumatoid arthritis obtained 4 months following successful management with simultaneous subtalar arthrodesis and total ankle arthroplasty.

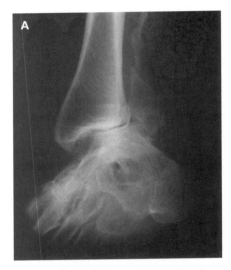

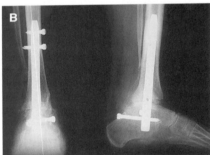

Figure 5 Preoperative (**A**) and postoperative (**B**) radiographs of a 62-year-old woman with poliomyelitis that was managed with distal fibular osteotomy and triple arthrodesis. On presentation, she had severe deformity and tibiotalar subluxation. The postoperative radiograph was obtained 3 months after realignment osteotomy and conversion of the triple arthrodesis to a pantalar arthrodesis using intramedullary nail fixation. The patient is currently ambulatory with a pain-free plantigrade foot.

cancellous bone graft are used after preparation of the arthrodesis site. Many orthopaedic surgeons use one talocalcaneal screw, but two talocalcaneal screws may minimize talocalcaneal rotation. These procedures are described elsewhere in this text.

When the ankle and subtalar joints are involved, but the transverse tarsal joints are relatively normal, the procedure of choice is tibiotalocalcaneal arthrodesis with a transfibular approach or intramedullary nail fixation (**Figure 1**). Nail fixation has the advantage of immediate rigid internal fixation with compression in a load-sharing capacity, providing collinear reduction of the distal extremity and high fusion rates (**Figure 2**). Alternative fixation methods include blade plate, cannulated screws, or a combination of internal and external fixation (**Figure 3**).

An alternative to tibiotalocalcaneal arthrodesis in the patient with ankle and subtalar arthritis is total ankle arthroplasty concurrently with or following subtalar arthrodesis. However, there is very little supporting literature. This procedure may have the theoretical benefit of maintaining ankle mobility after subtalar arthrodesis but is controversial (**Figure 4**).

In some situations, there may be a limited role for talectomy instead of pantalar fusion. Talectomy and slid-

ing fusion of the tibia to the very distal talus and midfoot (Blair procedure) have been used for patients with severe osteonecrosis of the talar body. Talectomy may be indicated primarily for the patient with complete talar body bone loss resulting from either osteonecrosis or, more commonly, talar body extrusion after trauma or neuropathic arthropathy. In these patients it may be better to fuse the tibia to the calcaneus with intramedullary rod fixation than it is to leave them unstable after talectomy with a pseudarthrosis that would require bracing on an indefinite, life-long basis.

Triple arthrodesis can restore excellent biomechanical alignment and function to the diseased hindfoot with a relatively normal ankle. For patients who have pantalar arthritis with limited ankle involvement, realignment triple arthrodesis incorporating bone graft may preserve ankle dorsiflexion and plantar flexion.

Pantalar arthrodesis is a technically demanding procedure that sacrifices any residual ankle and hindfoot motion. This procedure is somewhat akin to providing the patient with a sensate plantigrade prosthesis. Achieving plantigrade alignment in neutral dorsiflexion is critical for these patients because of the motion sacrificed (**Figure 5**). The procedure is a salvage technique for extremely disabling or limb-threatening pantalar arthritis, neuropathic joint destruction, and paralytic or flail extremities.

A controversial alternative to pantalar arthrodesis for the patient with pantalar arthritis is staged triple arthrodesis followed by total ankle arthroplasty. Total ankle arthroplasty and triple arthrodesis usually are not performed at the same surgical setting because of the risk of soft-tissue compromise and circulatory embarrassment.

Management of Complications

The risk of wound infection increases greatly in patients with neuropathy, a history of open trauma or surgical management, or a history of tobacco use.

Malunion of a pantalar arthrodesis may result in painful callosity and ulcer. The optimal position of arthrodesis is 3° to 5° of ankle and hindfoot valgus, neutral dorsiflexion, and external rotation symmetric with the contralateral uninvolved side. The second ray is aligned with the anteromedial crest of the tibia in most patients, and the first and fifth metatarsals strike the ground in synchrony.

The likelihood of talonavicular arthritis following ankle arthrodesis is increased, particularly following an ankle arthrodesis in equinus position. Fusion of the ankle in excessive dorsiflexion concentrates pressures on the heel at the beginning of the stance phase, contributing to heel pain or ulcer. When the ankle and subtalar joint are fused in neutral dorsiflexion, patients will have, on average, 10° of plantar flexion occurring in the midfoot. Patients who have 10° or more of equinus position at the ankle arthrodesis site may have a vaulting gait pattern and greater difficulty ambulating barefoot. Very little dorsiflexion is present in the midtarsal area after tibiotalocalcaneal arthrodesis. Therefore, neutral dorsiflexion is preferred to positions of equinus.

In a limb with tibiotalocalcaneal arthrodesis, loss of dorsiflexion or plantar flexion is minimal compared with a limb following ankle arthrodesis alone. Diminution of inversion and eversion, however, is at least 40% greater after tibiotalocalcaneal arthrodesis than with ankle fusion alone. Deficits in dorsiflexion, plantar flexion, inversion, and eversion are even greater after pantalar arthrodesis. Therefore, appropriate positioning of the foot and ankle in pantalar arthrodesis is important.

Realignment and rotational osteotomies through hindfoot, ankle, and subtalar fusion masses can be done in the salvage setting to manage malunion. These are technically demanding procedures but can be very gratifying for the patient with a stiff, malunited hindfoot. Nonunion is treated with pseudarthrosis débridement, bone grafting, and rigid fixation in the appropriate position and alignment.

References

Quill G: An approach to the management of ankle arthritis, in Myerson M (ed): *Foot and Ankle Disorders*. Philadelphia, PA, WB Saunders, 2000, pp 1059-1084.

Quill GE: Tibiotalocalcaneal and pantalar arthrodesis. *Foot Ankle Clin* 1996;1:199-210.

Coding

ICD-9 CODES

714.0   Rheumatoid arthritis

715.17   Osteoarthritis

727.06   Tenosynovitis

CPT CODES

27685   Lengthening or shortening of tendon, leg or ankle; single tendon (separate procedure)

27702   Arthroplasty, ankle; with implant ("total ankle")

27870   Arthrodesis, ankle, open

27871   Arthrodesis, tibiofibular joint, proximal or distal

28130   Talectomy (astragalectomy)

28220   Tenolysis, flexor, foot; single tendon

28225   Tenolysis, extensor, foot; single tendon

28705   Arthrodesis; pantalar

28715   Arthrodesis; triple

28725   Arthrodesis; subtalar

Oblique Calcaneal Osteotomy and Arthrodesis for Malunited Calcaneal Fracture

Michael M. Romash, MD

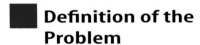

Definition of the Problem

Patient Presentation

The patient with a malunited calcaneal fracture will present with a stiff, painful foot. The pain will be centered about the sinus tarsi, fibulocalcaneal impingement area, and anterior ankle. The patient will describe difficulty walking on uneven terrain and will have difficulty fitting into a normal shoe.

The malunited calcaneal fracture causes multiple functional deficits. Shortening of the foot diminishes the lever arm for the triceps surae, making it inefficient in plantar flexion of the foot. With the loss of support for the posterior aspect of the talus, the foot becomes flat as the pedestal function of the calcaneus is lost. The talus then undergoes relative dorsiflexion and changes its relationship in the ankle joint. As a result, there may be anterior impingement between the tibia and the neck of the talus and limited ankle dorsiflexion. Dorsiflexion of the talus while the tarsal navicular remains in its normal position relative to the midfoot causes a subluxation at the talonavicular joint. The disruption of the posterior facet of the calcaneus results in a posttraumatic arthritis. The lateral, cephalad, and anterior displacement of the tuberosity fragment can cause direct impingement against the fibula and peroneal ten-

dons (**Figure 1**). Displacement of the calcaneal tuberosity also causes widening of the foot and loss of its height, making standard shoe wear very difficult because a flat, short, and wide foot will impinge the malleoli on the normal counter of a shoe. The disruption of the three-dimensional (3-D) spatial arrangement of the subtalar, calcaneocuboid, and talonavicular joints will disrupt coordinated multicentric motion through these joints.

Physical Examination

Physical examination will reveal a shortened, wide heel that may be inverted. Subtalar motion will be severely limited, and ankle dorsiflexion may be limited. The patient will walk with an antalgic gait. The ability to do a single-leg toe raise will be diminished as a result of triceps surae weak-

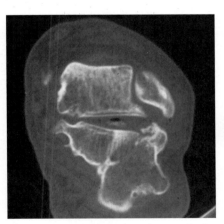

Figure 1 Coronal CT scan shows subtalar arthritis and fibular impingement.

ness. There will be no sulcus or step-off at the tip of the fibular malleolus because of fibulocalcaneal impingement, and the peroneal tendons will be displaced. Tenderness is common in the sinus tarsi and at the fibulocalcaneal region, and possibly at the calcaneocuboid joint. The patient should not use tobacco.

Differential Diagnosis

- Sural nerve entrapment
- Malunited talar fracture
- Complex regional pain syndrome
- Posterior tibial nerve entrapment

Additional Work-up

CT in coronal, axial, and sagittal planes as well as 3-D volumetric reconstruction should be ordered. Noninvasive peripheral vascular studies will confirm the vascular status of the limb. Electromyography and nerve conduction velocity studies may be helpful.

The Solutions

Treatment Options and Rationale

Surgical treatment of the malunited calcaneal fracture must address all of the patient's functional losses. It should ablate the arthritis and restore

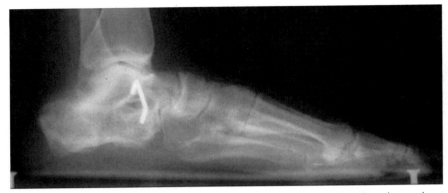

Figure 2 Lateral radiograph following subtalar arthrodesis done in situ. Note the resultant abnormal architecture and talar inclination.

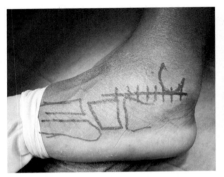

Figure 3 Skin incision over the sinus tarsi. (Reproduced with permission from Romash MM: Calcaneal osteotomy and subtalar arthrodesis for malunited calcaneal fracture, in Kitaoka H (ed): *Master Techniques in Orthopaedic Surgery: Foot and Ankle*, ed 2. Philadelphia, PA, Lippincott Williams & Wilkins, 2002.)

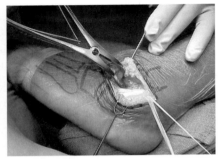

Figure 4 The lateral aspect of the subtalar joint opened and spread with a baby Inge lamina spreader.

the architectural relationships of the hindfoot to the midfoot. That is, surgical correction should reestablish both the height of the calcaneus and the normal inclination of the talus and its relationship to the navicular. Finally, it is important to relieve the fibular impingement and concomitantly narrow the heel.

Arthrodeses in situ, whether they are subtalar or triple arthrodeses, have limited success. These procedures do not restore the height of the calcaneus and its relationship to the other tarsal bones. A limited procedure to diminish the width of the heel by removing bone about the peroneal tendons and fibula would also have limited success because the posttrau-

matic arthritis and architectural derangement of the foot are not corrected (**Figure 2**).

A malunion in which the posterior facet is driven directly downward into the body without a significant primary oblique fracture or lateral shift of the tuberosity is not appropriately treated by a reconstructive osteotomy. Better treatment of this situation may be an interpositional distraction bone block arthrodesis because no corrective medial shift of the tuberosity is needed, and only calcaneal height need be restored.

Loss of more than 1.5 cm of height is also a contraindication for the reconstructive osteotomy because the magnitude of the shift is limited by the geometry of the osteotomy and the size of the calcaneus. If greater correction is to be obtained, an interposition

bone block arthrodesis should be considered.

Author's Preferred Treatment and Rationale

The procedure described here corrects the deformity of the malunited calcaneal fracture by re-creating the primary oblique shearing fracture with an osteotomy. This restores height and length to the heel and decompresses the lateral side by shifting the tuberosity away from the fibula. Addition of the subtalar arthrodesis ablates the subtalar arthritis.

The ideal patient for this procedure has a painful malunion of a calcaneal fracture in which there has been loss of calcaneal height and lateral displacement of the tuberosity fragment. The tuberosity fragment should be implicated in fibulocalcaneal impingement, and its primary displacement should be along the primary fracture line, which is the plane of the proposed osteotomy. Joint depression-type fractures have better results with this treatment than tongue-type fractures in which there is significant cephalad displacement of the tongue fragment.

PREOPERATIVE PLANNING

Preoperative evaluation for this particular surgical procedure focuses on the patient's symptoms and radiographic evaluation. The patient's pain should be of a degree to justify the procedure. In addition, problems such as difficulty with shoe wear because of impingement on the malleoli or decreased ankle motion should be noted. Pain at the anterior ankle suggests anterior impingement; pain at the sinus tarsi suggests subtalar arthritis; pain at the subfibular region indicates possible impingement of the peroneal tendons or direct fibulocalcaneal impingement; and pain at the calcaneocuboid joint indicates direct fracture involvement and arthritis. Sural nerve entrapment is another potential source of pain.

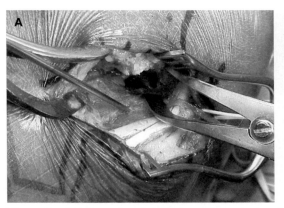
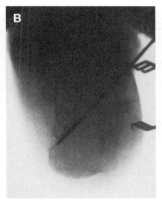
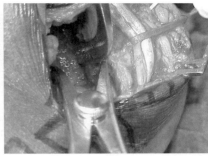

Figure 5 **A,** Fracture line. A Steinmann pin marks the obliquity of the fracture. **B,** Intraoperative radiograph confirms the placement of the Steinmann pin.

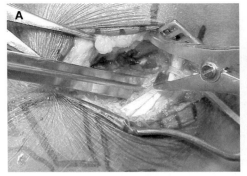
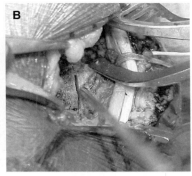

Figure 6 The calcaneus is osteotomized in the plane of the previous fracture. **A,** Osteotomy is performed along the Steinmann pin. **B,** The completed osteotomy, with no shift.

Figure 7 Baby Inge lamina spreader placed between the osteotomy fragments, widening the gap between the fragments and providing soft-tissue stretch to facilitate the tuberosity shift. (Reproduced with permission from Romash MM: Calcaneal osteotomy and subtalar arthrodesis for malunited calcaneal fracture, in Kitaoka H (ed): *Master Techniques in Orthopaedic Surgery: Foot and Ankle*, ed 2. Philadelphia, PA, Lippincott Williams and Wilkins, 2002.)

Radiographic evaluation is similar to that for the acute calcaneal fracture. Important radiographic findings include the loss of Böhler's angle, dorsiflexion of the talus noted by loss of the normal talar inclination angle, disruption of the alignment of the talonavicular joint on the lateral projection, and anterior tibiotalar impingement that may be seen on a dorsiflexion view. CT will demonstrate the lateral shift of the tuberosity, fibulocalcaneal impingement, and subtalar and calcaneocuboid arthritis.

If the calcaneocuboid joint is involved in the fracture it also may need to be arthrodesed at the time of surgery. In an equivocal instance, a technetium Tc 99m bone scan may help identify the presence of calcaneocuboid arthritis. If the calcaneocuboid joint shows activity

on the bone scan, it should probably be arthrodesed.

SURGERY

Appropriate small surgical instruments, including No. 15 scalpel blades, small tenotomy scissors, Freer elevators, small key elevators, and Joker elevators are necessary. Joseph skin hooks (10-mm wide), Ragnell retractors, somewhat larger 90° retractors such as Mason's or Army-Navy, and a baby Inge lamina spreader are used. A small drill with a wire driver, Kirschner wires (K-wires), and Steinmann pins are helpful. A small fragment screw set is also used. Particularly helpful are small curved osteotomes and motorized burrs to denude the subtalar cortical and articular surfaces. A pneumatically powered osteotome also is

useful in decortication and preparation of the bony surfaces to be arthrodesed. A cannulated cancellous 7-mm screw for tuberosity fixation and cannulated 4.5- or 4.0-mm screws fix the osteotomy. An anterior cruciate ligament guide is used to place the guide wire for the 7.0-mm cannulated screws.

The patient is placed in a lateral debucitus position with the affected limb on a bolster facing toward the surgeon. This position allows easier passage of the final fixation screw through the tuberosity of the calcaneus into the talus. Both the extremity up to the thigh and the ipsilateral iliac crest are sterilely prepared and draped, and a pneumatic tourniquet is placed about the thigh.

After exsanguination and tourniquet inflation, a longitudinal incision is made centered over the sinus tarsi (**Figure 3**), allowing access to the anterior process, body, and posterior facet of the calcaneus. This incision may be extended posteriorly for more exposure. The extensor digitorum brevis is reflected, and the fat in the sinus tarsi is excised as necessary. The lateral ligament structures between the talus and calcaneus are incised deep to the retracted peroneal tendons, moving from anterior to poste-

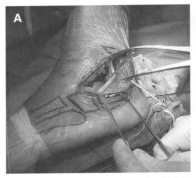

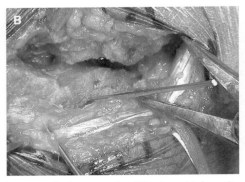

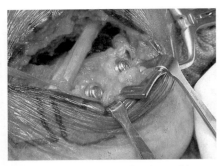

Figure 9 Osteotomy, fixation with two screws.

Figure 8 **A,** Osteotomy shifted with lamina spreader between tip of fibula and tuberosity fragment. **B,** Shift of osteotomy held by "deadman" K-wire.

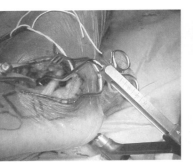

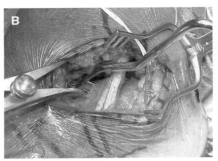

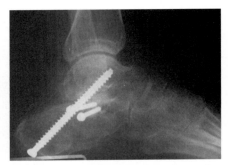

Figure 11 Lateral view of axial transfixation with the screw in place.

Figure 10 **A,** Anterior cruciate ligament guide applied for placement of guide pin. **B,** Tip of the cannulated screw guide pin in sustentacular fragment. (Reproduced with permission from Romash MM: Calcaneal osteotomy and subtalar arthrodesis for malunited calcaneal fracture, in Kitaoka H (ed): *Master Techniques in Orthopaedic Surgery: Foot and Ankle*, ed 2. Philadelphia, PA, Lippincott Williams & Wilkins, 2002.)

rior (**Figure 4**). A baby Inge lamina spreader in the sinus tarsi between the talus and calcaneus provides distraction of the joint and exposure to the sustentaculum tali.

At this point, the displaced articular surface of the posterior facet is exposed. The scarring within the joint is removed with a pituitary rongeur. Once the posterior facet surface has been uncovered, the site of the primary fracture line, which runs obliquely across the calcaneus from dorsolateral to plantar medial and anterolateral to posteromedial, can be identified.

Remaining articular cartilage and cortical surfaces are removed from the subtalar surfaces of the talus and calcaneus. Special care is taken to reach the sustentaculum tali of the calcaneus and to include the undersurface of the talar neck. Small curved

osteotomes and a powered burr or pneumatic osteotome are particularly helpful in preparing the subtalar arthrodesis surfaces.

A Steinmann pin is then placed across the calcaneus in the plane of the primary fracture line (**Figure 5**). The position of this pin is confirmed intraoperatively by an axial radiograph. Once the pin position is satisfactory, the calcaneus is osteotomized in the plane of the previous fracture. This osteotomy frees the tuberosity from the sustentaculum (**Figure 6**, *A*), and exits the calcaneus anteriorly through the lateral wall. Posteriorly and inferiorly it exits through the medial wall of the calcaneus beneath and posterior to the neurovascular bundle (**Figure 6**, *B*). The tuberosity fragment is then released as necessary to permit displacement.

The most difficult part of the surgery is shifting the tuberosity fragment relative to the sustentacular fragment. It is helpful to obtain provisional fixation of the sustentacular fragment to the talus with screws, Steinmann pins, or K-wires that are placed through the lateral body of the talus and into the sustentacular fragment. This fixation will stabilize the sustentacular fragment and prevent its motion as the tuberosity is manipulated.

It often is helpful to use osteotomes as levers to distract the tuberosity from the sustentaculum. Baby Inge lamina spreaders are placed in the osteotomy and opened (**Figure 7**), thereby distracting the fragments relative to each other. This soft-tissue stretch facilitates the shift of the tuberosity. Also, a Steinmann pin often is placed through the tuberosity from anterolateral to posteromedial, parallel to the plane of the osteotomy, to provide control of this fragment as the shift is done. A baby Inge lamina

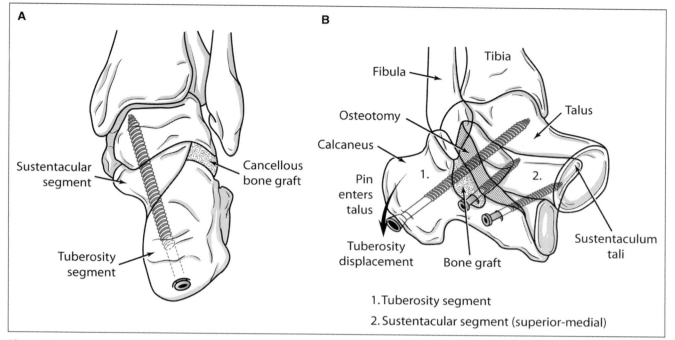

Figure 12 Diagrams of construct. **A,** Axial view. (Reproduced with permission from Romash MM: Calcaneal osteotomy and subtalar arthrodesis for malunited calcaneal fracture, in Johnson K (ed): *Master Techniques in Orthopaedic Surgery: Foot and Ankle.* Philadelphia, PA, Raven Press, 1994.) **B,** Lateral view. (Adapted with permission from Romash MM: Reconstructive osteotomy of the calcaneus with subtlar arthrodesis. *Clin Orthop* 1993;228:157-167.)

spreader between the sustentaculum and the tuberosity fragment will help push the tuberosity into its new position. Even placing an Inge lamina spreader between the tip of the fibula and the tuberosity posteriorly will help affect the shift. Shifting the tuberosity and placing a 0.62-in K-wire across the superior surface of the tuberosity into the exposed wall of the sustentaculum will act as a "deadman" stop, which can facilitate further shifting (**Figure 8**). If necessary, an external fixation-type distractor can be applied between the tibia and the tuberosity fragment to help move the tuberosity fragment into its new position. Plantar flexion of the midfoot and talus helps affect the appropriate translation and rotation of the tuberosity fragment. Because of the obliquity of the osteotomy from dorsolateral to plantar medial, the tuberosity fragment will move away from its impinging location on the peroneal tendons and the fibula as it is displaced. A

space will be created under the lateral aspect of the talus and the lateral aspect of the shifted tuberosity fragment.

Once the shift has been obtained, transverse fixation through the lateral wall of the calcaneus into the sustentaculum tali is done with small fragment screws or cannulated 4.0- or 4.5-mm screws (**Figure 9**). The neutral position of inversion and eversion of the subtalar joint is then established and noted for final fixation of the subtalar joint. Next, a large cannulated 7-mm screw is placed through the tuberosity and the sustentacular fragment and into the body of the talus. This screw can be placed with direct visualization, as well as with a radiographic control arm. An anterior cruciate ligament reconstruction drill guide will help position this guide wire (**Figure 10**). Once satisfactory position has been obtained, fixation is secured (**Figure 11**). The dead space created laterally under the talus is packed with morcellized cancellous

bone graft from the ipsilateral iliac crest. The repositioned tuberosity is not structurally dependent on the bone graft for maintenance of this position (**Figure 12**). The wound is closed using absorbable suture in the subcutaneous tissue and nylon mattress sutures for the skin.

POSTOPERATIVE MANAGEMENT

Postoperative management is similar to that used for the surgically treated acute calcaneal fracture. The patient is initially placed in a short leg cast over an A-V Impulse System foot pump (Novamedix, Mansfield, MA). After about 3 days, the cast is changed, and the foot is maintained in a non–weight-bearing status for 8 to 12 weeks. When casting is discontinued, graduated weight bearing and ankle range-of-motion exercises are begun.

The result depends to a large degree on obtaining a solid subtalar arthrodesis with the calcaneus narrowed and the tuberosity in an improved position. As with a subtalar arthrodesis alone, the subtalar motion is lost, and adaptation of the hindfoot to uneven ground surfaces is difficult. Pain relief is emphasized as the primary goal of treatment. Restoration of heel height and possible improvement in shoe wear are secondary goals.

Management of Complications

All the complications of a realignment with arthrodesis—infection, loss of correction, incomplete correction, and nonunion—may occur. Infection is avoided by use of antibiotics during the surgical procedure and for 24 hours afterward. Surgical technique to prevent tissue ischemia and use of a compression dressing with an A-V Impulse System foot pump have all helped to decrease the incidence of possible infection.

Pseudarthrosis has not been a problem, probably because of the large area of the arthrodesis site in the subtalar joint and the use of bone graft along with stable fixation.

Inadequate realignment is probably the most common postoperative problem. Use of preoperative radiographs and CT to obtain a thorough understanding of the fracture position allows proper planning of the appropriate tuberosity displacement. In patients with complex secondary fracture lines, the realignment will not be ideal but should be improved.

Fixation devices have not broken with bone block procedures and early weight bearing. I believe this is because the final construct does not depend on a graft bone block for stability or correction.

Neurologic injury to the posterior tibial nerve, medial plantar nerve, or lateral plantar nerve has not been a problem with either this procedure or the procedure for treating an acute calcaneal fracture. The osteotomy exits the medial calcaneus posteriorly and inferiorly to the neurovascular structures.

References

Bradley SA, Davies AM: Computerized tomographic assessment of old calcaneal fractures. *Br J Radiol* 1990;63:926-933.

Carr JB, Hansen ST, Benirshke SK: Subtalar distraction bone block fusion for late complications of the os calcis fractures. *Foot Ankle* 1988;9:81-86.

Hansen ST Jr: Calcaneal osteotomy in multiple planes for correction of major postraumatic deformity, in *Functional Reconstruction of the Foot and Ankle*. Philadelphia, PA, Lippincott, Williams & Wilkins, 2000, pp 380-383.

Romash MM: Reconstructive osteotomy of the calcaneus with subtalar arthrodesis for malunited calcaneal fractures, in Kitaoka H (ed): *Master Techniques in Orthopedic Surgery: Foot and Ankle*, ed 2. Philadelphia, PA, Lippincott Williams & Wilkins, 2002.

Romash MM: Reconstructive osteotomy of the calcaneus with subtalar arthrodesis for malunited calcaneal fractures. *Clin Orthop* 1993;290:157-167.

Coding

ICD-9 CODES

715.17   Osteoarthrosis, localized, primary, ankle and foot

719.97   Unspecified disorder of joint, ankle and foot

733.81   Malunion of fracture

CPT CODES

28300   Osteotomy; calcaneus (eg, Dwyer or Chambers type procedure), with or without internal fixation

28725   Arthrodesis; subtalar

Malunited Triple Arthrodesis

Elly Trepman, MD

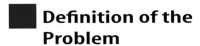

Definition of the Problem

Patient Presentation

The patient who has a malunion of a triple arthrodesis will have previously undergone arthrodesis for hindfoot arthritis (primary, posttraumatic, or rheumatoid), diabetic Charcot neuroarthropathy, tarsal coalition, clubfoot, or other congenital deformity. The malunion may have resulted from inadequate correction of deformity, difficulty in assessing alignment during surgery, failure of fixation, loss of correction from poor bone quality, infection, or noncompliance with the postoperative non–weight-bearing regimen. Nonunion may be present secondary to inadequate excision of the articular surfaces, loss of fixation, infection, or smoking.

The patient with a malunion of a triple arthrodesis presents with pain and difficulty with ambulation. Lateral ankle pain with a varus deformity or medial ankle pain with a valgus deformity may result from rubbing of the prominent malleoli against the shoe. Hindfoot pain may be associated with micromotion at the nonunion site or infection. Midfoot and forefoot pain may occur from the abnormal pressure distribution under the foot, such as direct pressure and callus at the lateral fifth metatarsal tuberosity associated with hindfoot varus deformity. The patient with diabetic neuropathy may present with an ulcer. Fitting of shoes may be difficult because of the deformity, and both standing and walking may be severely restricted by the pain. With hindfoot varus malunion, inversion instability and giving way may occur. The pain and increased energy demands of walking with a deformed foot may result in fatigue and limitation of vocational and recreational activities.

Physical Examination

Physical examination reveals that the patient walks with difficulty or not at all. The patient may be sitting in a wheelchair or may have limped into the office with crutches, canes, or an ankle-foot orthosis. Previous surgical scars are noted for location, quality of skin, and evidence of previous infection or dehiscence. Scars are percussed and may be sensitive to touch if a neuroma is present. The ankle joint may have limited motion and pain or crepitus resulting from trauma, rheumatoid arthritis, or mechanical degeneration adjacent to the fused hindfoot, which is aggravated by the malalignment. The subtalar and Chopart's (talonavicular and calcaneocuboid) joints are ankylosed and may be tender to palpation or painful, with crepitus noted with mechanical maneuvers (inversion, eversion, abduction, adduction). Arthritis may also be present in the midfoot and forefoot.

The key to evaluation and treatment is the assessment of alignment. The posterior calcaneal tuberosity, viewed from behind, may be malaligned in varus or valgus position as a result of malunion of the subtalar joint or collapse of the talocalcaneal complex. The varus (inverted) or valgus (everted) position of the midfoot and forefoot may be a result of malunion of the subtalar joint, Chopart's joints, or the entire triple joint complex. Varus deformity of the hindfoot may result in prominence, intractable keratoses, and tenderness at the lateral base of the fifth metatarsal and under the lateral (usually fourth and fifth) metatarsal heads (**Figure 1**). Valgus deformity of the hindfoot may be associated with prominence, keratoses, and tenderness under the navicular, first metatarsocuneiform joint, and sesamoids; furthermore, there may be a dorsiflexion deformity of the medial midtarsal or tarsometatarsal joint region. Deformity is often manifested by molding and wear patterns evident in the shoe and orthosis.

Initial radiographic examination includes a weight-bearing AP view of the foot, a weight-bearing lateral view of the foot and ankle, a non–weight-bearing oblique view of the foot, and non–weight-bearing AP and mortise views of the ankle (**Figure 2**). The subtalar and Chopart's joints are assessed for residual articular (subchondral bone) surfaces present with some nonunions. Signs of infection may include osteolysis, sclerosis (sequestrum), or soft-tissue swelling. Bone and joint malalignment are correlated with the clinical deformity. With varus malunion of a hindfoot arthrodesis, there may be medial talonavicular subluxation, lateral prominence of

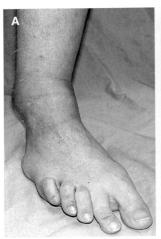
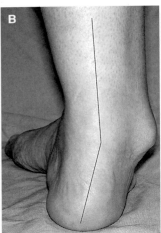
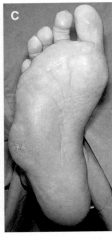

Figure 1 Anterior (**A**) and posterior (**B**) clinical photographs of a 40-year-old woman with a 27-year history of rheumatoid arthritis who had undergone a right triple arthrodesis 9 years previously. **C**, A large prominence was noted along the plantar base of fifth metatarsal region with associated keratosis, and a keratosis was present under the fourth and fifth metatarsal heads.

the fifth metatarsal tuberosity, and adduction of the metatarsals. With valgus malunion, there may be lateral talonavicular subluxation, medial prominence of the medial cuneiform, and abduction of the metatarsals. Fixation devices, if present, are assessed for hardware failure or osteolysis ("windshield wiper effect").

Technetium Tc 99m bone scans may reveal increased uptake with nonunion, arthritis in adjacent joints, or infection. Infection may be further evaluated with gallium- or indium-labeled leukocyte scintigraphy. CT may be useful in the assessment of bony malalignment, bone deficiency, residual articular surfaces, and infection (sequestrum) (**Figure 3**). Gadolinium-enhanced MRI may be useful in the evaluation of infection, and bone edema on an MRI scan may result from abnormally increased mechanical stresses or infection.

Differential Diagnosis
- Incomplete excision of articular surfaces
- Failure of fixation
- Limited fixation with poor bone stock

- Patient noncompliance with a postoperative non–weight-bearing regimen
- Immunocompromised patient (steroids, methotrexate, immune deficiency)
- Nutritional deficiency
- Infection
- Wound dehiscence
- Rheumatologic disease (rheumatoid arthritis, vasculitis)
- Osteoarthritis (primary or posttraumatic)
- Ischemia
- Charcot arthropathy
- Charcot-Marie-Tooth disease
- Stroke

Additional Work-up
Laboratory studies include white blood cell count, erythrocyte sedimentation rate, and C-reactive protein, which may be elevated with infected nonunion. Compromised nutritional status of the patient, reflected by a low white blood cell count and serum albumin level, may be a contributing factor to nonunion.

The Solutions

Treatment Options and Rationale
SURGICAL APPROACH
The patient is positioned supine, with a roll behind the ipsilateral hip to internally rotate the lower extremity, allowing access to both the lateral and dorsomedial hindfoot. The surgical approach may be dictated, in part, by the location and age of the previous scars. The creation of a narrow skin bridge between a new incision and an old scar, or of a triangular area of skin where a new incision crosses an old scar, may increase the postoperative risk of wound dehiscence. This risk may be lower if the old scar is from the distant past, but specific time guidelines are unavailable. If the skin adjacent to a previous scar appears unhealthy, then parallel or crossing scars are usually avoided. However, exposure through an old scar that is in a poor location may compromise the potential to achieve the required correction. In this situation, the surgeon must make a clinical judgment about selecting a surgical approach that will enable the exposure required and minimize potential wound problems.

The most direct surgical approach to the subtalar and calcaneocuboid joints is from a straight incision starting at one finger width below the tip of the lateral malleolus, along a line toward the base of the fourth metatarsal, ending at the cuboid. The main risk of this approach is to the dorsolateral cutaneous nerve, which, even if avoided and protected, may contribute to postoperative neuritis secondary to bruising or scarring. The extensor digitorum brevis is elevated from the calcaneus, and the subtalar ligaments are transected and débrided along the dorsal calcaneus from the calcaneocuboid joint to the posterior facet of the subtalar joint. Dissection may be complicated by ankylosis and extensive scar tissue present from previous surgery.

The talonavicular joint is approached from a longitudinal incision along the dorsomedial hindfoot, just medial to the tibialis anterior tendon. The dorsalis pedis artery and deep peroneal nerve are located lateral to the tibialis anterior tendon, and care with blunt-tipped retractors may reduce the risk of neurovascular injury. The similar curvature and the close proximity of the talonavicular and naviculocuneiform joints may confound the correct identification of the talonavicular joint. Fluoroscopic identification of the talonavicular joint with an instrument in the joint may be prudent before joint débridement if there is doubt about the correct identity of the joint.

INTRAOPERATIVE ASSESSMENT

A malunion without nonunion is identified from the contours of the exposed bony surfaces in conjunction with knowledge from the preoperative CT scan. With a varus malunion, the lateral wall of the calcaneus is in varus malalignment relative to the lateral wall of the talus, and there may be a medially displaced step-off at the calcaneocuboid and talonavicular joints. With a valgus malunion, the lateral wall of the calcaneus is in valgus malalignment relative to the lateral wall of the talus, and there may be a laterally displaced step-off at the calcaneocuboid and talonavicular joints. If the anatomy is grossly distorted, correct identity of the former joint levels may be facilitated with intraoperative fluoroscopy with the tip of a clamp or elevator adjacent to the edge of the arthrodesis.

If the preoperative studies suggest the presence of a nonunion, it is entered with various-sized straight or curved curets, blades, or elevators (**Figure 4**). Osteotomes may be used to excise the cortical shell that may surround and obscure

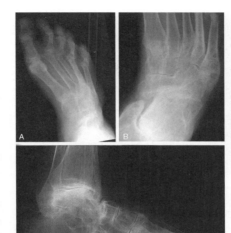

Figure 2 Initial AP (**A**), oblique (**B**), and lateral (**C**) radiographs of the foot in the patient shown in Figure 1. Note the previous triple arthrodesis with evidence of nonunion of the posterior subtalar joint and malunion of the calcaneocuboid and talonavicular arthrodesis. Medial subluxation of the navicular relative to the talar head is noted (**B**) associated with forefoot adduction (**A**). Arthritis of the fifth metatarsocuboid joint is noted with soft-tissue swelling adjacent to the hypertrophic base of the fifth metatarsal.

the underlying nonunion. A clear understanding of the deformity and the location of the nonunion surfaces, documented with a preoperative CT scan (**Figure 3**), may improve ease in finding the nonunion.

The nonunion may contain fibrous tissue, fluid, sclerotic bony surfaces, and residual articular cartilage or arthritis. A Gram stain, culture of swabs and tissue, and histologic evaluation may help exclude the presence of infection. If these tests are positive, the culture results may help direct postoperative antibiotic management. When there are no gross signs of infection, the surgeon may elect to continue with the reconstruction at the same time. However, if there is gross pus, then a two-stage approach is indicated. In the first stage, the infection is eradicated with débridement, irrigation, and placement of

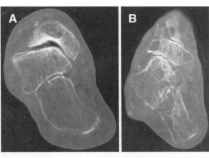

Figure 3 Coronal (**A**) and transverse (**B**) CT scans confirm nonunion of the posterior subtalar and talonavicular arthrodesis, ankle arthritis, varus malalignment of the calcaneus, and medial subluxation of the navicular.

antibiotic-impregnated methylmethacrylate beads followed by postoperative antibiotics; in the second stage, the beads are removed, repeat cultures are done, and the realignment-arthrodesis reconstruction is done.

CORRECTION OF ALIGNMENT AND PREPARATION OF ARTHRODESIS

The sequence of correction of alignment is from proximal to distal. Malunion with isolated heel varus deformity may be managed with a Dwyer laterally based closing wedge osteotomy. However, more commonly, malalignment is present not only within the hindfoot but also between the hindfoot and midfoot, necessitating correction at both levels. The talocalcaneal site is realigned followed by the Chopart region.

The malunion or nonunion is débrided of fibrous tissue, residual cartilage, and dense cortical bone with curets and osteotomes. After the fusion or pseudarthrosis is broken up and there is increased mobility among the calcaneus, talus, cuboid, and navicular, the bones can be further separated with a baby Inge lamina spreader to allow for thorough débridement. The goal at this stage is to completely separate the calcaneus, talus, cuboid, and navicular and to expose healthy cancellous bone. This will permit reduction and realignment of the bones relative to each other to achieve a neutral, plantigrade foot and a solid union.

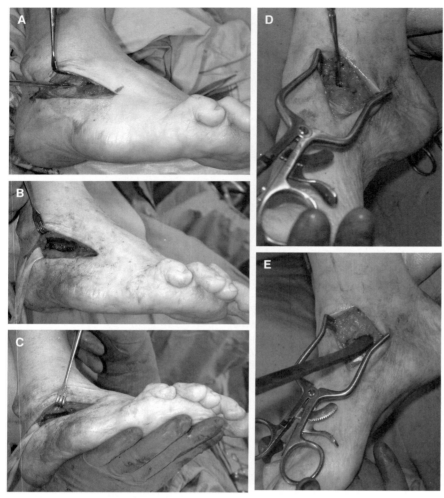

Figure 4 **A,** At surgery, the posterior subtalar nonunion is indicated with a scalpel blade easily placed in the space between the talus and calcaneus. **B,** The subtalar gap after osteotomy and wedge resection; the lateral width of the wedge excised was 4 to 5 mm. **C,** The subtalar gap was closed to move the heel from varus to slight valgus alignment. **D,** The talonavicular nonunion is indicated by an elevator between the talar head and navicular. **E,** After osteotomy of the calcaneocuboid arthrodesis, débridement of the talonavicular nonunion and soft-tissue release about the calcaneocuboid and talonavicular joints, the midfoot and forefoot were reduced from adduction to neutral position.

The calcaneus should be mobile enough to allow it to be corrected to 0° to 5° of valgus position when viewed from the back of the leg; this assessment is done intraoperatively by lifting the supine leg upward and viewing the posterior aspect of the leg from underneath. The navicular and cuboid should be mobile enough to allow the midfoot and forefoot to be corrected to a neutral, plantigrade position relative to the corrected hindfoot.

If reduction of a malunion cannot be achieved after separation of the bones, or if a solid nonunion is present, then a wedge of bone may be excised from the convexity (apex) of the deformity to allow correction of alignment. Subtalar wedge excision is the most direct and simplest technique to achieve realignment. An alternative to wedge excision is bone-block lengthening, with a wedge of iliac crest bone inserted to lengthen

the concave side of the deformity. Risks of bone-block lengthening include bone graft donor site morbidity, dehiscence because of increased wound tension (potentially avoided with a gently curved or shallow S-shaped incision), and nonunion at the surfaces of the bone block. Nevertheless, bone-block lengthening may be indicated in cases of bone deficiency, loss of hindfoot height, and associated anterior ankle impingement. Another alternative to wedge excision of a subtalar varus malunion is a laterally based closing wedge osteotomy of the posterior calcaneal tuberosity. This procedure is technically less complex than a wedge excision of the subtalar nonunion but may create a zigzag deformity consisting of varus subtalar malunion and valgus tuberosity malalignment, with loss of hindfoot height at both levels and associated anterior ankle and lateral malleolar impingement.

The subtalar wedge excision is done with an oscillating power saw or flat osteotomes. The saw may generate heat that may render bone cells nonviable, but cooling the saw blade with irrigating fluid may minimize this problem. The saw is most helpful in areas of highly sclerotic bone. A series of osteotomes of varied sizes is used to excise sequential slivers of bone until satisfactory correction of alignment is achieved. Care at the medial subtalar cortex is required to reduce the risk of posterior tibial neurovascular injury or injury to the flexor hallucis longus tendon, and if a saw is used, the medial corticotomy may be completed with an osteotome to avoid thermal and direct neurovascular or tendon injury from the saw blade.

The Chopart wedge excision osteotomy is facilitated by placing Kirschner wires (K-wires) perpendicular to the longitudinal axes of the hindfoot and midfoot-forefoot complex and making the wedge osteotomy parallel to the K-wires. The gap thus created is then closed down, bringing the K-wires parallel to each other to reduce the midfoot-forefoot complex to the hindfoot. Midfoot-forefoot correction may require rotation in addition to correction in the abduction-adduction direction, and it is important to assess for rotational deformity to avoid residual postoperative forefoot varus or valgus deformity. Soft-tissue release or excision of more bone may be required in addition to osteotomy to permit complete rotational correction.

The exposed cancellous arthrodesis surfaces (talocalcaneal, talonavicular, and calcaneocuboid) are further prepared by using a small osteotome to make multiple "fish scales" on the surfaces and a small drill bit to make multiple drill holes. The increased bony surface area and the communication of the arthrodesis surface with healthy deeper bone improve the potential for solid union. An Achilles tendon lengthening is done if the foot and ankle are not easily dorsiflexed beyond neutral.

FIXATION

The sequence of fixation is from proximal to distal. The talocalcaneal arthrodesis is fixed first, and then the Chopart fusion is fixed.

The calcaneus is held in the desired (0° to 5° of valgus) alignment and is fixed to the talus. A 7.3-mm, self-tapping, partially threaded cannulated screw is commonly used for talocalcaneal fixation. Some surgeons prefer placement of the screw from the dorsal talar neck to the calcaneal body and tuberosity (talocalcaneal screw); others place the screw from the posterior calcaneal tuberosity to the talus (calcaneotalar screw). If fixation is rigid, a single screw is sufficient, although some surgeons prefer to use two screws.

The talonavicular and calcaneocuboid joints are fixed with 3.5- to 4.5-mm cannulated screws or bone staples. Excessive forefoot abduction is avoided by fixing the talonavicular before the calcaneocuboid fusion; excessive forefoot

adduction is avoided by fixing the calcaneocuboid before the talonavicular fusion. Neutral alignment of the midfoot-forefoot complex relative to the hindfoot is preferred. External fixation may be considered in cases of infection, wound and flap problems, poor bone stock, and complex deformity.

Sufficient cancellous bone graft is usually available from the distal tibia. The graft is taken through a cortical window made in the anteromedial distal tibial metaphyseal flare, and the cortical window is replaced before wound closure. The proximal tibia or iliac crest may be considered as alternate sources of bone graft. The iliac crest may be used if a tricortical structural bone graft is required. Wounds are closed in layers with sutures, and suction drains are used if dead space is present or if excessive postoperative bleeding is anticipated. A local anesthetic block placed at the completion of surgery may be helpful for postoperative analgesia.

AFTERCARE

Patients remain in the hospital for 2 to 3 days for parenteral analgesics. The leg is splinted with a well-padded plaster U-splint with a plantar plate, which is changed 1 to 2 days after surgery. The patient ambulates with crutches or a walker, bearing no weight on the surgically corrected side. Some patients with severe contralateral arthritis or deformity use a wheelchair. The splint is changed weekly for the first month because of the potential risk of wound maceration and dehiscence, but some surgeons review the patient at 2 and 6 weeks after surgery. When the wound is healed and swelling decreased, skin sutures are removed (2 to 4 weeks after surgery) and an anteriorly univalved fiberglass cast is applied.

Radiographs are obtained at 1 to 2 weeks, 6 weeks, and 12 weeks after surgery. If alignment is stable and early callus is noted, partial weight bearing is begun at 6 weeks after sur-

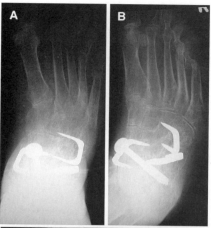
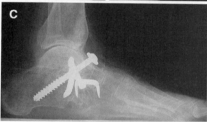

Figure 5 AP (**A**), oblique (**B**), and lateral (**C**) radiographs obtained 6 months after revision triple arthrodesis show satisfactory alignment and consolidation of the arthrodesis.

gery. At 12 weeks or when union appears solid on radiographs, full weight bearing in a removable walker boot is begun; the boot is tapered to an ankle stirrup brace and shoes when the patient is comfortable and gait is steady (**Figures 5** and **6**). An external electrical bone stimulator may be considered for difficult revision fusion cases, but an implanted electrical bone stimulator is rarely used.

Author's Preferred Treatment and Rationale

A high thigh tourniquet is used. A sheet roll made from two flannel sheets is placed behind the ipsilateral buttock to internally rotate the lower extremity to neutral position. After the sterile field is prepared, a thick cotton laparotomy sheet is placed behind the calf to elevate the leg, thus providing freedom of foot movement during débridement, osteotomy, and

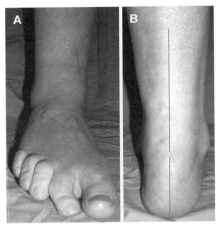

Figure 6 Anterior (**A**) and posterior (**B**) clinical photographs obtained 6 months after revision triple arthrodesis show neutral heel and forefoot alignment. The patient reported marked improvement of pain and ambulatory function compared with her preoperative status.

fixation. A prophylactic antibiotic is given intravenously before surgery.

For débridement of a nonunion, I prefer curets instead of a motorized burr. With the curet, tactile loss of pressure is more easily felt and controlled as the curet falls into the nonunion space, and no heat is generated. Alignment is usually corrected with subtalar and Chopart's wedge excision; bone-block lengthening of the subtalar fusion is rarely done. The power saw is used for the wedge excision, and the corticotomy of the far cortex is completed with an osteotome.

I prefer talocalcaneal screw fixation for the subtalar arthrodesis. The surgeon holds the heel in the corrected position between the thumb, index, and middle fingers of the nondominant hand, with the index finger just lateral to the sagittal plane of the tuberosity at the posteroplantar aspect of the heel. The ankle is held in dorsiflexion, and the tibialis anterior is retracted laterally. The guide pin is drilled from the distal portion of the dorsal talar neck to avoid impingement of the screw head at the anterior ankle. The surgeon uses propriocep-

tion to drill the guide pin directly toward the nondominant index finger, which is moved away from the heel after the pin is felt to enter the calcaneus. Aiming just lateral to the sagittal plane of the tuberosity decreases the potential for screw penetration from the concave medial calcaneal wall. Pin position and length are evaluated with lateral and axial C-arm fluoroscopic images. After measurement of length with the depth gauge, the pin is driven out the back of the heel and held with a clamp to avoid pin extrusion when the cannulated drill is removed. Alignment is again checked from behind the heel. The screw track is made with the cannulated drill over the guide pin, and the screw is placed with a washer to avoid settling of the screw head into the soft bone of the dorsal talar neck. Fluoroscopy (lateral and axial) is used to check correct screw position within the bone (with screw threads fully in the calcaneus), screw length, and bony alignment.

The advantage of talocalcaneal fixation is that it is easier to place the screw threads (including longer thread length) across the arthrodesis plane when aiming from a smaller bone (talus) to a larger bone (calcaneus) and from the front of the supine patient toward the floor than with a calcaneotalar screw. When the screw insertion site is distal along the talar neck, anterior ankle impingement of the screw head is unlikely.

Disadvantages of calcaneotalar fixation include the difficulty of ensuring that all screw threads are across the arthrodesis site in the talus, which is smaller than the calcaneus, necessitating a shorter thread length. Calcaneotalar screw placement may be more awkward because the surgeon must aim from behind the supine patient upward. Furthermore, screw penetration into the ankle joint, which is a risk of calcaneotalar screw placement, is avoided with the talocalcaneal screw.

Heel alignment is evaluated clinically during osteotomy, realignment, and fixation by elevating the leg and viewing the back of the leg with the foot and ankle held in neutral dorsiflexion. Alignment of the forefoot relative to the hindfoot is evaluated clinically from the anterior, plantar, and dorsal views with the foot and ankle held in neutral dorsiflexion. Residual equinus is assessed clinically from the lateral and medial sides with the knee in full extension and may be corrected with a triple hemisection lengthening of the Achilles tendon or a gastrocnemius slide procedure.

Management of Complications

Complications occur in 25% of patients treated with revision of a failed triple arthrodesis. General risks of surgery include anesthetic problems, infection, wound dehiscence, neurovascular injury, and thrombophlebitis. Infection is managed with wound culture, débridement as needed, and antibiotics. Wound drainage or dehiscence is managed with half-strength povidone-iodine dressings and oral antibiotics, with weekly wound checks until dehiscence is resolved, or skin grafting. Residual swelling is controlled with graded-pressure support hose.

Neuritic pain or paresthesias are managed with amitriptyline (starting with 10 mg orally before bedtime, increasing the dose by 10 mg increments every 2 to 4 weeks until symptoms resolve or until drowsiness develops that may preclude further use of the drug at the increased dose). If symptoms persist despite amitriptyline, gabapentin may be considered. Prophylaxis against thrombophlebitis, which is optional, is with low-dose aspirin (81 mg once daily), heparin (5,000 U subcutaneously every 12 hours), or a contralateral intermittent compression boot, but other measures such as warfarin may be considered if there is a previous history of thromboembolic disease.

Smoking may increase the risk of nonunion. Therefore, if the patient has a history of smoking, surgery is not done until after the patient has completely quit. Management of recurrent nonunion or delayed union may include revision surgery, bone grafting, and supplementation with an external or implanted electrical bone stimulator. Malunion or recurrent deformity may be treated with bracing or revision surgery. Persistent pain from prominent fixation hardware may be alleviated with hardware removal. Mild residual deformity may be successfully managed with an orthotic insole, rocker-bottom shoe modification, physiotherapy, or movement reeducation (Feldenkrais Method).

References

Haddad SL, Myerson MS, Pell RF, Schon LC: Clinical and radiographic outcome of revision surgery for failed triple arthrodesis. *Foot Ankle Int* 1997;18:489-499.

Ishikawa SN, Murphy GA, Richardson EG: The effect of cigarette smoking on hindfoot fusions. *Foot Ankle Int* 2002;23:996-998.

Mäenpää H, Lehto MUK, Belt EA: What went wrong in triple arthrodesis? An analysis of failures in 21 patients. *Clin Orthop* 2001;391:218-223.

O'Malley DF, Conti SF: Results of distal tibial bone grafting in hindfoot arthrodeses. *Foot Ankle Int* 1996;17:374-377.

Coding

ICD-9 CODES

733.8   Malunion and nonunion of fracture

733.82   Nonunion of fracture

736.71   Acquired equinovarus deformity

736.72   Equinus deformity of foot, acquired

736.75   Cavovarus deformity of foot, acquired

CPT CODES

28320   Repair, nonunion or malunion; tarsal bones

28715   Arthrodesis, triple

28725   Arthrodesis; subtalar

CPT copyright © 2003 by the American Medical Association. All Rights Reserved.

Osteonecrosis of the Talus

Saul G. Trevino, MD

■ Definition of the Problem

Patient Presentation

Although osteonecrosis of the talus is present in most talar neck fractures, many patients will have only minor symptoms. Early on, the patient may be asymptomatic or have no radiographic changes suggesting osteonecrosis. The usual outcome of osteonecrosis of the talus is the development of arthritis of the ankle, the subtalar joint, or both. Significant shortening or deformity can occur from collapse of the talar body. Most patients will present with an equinovarus deformity of the foot with limited motion at both the ankle and subtalar joints.

Physical Examination

The physical examination should focus on identifying the joint or joints that are symptomatic. Because of the nature of talar fractures, posttraumatic changes are common in both articular sides of the talus. Selective anesthetic blocks can be performed to identify the involved joints. The transverse tarsal joints can also be involved. Any equinus deformity can be corrected with an Achilles tendon lengthening. Prior incisions should be noted, as well as any prior skin sloughs or delayed healings. The surgeon, at times, may select a posterior approach for an ankle, subtalar, or tibiotalocalcaneal fusion if previous incisions jeopardize anterior approaches.

Radiographic evidence of osteonecrosis usually occurs within the first 8-week period. Radiographic evaluation includes bilateral weight-bearing AP and lateral views of the ankles and feet. With hindfoot deformities, a Morrey view (hindfoot alignment view) will help visualize the degree of varus or valgus malalignment. MRI is useful to assess the stage of osteonecrosis using the Ficat and Arlet classification as modified for the ankle (**Table 1**). Small or large areas of nonhomogeneous signal surrounded by a band of low signal with a potential second band of high signal indicate areas of osteonecrosis and are known as a "double-line sign." This signal pattern is believed to be a precursor to subchondral fractures of the femoral head, and it may be useful as an indication for a core decompression procedure. The size of the subchondral infarct is a factor for potential subcortical collapse. The use of titanium screws in the treatment of talar fractures facilitates future MRI evaluation by minimizing signal changes from the metal.

Differential Diagnosis

- Trauma
- Hypercortisolism
- Renal transplant
- Alcoholism or pancreatitis
- Dysbaric conditions
- Irradiation
- Collagen vascular disorders

Additional Work-up

In addition to routine radiographic studies, MRI is useful to clarify the extent of osteonecrosis. Several authors have reported that MRI changes can be noted as early as 3 weeks after injury. A prospective study of 21 consecutive cases of talar neck fractures showed a positive correlation of osteonecrosis with MRI if the plain ra-

Table 1   Staging of Osteonecrosis of the Talus According to Ficat and Arlet (1950)

Stage	Radiographic Appearance
I	Normal
II	Cystic and/or osteosclerotic lesions, normal contour of talus, no subchondral fracture
III	Crescent sign or subchondral collapse
IV	Joint space narrowing, secondary distal tibial changes (cysts, marginal osteophytes, and destruction of the cartilage)

(Adapted with permission from Mont MA, Schon LC, Hungerford MW, Hungerford D: Avascular necrosis of the talus treated by core decompression. *J Bone Joint Surg Br* 1996;78:827-830.)

diographs demonstrated more than 50% involvement of the talar dome. If less than 50% of the talar body was involved, the MRI correlated poorly.

The Solutions

Treatment Options and Rationale

INDICATIONS AND CONTRAINDICATIONS

Treatment of osteonecrosis of the talus depends on both the extent and cause of the condition. The most common cause is related to fractures and dislocations of the talus. The occurrence of osteonecrosis related to talar neck fractures varies from 0% to 100%, depending on the displacement of the talar body. The difficulty is that the extent of the osteonecrosis is quite variable, and the progression is unpredictable; thus, each instance must be individualized. Other causes include steroid use, Charcot arthropathy caused by diabetes, vascular occlusion (alcoholism, fatty emboli, and Gaucher's disease), and sepsis.

Treatment is predicated by the stage of the disease and the severity of the symptoms. A positive Hawkins sign is defined as the presence of disuse osteoporosis on an AP view of the ankle approximately 6 to 8 weeks postinjury. A positive sign indicates normal vascularity of the talus. In the most comprehensive series regarding the prognosis of the onset of osteonecrosis, 23 of 49 patients had positive Hawkins signs. Only one patient with a positive Hawkins sign developed osteonecrosis. Of the 27 patients who did not have a positive Hawkins sign, 77% had osteonecrosis. These fractures can heal in the presence of osteonecrosis; however, it can take up to 36 months for the dead bone to be replaced.

Methods of avoiding talar body collapse are controversial. Most studies show that non–weight-bearing status for a prolonged period gives the best results, but it is unknown whether this approach will prevent collapse. In one report, 6 of 13 patients had talar body collapse even though they were not bearing weight. A patella-bearing caliper was developed for off-loading during ambulation. Unfortunately, non–weight-bearing calipers are poorly tolerated, and they seldom are used. Custom fabricated patellar-tendon bearing braces are a better alternative to the caliper. In another report, the best results were obtained with patients who did not bear weight for 8 months. However, patient compliance with such an extended period of non weight bearing is an issue.

Types of osteonecrosis can be divided into three groups. Group I includes the smallest lesion, which can present as an osteochondral lesion with an underlying necrotic bed. Group II includes partial osteonecrosis involving less than 50% of the talar body that can be singular or multiple. Group III involves most of the talar body or, in rare circumstances, the en-

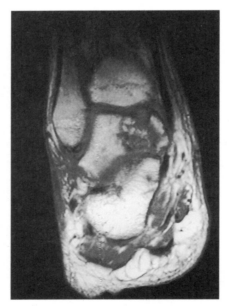

Figure 1 AP MRI scan showing involvement of 40% of the talar body with evidence of collapse of the cortical rim.

tire talus (**Figure 1**). Treatment of group I lesions can consist of débridement with either drilling or microfracture. Larger lesions or group I lesions that have not responded to débridement are treated with either an osteochondral autograft transfer system (OATS), autogenous cultured chondrocytes (Carticel procedure), or an allograft.

The treatment of group II lesions is dictated by the extent and location of the lesion. Early in the course of this disease, a trial of a patellar-tendon bearing-type orthosis is indicated. The length of treatment depends on the patient's needs and the surgeon's philosophy. One surgical option is a core decompression of the talar body before any collapse is seen radiographically. A more standard option is a hindfoot fusion, which can be limited to one or two joints depending on the initial evaluation (**Figure 2**). Hindfoot fusions in the presence of osteonecrosis require a much longer time to fuse than the usual 10 to 16 weeks when there is no osteonecrosis.

Group III lesions are more problematic as a result of the potential loss of the entire talus, given the impossibility of incorporating the usual viable head and neck into a standard arthrodesis. The outcome of a successful tibiocalcaneal fusion is markedly limited in regard to gait because of the marked loss of motion.

The contraindications for surgical treatment are few. Relative contraindications are history of smoking, active infection, prior pin tract infections, and noncompliance, especially in regards to prolonged immobilization and non–weight-bearing status. Dysvascularity is a contraindication to surgery and requires consultation for possible revascularization.

PREOPERATIVE PLANNING

Complications are common with multiple joint fusions. Patients should be advised about prolonged healing time, nonunions, infection, and, in some in-

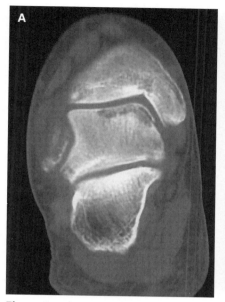 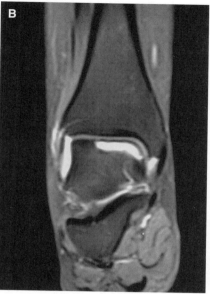 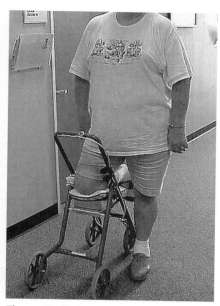

Figure 2 **A,** CT scan revealing an isolated osteonecrosis of the talus involving the medial talar dome. **B,** T2-weighted MRI scan revealing the same lesion with more extensive signal changes involving almost 60% on the AP view.

Figure 3 Patient using a kneeling device to unweight the treated leg during the non–weight-bearing period.

stances, the potential for amputation if the procedure is unsuccessful. They should also be advised of the adverse effects of smoking on healing, as well as the possible need for autogenous graft and/or allograft, depending on the size of the defect. Patients should be counseled about the expected goals of such an extensive fusion and also the potential need of bracing and/or shoe modification. A kneeling device that allows the patient to mobilize without crutches is useful for the prolonged non–weight-bearing period. This is especially true for patients with diabetes mellitus or neuropathy. (**Figure 3**).

SURGERY
Core decompression is indicated for patients who have radiographic evidence of stage I or II osteonecrosis according to the Ficat staging system (**Table 1**). This stage represents retention of the normal contour of the talus with no evidence of a subchondral fracture or arthritis. The decompression can be performed as a simple outpatient procedure with the patient un-

der an ankle block. It can be performed either arthroscopically or with a standard anterolateral or anteromedial open approach. The approach is dictated by the location of the lesion on MRI. Medial lesions can be readily accessed arthroscopically with a retrogade approach. Under fluoroscopic guidance, a 4-mm cannula is inserted through a portal or incision of choice. A bone biopsy specimen is obtained to verify the pathology of the lesion. One or two cores are taken, depending on the size of the lesion. Postoperatively, the patient is restricted to 40 lb partial weight bearing for a 6-week period followed by full weight bearing as tolerated. The patient is then followed with repeat radiographs and MRI in 3 to 6 months. The goal of this procedure is to lessen the vascular hypertension, aid in revascularization, and prevent future collapse of the talus.

ARTHRODESIS OF THE ANKLE
The arthrodesis can be stabilized using screw or plate fixation or an intramedullary nail. In the presence of an active or previous infection, the use of an external fixator such an Ilizarov

frame is acceptable. The patient undergoes general or spinal anesthesia, which can be supplemented with a popliteal block to minimize pain and allow for the procedure to be performed on an outpatient basis. The patient is placed in a supine position with a bolster under the ipsilateral hip. The preparation should be performed sterile above the knee so as to be able to judge the alignment of the lower extremity to the fusion. An ankle tourniquet is used routinely in all procedures. After exsanguination of the lower extremity, a posterolateral incision is made approximately 8 cm above the tip of the fibula (**Figure 4**). This incision is placed just posterior to the fibula to have adequate space for an anteromedial incision. Full-thickness flaps are developed both anteriorly and posteriorly. In 15% of the patients, a communicating branch of the sural nerve combines with the superficial peroneal nerve distal to the fibula. In thin patients, it can be identified by plantar flexion and inversion of the foot. This branch needs to be identified and protected

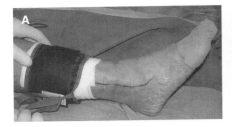

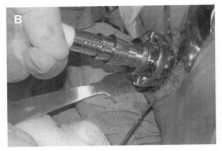

Figure 4 **A,** The location of the proposed incision for a standard ankle or pantalar arthrodesis. **B,** A small acetabular reamer is used to obtain large amounts of morcellized bone from the lateral malleolus.

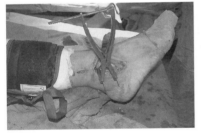

Figure 5 A joint distractor using pins is helpful for increasing the exposure for hindfoot fusions.

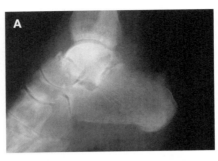

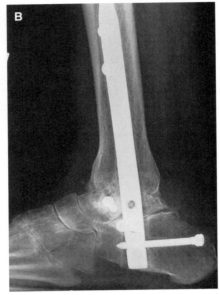

Figure 6 **A,** Preoperative radiograph of an 80-year-old woman with untreated Hawkins II fracture of the talar neck with subsequent malunion and osteonecrosis. **B,** One-year follow-up after use of a retrograde intramedullary rod with locking screws. Note partial consolidation of the subtalar joint.

of any necrotic bone. The cartilaginous surface of the tibia is first denuded with the use of osteotomes and curets. Aids in distracting the ankle are smooth and toothed lamina spreaders. The smooth version has a tendency to be unstable while the toothed version tends to be difficult to insert. I prefer the Hintermann distractor (Newdeal, Vienne, France). Small 0.62–in Kirschner wires are placed in the talus and tibia, respectively, to enhance visualization and débridement (**Figure 5**). The type of arthrodesis will now be determined by the extent of the talar necrosis found at the time of surgery.

For patients with minimal necrosis, a standard tibiotalar arthrodesis can be performed with supplementation of autogenous graft. For patients in whom significant amounts of the talar body are removed, modification of the fixation is required. This modification will also entail a subtalar arthrodesis because of potential damage to the joint from the débridement (**Figure 6**). In these patients, the lateral incision is made as distal as possible to facilitate exposure of the subtalar joint.

In patients with more extensive necrosis, the entire talar body is removed. A modified Blair-type fusion is performed by removing enough bone to dock the tibia onto the calcaneus and onto the residual neck of the talus. To facilitate this reduction, an anteromedial ankle incision is made parallel to the anterior tibial tendon. As much of the distal portions of the medial malleolus are removed as needed to achieve bony apposition. Large amounts of bone graft are useful, especially in patients with neuropathy. Needed bone can be obtained from the distal fibula, iliac crest, or Gerdy's tubercle. For neuropathic joints, it is more feasible to use fresh-frozen femoral head allograft. Using a small acetabular reamer, large amounts of shavings can be extracted from the femoral heads. To limit infection in

with the posterolateral approach. An incision is made directly on the fibula to allow for subperiosteal dissection of the distal 4 cm of this bone. The lateral malleolus is then protected with Homan retractors to avoid damage to the peroneal tendons.

Autogenous bone from the lateral malleolus is obtained with the smallest acetabular reamer. The bone graft is then stored in a sterile container until ready for use. Allograft is a possible alternative but is less successful in these difficult cases. Its use is indicated for large deficits, morbidly obese patients, or if the surgeon

wishes to preserve the fibula to allow for possible conversion to a total ankle replacement at a later date. This latter possibility is unlikely for severe cases of osteonecrosis.

Minimizing the removal of bone from the distal fibula allows for retention of the anterior tibiofibular ligament, which aids in the stability of the proximal tibia and fibula and helps prevent postoperative stress fractures. Removal of the fibula proximal to the lateral malleolus is more likely to promote stress fractures or stress reactions. Inspection of the joint will determine the exact location and extent

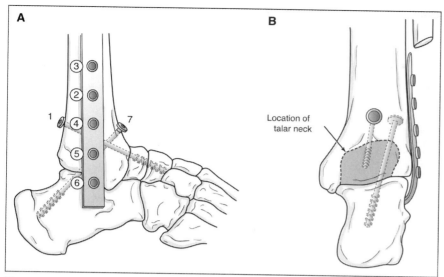

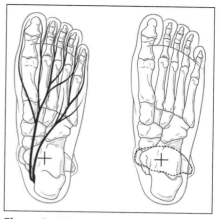

Figure 8 Plantar incision; the relationship between the lateral plantar nerve and the entrance for intramedullary nailing. (Adapted with permission from Kile TA: Tibiotalocalcaneal arthrodesis, in Kitaoke HB (ed): *Masters Techniques in Orthopaedic Surgery*, ed 2. Philadelphia, PA, Lippincott Williams & Wilkins, 2002, pp 551-558.)

Figure 7 Procedure for blade plate pantalar arthrodesis. **A,** Lateral view. Note the numbered order of screws. **B,** Posterior view. Note the alignment of the transfixing cancellous screws into the talus and calcaneus, which supplement rotational stability. (Adapted with permission from Trevino SG: Surgical treatment of the Charcot foot and ankle, in Kelikian A (ed): *Surgical Treatment of the Foot and Ankle*. Stamford, CT, Appleton & Lange, 1999, pp 147-175.)

patients with diabetes mellitus, the shavings from each femoral head are mixed with 500 mg of vancomycin and 360 mg of tobramycin powder in a metal basin. Any excessive fat from the marrow is removed by wringing the composite in a small towel. This procedure will prevent the shavings from floating out of the arthrodesis site.

The type of implant used depends on the cause of the osteonecrosis. For posttraumatic injuries, tibiocalcaneal fusions are easily accomplished using an intramedullary rod with compression. For neuropathic joints, compression is best obtained using a 90° titanium blade plate. Unfortunately, the intramedullary nail fixation frequently fails at the interface of the distal interlocking screws because of the osteoporotic condition of the calcaneus.

Author's Preferred Method and Rationale
MODIFIED TIBIOCALCANEAL FUSION WITH THE 90° BLADE PLATE

A universal AO femoral distractor or compressor is used on the medial side to achieve tibiocalcaneal reduction. Under fluoroscopic control, AP and lateral alignment is verified. Compression with the above device achieves temporary fixation and facilitates compression of the blade plate without causing angulation of the reduction during fixation. Temporary fixation of the tibia to the neck of the talus is achieved with a 2.8-mm guide wire from the posterolateral tibia. It may be necessary to extend the guidewire to the navicular for adequate fixation. After appropriate pin placement, a 7.3-mm partially threaded titanium cannulated screw is used to obtain the initial fixation between the tibia and the foot.

At this time the standard techniques for the 90° titanium blade plate are used. The entry point of the blade plate is at the junction of the lower and middle thirds of the calcaneus. The blade is parallel to the sole of the foot. The blade length is determined with a depth gauge and is usually between 30 and 40 mm with a 6- to 8-hole plate. The peroneal tendons are in close proximity and need to be pro-

tected from damage while positioning the blade plate. Once the proper position of the plate in the calcaneus is determined, the near cortex is prepared with multiple drill holes created with a 2.5-mm drill bit, thus creating the oval-shaped defect in the cortical area. The titanium plate is then contoured to the lateral tibia with a plate bender. Care is taken not to overcorrect the bend so that the titanium is not weakened. After inserting the blade portion of the plate, compression is achieved at the plate portion by an AO tensioning device or a push-pull technique. The latter technique uses a 4.5-mm cortical screw and a No. 1 Verbrugge clamp (Sklar Instruments, West Chester, PA). The Verbrugge clamp is a bone-holding forcep with one ragged end and one smooth end. The ragged end is placed over a protruding 4.5-mm cortical screw around 1.5 cm from the end of the plate. The smooth portion is placed in the most proximal portion of the plate and allows for compression of the plate to the screw. Further compression is accomplished using the distal compression holes of the plate. After completion of plate fixation, a final

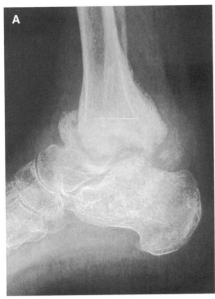

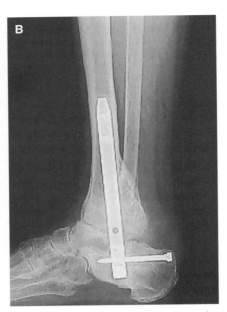

Figure 9 **A,** Preoperative radiograph of a 55-year-old woman with diabetes mellitus who has osteonecrosis of the talus secondary to Charcot arthropathy. **B,** Lateral view also demonstrates nonunion of the subtalar joint.

cannulated 7.3-mm screw is inserted from the anterior aspect of the tibia into the tuberosity of the calcaneus; thus, rotation is controlled as is fixation of the foot to the tibia (**Figure 7**).

TIBIOCALCANEAL FUSION USING AN INTRAMEDULLARY ROD

A transverse incision in line with the transmalleolar axis is made at the junction of the middle and anterior thirds of the heel pad (**Figure 8**). Reduction between the foot and the tibia is checked visually and fluoroscopi-

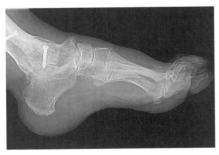

Figure 10 Severe equinus deformity secondary to malunited arthrodesis for osteonecrosis of the talus. Note the degenerative midfoot secondary to forefoot cavus compensation.

cally. An off-centered Steinmann pin can be used for temporary fixation. Blunt dissection is performed in a transverse plane to protect the lateral plantar nerve. A threaded, tipped guide pin is advanced through the calcaneus into the center of the tibia and verified with fluoroscopy in both planes. The medullary canal of the tibia is often medial to the calcaneal insertion site. To improve proper alignment, the subtalar joint is débrided thoroughly, and, if necessary, the capsular structures on the medial aspect of the talus can be divided to allow medial subluxation. Further adjustments in alignment can occur by selective débridement of the articular surface of the medial malleolus as well as resection of its distal portion to allow for better compression. Visual verification of sagittal alignment is made from a lateral view, which is more accurate than a medial view. Optimal alignment is 5° of valgus, external rotation similar to that of the opposite leg, and the ankle at neutral; however, with a tibiocalcaneal fusion, the surgeon must compensate

for any tibia vara so that the foot is plantigrade. This compensation may require more eversion than 5°. Before reaming, the harvested bone graft is placed medially and laterally. Some graft is reserved for the end of the procedure. Once reaming has started, no significant changes can be made in this alignment.

The proper functioning of the nail construct must be checked before the nail is implanted. The drill should fit nicely with the corresponding holes in the nail. The surgeon reams either to the selected nail diameter or 0.5 mm less. Underreaming ensures a tight fit with the calcaneus and tibia but may result in difficulty in placement. I am currently using the Biomet arthrodesis nail (Biomet, Inc, Warsaw, IN), which allows for compression and AP calcaneal screw placement. The most common size nails used are 10 to 12 mm in diameter and 15 cm in length.

When using a nail that offers distal compression, the surgeon needs to factor in the potential distance that will be reduced once compression is applied. The nail is driven so that its distal end lies within the calcaneus to provide this relief factor. The rod is rotated internally to avoid the fibula. The compression device is then attached. The attached jig is rotated until proper depth is confirmed by image intensification. With extensive loss of the talar body, no locking screw can be placed in the talus; however, the Biomet nail allows for both a lateral to medial interlocking screw and, more importantly, a posterior to anterior locking screw. After placement of the lateral to medial screw, the attached drill guide is rotated 90° degrees for placement of the posterior to anterior screw.

The postoperative protocol is the same for all procedures. The patient will be immobilized for a least 6 weeks in a non–weight-bearing cast. Patients with neuropathy require 3 to 4 months. This period is followed with

6 weeks in a weight-bearing cast. After determination of clinical healing, the patient is converted to a walking boot to prevent stress fractures from the implant. The time schedule is lengthened for patients with neuropathy. For this group of patients, immobilization in a diabetic brace is indicated postoperatively. The brace consists of a double upright with a fixed ankle attached to a rocker-bottom shoe modified with an extended shank. In normal patients, shoe modifications are common, especially with a tibiocalcaneal fusion. A rocker-bottom shoe with the apex placed over the proximal one third of the foot and an extended shank enables an improved gait.

Management of Complications

The most common complication is delayed fusion or a nonunion. In instances where the patient remains symptomatic and has radiographic evidence of nonunion, ultrasound or electromagnetic stimulation is considered (**Figure 9**). If no improvement is noted 3 months after using stimulation, regrafting of the arthrodesis site or converting a tibiotalar fusion to a tibiocalcaneal fusion should be considered. Intramedullary retrograde nailing is associated with major complications in up to 30% of patients, including nonunion at either the ankle or subtalar site, protrusion of the nail, and stress fractures above the implant. Prevention of these complications includes use of autogenous bone graft, using a nail with a compressive device, or consideration of a blade plate as an alternative to the nail for patients with neuropathy.

Malunions can occur due to the technical difficulty in correcting the equinovarus deformity, the limited acceptable position of a tibiocalcaneal fusion, and the need to avoid varus positioning. Normally the acceptable position for ankle arthrodesis is neutral at the ankle, 5° of valgus, and external rotation similar to that of the opposite extremity. However, in the presence of any excessive tibia vara, the correct position is 10° to 15° of valgus of the heel to compensate for the malalignment of the lower leg (**Figure 10**).

Superficial infections are common and can be controlled with either oral or intravenous antibiotics, depending on the severity. Infection of an intramedullary rod requires removal of the rod, intravenous antibiotics, and possible antibiotic bead placement in the medullary cavity. My protocol is to treat the patient with 2 weeks of culture-specific intravenous antibiotics followed by 4 weeks of oral antibiotics. The antibiotic beads are retained for a minimum of 6 weeks or until revision. Use of an intramedullary rod or blade plate after infection is not recommended. Once the infection is controlled, placement of an external fixator and repeat arthrodesis can be considered.

References

Dennison M, Pool R, Simonis R, et al: Tibiocalcaneal fusion for avascular necrosis of the talus. *J Bone Joint Surg Br* 2001;83:199-203.

Kitaoka H, Patzer G: Arthrodesis for the treatment of arthrosis of the ankle and osteonecrosis of the talus. *J Bone Joint Surg Am* 1998;80:370-379.

McGarvey W, Trevino S, Baxter D, et al: Tibiotalocalcaneal arthrodesis: Anatomic and technical considerations. *Foot Ankle Int* 1998;19:363-369.

Mont MA, Schon LC, Hungerford MW, Hungerford D: Avascular necrosis of the talus treated by core decompression. *J Bone Joint Surg Br* 1996;78:827-830.

Coding

ICD-9 CODES

716.17   Posttraumatic arthritis of the ankle and/or foot

733.44   Avascular necrosis of the talus

825.21   Fracture talus

CPT CODES

20900   Bone graft, minor

20902   Bone graft, major

27870   Ankle arthrodesis, any method

28130   Talectomy

28705   Pantalar arthrodesis

28725   Subtalar arthrodesis

Osteonecrosis of the Navicular

George J. Haidukewych, MD

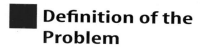 Definition of the Problem

Patient Presentation

Patients typically present with pain in the midfoot and hindfoot that is aggravated by activity, especially on uneven ground, and improved by rest. Pain frequently occurs bilaterally and is especially common in women. Unilateral pain and deformity are also possible.

Physical Examination

Patients typically have tenderness over the talonavicular and/or naviculocuneiform joints and an antalgic gait. Occasionally, synovitis or an effusion in the talonavicular and naviculocuneiform joints will be present. Examination will reveal tenderness with subtalar motion, and patients will resist subtalar motion secondary to pain or arthritis. Pes planus and hindfoot valgus deformities are frequently seen as well. However, post-traumatic osteonecrosis of the navicular has been associated with a varus hindfoot. Patients are typically able to perform a single heel rise but may have pain associated with this maneuver.

Differential Diagnosis

- Insufficiency fracture of the navicular
- Healing acute fracture of the navicular
- Stress reaction of the navicular
- Neoplasia
- Osteomyelitis

Additional Work-up

Weight-bearing AP, lateral, and oblique radiographs of the foot should be obtained. The classic radiographic changes of osteonecrosis include loss of volume of the navicular, commonly seen in the lateral aspect, and increased bone density. The lateral aspect of the navicular is typically involved, but the medial aspect or even the entire bone may be involved (**Figure 1**).

Understanding the blood supply to the navicular is important in understanding the disease process. Because of the extensive amount of articular cartilage, the arterial blood supply is limited to a branch of the dorsalis pedis artery, the medial plantar branch of the posterior tibial artery, and a network of arteries from both the dorsal and plantar arteries that supplies the tuberosity. Microangiographic studies have demonstrated a largely avascular zone in the central third of the navicular. This may contribute to nonunions, stress fractures, and osteonecrosis.

Progressive collapse with bony destruction can be seen, often with dorsal protrusion and fragmentation of either a portion or the entire navicular. The collapse results in the so-called "common-shaped" navicular, characteristic on radiographs of patients with osteonecrosis. With severe collapse, the head of the talus will articulate with the cuneiforms.

Advanced imaging studies such as CT and MRI can also be helpful. Typical findings on CT include sclerosis of the lateral aspect of the navicular and frag-mentation with dorsal protrusion. MRI may be indicated for patients with normal radiographs and pain and deformity of unknown etiology. The advantage of MRI is the improved visualization of the associated tendons and bony structures. Osteonecrosis of the navicular appears as homogenous loss of signal intensity in the bone marrow on T1-weighted images. T2-weighted images frequently show focal loss of signal intensity in the affected area. Neither study, however, is perfect: on the CT scan there is frequently a discrepancy in the degree of sclerosis; on the MRI, the extent of the signal loss is variable. The MRI findings, however, are diagnostic for this condition.

Osteonecrosis of the navicular can be categorized as either primary or secondary, depending on the etiology. Primary disease is seen in idiopathic osteonecrosis of the navicular. Secondary disease is seen in patients with a known process that can cause osteonecrosis such as renal failure, rheumatoid arthritis, systemic lupus erythematosus, or trauma. This entity is distinct from Köhler's disease, which is seen in children. The cause of Köhler's disease has been hypothesized to include normal variations in the ossification centers, disturbances of the endochondral bone formation, and an ischemic necrosis of bone. However, Köhler's disease is not associated with clinical abnormalities and frequently is associated with minor symptoms. In sharp contrast, osteonecrosis of the navicular in adults is as-

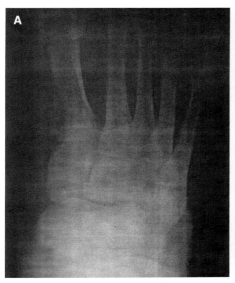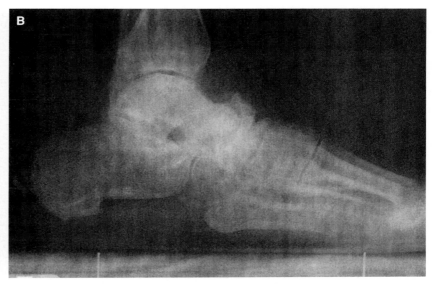

Figure 1 AP (**A**) and lateral (**B**) radiographs show destruction of the navicular, with dorsal protrusion and fragmentation.

sociated with significant pain and functional limitations. The underlying etiology has not been identified, but it is believed that an underlying stress reaction may be contributory.

----■

■ The Solutions

Treatment Options and Rationale

The natural history of the disease is not known; however, most patients are sufficiently symptomatic so that nonsurgical care is rarely satisfactory. There are no published data available on the results of nonsurgical treatment or guidelines for clinicians regarding this approach. A trial of immobilization with a removable boot may provide temporary relief, as may an orthosis that limits inversion/eversion and improves hindfoot alignment.

Surgical treatment is focused primarily on fusion of the involved joints, including fusion of the talonavicular joint and/or the naviculocuneiform joints, as indicated. Imaging studies may help define the involved joints and guide treatment. If identifying which joints require fusion is difficult, fluoroscopically guided injection of a local anesthetic can assist in visualizing the joints that are most symptomatic.

The results of talonavicular arthrodesis have been reported, but not specifically for this clinical problem. In a recent review of 16 patients who underwent talonavicular arthrodesis for osteoarthritis, previous fractures, systemic lupus erythematosus, and flatfoot deformities, 15 achieved a solid union and had marked improvement in ankle and hindfoot scores. However, the authors noted that after more than 4 years, clinically significant degenerative changes were noted in the adjacent joints.

Other authors have reported on the efficacy of performing talonavicular arthrodesis in combination with a calcaneocuboid arthrodesis. The rationale for this approach was that simultaneous fusion would be superior biomechanically by decreasing the stress placed on the talonavicular arthrodesis site. In another study in which double arthrodesis was performed on 16 feet, solid union was achieved in 15 of the 16 feet. Asymptomatic nonunion occurred in one patient; six had degenerative ankle arthritis, and seven had osteoarthritic changes in the naviculocuneiform. Another report on double arthrodesis in 24 patients reported satisfactory results in 83% of patients. These authors also noted that progression of arthritis in adjacent joints was common but usually asymptomatic. They also stated that the addition of a calcaneocuboid arthrodesis provided further stability to the transverse tarsal complex. Other authors have recommended this technique in obese patients.

Author's Preferred Treatment and Rationale

The current approach used for osteonecrosis of the navicular begins with a trial of nonsurgical treatment. Bracing with an articulating ankle-foot orthosis to allow ankle motion but limited inversion/eversion is attempted and continued as long as the patient reports satisfactory relief. If nonsurgical treatment fails, surgical treatment is recommended. An isolated talonavicular arthrodesis and/or a naviculocuneiform arthrodesis is preferred. Occasionally, in obese patients, a calcaneocuboid arthrodesis is performed in conjunction with the talonavicular arthrodesis.

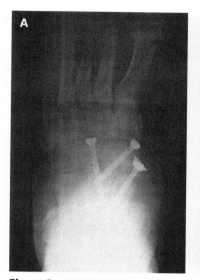
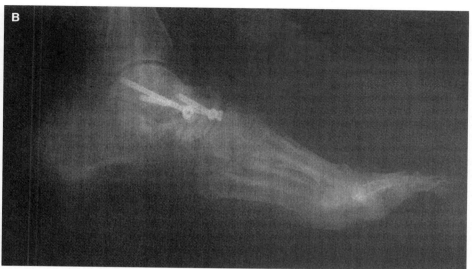

Figure 2   AP (**A**) and lateral (**B**) radiographs show a talonavicular arthrodesis with cannulated screw fixation.

For a talonavicular arthrodesis, the patient is placed supine on the operating room table after anesthesia is administered. An incision is made medially over the talonavicular joint and extended to the naviculocuneiform joint, if necessary. Dissection is carried through the skin and down to the capsule. The capsule is then incised, exposing the talonavicular joint. Frequently, a portion of the navicular tuberosity is removed to expose the talonavicular joint. The necrotic bone is removed with a rongeur or a burr. The arthrodesis site is prepared using curets and osteotomes until the bleeding bone is identified. Multiple small drill holes are made on the opposing surfaces, as needed. If the resulting defect is large, autogenous iliac crest bone graft can be used. The foot is then positioned in a plantigrade position with 5° of valgus of the hindfoot

and the talonavicular joint in neutral alignment. Guide pins are placed from the navicular into the talus. Positioning is verified with fluoroscopy, and partially threaded 4.0- or 5.0-mm cannulated screws are placed, depending on the size of the patient (**Figure 2**). Great care is taken to avoid abduction/adduction deformity of the midfoot during placement of the screws. The wound is then closed in layers, and the patient is placed in a compressive dressing with a plaster splint. The patient is then placed into a short leg cast and kept on non–weight-bearing status for 6 weeks. At that time, if there is radiographic evidence of progressive consolidation of the arthrodesis site, partial weight bearing in a short leg cast is recommended for another 6 weeks. At 3 months, casting is discontinued if there is radiographic evidence of fusion.

Management of Complications

The most common complications of these procedures are malunion and nonunion. Nonunions can be salvaged by revision with autologous bone grafting and stable internal fixation. If the alignment is acceptable, a slot is created and an inlay bone graft is used.

Malalignment of this joint usually involves malpositioning of the hindfoot and the forefoot; salvage is possible with realignment and triple arthrodesis. The best treatment, however, is prevention. Therefore, we recommend careful intraoperative imaging to evaluate the position of the arthrodesis.

The author wishes to acknowledge the contribution of Norman S. Turner, MD, in the creation of this chapter.

References

Brailsford JF: Osteochondritis. *Br J Radiol* 1935;119:87-134.

Chen CH, Huang PJ, Chen TB, et al: Isolated talonavicular arthrodesis for talonavicular arthritis. *Foot Ankle Int* 2001;22:633-636.

Clain MR, Baxter DE: Simultaneous calcaneocuboid and talonavicular fusion. Long-term follow-up study. *J Bone Joint Surg Br* 1994;76:133-136.

Fogel GR, Katoh Y, Rand JA, Chao EY: Talonavicular arthrodesis for isolated arthrosis. 9.5 year results and gait analysis. *Foot Ankle* 1982;3:105-113.

Haller J, Sartoris DJ, Resnick D, et al: Spontaneous osteonecrosis of the tarsal navicular in adults: Imaging findings. *AJR Am J Roentgenol* 1988;115:355-358.

Mann RA, Beaman DN: Double arthrodesis in the adult. *Clin Orthop* 1999;365:74-80.

Coding

ICD-9 CODE
715.37   Osteoarthritis, localized, foot

CPT CODES
28740   Midtarsal single joint

20900   Bone graft, minor or small

20902   Bone graft, major or large

CPT copyright © 2003 by the American Medical Association. All Rights Reserved.

Lisfranc Joint Injuries

Thomas H. Lee, MD

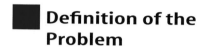

Definition of the Problem

Patient Presentation

After acute tarsometatarsal (TMT) injuries, patients present with midfoot pain, swelling, and the inability to bear weight. A high index of suspicion is required to consistently identify Lisfranc joint injuries. Many of these injuries occur in patients with multiple traumatic injuries; these injuries should be suspected in any patient who reports midfoot pain or has unexplained or excessive swelling. In one series up to 20% of these injuries were missed.

Injuries of the Lisfranc joints are relatively uncommon, with a reported incidence of one per 55,000 persons. Other studies report a rate of one Lisfranc injury per 5,500 fractures treated. TMT injuries can occur by direct or indirect mechanisms. A direct blow to the TMT joint, as may occur during a crush injury, will often result in a very severe soft-tissue injury with ligamentous and bony disruption.

The most common mechanism of injury is indirect. Most of the indirect mechanisms described include loading of the plantar flexed foot with an associated abduction of the midfoot. An example of this is the rider who falls from a horse with the foot secured inside the stirrup. Another proposed mechanism occurs if the deforming force is primarily abduction. In this mechanism, the hindfoot is fixed and the forefoot is forcefully abducted, resulting in lateral displacement of the metatarsals and fractures at the base of the second and other metatarsals.

Physical Examination

Physical examination should focus on the integrity of the skin and tenderness in the midfoot. Careful palpation will often elicit pain along the TMT joints that is exacerbated by pronation and supination of the forefoot. Tense swelling of the foot compartments may indicate a compartment syndrome and mandates measurement of foot compartment pressures.

The initial radiographic examination of the suspected Lisfranc injury should include AP, lateral, and 30° oblique views of the injured foot. These radiographs should be obtained with the patient weight bearing, when possible, and then compared with radiographs of the contralateral uninjured foot. Three consistent anatomic patterns must be systematically reviewed in all radiographs to reliably detect midfoot injuries: (1) On the AP view, the medial border of the second metatarsal forms a continuous line with the medial border of the middle cuneiform. (2) On the 30° oblique view, the medial border of the fourth metatarsal forms a continuous line with the medial border of the cuboid. (3) On the lateral view, no evidence of plantar or dorsal displacement of the metatarsals relative to the cuneiforms should be evident.

Other signs that raise suspicion for a midfoot injury include a fleck of bone in the 1-2 intermetatarsal base, which represents an avulsion fracture of the Lisfranc ligament or an impaction fracture of the cuboid (nutcracker injury).

Differential Diagnosis
- Midfoot sprain
- Midfoot fracture-dislocation (Lisfranc)
- Metatarsal fractures

Additional Work-up

If an injury is suspected but not confirmed by initial radiographic views, stress views under anesthesia, CT, or MRI should be considered. MRI has the advantage of showing bony edema patterns, cross-sectional images of the Lisfranc ligament, and any soft-tissue interposition between fracture fragments.

The Solutions

Treatment Options and Rationale

Nonsurgical treatment of Lisfranc injuries, consisting of closed reduction and casting, has had poor results as reported in the literature. If an instability pattern is not obvious with standard radiographic views but the mechanism of injury and clinical presentation raise suspicion for midfoot

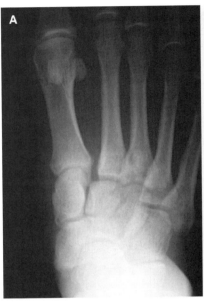
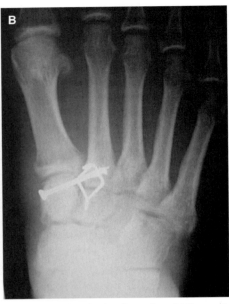

Figure 1 **A,** Partial incongruity lateral dislocation. Note that the line from the middle cuneiform to the second metatarsal is disrupted but the line from the medial cuboid to the fourth metatarsal remains well aligned. **B,** Open reduction and internal fixation has realigned the second metatarsal base. The second metatarsal base is stabilized by a Lisfranc screw and an extra-articular staple. The staple may be replaced by a single screw from the second metatarsal to the middle cuneiform.

injury, CT, MRI, or stress testing is mandatory. Any instability of the TMT joint warrants internal fixation (**Figure 1**).

A Lisfranc sprain refers to injury of the Lisfranc ligament without demonstrable shift of osseus relationships. Treatment of these injuries is controversial, with some advocating initiating treatment with a non–weight-bearing cast and progressing to a weight-bearing cast when tenderness has subsided. These sprains generally result in significant morbidity, and there is increasing support for temporary percutaneous screw stabilization of the midfoot.

Author's Preferred Treatment and Rationale

Almost all recent studies advocate surgical treatment of Lisfranc dislocations. Open reduction and stable temporary internal fixation using screws is the most reliable means of restoring and maintaining joint congruity. We believe that closed reduction and per-

cutaneous pinning is inadequate to stabilize the medial three rays because of wire migration. Pin fixation of the lateral two rays is an accepted technique, provided the medial rays are stable. If they are unstable, screws are required.

Surgical exposure of Lisfranc joints is difficult to achieve. The traditional technique is to expose the joints through multiple longitudinal incisions. One incision is centered over the second metatarsal, one is medial to the first TMT joint, and one is over the fourth intermetatarsal space.

The second TMT joint is approached using the extensor hallucis brevis (EHB) muscle belly as a guide. The surgical plane is established medial to the muscle belly and developed to its musculotendinous junction. While retracting the EHB laterally, the deep peroneal nerve and dorsalis pedis artery are identified and protected. The dorsalis pedis artery should be mobilized carefully to preserve its per-

forating branch that enters the 1-2 intermetatarsal space.

Once appropriate intervals are established, capsulotomies are performed starting at the first TMT and working medial to lateral. Fluoroscopy is useful to prevent inadvertent exposure of the naviculocuneiform joints instead of the TMT joints.

The second TMT joint is reduced and temporarily stabilized while a cannulated screw is passed, under fluoroscopic guidance, from the medial cuneiform into the base of the second metatarsal. This screw must be sufficiently plantar to allow a dorsal screw starting in the second metatarsal to pass to the middle cuneiform. Although screws are the best form of fixation, alternative fixation (staples) may be used to minimize articular cartilage damage (**Figure 1**). Additional screws are passed across the first and third TMT joints as dictated by the injury pattern. The fourth and fifth TMT joints are stabilized with 0.62-in Kirschner wires (K-wires) if they are relatively stable. If they are grossly unstable, screws should be passed from the metatarsals into the cuboid.

With severe abduction or adduction injuries the lateral column (cuboid) or medial column (medial cuneiform) can be crushed (nutcracker injury). In this scenario the Lisfranc joints are fixed as described. An external fixator is applied laterally or medially to bring the column out to proper anatomic length. The articular surface is elevated through the fracture, and the dead space is filled with morcellized (or fragments of) bone graft. The external fixator is left in place for 6 weeks (**Figure 2**).

In severe Lisfranc fracture-dislocations with comminuted intra-articular fractures, anatomic restoration and articular congruity cannot always be reestablished. In this situation a dorsal bridge plate may be inserted, with screws placed in the metatarsal shaft and cuneiforms and/or cuboid.

The patient cannot bear weight

for 6 weeks, after which time a gradual increase in weight bearing is allowed as tolerated. If present, lateral column K-wires are removed at 6 weeks because of an increased risk of wire breakage in the mobile lateral rays. Screws are removed at 4 to 6 months.

Management of Complications

An anatomic reduction of the Lisfranc joint is imperative to, but does not guarantee, a good result. It is a mistake to look at radiographs of Lisfranc complex disruptions and view them as isolated radiographic abnormalities because this ignores the tremendous soft-tissue disruption that accompanies the injury and does not accurately reflect the articular injury. Neither injury type nor radiographic findings have been predictive of symptomatic posttraumatic arthroses. Although fracture or residual incongruity of the lateral TMT joints is rare, an impaction injury is the likely source for later joint degeneration. The reported incidence of symptomatic posttraumatic arthritis after Lisfranc injury is as high as 58%. Despite anatomic reduction, common symptoms after injury at the TMT joints include forefoot stiffness, loss of the metatarsal arch, and intrinsic contracture. Symptoms have been reported to improve for up to 4 years following injury and/or surgical repair.

A delayed diagnosis is relatively common in Lisfranc injuries. As a result of the poor prognosis associated with an unreduced Lisfranc fracture-dislocation, a delayed attempt at open reduction with internal fixation should be considered. The literature supports the conclusion that the best prognosis will be achieved if the reduction is achieved within 6 weeks of injury, but there are reports of reduction of ligamentous Lisfranc injuries up to 1 year postinjury.

The results of arthrodesis of the TMT joints for the arthritic sequela following traumatic injury have been

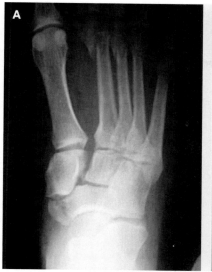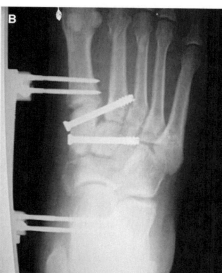

Figure 2 **A,** Partial incongruity medial column disruption with shortening of medial column and navicular fracture. **B,** Medial column instability pattern through the middle and medial cuneiform and first and second metatarsal stabilized with internal fixation. An external fixator has been applied medially to allow the navicular to heal out to length.

reported. Anatomic reduction of the TMT joints before fusion is essential and is the most significant prognostic factor. The major function of the TMT joint complex is the regulation and redirecting of loading forces during weight bearing. In situ fusion without realignment does not adequately restore the biomechanical role of the midfoot.

Posttraumatic arthritic changes noted on radiographs have little relationship to functional impairment. To rationalize this apparent discrepancy between radiographic appearance and clinical significance we recommend a midfoot differential injection. A fluoroscopically guided differential injection of the TMT joints is diagnostic, therapeutic, and prognostic. Patients with posttraumatic midfoot arthritis who achieved complete or near-complete pain relief with the differential injection had an average of 1.5 months of pain relief. A positive test was the most significant factor associated with outcome following surgery as measured by the American Orthopaedic Foot and Ankle Society midfoot scale.

We recommend the test be performed when there is doubt that the midfoot joints are causing most of the patient's pain.

The small incidence of reported symptoms in the lateral column (6% to 25%) is consistent throughout published series on posttraumatic midfoot arthritis. In a report on 49 midfoot joint fusions in 16 patients, the pain focus for most patients was found to be the first through third TMT joints; the fourth and fifth TMT joints were minimally symptomatic. When the lateral column has been confirmed as the source of pain, we recommend a motion-sparing surgical alternative for the fourth and fifth TMT joints. A resection arthroplasty with a soft-tissue interpositional arthroplasty has been shown to provide pain relief yet preserve motion in the mobile lateral rays.

The author wishes to acknowledge the contribution of Gregory G. Berlet, MD, in the creation of this chapter.

■ References

Berlet GC, Davis WH, Anderson RB: Tendon arthroplasty for basal fourth and fifth metatarsal arthritis. *Foot Ankle Int* 2002;23:440-446.

Hardcastle PH, Reschauer R, Kutscha-Lissberg E, Schoffmann W: Injuries to the tarsometatarsal joint: Incidence, classification and treatment. *J Bone Joint Surg Br* 1982;64:349-356.

Kuo RS, Tejwani NC, Digiovanni CW, et al: Outcome after open reduction and internal fixation of Lisfranc joint injuries. *J Bone Joint Surg Am* 2000;82:1609-1618.

Myerson MS, Fisher RT, Burgess AR, Kenzora JE: Fracture dislocations of the tarsometarsal joints: End results correlated with pathology and treatment. *Foot Ankle* 1986;6:225-242.

Sangeorzan BJ, Veith RG, Hansen ST Jr: Salvage of Lisfranc's tarsometatarsal joint by arthrodesis. *Foot Ankle* 1990;10:193-200.

Coding

ICD-9 CODES

825.23   Fracture of cuboid, closed

825.24   Fracture of cuneiform, foot

825.39   Fracture of other tarsal and metatarsal bones, open; other

845.11   Sprains and strains of ankle and foot, tarsometatarsal (joint) (ligament)

CPT CODES

20690   Application of a uniplane (pins or wires in one plane), unilateral, external fixation system

28122   Partial excision (craterization, saucerization, sequestrectomy, or diaphysectomy) bone (eg, osteomyelitis or bossing); tarsal or metatarsal bone

28465   Open treatment of tarsal bone fracture (except talus and calcaneus), with or without internal or external fixation, each

28615   Open treatment of tarsometatarsal joint dislocation, with or without internal or external fixation

Rheumatoid Forefoot

Jason H. Calhoun, MD

■ Definition of the Problem

Patient Presentation

The patient presentation for rheumatoid forefoot depends on the severity and duration of the disease. Initial signs and symptoms of systemic rheumatoid arthritis (RA) include fatigue, joint pain and stiffness, symmetric joint swelling, muscle wasting, weight loss, fever, and rheumatic nodules and rashes. The patient with RA affecting the forefoot may initially present with tenderness or pain in the forefoot, morning stiffness that lasts for more than 1 hour, and symmetric swelling of the joints.

With disease progression, synovial inflammation, swelling, and joint erosion lead to deformities of the forefoot. Usually, the lateral metatarsophalangeal (MTP) joints are affected first, but the more medial joints are also eventually affected. Claw toes often occur secondary to MTP joint involvement (**Figure 1**). The MTP joints become unstable because of ligamentous laxity that results from chronic synovitis. The proximal phalanx initially hyperextends and most commonly develops a lateral drift. As the deformity progresses, the proximal phalanx becomes dislocated dorsally, and the metatarsal heads eventually become more prominent on the plantar surface of the foot. The load bearing of the metatarsal heads in-

creases as they become more prominent, leading to overload and pain.

In addition, the metatarsal fat pad migrates distally as the toes displace dorsally, leaving behind much thinner, non–weight-bearing skin to cover the metatarsal heads. This deficiency in metatarsal padding is also a source of pain because heavy, painful calluses and bursae often form. Ligamentous laxity also leads to forefoot widening as the metatarsals spread. The widening of the intermetatarsal angles leads to hallux valgus as the great toe pronates and drifts laterally (**Figure 2**). As this deformity becomes more pronounced, a painful bursa often develops over the medial first metatarsal head.

Finally, laxity at the first tarsometatarsal joint leads to joint elevation and instability. This is accentuated by heel cord tightness and hindfoot valgus. As the load-bearing capacity of the first ray decreases, increasing forces are transmitted to the lateral metatarsals and midfoot, which contributes to painful overload.

Physical Examination

Examination of a patient with suspected rheumatoid forefoot should include a complete medical history and a family history of arthritis or degenerative diseases. The physical examination should include an evaluation of the patient's entire body, noting affected areas (eg, skin, gastrointestinal tract, joints) and whether there is fe-

ver or local cellulitis. In particular, a thorough examination of the lower extremities is necessary. In the early stages of disease, the forefoot is often tender and swollen around the joint. Pain is often caused by palpation, movement of the MTP joints, compression by squeezing the first and fifth metatarsal heads together, and dorsal-plantar compression of individual joints. The patient's gait should be evaluated for decreased MTP joint motion, especially at the first MTP joint. Weight bearing through the first ray is often decreased as the great toe deviates laterally. The deformity of the first MTP joint decreases the function of the great toe. The great toe often maintains its flexibility but loses its function.

The American Rheumatism Association has developed criteria for the diagnosis of RA. At least four of the following must be present to make the diagnosis of RA: (1) morning stiffness lasting at least 1 hour and present for 6 weeks or more; (2) swelling in at least three joints lasting 6 weeks or more; (3) swelling in the wrist, metacarpophalangeal, or proximal interphalangeal (PIP) joints for 6 weeks or more; (4) symmetric joint swelling; (5) characteristic radiographic changes in the hand, including erosions or unequivocal bony decalcification; (6) the presence of rheumatoid nodules; and (7) positive serum rheumatoid factor. Signs of systemic arthritis include fever, fatigue, rash, and

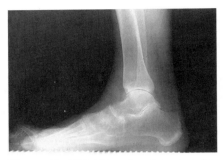

Figure 1 Weight-bearing lateral radiograph showing a claw toe deformity in a patient with rheumatoid arthritis.

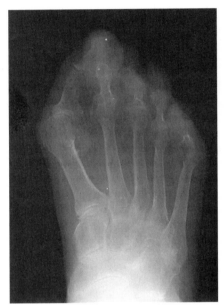

Figure 2 AP view showing characteristic splaying of the metatarsals and hallux valgus.

generalized joint pain, swelling, and stiffness.

Differential Diagnosis
- Osteoarthritis
- Inflammatory arthritis
- Gout
- Systemic lupus erythematosus
- Psoriatic arthritis connective tissue disease
- Viral infection
- Inflammatory bowel disease

Additional Work-up
RADIOGRAPHY
To sufficiently evaluate the foot and ankle with radiographs, weight-bearing AP and lateral views, along with oblique views, should be obtained. Radiographic findings early in the disease process include periarticular osteoporosis, soft-tissue swelling, and joint space narrowing. In later stages of the disease (> 3 years), joint and subchondral erosions of the metatarsal heads and the bases of the phalanges may be noted. Other findings on radiographs include MTP joint dislocations, hammer toes, and hallux valgus. In late stages of severe RA, changes consistent with secondary osteoarthritis, such as osteophyte formation, subchondral sclerosis, and joint ankylosis may be evident.

LABORATORY TESTS
Laboratory tests can be helpful but are not often diagnostic because patients with RA often present with an array of symptoms and problems. Rheumatoid factor, increased levels of C-reactive protein, an elevated erythrocyte sedimentation rate, and decreased levels of complement proteins may be detected in blood samples from patients with RA. Laboratory tests might be useful in ruling out septic arthritis, viral infection, or inflammatory bowel syndrome.

■ The Solutions

Treatment Options and Rationale
Surgical treatment is reserved for the later stages of RA. Although synovectomy and soft-tissue procedures are advocated by some orthopaedists, these procedures generally are not successful because the pain from inflammation and the deformities will progress until the joints are "burned out." Surgical treatment of the forefoot is based on the overall activity level of the patient. More active patients require frequent procedures to relieve pain such as RA nodule removal, aspiration and injections, soft-tissue procedures, and joint reconstruction. Increased function is the goal of these procedures. However, for more disabled patients, pain relief is the principal goal of treatment; the primary surgical options for relieving pain are fusion and joint resection. The patient can be educated with regard to "how much the toe moves now," so that fusion for pain relief, rather than for improved motion, is better understood.

Author's Preferred Treatment and Rationale
SYNOVECTOMY
A synovectomy is performed through a dorsal longitudinal incision over the involved joint or in the interspace for involvement of adjacent joints. A properly placed tourniquet is used for this procedure. The dissection is from the extensor tendon to the extensor hood and into the joint. The hypertrophic synovial tissue is removed with a knife and rongeur from the dorsal to lateral to plantar aspect while the toe is in traction. The joint capsule is closed with No. 3-0 to 4-0 resorbable sutures, and the skin is closed with interrupted nonabsorbable or resorbable sutures. Nonadhering, absorbable, soft dressings and mild compression with a securely taped 2-in elastic bandage are used after surgery. Ambulation is permitted as tolerated while the patient is in a postoperative shoe. The dressing is changed every other week for up to 4 to 6 weeks. The sutures are removed with good skin healing, usually at 2 to 4 weeks.

HAMMER AND CLAW TOE CORRECTION
Hammer toe or claw toe correction is indicated for rigid dorsal PIP joints or

plantar metatarsal head prominence and pain. Nonsurgical treatment options include the use of extra-depth shoes with increased padding. Mild deformities can be manipulated and pinned for 6 weeks. Moderate deformities can be corrected with closed osteoclasis, by PIP joint manipulation into hyperextension, and pinning. Osteoclasis alone is usually reserved for correcting the toes at the time of metatarsal head resection after manipulation. The toes should be pinned in full extension with an intramedullary pin placed into the metatarsal bases.

Open PIP resection and fusion is commonly used for rigid PIP deformities that are not responsive to nonsurgical methods, simple manipulation, or osteoclasis. A contracted, but correctable MTP joint with an extensor tendon contracture often accompanies the PIP joint deformity. A longitudinal skin incision is made to release the long and short extensors at the MTP joint. Tendon lengthening is usually not necessary as the tendon typically regrows. Only the skin is closed with interrupted sutures.

PIP joint fusion is performed through an oval incision centered on the proximal phalanx distal condyle with the PIP joint in forced flexion (**Figure 3**). An oval incision is made through the skin and extensor mechanism, exposing the dorsal half of the distal condyles on the proximal phalanx and the proximal condyles on the middle phalanx. The collateral ligaments are released with a small Freer periosteal elevator or scalpel, with the neurovascular bundles protected. Enough of the proximal and middle phalanges are removed to allow the joint reduction and toe shortening necessary to avoid recurrence. The length of the toes is adjusted through the bony resection so that each lateral toe is slightly shorter than the adjacent toe (ie, the third toe is slightly shorter than the second toe). A 0.062-in Kirschner wire (K-wire) is used for toes two, three, and four, and

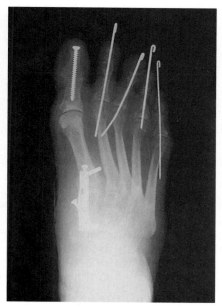

Figure 3 AP view showing PIP joint fusions.

a 0.045-in K-wire is used for the fifth toe. The wire is placed into the middle phalanx and, with the distal interphalangeal joint in forced hyperextension, drilled through the distal tuft and through the skin. The wire is grabbed distally and drilled out until just visible in the middle phalanx. The PIP joint is reduced in slight hyperextension, and the MTP joint is reduced in slight flexion. The pin is then drilled through the proximal phalanx across the MTP joint and into the metatarsal. It is not essential that the pin be placed inside the metatarsal; the pin can be left along the metatarsal as long as it is not plantar prominent. Pins that engage the metatarsal, however, are less likely to loosen. The distal pin is then bent with needle nose pliers into a U and the wire cut so that a J is left. The pin is then tapped in proximally so that it is just touching the skin.

The PIP joint is closed with three stitches of nylon. The middle suture is a horizontal mattress skin stitch that secures the skin, capsule, and tendon proximally and distally. The incision is then dressed using a nonadhering

dressing, gauze, or soft roll around the toe, and the dressing is held in place with an elastic bandage. A 0.5-in adhesive tape is placed over the pin in a U fashion, from dorsal to plantar, to prevent the pin from becoming dislodged. The tape should not be so tight as to force the pin into the skin, and it should be pinched over the tip of the pin to act as a bumper. Ambulation is allowed as tolerated with a postoperative shoe. The dressings are changed 2 weeks after surgery at which time smaller dressings or adhesive strips can be applied. The tape bumper is kept in place until the pin is removed 6 weeks after surgery. Pin removal is usually possible without local anesthesia with a hemostat, needle driver, or small pliers. Active and passive MTP joint motion, but not PIP joint motion, is started 6 weeks after surgery.

Slight overcorrection of the deformity and careful dissection of the PIP joint, in which the resection is square and well reduced, are also necessary. Approximately 85% of the PIP joint resection arthroplasties will fuse, but fibrous union is not problematic if the deformity has been corrected and the toe has been adequately shortened.

LESSER MTP JOINT RESECTION ARTHROPLASTY

Dislocation deformities of the MTP joint may require resection of the bases of the phalanges and/or metatarsal head resection. Fusion of the second through fifth MTP joints is difficult and usually not indicated. Resection of the phalangeal base is indicated when most of the pain at the MTP joints and plantar metatarsal head is caused by the dislocated proximal phalanx pushing the metatarsal head into the sole or if the toe is in severe valgus. If a single MTP joint is resected, then a dorsal longitudinal incision can be used. When two or more MTP joints are involved, resection of all four MTP joints is often recommended because the other hammer toes follow the first ones (**Figure 4**). For all four

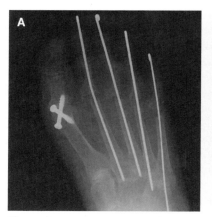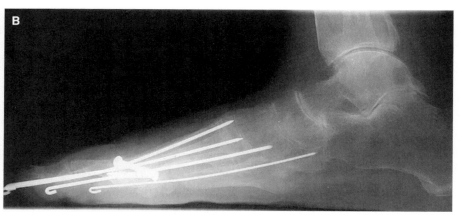

Figure 4 **A,** AP view showing first MTP joint fusion, resection of metatarsal heads two through five, and PIP joint resection arthroplasty with percutaneous pinning of toes two through five. **B,** Lateral view showing first MTP joint fusion, resection of metatarsal heads two through five, and PIP joint resection arthroplasty with percutaneous pinning of toes two through five.

MTP joints, two dorsal incisions are made similar to those for synovectomy. One incision is made between the second and third toes and the other between the fourth and fifth toes. The extensor tendon is then incised, with care taken to protect the medial and lateral digital nerve and vessels, and the base of the proximal phalanx is resected with a small bone cutter or rongeur. A 0.062-in K-wire is then drilled through the proximal phalanx distally and then retrograde to correct and hold the deformity for 6 weeks. Only the skin is closed, and hemostasis is obtained after the tourniquet is released. A PIP joint resection or osteoclasis may be indicated but usually enough of the base of the proximal phalanx can be resected to reduce the claw toe. The incision is dressed with a nonadhering dressing, gauze, or soft roll, elastic bandage, and tape to hold the pin. Dressings, sutures, and pins are treated as described previously.

With severe plantar metatarsal head pain and prominence, the same dorsal incisions are used, but some surgeons prefer to make transverse or plantar incisions. The metatarsal head is resected with a small rongeur or bone cutter. The four metatarsals must be resected in a gently curved or lateral sloping fashion so that the lateral rays are not prominent. The toes are then pinned and the wounds

treated as described above. Complications occur in about 10% of patients and include bleeding, nerve injury, recurrence, and spurs.

GREAT TOE SURGERY

Severe first MTP joint hallux valgus is generally treated with fusion and lesser toe resection arthroplasty. Some surgeons advocate resection of the first metatarsal head or proximal phalanx base, or first MTP joint Silastic or metal arthroplasty, but most of these procedures are not as successful as fusion. Traditional procedures for hallux valgus correction, such as the modified McBride bunionectomy, tend to fail because of soft-tissue incompetence around the first MTP joint.

The approach for first MTP joint fusion (**Figure 4**, *A*) is a longitudinal incision between the extensor tendon and dorsal medial cutaneus nerve. As in standard bunion surgery, care of the dorsal medial cutaneus nerve is essential to prevent neuroma. Hardware placement should not press the nerve against the shoe. Dissection into the joint is performed with a scalpel. The incision in the capsule is made parallel to the skin incision. The capsule is then elevated from the metatarsal head and proximal phalanx both medially and laterally. A No. 2-0 silk suture is used to secure the capsule to

the skin to protect the nerve medially and to protect the extensor tendon laterally. The extensor tendon is usually not cut or lengthened. The joint is entered, and the entire cartilage of the metatarsal head is exposed. Additional traction is achieved using Senn, Ragnell, or Hayes retractors. With the head exposed, a rongeur is used to resect the cartilage, subchondral bone, spurs, and medial prominence to obtain a smaller, rounded, 2- to 4-mm shorter metatarsal head. Many systems provide reamers to shape the metatarsal head. These can enhance bony contract and, therefore, aid in obtaining early fusion. The medial prominence can be removed with a small saw but is usually soft enough to be resected with a rongeur; this tissue can then be saved for bone graft. Obtaining a good cancellous metatarsal head is essential. The cartilage and subchondral bone of the base of the phalanges is removed by using a small curet to puncture the center of the proximal phalanx through subchondral bone. A small, straight rongeur is used to remove the cartilage and subchondral bone. The phalanx is then reduced to the metatarsal head with about 10° to 15° valgus, correction of pronation, and 15° of dorsiflexion of the phalanx to the sole or 30° to 35° of dorsiflexion of the phalanx to the metatarsal. The valgus position is important to prevent overload of the interphalangeal joint of the great toe.

After fusion of the great toe MTP joint, the 1-2 intermetatarsal angle will gradually decrease, so too much valgus in the fusion may lead to impingement or crossover with the second toe. Fixation can be achieved with screws, plates, or multiple K-wires. We prefer the crossed, cannulated 4.0-mm screw technique. The guide wires are placed dorsal medially to plantar laterally. Both proximal and distal radiographs are obtained with a hard surface (sterile basin) under the foot for plantigrade positioning of the radiograph to judge dorsiflexion. A small amount of cancellous bone graft is placed between the phalanx and metatarsal, and the screws are measured and placed compressing the bones. Hemostasis is obtained after releasing the tourniquet. The No. 2-0 silk skin capsule retention suture is removed. Excess capsule is resected with a scalpel and closed with No. 2-0 to 3-0 absorbable suture. Skin edges are closed with interrupted No. 3-0 to 4-0 nonabsorbable suture, a nonadhering dressing, and a bunion-type dressing of 2-in soft roll or gauze, 2- to 4-in elastic bandage, and adhesive tape.

Ambulation may be allowed, but patients should be instructed to avoid putting pressure on the great toe while walking in a postoperative shoe. Dressings are changed every 2 weeks for 6 weeks. Sutures are removed 2 to 4 weeks after good skin bridging. Radiographs are taken at 6 weeks, then at 3- to 4-month intervals to assess fusion. Shoes with wide toe boxes and rigid soles (inexpensive larger sneaker) should be worn for 6 to 12 weeks after surgery or until fusion is demonstrated on radiographs and physical examination.

Management of Complications

Bleeding, infection, and wound dehiscence may occur. The latter can be avoided by leaving the sutures in until the skin bridges. The development of hematomas can be avoided or minimized by releasing the tourniquet during the operation to ensure good hemostasis and by using appropriate dressings and pressure postoperatively. Wound dehiscence and infection may require wound care, culture to identify the pathogens, and use of appropriate antibiotics. Occasionally, an additional operation is required. Nonunion or hardware failure can occur in patients with osteoporosis or poor fixation, or in those who are overly active. Another operation may be needed to relieve pain or to correct a deformity. Malposition can cause great toe pain from plantar flexion, dorsiflexion, varus, or valgus. Painful hardware can occur from screw or plate prominence.

With synovectomy, the complication of dorsal cutaneous nerve injury is avoided with careful dissection and removal of the synovium. This injury is usually limited to a small area, and numbness is not a significant problem. Scar neuromas may require excision if significant problems develop after 1 to 2 years. Recurrence of proximal neuromas can be a problem.

Complications of hammer and claw toe correction also include distal nerve injury that may present as mild numbness but seldom neuroma. Ischemia and gangrene are avoided by careful dissection and sufficient shortening of the toe. When the PIP joint has been contracted for a long time, straightening it without shortening can injure or cause spasm of the digital arteries. Thus, it is essential to release the tourniquet while closing the incisions to ensure that the toes are pink. If adequate capillary refill does not return, the pin should be removed and further shortening of the toe performed. The surgeon should not leave the operating room until the toes are pink. Recurrence of PIP or MTP joint contractions and medial or lateral spurs occur in approximately 10% of patients; therefore, it is essential that patients have a clear understanding of potential complications and have provided the appropriate informed consent.

The author wishes to acknowledge the contribution of Richard T. Laughlin, MD, in the creation of this chapter.

References

Couglin MJ: Rheumatoid forefoot reconstruction: A long-term follow-up study. *J Bone Joint Surg Am* 2000;82:322-341.

Kerr LD: Arthritis of the forefoot: A review from a rheumatologic and medical perspective. *Clin Orthop* 1998;349:20-27.

Smyth CJ, Janson RW: Rheumatologic view of the rheumatoid foot. *Clin Orthop* 1997;340:7-17.

Tillmann K: Surgery of the rheumatoid forefoot with special reference to the plantar approach. *Clin Orthop* 1997;340:39-47.

Vandeputte G, Steenwerckx A, Mulier T, Peeraer L, Dereymaeker G: Forefoot reconstruction in rheumatoid arthritis patients: Keller-Lelievre-Hoffmann versus arthrodesis MTP1-Hoffmann. *Foot Ankle Int* 1999;20:438-443.

Coding

ICD-9 CODE
714.0   Rheumatoid arthritis

CPT CODES
28088   Synovectomy, tendon sheath, foot; extensor

28160   Lesser metatarsophalangeal joint resection arthroplasty

28285   Correction, hammertoe (eg, interphalangeal fusion, partial or total phalangectomy)

28750   Arthrodesis, great toe; metatarsophalangeal joint

28755   Correction, open proximal interphalangeal resection and fusion

Freiberg's Infraction

Michael J. Shereff, MD

◼ Definition of the Problem

Patient Presentation

The typical patient with Freiberg's infraction is a young woman with a vague history of activity-related forefoot pain. Often there is no history of trauma. Although Freiberg's infraction can occur in either sex, women appear to be affected more frequently than men. This is in contrast to all other osteochondroses, which are more common in men. Freiberg's infraction most often affects individuals in adolescence through the second decade of life, although it can be observed at any age. Younger patients typically present with acute symptoms, whereas older patients may present with more chronic arthritic pain and experience episodic exacerbations related to weight-bearing activities. Although the second metatarsal is the most commonly affected, Freiberg's infraction may involve any of the metatarsals. Usually there is only a single lesion in one foot. In approximately 10% of patients with Freiberg's disease, similar lesions will develop in the opposite foot, but both feet usually are not affected concurrently.

Physical Examination

Physical examination often reveals a painful and limited passive range of motion of the involved metatarsophalangeal (MTP) joint. There may be pain on direct palpation of the metatarsal head. Swelling, synovitis, and an effusion may be present. In older patients with long-term involvement, a callus may develop plantar to the affected metatarsal head. Occasionally, patients are completely asymptomatic with changes noted only on radiographs obtained for other purposes. Whether these patients later become symptomatic is not known.

The appearance on radiographs can be quite variable depending on the stage of the disease. In the early stages of the disease, only sclerosis and widening of the joint space may be evident on radiographs, specifically on oblique views (**Figure 1**). In later stages of the disease, various degrees of collapse or fragmentation of the metatarsal head may be observed. Secondary or later degenerative changes include joint space narrowing, osteochondral loose bodies, and hypertrophy of the metatarsal shaft (**Figure 2**). Long-term involvement can lead to complete joint destruction and collapse.

Differential Diagnosis

- Synovitis
- Inflammatory arthritis
- Metatarsalgia
- Morton's neuroma
- MTP joint instability
- Metatarsal stress fracture

Additional Work-up

Usually the history, physical examination, and radiographs are sufficient to

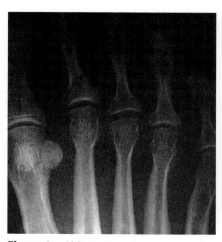

Figure 1 Oblique view demonstrates flattening of the third metatarsal head in early stage Freiberg's infraction.

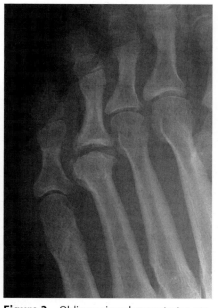

Figure 2 Oblique view demonstrates secondary arthrosis of the fourth MTP joint with joint destruction and loose body formation in later stage Freiberg's infraction.

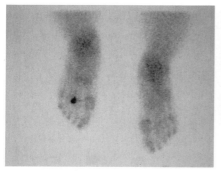

Figure 3 Bone scan demonstrates increased uptake at the third metatarsal head in a patient with symptomatic Freiberg's infraction.

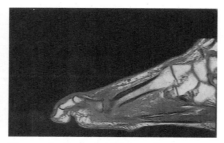

Figure 4 Sagittal MRI scan demonstrates synovitis and osteonecrosis of the dorsal aspect of the metatarsal head with hypertrophy of the metatarsal shaft.

make the diagnosis. Bone scintigraphy may be useful in ruling out another diagnosis, such as a stress fracture, or for localizing the source of vague, poorly localized forefoot pain. Changes on bone scintigraphy specific for Freiberg's infraction might include photopenia in the early (avascular) stages and intense uptake in the later (reparative) stages as the metatarsal head is revascularized (**Figure 3**). MRI may be helpful in evaluating the degree of involvement of the metatarsal head and for preoperative planning if an osteotomy is being considered (**Figure 4**).

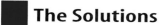

The Solutions

Treatment Options and Rationale

A period of appropriate nonsurgical management is indicated for all patients with Freiberg's infraction. The goal is to rest the joint to allow resolution of inflammatory and mechanical irritation. For adolescents with an acute onset of pain, swelling, and limited motion, nonsurgical measures typically are effective initially. Symptoms often slowly subside with time. The use of a good supportive, rubber-soled shoe can help dissipate impact

loading during the stance phase of gait. A soft, flexible insert with a metatarsal pad may alleviate increased pressures associated with weight bearing on the affected metatarsal. Activity modification with avoidance of high-impact activities or a trial of limited or protected weight bearing may be beneficial in some patients. For patients with severe disease, a non–weight-bearing short leg cast may be indicated as an acute measure.

In older adults with chronic symptoms secondary to degenerative changes, less restrictive options such as shoe modifications (including an inflexible rocker sole) and anti-inflammatory medications may suffice. Modification of activities during exacerbations may help limit pain and swelling. Some physicians have advocated using a limited series of steroid injections.

Progression of the disease is variable, both in terms of time course and severity. Adolescents who do not respond to nonsurgical measures and adults with advanced degenerative changes may benefit from surgery. Several surgical techniques for Freiberg's disease have been described. Simple débridement and loose body removal was originally described by Freiberg. Other procedures have included synovectomy, osteotomy, bone grafting, core decompression, metatarsal head arthroplasty, metatarsal shortening, proximal phalanx hemiphalangectomy, and joint arthroplasty. Although several

options exist, some procedures may be more appropriate than others depending on the stage of the disease, the patient's age, and the patient's presenting symptoms. For adolescents in whom nonsurgical measures have failed and for those without advanced degenerative changes, simple débridement may be indicated. Débridement includes removal of osteochondral fragments, débridement of avascular bone, and reshaping of the metatarsal head. A synovectomy can be included if hypertrophic synovium is encountered. For patients with late collapse of the metatarsal head and secondary degenerative changes, simple débridement may not suffice. For these patients, treatment options are similar to those for patients with other types of MTP arthritis. One option is a DuVries-type resection arthroplasty of the metatarsal head, which serves to decompress the inflamed joint by removing the damaged articular surface. Although this procedure is effective in reducing pain, there is concern about transfer lesions and MTP joint stiffness developing postoperatively.

Total small joint arthroplasty has also been described. Potential benefits compared with resection arthroplasty include maintenance of metatarsal length, improved joint motion, and better weight distribution. However, problems inherent to the use of implants include destructive synovitis, infection, and dislocation. Newer implants specifically designed for the foot may prove better than previous designs, but there are no long-term data regarding these implants.

Various osteotomies have been used. Osteotomies are intended to preserve the MTP joint and joint function, thereby avoiding the potential for stiffness and transfer lesions that sometimes occur with resection arthroplasty. The dorsal closing wedge osteotomy is a dorsiflexion osteotomy made at the level of the metatarsal neck. The basic premise is that the intact cartilage on the plantar surface of the metatarsal head is redirected to articulate with the articular surface of the proximal phalanx. In this way, motion at the MTP joint is preserved. Encouraging results have been reported for a few small series of patients. Metatarsal shortening osteotomy is also used for Freiberg's infraction. In theory, by shortening the metatarsal proximal to the MTP joint, overload of the affected metatarsal and symptoms are reduced. Various techniques for shortening and fixation also have been described. The horizontal distal metatarsal osteotomy is a potential treatment option. This osteotomy may prove to be effective, but experience with this procedure for treatment of symptomatic Freiberg's infraction is limited at this time.

Resection of the proximal portion of the proximal phalanx, when combined with partial syndactylization of an adjacent toe, can be effective in providing relief of symptoms in patients with advanced degenerative changes who have not had improvement with more simple procedures. Unlike some other procedures, partial phalangectomy addresses the degenerative changes that often are present on the articular surface of the proximal phalanx in addition to decompression of the MTP joint. Partial phalangectomy is combined with syndactylization to minimize the potential for postoperative instability of the toe.

If nonsurgical management fails, a less joint-altering procedure, such as a simple débridement with synovectomy, should be the initial consideration for younger patients or those with early stage disease. Joint-altering procedures or those that alter forefoot relationships should be reserved for patients in whom other forms of treatment have failed.

Author's Preferred Treatment and Rationale

DÉBRIDEMENT WITH SYNOVECTOMY

Indications There are two indications for this treatment: (1) symptom-

atic Freiberg's infraction (osteonecrosis) of a lesser metatarsal head with synovitis of the MTP joint that persists despite nonsurgical management and (2) early degenerative arthrosis of the MTP joint secondary to Freiberg's infraction of the metatarsal head.

Contraindications Patients with severe arthrosis and joint destruction secondary to Freiberg's infraction may be better treated with a procedure addressing arthrosis of the MTP joint. Patients with mild symptoms or those who have requirements for reduced activity may often be effectively treated nonsurgically.

Surgical Technique The skin incision is made dorsally and is centered over the MTP joint (**Figure 5,** *A*). The subcutaneous tissue is then divided in-line with the skin incision. The extensor digitorum longus tendon is identified and retracted. Alternatively, if an extension deformity is present at the MTP joint, the tendon may be released or Z-lengthened. The MTP joint capsule is incised, exposing the metatarsal head. The capsule and periosteum are reflected to expose the base of the proximal phalanx and the metatarsal head (**Figure 5,** *B*). If hypertrophic synovium is encountered,

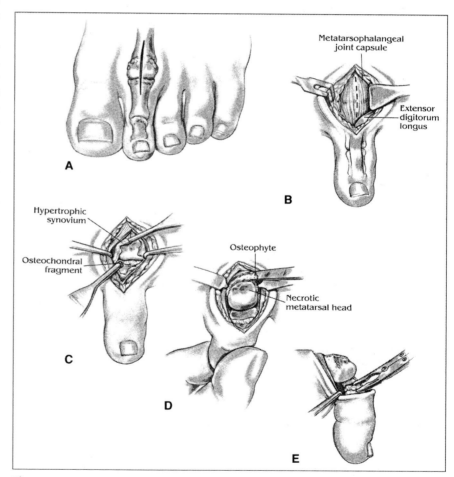

Figure 5 Débridement arthroplasty for osteonecrosis of the metatarsal head. **A,** A dorsal longitudinal incision is centered over the MTP joint. **B,** Longitudinal capsulotomy. **C,** Synovectomy and removal of the osteochondral fragments. **D,** Excision of osteophytes of the metatarsal head. **E,** Resection of osteophytes at the base of the proximal phalanx. (Reproduced with permission from Shereff MJ (ed): *Atlas of Foot and Ankle Surgery.* Philadelphia, PA, WB Saunders, 1993, p 151.)

it is sharply incised, and a complete synovectomy of the MTP articulation is performed, removing any osteochondral fragments or loose bodies from the joint (**Figure 5**, *C*). The MTP joint is hyperflexed to better visualize the metatarsal head (**Figure 5**, *D*). Any osteophytes encountered are resected. Areas of necrotic bone or cartilage are débrided. The articular surface of the proximal phalanx is inspected, any osteophytes are resected, and the base of the phalanx is reshaped as needed (**Figure 5**, *E*). The wound is irrigated and closed in the usual manner.

Postoperative Care In the immediate postoperative period, patients are allowed to bear weight on the heel in a stiff-soled postoperative shoe. Su-

tures are removed 2 to 3 weeks after surgery. Gentle range-of-motion exercises are encouraged.

PARTIAL PHALANGECTOMY AND SYNDACTYLIZATION

Indications This procedure is indicated for patients with (1) symptomatic arthrosis and destruction of the MTP joint secondary to Freiberg's infraction who have failed to respond to nonsurgical management, (2) continued symptoms and progressive arthrosis despite previous débridement and synovectomy, and (3) significant arthrosis involving the base of the proximal phalanx.

Contraindications Patients with mild symptoms or reduced activity re-

quirements may often be effectively treated with nonsurgical interventions. Patients with early Freiberg's infraction without collapse and arthrosis may be considered for débridement with synovectomy.

Surgical Technique A triangular web incision is outlined on the skin with a skin marker starting along the lateral aspect of the toe (**Figure 6**, *A*). The incision is outlined just dorsal to the midline from the base of the web to the level of the proximal interphalangeal joint. This mark is then extended plantarward back toward the base of the web. The mark is then transferred to the adjacent toe by squeezing the toes together while the ink is still wet. The incision is marked proximally

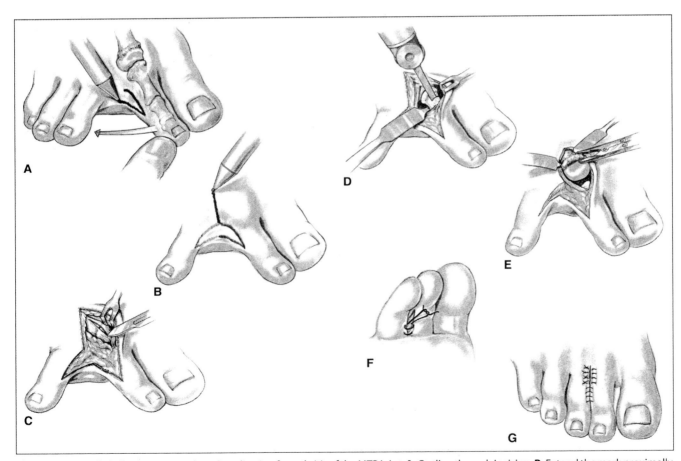

Figure 6 Partial phalangectomy and syndactylization for arthritis of the MTP joint. **A,** Outline the web incision. **B,** Extend the mark proximally as a dorsal longitudinal incision. **C,** Longitudinal capsulotomy. **D,** Resection of the proximal portion of the proximal phalanx. **E,** Resection of the osteophytes of the metatarsal head. Closure of the web incision begins on the plantar surface (**F**) and progresses to the dorsum of the toe (**G**). (Reproduced with permission from Shereff MJ (ed): *Atlas of Foot and Ankle Surgery*. Philadelphia, PA, WB Saunders, 1993, pp 155-157.)

as a dorsal longitudinal incision between the metatarsal heads (**Figure 6**, *B*).

The skin and subcutaneous tissue are excised as outlined. The incision is extended proximally as a dorsal longitudinal incision between the metatarsal heads. The subcutaneous tissue between the metatarsal heads is incised. The skin and subcutaneous tissue are reflected medially to expose the dorsal aspect of the affected proximal phalanx and the metatarsal head, if needed.

The periosteum and capsule are incised longitudinally (**Figure 6**, *C*). The base of the proximal phalanx is exposed subperiosteally. If needed, the metatarsal head is exposed. The proximal portion of the proximal phalanx is removed with the use of a microsagittal saw (**Figure 6**, *D*). Osteophytes associated with metatarsal head are excised and reshaped as necessary with a rongeur (**Figure 6**, *E*).

The web incision is closed with interrupted buried No. 3.0 chromic suture (**Figure 6**, *F*). The closure is started on the plantar surface and progresses to the apex of the syndactyly. Closure then progresses on the dorsum of the toe. Proximal to the web, the skin closure is performed in an interrupted vertical mattress fashion using No. 4.0 nylon suture (**Figure 6**, *G*).

Postoperative Care It may be beneficial to have patients avoid weight bearing and use crutches postoperatively to avoid tension on the syndactylization and promote wound healing. Sutures are removed 2 to 3 weeks postoperatively. Once the wound is healed, partial weight bearing is initiated on the heel in a stiff-soled postoperative shoe.

Management of Complications

Persistent or recurrent symptoms are the most common complications following débridement with synovectomy. Although débridement with synovectomy may relieve symptoms, it may not halt the underlying disease process and secondary arthrosis of the MTP joint may subsequently develop in some patients.

Resection of the base of the proximal phalanx with partial phalangectomy may result in a cock-up deformity or instability of the toe. Therefore, partial syndactylization to the adjacent toe is recommended. In addition, patients should continue only partial weight bearing until the wound is healed.

The author wishes to acknowledge the contribution of Matison I. Boyer, MD, in the creation of this chapter.

References

Freiberg AH: Infraction of the second metatarsal bone: A typical injury. *Surg Gynecol Obstet* 1914;19:191-193.

Helal B, Gibb P: Freiberg's disease: A suggested pattern of management. *Foot Ankle* 1987;8:94-102.

Katcherian DA: Treatment of Freiberg's disease. *Orthop Clin North Am* 1994;25:69-81.

Coding

ICD-9 CODE
732.5   Juvenile osteochondrosis of foot; Osteochondrosis (juvenile) of second metatarsal, (of Freiberg)

CPT CODES
28022   Arthrotomy, including exploration, drainage, or removal of loose or foreign body; metatarsophalangeal joint

28072   Synovectomy, metatarsophalangeal joint, each

28126   Resection, partial or complete, phalangeal base, each toe

28280   Syndactylization, toes (eg, webbing or Kelikian-type procedure)

SECTION 6
Athletic Injuries

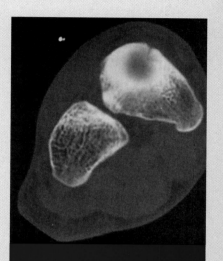

James A. Nunley, MD
Editor

Osteochondral Lesions of the Talus

Pierce E. Scranton, Jr, MD

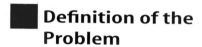

Definition of the Problem

Patient Presentation

Patients presenting with an osteochondral lesion of the talus (OLT) are usually athletic or, if not, have a history of a significant ankle injury within 1 or more years before the onset of symptoms. I have seen patients ranging in age from 17 to 74 years. Most patients are between ages 20 and 40 years, with men more commonly affected (ratio, 1.6:1).

Ankle sprains are by far the most common injuries leading to OLT. An ankle fracture or a fall from height with impaction also can cause OLTs. At least 90% of ankle sprains involve a plantar flexed foot forcibly supinating to injure the anterior talofibular ligament, making medial talar dome injuries the most common OLTs. As the plantar flexed foot and talus subluxate or dislocate with supination, the posteromedial corner of the talus strikes the tibial plafond. Damage to the articular surface can occur either in the form of a chondral bruise, chondral cracks, a shearing of the corner of the talus with intact chondral attachments, or outright fracture of the corner of the talus. Beneath the articular talar surface the talar body's marrow will also absorb some of this force, leading to edema, seen on MRI, that may or may not lead to vascular compromise and necrotic collapse. If ankle motion and weight bearing are not restricted, synovial fluid under pressure will intrude through any talar articular defect and may create an expanding ta-

lar cyst. Large cystic or necrotic areas in the bone below the articular defect are called type V lesions.

Transition from an acute ankle injury to symptomatic OLT takes time. It may take months or even more than a year for symptoms of the original ankle sprain to abate and new symptoms appear. The new symptoms vary and may include a sharp pain, a catching or clicking sensation, or a sudden pain with certain ankle movements during sport or strenuous activity. Because initial physical examination and radiographs can be interpreted as normal, patients are advised that they probably have residual scar tissue from the old ankle sprain, and physical therapy or continued patience is prescribed. Exercise and a continued intrusion of synovial fluid into the defect can lead to an aggravation of pathology or the persistence of symptoms, resulting in suspicion of an OLT. Proper MRI usually will confirm the diagnosis.

Physical Examination

Physical examination of the ankle of a patient with an OLT may reveal no abnormalities. The original ankle sprain may have healed completely, and there may be no evidence of ankle ligament instability, joint effusion, or synovitis. It is useful to do a comparative examination of both ankles. The medial and lateral corners of the talar dome should be palpated with the ankle maximally plantar flexed. The ankles should be dorsiflexed and plantar flexed under pressure while attempting to evert and

invert the joint in an effort to provoke snapping or catching on the talar defect. Advanced lesions will have some synovitis or an effusion, especially after activity. However, a small effusion can drain into the inferior and posterior ankle recesses as well as into the subtalar joint and sinus tarsi and will not be obvious. A posteromedial or posterolateral defect generally will have no obvious physical findings.

Differential Diagnosis

- Syndesmosis injury
- Bassett's lesion
- Bands of intra-articular anterolateral fibroid scar
- Subluxating or dislocating peroneal tendons
- Longitudinal tear of peroneal tendons
- Tear or avulsion of the peroneus longus
- Fracture or disruption of the os trigonum
- Malleolar avulsion fracture
- Cervical or interosseous subtalar ligament injury
- Anterior process fracture of the calcaneus
- Lateral shoulder fracture of the calcaneus
- Reactive neurodystrophy

The author of the departments with which he is affiliated have received something of value from a commercial or other party related directly or indirectly to the subject of this chapter.

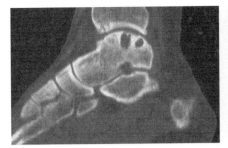

Figure 1 The lateral CT scan of a type V OLT. Fragmentation of the articular surface was discovered at surgery.

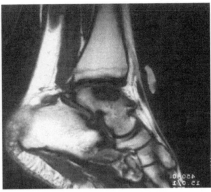

Figure 2 A lateral T1-weighted MRI scan of a 17-year-old football player's ankle 3 months after an ankle sprain. Massive marrow edema is seen, but no cystic defect is seen in the articular surface. Treatment consisted of 0.62-mm pin drilling and immobilization for 3 weeks.

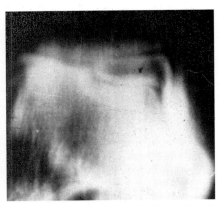

Figure 3 An arthrogram of a large Berndt and Harty type IV lesion that requires stabilization.

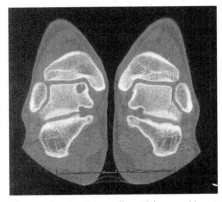

Figure 4 A structurally stable type V cyst with one small articular defect that was treated by introducing a drill bit through the defect and creating multiple drill holes with the tailings staying as graft within the cyst.

Additional Work-up

When radiographs suggest an OLT, obtaining plantar flexion-dorsiflexion mortise views can be helpful. A posteromedial OLT may be hidden in a straight mortise view but can be seen in plantar flexion. A technetium Tc 99m bone scan at this time will indicate whether localized bony pathology is present. Soft-tissue pathology, such as split or subluxating peroneal tendons or intra-articular scar tissue, will not be positive on the bone scan. If an OLT is noted, either by radiographs or bone scan, the next step is to obtain more definitive imaging using either CT or MRI; in some patients both studies are needed.

Both CT and MRI have advantages and disadvantages. CT shows only bony pathology (**Figure 1**) and does not show articular surface damage; therefore, it cannot provide all the information necessary for surgical planning. MRI shows articular defects and bony pathology, but its sensitivity to bone edema can cause misinterpretation of the extent of the pathology (**Figure 2**). Both MRI and CT require some circumspection in determining the extent of damage.

Depending on the surgeon's access to imaging modalities and the location of a lesion, diagnostic arthroscopy at the time of surgery may be used for accurate appraisal of intra-articular pathology and articular surface damage.

The Solutions

Treatment Options and Rationale

Treatment options should follow a gradation of intervention depending on the severity of the OLT and the chronicity of symptoms.

Author's Preferred Treatment and Rationale

ACUTE LESIONS

Acute lesions classified as Berndt and Harty stages I and II (seen on MRI only) require 3 weeks of immobilization. Stages III and IV should be treated by a boot walker with no weight bearing for 3 weeks followed by weight bearing for another 3 weeks. MRI is used to visualize combination pathology associated with an ankle injury; however, it should not be ordered routinely.

CHRONIC SYMPTOMATIC LESIONS

Chronic symptomatic lesions require surgical treatment. Painful Berndt and Harty OLT stages I and II that do not have type V lesions beneath them will benefit from arthroscopic débridement with drilling or microfracture, followed by 3 weeks in a boot walker without weight bearing and another 3 weeks with weight bearing. Graduated rehabilitation follows.

If the OLT is Berndt and Harty stage III or IV, the surgeon must determine the course of treatment based on the size of the lesions, the quality of bone, and the presence or absence of an underlying type V lesion. The large type IV lesion seen in **Figure 3** can be treated arthroscopically either by internal fixation with a Herbert screw or biodegradable pegs. Loose or fragmented stage IV lesions can be treated by débridement only unless there is a substantial defect, in which case an osteochondral autologous transplant (OATS) is needed.

Symptomatic Berndt and Harty stages I through IV lesions with type V lesions in the underlying bone require more extensive planning and treatment. If the lesion is 6 mm or less, structurally stable, and well contained (**Figure 4**), I have been successful in arthroscopically drilling into the center of the cyst with a drill bit. The cystic defect is located using a blunt probe to press on the weakened articular surface, and a 0.62-mm pin is used to confirm its location before drilling into the cyst. Multiple drill holes into the underlying bone are created through one articular entry point, and the tailings of the drilling are left in the cyst where they act as a graft. The ankle is then immobilized for 3 weeks without weight bearing, followed by 3 weeks of weight bearing. If the defect is small, simple drilling with a 0.62-mm pin followed by immobilization is adequate. Finally, a posteromedial lesion can be approached either by transmalleolar drilling or by retrograde drilling using appropriate arthroscopic guides.

If the lesion is on the tibial side (**Figure 5**), the same arthroscopic guides can be used for outside-in drilling of the defect. Outside-in drilling with supplementary grafting when indicated has been reported by Ferkel.

I believe large symptomatic type V lesions that are 7 mm or greater will require an OATS, which involves harvest of an autologous osteochondral graft from the ipsilateral or contralateral knee (ipsilateral preferred). Especially large lesions, greater than 1.2 cm, require either nesting of multiple grafts or one large fresh allograft.

In some patients, OATS in the ankle can be placed arthroscopically. However, the arthroscopy is so technically demanding that an arthrotomy is preferable. Anteromedial, anterolateral, and posterolateral lesions may all be treated by anterior arthrotomy, open grafting, and harvesting the donor graft from the ipsilateral knee. Anterior impingement spurs are not un-

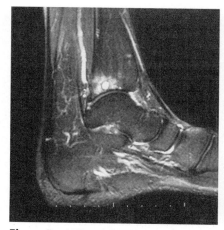

Figure 5 A T2-weighted lateral MRI scan of a symptomatic posteromedial tibial type V lesion.

common in association with OLT lesions in athletes; removing them at the time of arthrotomy will facilitate exposure. Having a surgical assistant maximally plantar flex the ankle will reveal middle talar lesions (**Figure 6**).

A fibular osteotomy with an anterior syndesmosis release to move the fibula posteriorly and facilitate exposure might be considered necessary for posterolateral lesions (**Figure 7**, *A*). However, release of the anterior talofibular ligament as in a Bröstrom procedure will allow the talus to subluxate or almost dislocate anteriorly (**Figure 7**, *B*).

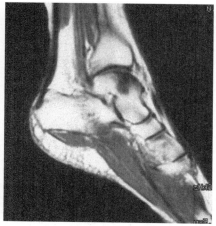

Figure 6 Lateral MRI scan of a type V middle OLT. This lesion can be treated by an anterior ankle arthrotomy with the patient under anesthesia and an assistant providing maximum plantar flexion.

Posteromedial lesions frequently require a medial malleolar osteotomy, which is technically demanding and must be precise. A medial longitudinal incision is used to expose the entire medial malleolus. A cannulated screw system may be used to predrill the medial malleolus (**Figure 8**, *A*). The anterior and posterior corners of the ankle joint are visualized. A micro oscillating saw is used for a 45° osteotomy, stopping short of the joint. The osteotomy is completed with an osteotome, and the medial

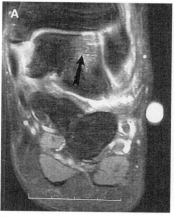 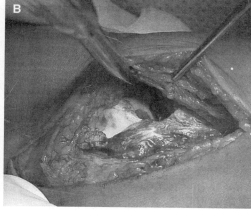

Figure 7 **A,** AP T2-weighted MRI scan showing a posterolateral type V OLT lesion next to the fibula. **B,** An anterolateral arthrotomy with transection of the anterior talofibular ligament allows the entire talus to subluxate anteriorly, exposing the posterolateral lesion.

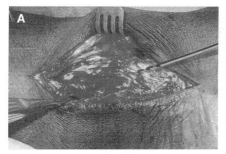
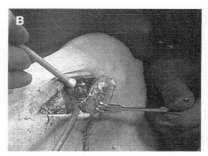
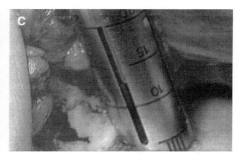

Figure 8 **A,** The medial malleolus has been exposed, and a blunt Homan retractor protects the posterior tibialis and flexor hallucis longus tendons. The cannulated drill is ready for the first of two medial malleolar drill holes. **B,** A medial malleolar osteotomy has been performed, and the malleolus is reflected inferiorly. The sizing rod is used to estimate the diameter of the type V lesion. **C,** The coring device for removing the type V OLT cystic area. Alternatively, it may be drilled.

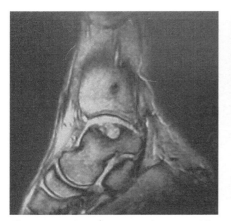

Figure 9 A large type V OLT best suited for an OATS rather than drilling or microfracture.

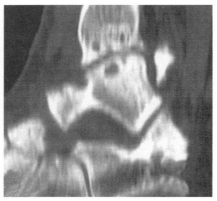

Figure 10 Posttraumatic tibial and talar cystic degeneration in a 17-year-old patient who is a suitable candidate for an en bloc ankle allograft.

malleolus is reflected inferiorly, exposing the talar OLT (**Figure 8**, *B*). The lesion is sized, drilled or cored, and then grafted (**Figure 8**, *C*). Two 40-mm cannulated screws are placed in the predrilled holes, reducing the medial malleolus. Closure is routine, and a compression dressing and boot walker are applied.

Aftercare depends on the size of the lesions and security of the graft and malleolar fixation, if performed. In my experience, a patient with a single, well-secured graft, 8 to 10 mm in diameter, should remain on crutches, immobile for 3 weeks, without weight bearing but mobile for the second 3 weeks, and fully weight bearing but in a boot walker the third 3 weeks. Multiple nested grafts add 3 weeks to each period for a total of 18 weeks.

TREATMENT ALTERNATIVES

Much decision making is based on the pathology present, the duration of symptoms, and the time between injury and diagnosis. For example, a patient who has a 12-mm talar cyst with articular damage (**Figure 9**) that is not discovered until 18 months after an ankle sprain probably will not do well with 3 weeks of cast immobilization. That patient is not likely to do well with simple drilling either. Bone grafting can be attempted using cancellous graft from either the distal tibial metaphysis or the iliac crest. At best, this bone grafting leaves an articular defect that hopefully will scar over with fibrocartilage.

Some lesions involve more surface avulsion or sloughing of the ar-

ticular surface. In these instances, an autologous cartilage transplantation (Carticel procedure) makes the most sense. This surgery requires great technical skill, two separate procedures, and at least 3 months on crutches. Large lateral lesions will require substantial exposure and a lateral malleolar osteotomy.

The final option for large lesions (**Figure 10**) is allograft replacement. Partial talar matches, a whole talus, or entire talotibial replacement grafts have been reported. This work is necessary in the exploration of treatment options for a younger patient who otherwise might be forced to undergo an ankle arthrodesis.

Management of Complications

Complications associated with treatment of OLT tend to be rare, occurring because there is a lack of technically expert treatment, secure fixation, and/or patient compliance. Aside from the usual unlikely risks of wound infection, dehiscence, neurovascular injury, and deep venous thrombosis, some complications are unique to OATS.

Two considerations should be noted with respect to the ipsilateral knee donor site. A superolateral knee arthrotomy for graft harvest at the lateral trochlea is associated with postoperative chondromalacia and degenerative patellofemoral joint disease. As a consequence, if the lateral knee arthrotomy is used, a lateral retinacular release to decompress the patellofemoral joint is advisable before skin closure. I have not had problems with arthroscopic harvest from the trochlea region. Other than an immediate postoperative knee effusion that resolves, this trochlear site is suitable for up to three grafts of 7 mm, 7 mm, and 6 mm.

The malleolar osteotomy is another area of concern. The malleolar holes must be drilled before the osteotomy. Questions of fixation stability have led some surgeons to recommend a chevron-like malleolar osteotomy. I have found that predrilled holes, followed by use of a reduction clamp at the time of screw fixation have successfully led to anatomic reduction. Most important is the angle of the malleolar osteotomy. If it is too superficial or longitudinal, the talar defect cannot be visualized; if it is too horizontal, graft insertion under the overhanging ledge of tibia is not possible. Fluoroscopic visualization of the ankle before osteotomy can be important if there is any doubt about exposure.

The final nuance concerning OATS is the matching of the recipient

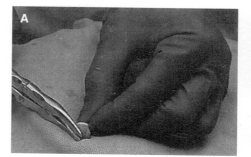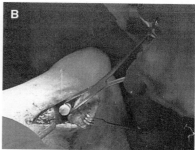

Figure 11 **A,** A rongeur is used to taper the distal end of an OATS where the initial insertion may start at a slight angle. **B,** A mosquito clamp is used to insert the donor graft with a tapered leading edge into the talar recipient hole.

hole to the donor hole. This must be an exact match. If the recipient talar hole is 10 mm deep, and the donor graft is 11 mm, it will protrude above the talar articular surface. The bone is hard and cannot be impacted into the recipient hole. Attempts to do this will destroy the chondral articular surface or cause it to shear off. In addition, when exposure is difficult the graft sometimes has to be inserted at a slight angle, especially when attempting to treat an OLT without performing a malleolar osteotomy when there is an overhanging rim of tibia. In this instance, it is best to carefully extrude

the graft from the donor tube, taper the leading insertion edge, (**Figure 11,** *A*) and then carefully introduce it into the recipient hole and impact it (**Figure 11,** *B*).

Finally, many OLTs involve defects on the shoulder or corner of the talus. The trochlear bone from the knee is ideal here, because its curve can match the curve of the talus. Here, too, the graft should be inserted under direct vision outside the donor tube to perfectly match the talar contour.

References

Al-Shaikh RA, Chou LB, Mann JA, Dreeben SM, Prieskorn D: Autologous osteochondral grafting for talar cartilage defects. *Foot Ankle Int* 2002;23:381-389.

Ferkel RD, Stone JW, Guhl JF: Articular surface defects, loose bodies, and osteophytes, in Ferkel RD (ed): *Arthroscopic Surgery: The Foot and Ankle*. Philadelphia, PA, Lippincott-Raven, 1996, pp 145-184.

Hangody L, Kish G, Karpati Z, Szerb I, Eberhardt R: Treatment of osteochondritis dissecans of the talus: Use of the mosaicplasty technique. A preliminary report. *Foot Ankle Int* 1997;18:628-634.

Scranton PE, McDermott JE: Treatment of type V osteochondral lesions of the talus with ipsilateral knee osteochondral autografts. *Foot Ankle Int* 2001;22:380-384.

Coding

ICD-9 CODES

718.17   Loose body in joint, ankle and foot

719.07   Effusion of joint, ankle and foot

719.47   Pain in joint, ankle and foot

719.77   Difficulty in walking, ankle and foot

733.10   Pathologic fracture, unspecified site

733.44   Aseptic necrosis of talus

CPT CODES

20902   Bone graft, any donor area; major or large

27705   Osteotomy; tibia

27899   Unlisted procedure, leg or ankle

00123T   is not listed under Category III codes. 0012T and 0013T are for the knee.

Failed Lateral Ankle Ligament Reconstruction

Thomas O. Clanton, MD

■ Definition of the Problem

Patient Presentation

Although failure of surgical stabilization of the lateral ligamentous complex of the ankle is uncommon, approximately 5% to 15% of patients who undergo a lateral ankle reconstruction proceed to failure requiring further intervention (**Figure 1**). Although there are more than 50 different lateral ankle reconstructive procedures, the most common involve either anatomic repair of the lateral ligaments or nonanatomic reconstruction with transfer of a local tendon.

Perhaps the most common cause for failure is recurrent instability. The symptoms may vary, but patients may describe a feeling of excessive looseness in the ankle or indicate that the ankle tends to give way or turn easily. The primary surgical procedure may have been inadequate, the patient may reinjure the ankle, or certain factors inherent to the patient, such as body weight, activity, or varus heel, may predispose the patient to a failed reconstruction.

Chronic pain that may be constant or related to activity is another indication of failure of lateral ankle reconstruction. This pain can be caused by pathology that was not adequately addressed in the reconstruction, new-onset pathology, or postoperative stiffness. Stiffness has several potential causes, but it is usually related to a nonanatomic reconstruction that, by its nature, restricts subtalar motion.

Studies of both anatomic and nonanatomic reconstructions, however, have shown that some patients report that their ankles feel "overly tight" after lateral ankle reconstruction.

A thorough history must be obtained to determine the cause of the poor result. In addition, it is important to obtain a record of the patient's primary procedure if possible. Helpful information includes the type of procedure performed, the status of the lateral ligaments, and which tendon (if any) was used in a transfer. This information is useful in planning a second reconstructive procedure. Knowledge of the primary procedure also helps determine if the preoperative pathology was adequately addressed. A procedure that addresses only the anterior talofibular ligament (ATFL) will not adequately stabilize an ankle with a subtalar component to its instability.

Physical Examination

Stress tests of the lateral ligaments should be positive in patients with re-

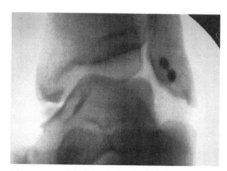

Figure 1 Radiograph obtained with intraoperative fluoroscopy demonstrates recurrent lateral ankle instability.

current instability. These include the anterior drawer maneuver to evaluate the ATFL and an inversion stress test to evaluate the calcaneofibular ligament (CFL). Evaluation of range of motion of the ankle and subtalar joints will identify patients whose lateral ankle ligament was overly tightened as a result of their original reconstructive procedure. As noted, these patients often experience pain, which may or may not be reproduced during ankle palpation. Nevertheless, a meticulous examination using a systematic sequence of palpation will often lead to the clinical diagnosis. Palpation over the course of the superficial peroneal or sural nerve may identify a Tinel's sign, suggestive of a neuroma or neuritis. Retrofibular tenderness associated with swelling and activity-related pain is a good indication that peroneal tendon pathology was not previously addressed or has recurred. The orthopaedic surgeon should also look for signs of generalized ligamentous laxity and/or connective tissue disorders.

Evaluation of hindfoot alignment is critically important. Varus alignment of the heel or plantar flexed first ray may predispose a ligament reconstruction to failure regardless of

The author or the departments with which he is affiliated have received something of value from a commercial or other party related directly or indirectly to the subject of this chapter.

the type of procedure previously performed. A fixed varus hindfoot deformity is an indication for a corrective osteotomy preceding or in conjunction with ligament reconstruction.

Differential Diagnosis
- Articular injury
  - Chondral and osteochondral fractures
- Nerve injury
  - Superficial peroneal
  - Posterior tibial
  - Sural
- Tendon injury
  - Peroneal (tear or dislocation)
  - Posterior tibial
- Other ligamentous injury
  - Syndesmosis
  - Subtalar
  - Bifurcate
  - Calcaneocuboid
- Impingement
  - Anterior tibial osteophyte
  - Anteroinferior tibiofibular ligament
- Miscellaneous conditions
  - Failure to regain normal motion (tight Achilles tendon)
  - Proprioceptive deficits
  - Tarsal coalition
  - Meniscoid lesions
  - Accessory soleus muscle
- Unrelated ongoing pathology masked by routine sprain
  - Undetected rheumatologic condition
  - Occult tumor

Additional Work-up
Plain radiographs should be obtained to evaluate potential bony pathology. Radiographs also help identify the placement of previous drill holes and prior use of hardware (**Figure 2**). Stress radiographs or fluoroscopy may aid in the diagnosis of recurrent instability or an overly tightened reconstruction.

Other diagnostic studies are frequently warranted in patients with complicated failed lateral ankle liga-

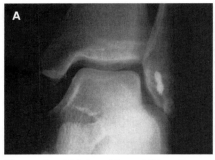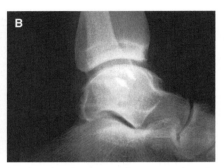

Figure 2　AP **(A)** and lateral **(B)** radiographs showing the placement of suture anchors in previously performed lateral ankle stabilization.

ment reconstructions. A technetium Tc 99m bone scan is particularly helpful when differentiating between soft-tissue and bony problems is difficult. MRI provides minimal information regarding the status of the lateral ligaments when there has been a previous lateral ankle ligament reconstruction; however, MRI can augment the work-up of a painful ankle. Intra-articular pathology, such as osteochondral lesions, can be diagnosed with MRI. Tears within the peroneus brevis or longus tendons can also be visualized on MRI scans. CT can determine the extent of an osteochondral lesion, but unlike MRI, clarity of the lesion is improved because bone edema is not a component of the CT image. For the failed lateral ankle reconstruction, CT scans are particularly helpful in defining previous bone tunnels. The location and direction of the tunnels are well visualized by this method. It is important for both the patient and the treating physician to recognize that this condition requires planning and preparation for all potential pathology.

The Solutions

Treatment Options and Rationale
Nonsurgical measures may be effective in the management of recurrent

ankle ligament instability. The goals of these measures include improving proprioception and strength in the affected ankle. Activity modifications, although often unacceptable to the active patient, aid the management of a failed reconstructive procedure. Other nonsurgical options include a shoe modification with a lateral flare and/or a wedge, an orthosis with a lateral heel wedge, or an ankle-foot orthosis. For many patients with symptomatic instability or pain following an attempt at ligamentous reconstruction, nonsurgical measures are difficult to accept as a long-term solution. Usually, these patients require a second attempt at surgical stabilization.

For recurrent instability after lateral ligament reconstruction, the decision must be made whether to perform an anatomic repair or a tenodesis procedure. A modified Broström repair can be performed if there is adequate remaining tissue, but the procedure should be planned as if there will not be enough tissue. Should insufficient tissue remain for a primary repair, an anatomic augmentation can be performed with an autograft or allograft tendon. Potential sources for an autograft include the hamstrings (semitendinosis or gracilis), plantaris, fascia lata, an extensor tendon to the third toe, and bone-patellar tendon-bone autograft. The tendons may be secured to bone via bone tunnels and sutures, staples, suture anchors, bioabsorbable screws, or metal interference screws.

A tenodesis procedure may also be used to treat recurrent instability. The status of the peroneus brevis tendon is critical because most tenodesis techniques harvest all or part of this tendon. The Chrisman-Snook modification of the Elmslie procedure has been the most commonly performed tenodesis technique. It was originally described with bone tunnels through the fibula that resulted in a nonanatomic reproduction of the ATFL or the CFL. Patients with combined ankle and subtalar instability have been successfully treated with this procedure. However, when the procedure is performed with tightening of the tendon graft as the heel and ankle are held in maximum eversion, the talocalcaneal joint is "captured," restricted in movement, and may cause persistent pain. In this situation, simply releasing the overly tight portion of the graft crossing the subtalar joint may be the only revision necessary. Careful intraoperative examination is crucial to the decision of whether or not to proceed to procedures other than a release.

A special category of failed ligamentous repair involves patients with excessive ligamentous laxity or connective tissue disorders. These disorders include rare genetic syndromes such as Marfan and Ehlers-Danlos, as well as the more common benign joint hypermobility syndrome. Although primary repair and nonanatomic tenodesis procedures have proved to be successful in the general population, the intrinsic ligamentous instability in these patients may preclude these techniques. Potential alternatives to standard repair in this hyperlax population include the use of allograft tendons or carbon fiber implants.

Author's Preferred Treatment and Rationale

For a patient with a failed lateral ankle ligament reconstruction who has symptoms of instability, I prefer re-

constructing the lateral ligament with a free tendon transfer using the semitendinosis or the gracilis tendon. The harvest of the graft tendon is performed in a manner similar to the method used for an anterior cruciate ligament autologous graft. A thigh tourniquet is applied with the patient supine on the operating room table with a bump under the ipsilateral buttock. Once the graft is harvested, it is prepared by sizing it for diameter and length. In general, the doubled semitendinosis is 9 to 11 cm long and approximately 5 to 6 mm in diameter. The gracilis is somewhat smaller. The graft is prepared using the same techniques as for an anterior cruciate ligament reconstruction.

While the graft is being prepared, the lateral ankle is exposed through one of two incisions selected on the basis of the underlying pathology. For patients whose problem is limited to the lateral ligamentous complex and its reconstruction, the incision can be a small curvilinear incision parallel and just distal to the anterior and distal border of the fibula. Careful dissection at the anterior part of the incision will avoid the lateral branch of the superficial peroneal nerve. The length of the incision should be limited to no further plantar than necessary to expose the peroneal tendon sheath to prevent injury to the sural nerve. For patients who have more extensive pathology, such as a peroneal tendon tear or anterior osteophytes, a more utilitarian longitudinal incision is made. The more extensive incision overlays the posterior border of the fibula and curves distally from the inferior fibula to the distal aspect of the sinus tarsi at the anterior process of the calcaneus. A flap is created anteriorly. This approach also requires caution to avoid injury to both the superficial peroneal nerve and the sural nerve.

With either approach, the ankle joint is exposed at the level of the plafond, and the anterolateral capsule is divided in midsubstance to preserve as much potentially useful tissue as

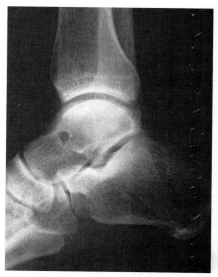

Figure 3 Radiograph showing the talar and calcaneal drill holes.

possible. Intra-articular pathology is also addressed. If the prior lateral reconstruction involved a tendon graft, it is identified, if possible. It is determined whether the tendon graft can be used, along with the existing capsule and/or inferior extensor retinaculum, as an augmentation to the planned reconstruction.

For proper graft placement, it is necessary to expose the insertion site of the ATFL on the talus, the distal fibula, and the insertion site of the CFL on the calcaneus. The surgeon then drills a hole with a 4.5- to 6.0-mm drill bit, depending on the size of the graft being used (**Figure 3**). When I use a 5.5-mm bioabsorbable interference fit screw for fixation, I use a 6.0-mm drill bit. Several manufacturers make bioabsorbable screws that vary from 4 to 11 mm. My experience is that the 5- to 5.5-mm size works best at the ankle. The Arthrex Bio-Tenodesis Screw system (Arthrex Corporation, Naples, FL) allows insertion of the tendon graft into the drill hole with an inserter and avoids the need for a through-and-through hole in the talus. This is a class 2 device indicated for "fixation of ligament and tendon graft tissue in surgeries of the... foot/ankle." The other option is drilling a hole in the talus to a depth of 25 to 30 mm and then passing sutures from the end of the tendon graft through the hole in the talus out the medial side of the foot with a long Keith needle. Then, with tension applied to the sutures pulling the tendon graft into the depth of the drill hole in the talus and the assistant holding tension on the opposite end of the tendon graft, an interference screw can be placed next to the tendon to secure the graft in the talus.

Once the graft is secure in the talus, an appropriately sized drill hole is made from the anterior distal fibula at the site of origin of the ATFL through the distal fibula and slightly proximal. This brings the drill hole out of the posterior fibula into the area of the proximal peroneal groove. With the more limited approach to the ankle, a separate 2-cm incision is made to insert a retractor to protect the peroneal tendons. A second drill hole is made in the fibula from the distal fibula at the site of origin of the CFL to the posterior fibula to exit same hole as previously drilled. This creates a V-shaped channel in the distal fibula. A suture passer is placed through the posterior fibular hole to exit the anterior hole. The sutures in the tendon graft are brought into the fibula creating a band to re-create an ATFL. The suture passer is next passed from the distal fibular hole to the posterior hole to retrieve the sutures in the tendon graft and is then passed out of the distal fibula. The drill is then used to create a hole in the calcaneus for the tendon graft. The depth of the hole should be

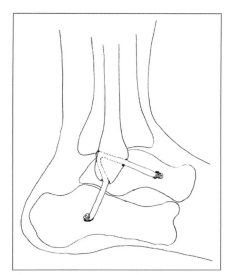

Figure 4 Lateral ankle stabilization using a free tendon graft and bioabsorbable interference fit screws.

sufficient to pull the entire length of the tendon graft into the bone tunnel in the calcaneus. The Keith needle is then used to drill through the calcaneus, exiting at the plantar medial heel. The tendon graft sutures can be passed through the calcaneus and out of the plantar medial heel. The ankle is examined and reduced with a bolster under the distal leg proximal to the heel. With an assistant holding the ankle in neutral dorsiflexion and plantar flexion and neutral inversion and eversion, tension is applied to the graft, and the bioabsorbable screw is placed within the bone tunnel next to the tendon graft to obtain an interference fit and secure the graft (**Figure 4**).

The ankle can be tested for stability and range of motion at this stage. I usually obtain stress radiographs on the operating table with the use of a mini-C arm. If there is insufficient stability, the screw in the calcaneus can be removed, the graft tension reconfirmed, and the screw replaced with the heel in slight eversion. The graft is secured with suture to the periosteum of the fibula at the entrance and exit holes. Additional stability can be added by imbricating the inferior extensor retinaculum or other local tissue or a former graft. After closure of the incision, the ankle is protected in a splint or boot. The patient should use crutches for the first 7 to 14 days after the procedure. After this initial period, the patient can progress from partial to full weight bearing and discontinue the use of crutches by the end of the fourth postoperative week. The trustworthy patient or athlete under supervision of an athletic trainer can be managed in a removable boot and started on active range of motion. A typical ankle rehabilitation program consisting of range of motion, strength, Achilles tendon stretching, and proprioceptive reeducation begins approximately 3 to 4 weeks postoperatively and progresses as tolerated by the patient. Any alterations to this general protocol are based on the patient's individual pathology.

Management of Complications
None

References

Clanton TO: Athletic injuries to the soft tissues of the foot and ankle, in Coughlin MJ, Mann RA (eds): *Surgery of the Foot and Ankle*, ed 7. St Louis, MO, Mosby, 1999, pp 1090-1209.

Hennrikus WL, Mapes RC, Lyons PM, Lapoint JM: Outcomes of the Chrisman-Snook and modified-Broström procedures for chronic lateral ankle instability. *Am J Sports Med* 1996;24:400-404.

Sammarco JS: Complications of lateral ankle ligament reconstruction. *Clin Orthop* 2001;391:123-132.

Sammarco JS, Carrasquillo HA: Surgical revision after failed lateral ankle reconstruction. *Foot Ankle* 1995;16:748-753.

Coding

ICD-9 CODES

718.57   Ankylosis of joint (fibrous), Ankle and foot; Ankle joint

718.97   Unspecified derangement of joint, ankle and foot

719.47   Pain in joint, Ankle and foot; Ankle joint

719.57   Stiffness of joint, Ankle and foot; Ankle joint

728.4   Laxity of ligament

845.00   Sprains and strains of ankle and foot, Ankle; Unspecified site

845.01   Sprains and strains of ankle and foot, Ankle; Deltoid (ligament) ankle

845.02   Sprains and strains of ankle and foot, Ankle; Calcaneofibular (ligament)

845.03   Sprains and strains of ankle and foot, Ankle; Tibiofibular (ligament), distal

845.09   Sprains and strains of ankle and foot, Ankle; Other

CPT CODES

20924   Tendon graft, from a distance (eg, palmaris, toe extensor, plantaris)

27685   Lengthening or shortening of tendon, leg or ankle, single tendon (separate procedure)

27690   Transfer or transplant of single tendon (with muscle redirection or rerouting); deep

27698   Repair, secondary, disrupted ligament, ankle, collateral (eg, Watson-Jones procedure)

Medial Ankle Instability

Beat Hintermann, MD

▇ Definition of the Problem

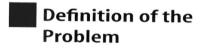

Patient Presentation

Patients with medial instability report a feeling of "giving way," especially in a medial direction, when walking on even ground, downhill, or down stairs; pain at the anteromedial aspect of the ankle; and sometimes pain at the lateral aspect of the ankle, especially during dorsiflexion of the foot. A history of chronic instability, manifested by recurrent injuries with pain, tenderness, and, occasionally, bruising over the medial and lateral ligaments indicates combined medial and lateral instability that is believed to result in rotational instability of the talus in the ankle mortise. Typically, injuries to the medial ankle ligaments occur during running down the stairs, landing on an uneven surface, and dancing while the body simultaneously rotates in the opposite direction.

Physical Examination

Medial ankle instability is diagnosed on the basis of the history and physical examination, including special maneuvers, and plain radiography. It is important to discover whether the patient has sustained a pronation (eversion) injury, ie, an outward rotation of the foot during simultaneous inward rotation of the tibia. In practice, however, the mechanism of injury is difficult to elucidate because patients often report having sustained one or more ankle sprains but are unable to clearly specify exactly what happened. Nevertheless, the orthopaedist should attempt to obtain a precise description of how the ankle sprain occurred.

With the patient bearing weight, the form and position of both feet are inspected for potential valgus malalignment, pronation deformity with and without internal rotation of the leg, asymmetry of the malleoli, and swelling of the medial and/or lateral ankle (**Figure 1**, *A*). Valgus malalignment of the hindfoot is defined as an asymmetric pronation deformity of the affected foot, with excessive hindfoot valgus, pronation of the foot, and often some internal rotation of the leg that disappears when the posterior tibial muscle is activated (**Figure 1**, *B*) and when the patient is standing on his or her toes (**Figure 1**, *C*). A patient with a tarsal coalition commonly will have hindfoot valgus with variable subtalar motion and overall decreased flexibility of the hindfoot.

Tenderness in the medial gutter is considered the hallmark of medial ankle instability, but the patient also may have pain along the anterior border of the lateral malleolus and along the posterior tibial tendon. Posterior tibial strength, however, is adequate; the examiner is unable to overcome the posterior tibial muscle with a maximum inversion effort. Posterior tibial weakness mandates a search for posterior tibial pathology.

The anterior drawer test is performed with the patient sitting on the edge of the table with the feet hanging and the knees flexed 90°. The orthopaedist stabilizes the tibia with one hand and attempts to draw the talus forward with the other hand. If the medial structures are incompetent, the displacement is an anterior translational movement that increases while the foot is internally rotated with respect to the tibia (rotatory instability). If the lateral ligaments also are incompetent, overall anterior translation can be increased further. Anterior displacement of the talus relative to the tibia on the injured side compared with the contralateral side or excessive displacement signifies a positive test.

Weight-bearing AP and lateral views are used to assess malalignment of the foot and to exclude bony pathologies. When a talocalcaneal coalition or bony fragmentation that involves the articular surfaces is suspected, CT is added. Increased plantar flexion of the talus (lateral talometatarsal angle) and/or internal rotation of the talus (dorsoplantar talometatarsal angle) on the injured side compared with the contralateral side or excessive displacement signifies a positive test for medial instability. A negative test, however, cannot exclude medial ankle instability, nor can stress radiographs. Thus, the orthopaedist might not rely on radiographs for making the diagnosis of medial ankle instability. MRI may be helpful to exclude pathology of the

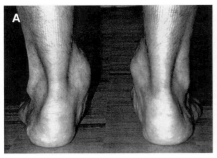 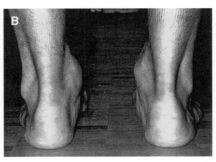 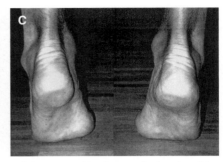

Figure 1   A 34-year-old male long-distance runner reports progressive giving way, pain in the medial gutter and on the anterior border of the fibula, and slight pain along the posterior tibial tendon 14 months after pronation injury of the left ankle. **A,** Note the asymmetric valgus deformity of the affected left foot with prominent medial malleolus and internal rotation of the tibia. **B,** Complete correction of the valgus deformity with activation of the posterior tibial muscle. **C,** Complete correction of the valgus deformity in the tiptoe position and some varus deformity caused by the lateral ankle ligament instability.

Table 1   Stages of Medial Instability of the Ankle

	Giving Way	Valgus/Pronation of Foot	Pain in Medial Gutter	Pain in Anterior Border of Fibula	Posterior Tibial Tendinitis	Deformity Fully Correctable
Stage 1	+	+	(+)	(+)	−	Yes
Stage 2	++	+	+	+	−	Yes
Stage 3	+++	++	++	++	+	No
Stage 4	++++	+++	+++	+++	++	No

posterior tibial tendon, but it does not show incompetence of the medial ligament structures.

Based on clinical and radiographic findings, medial ankle instability can be divided into four stages (**Table 1**).

Differential Diagnosis
- Posterior tibial tendon dysfunction
- Tarsal coalition
- Neurologic disorder causing pronation deformity

Additional Work-up
Ankle arthroscopy is a helpful tool for preoperative evaluation and planning. Because most ligament tears are located at their proximal insertion, this frequently can be seen as a completely free insertion area of the ligament on the fibula or the medial malleolus. The deltoid ligament is considered incompetent when it is tensioned as the foot is pronated (everted), but obviously no strong medial buttress is created with this maneuver (**Figure 2**). An excessive lifting away of the talus from the medial malleolus when pulling the foot anteriorly also is considered an indicator of deltoid ligament stretching.

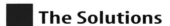

▉ The Solutions

Treatment Options and Rationale
Medial ankle ligament reconstruction is indicated for symptomatic mechanical instability that has persisted despite appropriate nonsurgical management. Because the involved ligaments usually are found to be elongated or disrupted there is a possibility of primary reconstruction. Direct late repair has the advantage of preserving normal anatomy and avoiding morbidity associated with autologous tendon grafts. The disadvantage of this technique is that it relies on previously damaged tissue for a strong repair. The outcome is expected to be good in the case of subtle deformity and/or malalignment. However, an isolated repair of the medial ankle ligaments might not sufficiently address a long-standing pronation deformity and valgus alignment that may have provoked complex changes in other structures of the foot, such as muscular imbalance, tendon dysfunction, and ligament and capsular distention. If the injured ligament structures are of poor quality, reinforcement by a free plantaris tendon graft should be considered.

Lateral ankle ligament reconstruction should be considered in the presence of additional lateral ankle in-

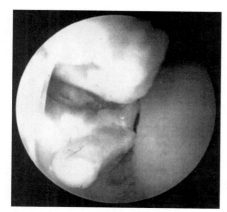

Figure 2 Arthroscopic assessment of the patient shown in Figure 1. Anterior view of the medial malleolus shows a completely free insertion area of the ligament and the distal scarred stump of the deltoid ligament.

stability found by clinical examination and confirmed by preoperative arthroscopy. In my experience, combined medial and lateral instability is common. This combination probably can be explained by the repetitive rotatory shift of the talus within the medial ankle mortise, which provokes overuse and attenuation of the lateral ankle ligaments. This hypothesis is supported by the high incidence of cartilage lesion seen on the medial talus and the consistently uniform injury pattern of the lateral ankle ligaments. Both the anterior talofibular ligament and the calcaneofibular ligament are detached from their inser-

tion on the anterior aspect of the distal fibula.

Shortening of the posterior tibial tendon may be advised for a long-standing pronation deformity that has led to degeneration and/or elongation of the tendon. If there is a detached accessory bone on the navicular bone (os tibiale externum), distal displacement and refixation is advised to restore the power of the posterior tibial muscle.

A calcaneal lengthening osteotomy is considered for both a severe long-standing valgus and pronation deformity and a severe attenuation or defect of the tibionavicular, tibiospring, and/or spring ligaments. Calcaneal lengthening osteotomy may also be indicated in the case of a preexisting valgus and pronation deformity of the foot (eg, when a valgus and pronation deformity is also present on the contralateral, asymptomatic foot) and/or chronic tarsal tunnel syndrome. As the calcaneal lengthening osteotomy corrects the foot deformity, it protects the reconstructed ligaments from overloading and allows the muscles to function more physiologically.

Talonavicular arthrodesis is considered when the medial ankle instability is so excessive that the patient cannot fully correct the pronation deformity (eg, when a significant defect

of the tibionavicular and spring ligaments is present). The need for a talonavicular arthrodesis, however, also is influenced by the patient's body habitus and activity pattern. For example, talonavicular arthrodesis might be recommended for an obese, sedentary patient who requires basically a pain-free and stable foot, whereas ligament reconstruction and bony correction might be recommended for professional athletes and those whose livelihood necessitates a full range of ankle motion.

Author's Preferred Treatment and Rationale

The choice of treatment of medial ankle instability depends on the clinical findings and is influenced by the patient's habitus and activity pattern. My rationale for the treatment options is shown in **Table 2**.

MEDIAL ANKLE LIGAMENTS: PROXIMAL TEAR

The anterior border of the medial malleolus is exposed by a short longitudinal incision between the tibiocalcaneal and tibiospring ligaments, where there usually is a small fibrous septum without adherent connective fibers between the two ligaments (**Figure 3**). After roughening of the medial aspect of the medial malleolus, a surgical an-

Table 2 Treatment of Symptomatic Medial Instability of the Ankle

	Surgery	Medial Ligament Repair	Lateral Ligament Repair	Calcaneal Lengthening Osteotomy	Posterior Tibial Shortening	Talonavicular Arthodesis
Stage 1	No	No	No	No	No	No
Stage 2	Yes	Yes	Yes*	No	No	No
Stage 3	Yes	Yes	Yes*	Yes†	Yes‡	No
Stage 4	Yes	No	No	No	No	Yes§

* If lateral ankle instability is present and arthroscopically confirmed.
† If long-standing instability/deformity exceeds 12 months.
‡ If significant elongation and/or degenerative changes of the tendon, and/or long-standing instability/deformity exceeds 12 months.
§ In the case of short-term instability/deformity (<6 months) and/or high sports demand treat as stage 3.

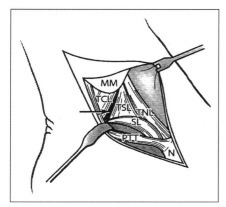

Figure 3 Anatomic exposure of the medial ankle ligament. MM = medial malleolus, N = navicular bone, PTT = posterior tibial tendon, SL = spring ligament, TNL = tibionavicular ligament, TSL = tibiospring ligament, TCL = talocalcaneal ligaments, arrow = small fibrous septum without adherent connective fibers between the TCL and TSL.

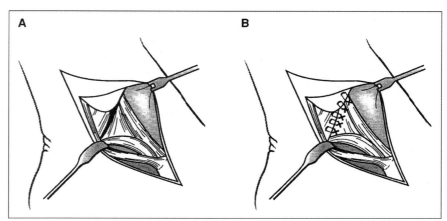

Figure 4 **A,** Proximal tear along the interval between the tibiocalcaneal and tibiospring ligaments involving the proximal insertion of both ligaments; in most patients the superficial fibers are intact, whereas the deep portions are disrupted. **B,** Transosseous suture of the tibiospring and tibionavicular ligaments to the medial malleolus and closure of the interval between the ligaments by No. 0 bioabsorbable sutures, thereby tensioning the spring ligament.

chor is placed 6 mm above the tip of the malleolus and is used to refix the tibionavicular and tibiospring ligaments to the medial malleolus and to shorten both ligaments (**Figure 4**). Additional No. 0 bioabsorbable sutures are used to close the interval between the tibiocalcaneal and tibiospring ligaments.

MEDIAL ANKLE LIGAMENTS: INTERMEDIATE TEAR

After separating the tibiospring and tibionavicular ligaments, the tibiospring ligament is sharply dissected from its insertion on the medial malleolus. A longitudinal incision is made to divide the tibionavicular ligament into two parts, with the cranial part including about two thirds of the ligament. The cranial part is prepared for being tightened and refixed to the navicular bone by an anchor, whereas the caudal part is prepared for being tightened and refixed to the medial malleolus and the tibiospring ligament, as described above (**Figure 5**).

MEDIAL ANKLE LIGAMENTS: DISTAL TEAR

A distal rupture and/or attenuation of the tibionavicular ligament consistently

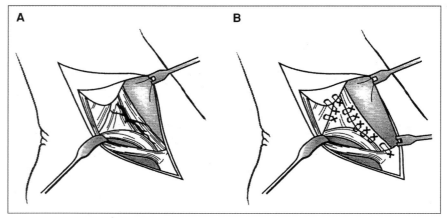

Figure 5 **A,** Intermediate tear of the tibiospring and tibionavicular ligaments. **B,** After Z-shaped incision to detach the tibiospring ligament from the medial malleolus and the cranial part of the tibionavicular ligament, the tibiospring ligament is tightened and reattached by transosseous sutures to the medial malleolus, and the main part of the tibionavicular ligament is tightened and reattached to the navicular bone. No. 0 bioabsorbable sutures are used to close the intervals, thereby tensioning the spring ligament.

is combined with a rupture of the spring ligament, whereas the tibiospring ligament is intact. The tibionavicular ligament is prepared to be tightened and refixed to the navicular bone by using an anchor. Two additional bioabsorbable sutures are used to repair the tear of the spring ligament (**Figure 6**).

MEDIAL ANKLE LIGAMENTS: FREE PLANTARIS GRAFT AUGMENTATION

If the injured ligament structures are of poor quality, the reconstruction of

tibiospring and tibionavicular ligaments is reinforced by a free plantaris tendon graft. Two converging 3.2-mm holes are drilled into the anterior border of the medial malleolus, 2 to 8 mm proximal to its tip. One arm of a forceps is introduced into the cranial hole and the other into the distal hole, and a tunnel is made by swivelling the forceps. A tunnel is created similarly in navicular bone. The plantaris tendon graft is introduced cranially to caudally into the tunnel of the malleolus, and again cra-

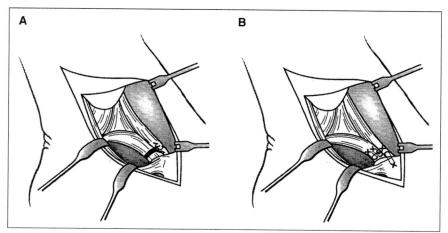

Figure 6 **A,** Distal rupture and attenuation of the tibionavicular ligament and vertical rupture of the spring ligament. **B,** Two bioabsorbable sutures are used to repair the tibiospring ligament and transosseous sutures to tighten and reattach the tibionavicular ligament to the navicular bone.

nially to caudally into the tunnel of the navicular bone. While the foot is kept in a neutral position, the ends of the transplanted tendon are sutured under slight tension with No. 0 bioabsorbable suture. The remaining ligaments are sutured to the tendon transplant, thereby creating a strong repair of the tibiospring and tibionavicular ligaments.

SHORTENING OF THE POSTERIOR TIBIAL TENDON

An osteotomy is performed to detach the distal posterior tibial tendon and a piece of bone from the navicular bone. If there is a detached accessory bone on the navicular (os tibiale externum), it is separated from the navicular. Care is taken to avoid damaging the ligamentous structures on the plantar aspect of the navicular. Starting almost at the distal insertion of the spring ligament, a second osteotomy is performed in the sagittal plane from proximally to distally, and the medial piece of approximately 8 to 12 mm is removed. While the foot is kept in a supinated position, the posterior tibial tendon is tightened and its bony attachment refixed to the navicular bone by one or two screws.

CALCANEAL LENGTHENING OSTEOTOMY

The calcaneal neck is exposed through a 3- to 4-cm long longitudinal incision. One Homan retractor is inserted into the sinus tarsi and another into the bottom of the calcaneus. Calcaneal osteotomy is performed along and parallel to the posterior facet of the subtalar joint, from lateral to medial, preserving the intact medial cortex. As the osteotomy is widened, the pronation deformity of the foot is seen to disappear. A tricortical graft from the iliac crest is fashioned to the length required (usually 4 to 6 mm) and placed into the osteotomy site.

TALONAVICULAR ARTHRODESIS

The talonavicular joint is exposed through a 4- to 5-cm long dorsomedial incision, and the cartilage is removed. While the foot is kept in plantigrade position, the joint is fixed by three 3.5-mm AO screws or three No. 4.0 I.CO.S. Screws (Newdeal SA, Vienne, France).

POSTOPERATIVE MANAGEMENT

The patient remains in a splint and is not allowed to bear weight until initial swelling has disappeared, usually after 1 week. Thereafter, a weight-bearing cast with a strong medial support of the longitudinal arch is used for 5 weeks, or in the case of talonavicular arthrodesis for 7 weeks, in the neutral position. After cast removal, a rehabilitation program focusing on range of motion, strengthening of the peroneal and posterior tibial muscles, and neuromuscular control is initiated. The physiotherapy continues until muscular strength and proprioception are restored.

Management of Complications

Intravenous or oral antibiotics are given for superficial infections. If there is a deep infection, the wound is opened and revised, and, based on the results of the culture and sensitivity, specific antibiotics are given.

If the patient's ankle or subtalar joints are stiff and all nonsurgical measures fail, arthroscopic or open arthrotomy may be necessary. If pain and restricted subtalar motion persist, open revision is advised. If the osteotomy or arthrodesis has not healed within 3 to 4 months, surgical revision and bone grafting are advised.

References

Hintermann B, Boss AP, Schäfer D: Arthroscopic findings in patients with chronic ankle instability. *Am J Sports Med* 2002;30:402-409.

Hintermann B: Biomechanics of the unstable ankle joint and clinical implications. *Med Sci Sports Exerc* 1999;31(suppl 7):S459-S469.

Hintermann B, Valderrabano V, Kundert HP: Lengthening of the lateral column and reconstruction of the medial soft tissue for treatment of acquired flatfoot deformity associated with insufficiency of the posterior tibial tendon. *Foot Ankle Int* 1999;20:622-629.

Milner CE, Soames RW: Anatomy of the collateral ligaments of the human ankle joint. *Foot Ankle Int* 1998;19:757-760.

Milner CE, Soames RW: The medial collateral ligaments of the human ankle joint: Anatomical variations. *Foot Ankle Int* 1998;19:289-292.

Coding

ICD-9 CODES

718.37   Recurrent dislocation of joint, ankle and foot

718.47   Contracture of joint, ankle and foot

719.47   Pain in joint, ankle and foot

719.77   Difficulty in walking, ankle and foot

845.00   Sprains and strains of ankle and foot, Ankle, unspecified site

CPT CODES

27695   Repair, primary, disrupted ligament, ankle; both collateral ligaments

27698   Repair, secondary disrupted ligament, ankle, collateral (eg, Watson-Jones procedure)

Subtalar Pain

Carol Frey, MD

Definition of the Problem

Patient Presentation

Chronic pain or instability after an inversion ankle injury may be the result of an undiagnosed or untreated injury to the subtalar joint. Chronic subtalar joint pain has most commonly been associated with sinus tarsi syndrome. Signs and symptoms of sinus tarsi syndrome include lateral foot pain, pain on palpation of the sinus tarsi, perceived hindfoot instability, and a common history of an inversion injury. The term sinus tarsi syndrome describes the location of the pain and is not an accurate diagnosis. The term is grouped with other causes of subtalar pain.

A thorough history and physical examination are important to determine the etiology of lateral foot and ankle pain. Most patients report a prior inversion injury to the ankle and hindfoot. Patients usually describe pain at the lateral aspect of the foot and note pain and a feeling of hindfoot instability when walking on uneven surfaces.

Physical Examination

Physical examination of the injured extremity may reveal ecchymosis at the medial border of the hindfoot (Battle's sign) and may be the first indication of an injury to the subtalar joint after an ankle sprain. There may be tenderness to palpation of the sinus tarsi. Pain and instability often can be relieved temporarily with an injection of local anesthetic into the sinus tarsi or subtalar joint.

Differential Diagnosis
- Fracture of the anterior process of the calcaneus
- Fracture of the os trigonum and Steida's process
- Subtalar joint instability
- Subtalar joint dislocation
- Tarsal coalition
- Degenerative joint disease
- Occult fracture
- Fracture of the lateral process of the talus
- Interosseous ligament tear/impingement
- Synovitis
- Tumor
- Infection

Additional Work-up

The subtalar joint is difficult to examine radiographically. An oblique view will show the anterior process of the calcaneus. The lateral view shows the subtalar joint and allows measurement of the critical angle of Gissane and Böhler's angle. The mortise view may also show the posterior subtalar joint. The posterior facet of the subtalar joint is best seen on a Broden view. This view is taken with the foot in dorsiflexion and medially rotated 15°. The x-ray beam is angled cephalad and directed at the lateral malleolus. The angle of the x-ray beam is increased from 10° to 40° to obtain the different Broden views of the subtalar joint.

CT has essentially replaced radiography in the evaluation of the subtalar joint. Obtaining 2- to 3-mm sections in two planes (axial and coronal) may demonstrate intra-articular and bony pathology.

MRI has been useful in delineating the soft tissues around the ankle and hindfoot. Pathologic changes in the sinus tarsi in patients with sinus tarsi syndrome may be seen on MRI scans. Findings may include (1) low signal intensity on both T1- and T2-weighted images consistent with fibrosis, (2) low signal intensity on T1-weighted images and increased signal intensity on T2-weighted images consistent with chronic synovitis and nonspecific inflammatory changes, and (3) multiple abnormal fluid collections consistent with synovial cysts. The findings also may be associated with injuries to the lateral ankle ligament complex.

Subtalar instability is difficult to demonstrate radiographically. Stress radiographs, arthrograms, and stress tomograms offer limited information. The most practical test is a standard stress test of the ankle joint, including the subtalar joint. A varus stress test may result in loss of parallel alignment in the facets of the posterior subtalar joint. Use of the anterior drawer test in patients with subtalar instability may result in anterior subluxation of the calcaneus with respect to the talus.

A bupivacaine arthrogram may confirm or rule out localization of pain to the subtalar joint. Fluoro-

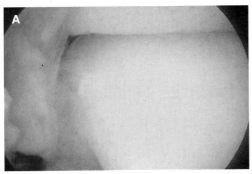 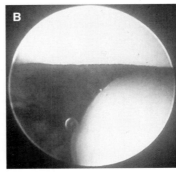

Figure 1 Instability of the subtalar joint demonstrated at arthroscopy. **A,** The lateral aspect of the posterior subtalar joint before varus stress. **B,** The joint after varus stress. The calcaneus glides medially under the talus. (Reproduced from Frey C: Injuries to the subtalar joint, in Pfeffer GB (ed): *Chronic Ankle Pain in the Athlete*. Rosemont, IL, American Academy of Orthopaedic Surgeons, 2000, pp 21-42.)

scopic confirmation of the injection with contrast may exclude the possibility that other communicating anatomic sites are a cause of pain.

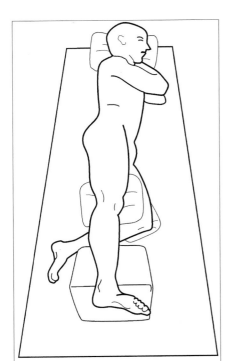

Figure 2 The patient is placed in the lateral decubitus position with the injured side up. (Reproduced from Frey C: Injuries to the subtalar joint, in Pfeffer GB (ed): *Chronic Ankle Pain in the Athlete*. Rosemont, IL, American Academy of Orthopaedic Surgeons, 2000, pp 21-42.)

The Solutions

Treatment Options and Rationale

Inversion injuries to the ankle and hindfoot are common. Most patients return to normal function within 4 to 8 weeks after appropriate treatment that includes rest, ice, compression, elevation, early mobilization and weight bearing, peroneal strengthening exercises, and proprioceptive retraining. However, 20% to 40% of patients continue to have residual pain and dysfunction despite adequate therapy. This pain and feeling of instability in many instances may be localized to the sinus tarsi and subtalar joint.

In addition to MRI, the advent of arthroscopy has greatly aided the diagnosis and treatment of subtalar pain (**Figure 1**). In a review of 49 subtalar arthroscopies, many of which were performed for presumed sinus tarsi syndrome, 74% were interosseous ligament tears, 14% arthrofibrosis, 8% degenerative joint disease, and 4% fibrous coalitions of the calcaneonavicular articulation. With an average follow-up of 4 years, 47% of patients had excellent results, 47% had good results, and only 6% had poor results with débridement. The results correlated with the type and severity of the injury.

Exploration of the subtalar joint and sinus tarsi, with possible débridement, may be considered when arthroscopy is not feasible or unsuccessful, as in patients with scarring from previous surgery or trauma.

Author's Preferred Treatment

Anterior, posterior, and middle portals are used for subtalar arthrosopy. The middle portal is essential for the evaluation of the sinus tarsi and its contents. Local, general, spinal, or epidural anesthesia can be used for the procedure. The patient is placed in the lateral decubitus position with the injured extremity facing up (**Figure 2**). Padding is placed between the legs,

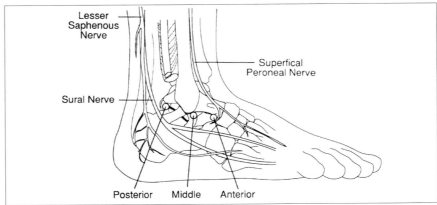

Figure 3 Portals and relevant anatomy for arthroscopic evaluation of the sinus tarsi and subtalar joint. (Reproduced from Frey C: Injuries to the subtalar joint, in Pfeffer GB (ed): *Chronic Ankle Pain in the Athlete*. Rosemont, IL, American Academy of Orthopaedic Surgeons, 2000, pp 21-42.)

and a bolster is placed distally under the injured extremity to suspend the foot and leg. A tourniquet is used.

The three portals are available for visualization and instrumentation of the subtalar joint. The anterior portal is placed 2 cm anterior and 1 cm distal to the tip of the lateral malleolus (**Figure 3**). The posterior portal is placed 1 cm proximal to the tip of the fibula and anterior to the Achilles tendon. The middle portal is placed under direct visualization, using an 18-gauge needle with outside-in technique. A 2.7-mm, 30° oblique arthroscope, and an arthroscopic pump are used for the procedure.

At the time of surgery, the surgeon is able to (1) remove loose bodies, (2) evaluate chondral and osteochondral fractures, (3) excise intra-articular adhesions, (4) perform an appraisal of articular cartilage damage after calcaneal or talar body fractures, (5) remove inflamed or excessive synovium, (6) excise torn or impinging soft tissue in the sinus tarsi and/or gutters, (7) fuse the joint, and (8) evaluate subtalar instability.

Open approaches to the subtalar joint may involve excision of the fat pad, detachment of the extensor digitorum brevis, and transsection of the ligaments of the sinus tarsi. Although the exact morbidity of this dissection is unknown, there are obvious theoretical advantages to preserving normal anatomy.

Management of Complications
Complications include neuritis of the superficial peroneal nerve, sinus tract formation, and wound infections. I reported five complications in 45 patients undergoing subtalar arthroscopy, including three patients with neuritis along branches of the superficial peroneal nerve and one case each of sinus tract formation and superficial wound infection. The wound infection occurred in the patient with the sinus tract formation. The three patients with neuritis were treated successfully with cortisone injections and physical therapy. The patient with the sinus tract formation and the superficial wound infection was treated sucessfully with antibiotics, wound care, and subsequent total contact casting. Overall, the complication rate was low and all problems resolved with nonsurgical treatment. As seen in ankle arthroscopy, the most common complication is a transient neurapraxia involving branches of the superficial peroneal nerve.

References

Frey C, Gasser S, Feder K: Arthroscopy of the subtalar joint. *Foot Ankle Int* 1994;15:424-428.

Heilman AE, Braly WG, Bishop JO, Noble PC, Tullos HS: An anatomic study of subtalar instability. *Foot Ankle* 1990;10:224-228.

Kjaersgaard-Andersen P, Wethelund JO, Helmig P, Soballe K: The stabilizing effect of the ligamentous structures in the sinus and canalis tarsi on movements in the hindfoot: An experimental study. *Am J Sports Med* 1988;16:512-516.

Klein MA, Spreitzer AM: MR imaging of the tarsal sinus and canal: Normal anatomy, pathologic findings, and features of the sinus tarsi syndrome. *Radiology* 1993;186:233-240.

Coding

ICD-9 CODES

355.5   Tarsal tunnel syndrome

355.9   Mononeuritis of unspecified site

707.09 Lateral gutter syndrome

718.87 Other joint derangement, not elsewhere classified; ankle and foot

726.79 Enthesopathy of ankle and tarsus, other

727.68 Rupture of tendon nontraumatic, other tendons of foot and ankle

728.4   Laxity of ligament

845.09 Sprains and strains of ankle and foot, other

CPT CODE

29898 Arthroscopy, ankle (tibiotalar and fibulotalar joints), surgical; debridement, extensive

Stress Fractures of the Tarsal Navicular

Todd A. Kile, MD

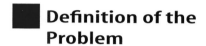

Definition of the Problem

Patient Presentation

Tarsal navicular stress fractures have derailed many promising athletic careers and remain a source of frustration for physicians and athletes alike. Poorly defined symptoms combined with minimal physical findings, which are rarely visible on radiographs, have allowed this problem to elude diagnosis, often leading to a significant delay in appropriate treatment.

Though first described by Towne and associates in 1970, few articles on navicular stress fractures have been published, making an objective analysis of appropriate treatment difficult. This may be due in part to a very low incidence as seen in one review of 142 stress fractures in athletes with only one fracture of the navicular (0.7%). However, many authors feel that this condition is frequently underdiagnosed, or missed entirely, with and without radiographs because this fracture is not suspected. Either way, much of our current treatment rationale is based on a relatively small number of reported cases with limited clinical and radiographic follow-up.

The pathophysiology of navicular stress fractures may be explained by a review of the vascular anatomy. With its extensive articular surfaces proximally and distally, the blood supply to the navicular is limited. Microangiographic studies have shown that the blood supply is most abundant within the tuberosity medially and at the dorsal and plantar surfaces of the lateral aspect, with a central area of relative avascularity. This arrangement seems to correspond with the location of the fractures at the junction of the lateral one third and the medial two thirds of the navicular. In addition, shear stresses and increased forces transmitted through the second metatarsal and middle cuneiform have been hypothesized.

Stress fractures of the navicular often are misdiagnosed as a result of the ill-defined nature of the pain and the difficulty in identifying the fracture on radiographs. A high index of suspicion is necessary to prevent delay in diagnosis and possible progression of an incomplete fracture to a complete fracture with displacement.

Symptoms include the insidious onset of vague pain over the dorsum of the medial midfoot or forefoot or along the medial aspect of the longitudinal arch. The pain may be described as an ill-defined soreness or cramping that is aggravated with exercise and relieved by rest. Little, if any, swelling or skin discoloration is noted by the patients.

In general, patients are younger than age 30 years, with one series having an average age of 21 years. Sixty-eight percent of the fractures occur in men, and 5% of the total number of fractures are bilateral. Patients' athletic activities usually involve explosive sporting events, such as track and field with jumping, sprinting, hurdling, and pole vaulting; football; and basketball, leading some authors to speculate that the injured foot is biomechanically unsuited to perform at these levels.

The average duration of symptoms before definitive diagnosis has been reported to be 4 months (range, 3 to 60 months). Reasons for this delay include lack of awareness on the part of the athletes and physicians, with distally radiating pain and normal radiographs frequently resulting in missed diagnoses.

Differentiating between stress fractures and overuse syndromes can be difficult but is made easier by noting that pain associated with stress fractures increases with activity, whereas pain associated with overuse syndromes follows the activity.

Physical Examination

The typical patient with a stress fracture of the navicular has minimal physical findings, requiring a higher degree of suspicion on the part of the treating physician. Tenderness to palpation may prove difficult to localize, but when present it is frequently located over the dorsal aspect of the talonavicular joint, as well as along the medial longitudinal arch. A significant percentage of patients are unable to localize their symptoms despite careful inspection and have no ecchymosis or swelling. However, limited ankle dorsiflexion, subtalar joint motion, or both has been noted in a high percentage of patients.

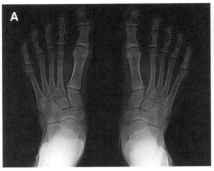
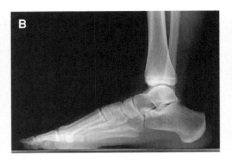
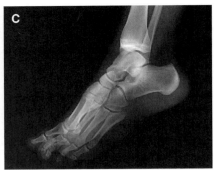

Figure 1 Normal weight-bearing AP **(A)**, lateral **(B)**, and oblique **(C)** radiographs of symptomatic patient who was later diagnosed with a navicular stress fracture.

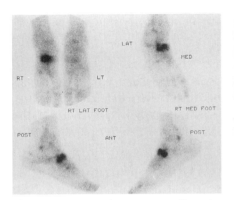

Figure 2 Positive bone scan outlines the symptomatic right navicular stress fracture. (Reproduced with permission from Khan KM, Fuller PJ, Brukner PD, et al: Outcome of conservative and surgical management of navicular stress fracture in athletes. *Am J Sports Med* 1992;20:657-666.)

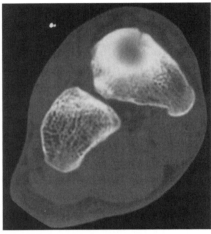

Figure 3 Axial CT scan shows a small partial fracture of the navicular. (Reproduced with permission from Khan KM, Fuller PJ, Brukner PD, et al: Outcome of conservative and surgical management of navicular stress fracture in athletes. *Am J Sports Med* 1992;20: 657-666.)

A review of the current literature reveals no evidence to support the theories that foot posture or type seems to predispose athletes to this injury. All types of feet are represented, ranging from pes planus with significant pronation to normal feet to rigid pes cavus.

A single limb hopping test may help to reproduce symptoms in a patient believed to have a navicular stress fracture who has minimal other findings. In those patients, imaging studies may be indicated.

Radiographic evaluation in the symptomatic athlete routinely begins with weight-bearing AP, lateral, and oblique views of the affected foot (**Figure 1**). Although comparison views of the contralateral foot may prove helpful, most stress fractures of the navicular are not seen on radiographs. Initial radiographs have been reported to be positive in only 18% of stress fractures, leading to frequent delays in diagnosis and treatment. This delay can allow an incomplete fracture, which may respond well to nonsurgical treatment, to progress to a complete or displaced fracture necessitating open reduction and internal fixation (ORIF) with possible bone graft. An arthrodesis may be needed if end-stage arthrosis develops.

In patients who have a history or physical examination consistent with a stress fracture of the navicular and normal radiographs, additional imaging studies may be necessary to confirm the diagnosis and guide treatment recommendations.

Differential Diagnosis

- Metatarsal stress fracture
- Plantar fasciitis
- Anterior tibial tendinitis
- Posterior tibial tendinitis (insertional)
- Spring ligament tear or rupture
- Compression neuropathy or neuritis (superficial versus deep peroneal, saphenous)
- Degenerative joint disease, midfoot (tarsometatarsal, intertarsal) versus hindfoot
- Lisfranc sprain or fracture, with or without subluxation

Additional Work-up

Radionuclide bone scanning is a reliable and sensitive screening examination for patients with suspicious symptoms and normal radiographs. Whether partial or complete, navicular stress fractures consistently demonstrate increased uptake on delayed imaging with technetium Tc 99m medronate sodium bone scan (**Figure 2**). In particular, the plantar views provide better visualization of the navicular and other midfoot bones than do the AP and lateral images.

While tomography has proven

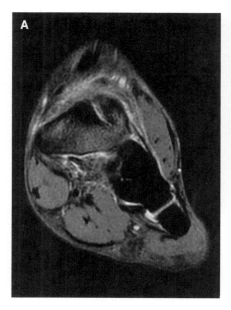

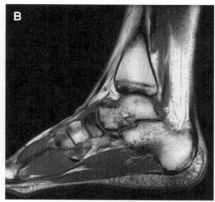

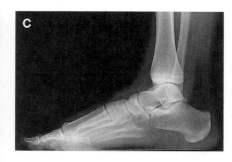

Figure 4 **A,** Coronal hindfoot T2-weighted MRI scan confirms a partial navicular stress fracture in an elite gymnast. **B,** Sagittal T1-weighted image reveals changes in signal intensity within the dorsal aspect of the navicular that seem to correspond with "normal" lateral radiograph **(C)** obtained the same day. Note the curvilinear radiolucency that parallels the signal changes seen on MRI.

useful in the past, CT has replaced plain tomography at most institutions and is the preferred imaging modality for identification of fracture type as well as preoperative planning. For visualization of these fractures, I routinely use helical CT with a bone algorithm and thin sections (0.5- to 1.25-mm thickness, 50% overlap) acquired in a coronal oblique plane, with mulitiplanar reconstructions in the axial, coronal, and sagittal planes.

Typically, an incomplete fracture involving the upper 5 mm of the navicular is seen linearly in the sagittal plane (**Figure 3**). However, these fractures can be missed for several reasons, including improper patient positioning, software and hardware issues, and the imaging protocol used. Moreover, if the scan does not include the entire dorsal cortex, the fracture can be missed. Complete fractures that extend from the dorsal to the plantar surface, with or without displacement, may be visible on radiographs.

MRI continues to evolve and can reveal subtle fractures not seen on CT due to better visualization of incomplete trabecular fractures and surrounding bone marrow edema (**Figure 4**). Areas of vascular irregularity, as seen in osteonecrosis, are also bet-

ter visualized on MRI. However, CT remains the imaging modality of choice for confirmation of navicular stress fractures, as well as for preoperative planning.

---■

The Solutions

Treatment Options and Rationale

Although navicular stress fractures were first described in 1970, few articles have been published, making an objective analysis of appropriate treatment difficult. This may be due in part to a very low incidence as seen in a review of 142 stress fractures in athletes with only one fracture of the navicular (0.7%). However, many authors feel that this condition is frequently underdiagnosed or missed entirely, with and without radiographs, because it is not suspected. Either way, much of the current treatment rationale is based on a relatively small number of reported occurrences with limited clinical and radiographic follow-up.

Most stress fractures of the nav-

icular are incomplete and respond well to nonsurgical treatment, consisting of 6 to 8 weeks of non–weight-bearing immobilization in a short leg cast. Similarly, patients with complete fractures that are not displaced have had a high union rate with a non–weight-bearing cast. In one series of 21 navicular stress fractures, all 10 patients (five partial and five complete fractures) healed when treated in this fashion. In another series, an 86% success rate (19 of 22 patients) was reported when non–weight-bearing cast immobilization was used as the first treatment and a 90% success rate when it was used as the second treatment.

A complete displaced fracture usually is treated with ORIF and may be augmented with fresh autologous cancellous bone graft. Rarely, in patients with advanced degenerative changes at the naviculocuneiform or talonavicular joints, or both, an arthrodesis may be needed to control pain and deformity.

Indications for surgical treatment include complete fractures that have failed to respond to nonsurgical management or have become displaced, incomplete fractures in which the fracture line extends more than halfway through the body of the navicular, or failure of nonsurgical treatment.

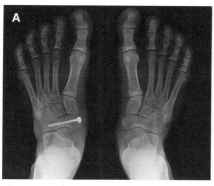
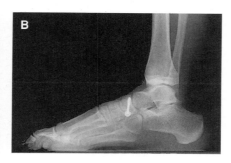

Figure 5 Weight-bearing AP **(A)** and lateral **(B)** radiographs obtained following percutaneous fixation of a symptomatic navicular stress fracture that was treated initially with non–weight-bearing cast immobilization but recurred with return to competitive gymnastics.

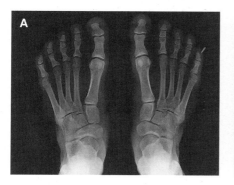
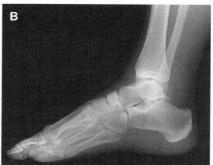
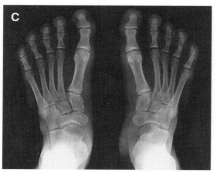
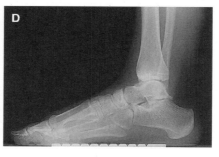

Figure 6 Weight-bearing AP **(A)** and lateral **(B)** radiographs obtained 6 months following hardware removal in a patient who has returned to competitive gymnastics and remains asymptomatic. Weight-bearing AP **(C)** and lateral **(D)** radiographs of the same patient approximately 20 months after surgery. Despite persistent radiographic abnormalities, she remains asymptomatic and was able to return to elite level competition.

In addition, elite athletes may elect surgical repair when faced with a significant delay or loss of career opportunities, even with an incomplete fracture.

Contraindications to ORIF include an incomplete fracture in a recreational or other noncareer athlete or a significantly displaced fracture with advanced degenerative changes. A patient with the latter problem may be best served with an arthrodesis.

Author's Preferred Treatment and Rationale

For young, athletic patients with atraumatic midfoot pain and normal radiographs, I usually obtain a limited technetium Tc 99m bone scan. A positive bone scan is followed by high-resolution helical CT.

If the patient has an incomplete fracture, 6 weeks in a short leg, fiberglass, non–weight-bearing cast generally will allow for early healing. A removable fracture boot is then prescribed, and the patient is gradually weaned as symptoms allow.

Complete nondisplaced fractures are first treated with non–weight-bearing cast immobilization. However, if that treatment fails to control the patient's symptoms or if an injury recurs, then a closed reduction and possibly ORIF may be indicated (**Figure 5**).

Finally, I recommend ORIF with bone grafting for a displaced fracture of the navicular. Generally, fresh autologous cancellous bone graft is harvested from the lateral aspect of the calcaneus or, depending on the volume needed, through a limited iliac crest incision.

It may be preferable to delay definitive surgical management of athletes, considering an arthrodesis for either chronic nonunion or advanced degenerative changes until their career decisions have been finalized. The limited motion or persistent pain following a fusion may preclude the elite athlete from resuming his or her usual activities.

SURGICAL TECHNIQUE
Closed Reduction With Percutaneous Screw Fixation Under miniature C-arm fluoroscopic control, guide pins from the 4.0- or 4.5-mm cannulated screw set are advanced across the fracture site, taking care to avoid intrusion into the talonavicular or naviculocuneiform joints. The pins are placed parallel to one another from dorsolateral to plantar medial. Once satisfactory position is confirmed, the screws are placed over the guide pins, and the fracture site is evaluated critically in all planes using the C-arm.

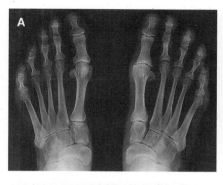
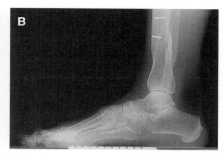
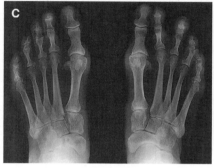
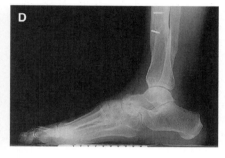

Figure 7   Weight-bearing AP **(A)** and lateral **(B)** radiographs in a patient with mild talonavicular arthrosis. AP **(C)** and lateral **(D)** views of same patient 4 years later with a complete displaced stress fracture of the navicular and end-stage degenerative joint disease of the talonavicular joint. An arthrodesis may be required as a salvage procedure to provide pain relief for this patient.

Open Reduction With Internal Fixation   A longitudinal incision is made over the dorsal aspect of the navicular just lateral to the neurovascular bundle. The fracture site may be difficult to visualize, particularly when the fracture is incomplete. Visualization of the junction of the medial two thirds and the lateral third of the navicular will generally help to locate the fracture; the miniature C-arm may be used as needed. Opening the talonavicular joint and distracting with longitudinal traction and plantar flexion of the foot allows confirmation of satis-factory reduction of the joint surfaces in displaced fractures.

When bone graft is needed, an inlay trough is created along the fracture, taking care to avoid damaging the articular surfaces. Fresh autologous cancellous bone is placed into the trough, and the fracture is stabilized with screws as described above.

Postoperative Management   Postoperative management begins with 1 to 2 days in a short leg modified Robert Jones compression dressing with stirrup splint, followed by 4 weeks in a fiberglass short leg non–weight-bearing cast. Depending on the fracture, an ad-ditional 4 weeks of a non–weight-bearing regimen may be prescribed. During this time the patient usually is placed in a fracture or cast boot for convenience.

At this point, the patient's physical therapist or the team's athletic trainer is intimately involved in the gradual return to activity, based on the severity of pain. Radiographs and CT scans have been used for evaluation of these fractures following treatment; however, neither has proved reliable because imaging studies may remain abnormal for several months to years following the injury (**Figure 6**). Custom orthotics may be prescribed for patients with significant forefoot or hindfoot malalignment or for relieving symptoms of other biomechanical abnormalities.

Management of Complications
Nonunion with persistent pain remains the most frequent complication associated with early nonsurgical treatment, particularly when the patient is not immobilized and is allowed to continue to bear weight. If the fracture remains nondisplaced, placing the foot in a non–weight-bearing cast for 6 to 8 weeks has been successful. The additional delay of further immobilization and lengthy rehabilitation may make this treatment option less desirable for the elite athlete. In established nonunions, an open bone graft with rigid internal fixation may be indicated.

Delay in diagnosis may predispose the patient to fracture displacement and severe degenerative changes with deformity, necessitating a fusion procedure for salvage of disabling midfoot or hindfoot pain (**Figure 7**).

—————————■

References

Coughlin MJ: Stress fractures of the tarsal navicular. *Tech Foot Ankle Surg*, in press.

Khan KM, Fuller PJ, Brukner PD, et al: Outcome of conservative and surgical management of navicular stress fracture in athletes. *Am J Sports Med* 1992;20:657-666.

Kiss ZS, Khan KM, Fuller PJ: Stress fractures of the tarsal navicular bone: CT findings in 55 cases. *AJR Am J Roentgenol* 1993;160:111-115.

Sanders R: Fractures of the midfoot and forefoot, in Coughlin M, Mann R (eds): *Surgery of the Foot and Ankle*, ed 7. St. Louis, MO, Mosby-Yearbook, 1999, pp 1575-1586.

Torg JS, Pavlov H, Cooley LH, et al: Stress fractures of the tarsal navicular. *J Bone Joint Surg Am* 1982;64:700-712.

Towne L, Blazina M, Cozen L: Fatigue fracture of the tarsal navicular. *J Bone Joint Surg Am* 1970;52:376-378.

Coding

ICD-9 CODE

733.95 Other disorders of bone and cartilage, Other and un-specified disorders of bone and cartilage, Stress fracture of other bone

CPT CODES

20902 Bone graft, any donor area; major or large

28456 Percutaneous skeletal fixation of tarsal bone fracture (except talus and calcaneus), with manipulation, each

28465 Open treatment of tarsal bone fracture (except talus and calcaneus), with or without internal or external fixation, each

29405 Application of short leg cast (below knee to toes)

29425 Application of short leg cast (below knee to toes); walking or ambulatory type

Surgical Correction of Posterior Ankle Pain in Athletes and Dancers

William G. Hamilton, MD

◼ Definition of the Problem

Patient Presentation

Patients have posterior ankle pain that results from plantar flexion, which typically occurs with activities such as kicking a soccer ball or ballet dancing on pointe. A careful work-up is necessary, however, to identify the source of pain so that an appropriate surgical procedure and incision can be selected. In general, there are three sources of posterior ankle pain in these patients: (1) posterior impingement on an os trigonum, trigonal process (Stieda's process), or soft-tissue structures in the posterolateral ankle; (2) chronic flexor hallucis longus (FHL) tendinitis in the posteromedial ankle; and (3) a combination of both syndromes (**Figure 1**). This chapter addresses only pain related to the ankle itself and not pain associated with the insertional Achilles tendon (Haglund's disease).

Physical Examination

The hallmark of posterolateral impingement is the plantar flexion sign, and forced plantar flexion will cause the posterior ankle pain described by the patient (**Figure 2**). This sign will be positive in patients with posterior impingement but not in those with Achilles tendinitis, peroneal tendinitis, FHL tendinitis, or other local conditions.

Patients with FHL tendinitis have posteromedial ankle pain related to motion of the FHL tendon within its sheath on the medial side of the os calcis, running from behind the ankle to the superior border to the sustentaculum tali. Tenderness and swelling over the sheath behind the medial malleolus are common, and symptoms are exacerbated by active and passive motion of the great toe. Masses on the tendon can often be felt when the tendon moves. If the condition is chronic, "hallux saltans" or triggering of the hallux may be present. Lateral radiographs obtained plantar grade and in maximum plantar flexion can be helpful.

Differential Diagnosis

- Shepherd's fracture of the posterolateral process of the talus
- Fracture of the posteromedial process of the talus
- Osteoid osteoma in the back of the ankle
- Occult hairline fracture of the posterior lip of the tibia
- Stress fracture of the posterior os calcis

Additional Work-up

Bone scans, CT, and MRI can help with the diagnosis, but they must be combined with the history and a careful physical examination because radiographs can show abnormalities that may not be related to the problem. Shepherd's fracture of the posterolateral process of the talus can often be seen on a lateral radiograph of the ankle (**Figure 3**), and a bone scan will be markedly positive behind the

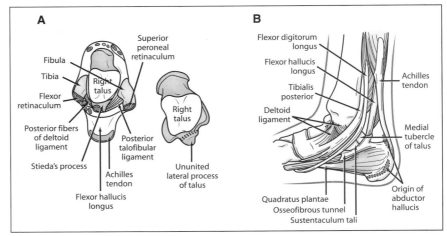

Figure 1 **A,** The posterior anatomy of the right ankle. **B,** The medial anatomy of the right ankle. (Adapted with permission from Boileau Grant JC: *A Method of Anatomy*, ed 6. Philadelphia, PA, Williams and Wilkins, 1958.)

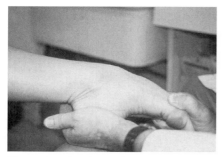

Figure 2   The plantar flexion test.

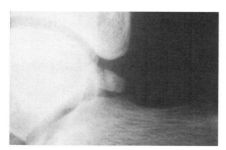

Figure 3   Shepherd's fracture of the posterior (Stieda's) process.

ankle. A fracture of the posteromedial process of the talus is very rare because the posteromedial process is usually quite small, but it can occur, usually as the result of a direct blow.

An injection of local anesthesia into the back of the ankle from the lateral side that dramatically relieves symptoms can confirm the diagnosis of posterior impingement. A diagnostic injection of local anesthesia might also help to determine the amount of the pain from posterior impingement and distinguish this pain from the pain of FHL tendinitis. Ultrasonography to confirm the placement of the needle should be performed when a diagnostic injection of the FHL sheath is administered.

■   **The Solutions**

Treatment Options and Rationale

Once the diagnosis has been made, nonsurgical treatments should be implemented in a stepwise process, beginning with the least complicated treatments and progressing to the most complicated treatments. In general, surgery is considered when other treatment options have failed. The presence of a tear or partial tear of the FHL tendon, however, would be an indication to explore the tendon before it ruptures, rather than pursue nonsurgical therapy.

Initial treatment usually includes activity modification ("Don't do what hurts until it doesn't hurt to do it anymore"), physical therapy, and the judicious use of anti-inflammatory medications. It is counterproductive, however, to use anti-inflammatory agents to simply mask the pain so that the athlete can keep doing the activity that initially caused the problem. If these interventions do not work, a removable boot to immobilize the first metatarsophalangeal joint will often improve the symptoms and force the athlete to allow the injury to heal. If the symptoms are caused by posterior impingement and this has been confirmed by diagnostic injection, a small amount of corticosteroid injected into the site of pain can often provide dramatic and permanent relief of the symptoms.

Author's Preferred Treatment and Rationale

If pain is caused by posterior impingement alone, the procedure of choice is a posterior cleanout and débridement performed from the lateral side. This procedure is easier, heals faster, and involves less dissection than the medial approach. However, the neurovascular bundle on the medial side lies directly over the FHL tendon and cannot be safely protected when working from the lateral side.

For chronic FHL tendinitis or the combination of both FHL tendinitis and posterior impingement, use of a medial approach is best so that the neurovascular bundle can be safely protected while the FHL tunnel is released and the os trigonum removed. Working laterally from the medial side can be done safely, but working medially from the lateral side should not be done.

INDICATIONS AND CONTRAINDICATIONS

Indications for surgery include persistent, disabling symptoms and the failure of nonsurgical therapy in a reliable patient with a secure diagnosis. Contraindications include lack of a secure diagnosis, no trial of nonsurgical therapy, neuropathy, poor circulation, the presence of infection, the presence or history of reflex sympathetic dystrophy, and an unreliable, hysterical, or unstable patient personality.

THE SURGICAL PROCEDURE

The lateral approach is performed with the patient prone or supine and under regional anesthesia with a thigh tourniquet. A headlamp, small thin osteotomes, Kerison rongeurs, and a 4-in bolster are helpful when performing this procedure. A 2-cm incision is made just posterior to the peroneal tendon sheath centered on the upper border of the os calcis (**Figure 4**, *A* and *B*). The sural nerve should be identified and avoided. The dissection is carried down along the back of the peroneal tendon sheath until the back of the ankle joint is identified. Frequently, the posterior facet of the subtalar joint is the first thing to be observed. When the posterior facet is identified, it can be traced proximally and will lead to the undersurface of the os trigonum or the posterior process. The os trigonum should be removed flush with the posterior edge of the talus. The soft tissues surrounding the os trigonum must be dissected from the bone for exposure before its removal. These soft tissues include the origin of the posterior talofibular ligament laterally, the sheath of the FHL tendon medially, the posterior ankle joint capsule dorsally, and the poste-

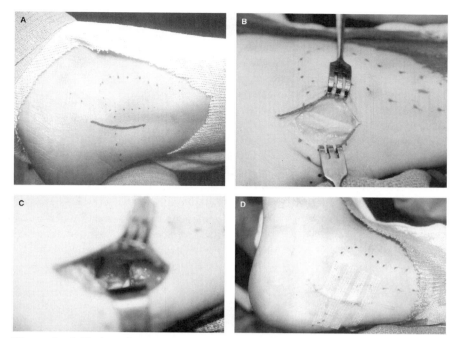

Figure 4 **A,** The lateral incision. **B,** Sural nerve through incision. **C,** Deep exposure. **D,** Wound closure.

rior talocalcaneal ligament plantarly. The FHL tendon can be seen in the depths of the wound, and it marks the medial limit of the dissection because

the posterior tibial nerve and artery lie just on the other side of the tendon and cannot be protected from the lateral side (**Figure 4**, *C*). When the bone

removal is complete, the wound should be inspected and palpated for other loose bodies or debris. When finished, the incision should be closed with the ankle in neutral dorsiflexion (**Figure 4**, *D*) so that the patient will not have trouble getting his or her heel down to the floor when bearing weight postoperatively. I usually discharge patients in a posterior plaster splint for a few days of elevation at home before converting them to a removable boot or postoperative shoe. After the wound is healed, patients undergo physical therapy with progressive exercises as tolerated.

The medial approach is more functional because the neurovascular bundle can be isolated and protected while working on the FHL tendon and exploring the posterior ankle. This approach is performed with the patient supine with a thigh tourniquet. A 3-cm incision is made directly over the neurovascular bundle posterior to the medial malleolus centered on the upper border of the os calcis (**Figure 5**, *A*). Care should be taken to avoid

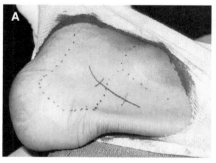
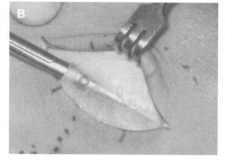
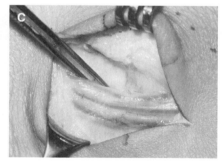
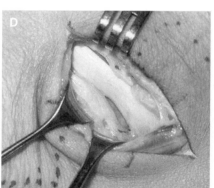
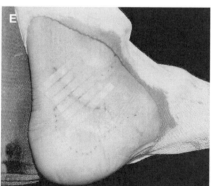

Figure 5 **A,** The medial incision. **B,** The laciniate ligament through the medial incision. **C,** Taking down the neurovascular bundle from the back of the medial malleolus. **D,** The FHL tendon lying beneath the neurovascular bundle (the tendon sheath has been opened). **E,** Wound closure.

damaging the neurovascular bundle while making the incision because the laciniate ligament protecting the neurovascular bundle is very thin at this level (**Figure 5**, *B*). The laciniate ligament is then divided, and the neurovascular bundle is taken down off of the back of the medial malleolus (**Figure 5**, *C*). A few small blood vessels crossing the field should be cauterized, then the neurovascular bundle can be protected with a blunt retractor. The FHL sheath lies directly beneath the neurovascular bundle. The FHL sheath is exposed and opened moving proximal to distal to the level of the sustentaculum tali where the FHL tunnel ends. The FHL tendon can now be inspected for damage and débrided or repaired as necessary (**Figure 5**, *D*). The trigonal process or os trigonum lies just lateral to the entrance of the FHL tunnel on the superior border of the os calcis. If posterior impingement is also present, the os trigonum can easily be removed with this exposure. The wound is then irrigated and closed in layers with the ankle in neutral dorsiflexion (**Figure 5**, *E*). No attempt is made to close the FHL sheath, and care should be taken to avoid damage to the neurovascular bundle during the closure. The patient is discharged in a posterior plaster splint with crutches for a few days of elevation before being placed in a removable boot until the wound is healed. Swimming and range-of-motion exercises can then be initiated. The patient continues to undergo progressive physical therapy as tolerated. The average recovery time is 2 to 3 months.

Management of Complications

Complications can occur with any surgical procedure. Fortunately, complications associated with the procedures described in this chapter are rare. Potential complications include damage to the sural nerve when using the lateral approach and damage to the neurovascular bundle with the medial approach.

References

Hamilton WG: Tendonitis about the ankle joint in classical ballet dancers. *Am J Sports Med* 1977;5:84-88.

Hamilton WG: Stenosing tenosynovitis of the flexor hallucis longus tendon and posterior impingement upon the os trigonum in ballet dancers. *Foot Ankle* 1982;3:74-80.

Hamilton WG, Geppert MJ, Thompson FM: Pain in the posterior aspect of the ankle in ballet dancers: Differential diagnosis and operative treatment. *J Bone Joint Surg Am* 1996;78:1491-1500.

Howse AJ: Posterior block of the ankle joint in dancers. *Foot Ankle* 1982;3:81-84.

Quirk R: Talar compression syndrome in dancers. *Foot Ankle* 1982;3:65-68.

Coding

ICD-9 CODE

727.06   Tenosynovitis of foot and ankle

CPT CODES

27612   Arthrotomy, posterior capsular release, ankle, with or without Achilles tendon lengthening

27680   Tenolysis, flexor or extensor tendon, leg and/or ankle; single, each tendon

CPT copyright © 2003 by the American Medical Association. All Rights Reserved.

Insertional Achilles Tendinopathy

W. Hodges Davis, MD

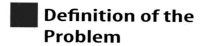

Definition of the Problem

Patient Presentation

Pain along the posterior aspect of the heel is a common presenting symptom associated with insertional Achilles tendinopathy. Although posterior heel pain may involve a variety of inflamed structures and prominent bone, patients with insertional Achilles tendinitis typically describe pain localized to the bone-tendon junction. This pain might be caused by acute and chronic injuries. Although insertional Achilles tendon injuries have been described as an overuse phenomenon, approximately 25% of patients who present with these injuries are not participating in athletic activities and do not have a history of trauma. Insertional Achilles tendinitis appears to affect both athletic and nonathletic patients, but these groups represent very different patient populations.

Athletes with insertional Achilles tendinopathy are usually young and active and tend to have pain related to athletic activity and overuse. Pain associated with repetitive jumping, push-off, and cutting activities is commonly observed in runners, dancers, and basketball and tennis players. This pain frequently limits athletic activities, but it usually does not substantially affect activities of daily living. Athletes with insertional Achilles tendinopathy typically experience discomfort at initiation and completion of athletic activity. A

lack of general conditioning, inadequate preparation for activity, working out on uneven or slippery terrain, and sudden changes in the training regimen have been associated with injuries of the Achilles tendon. Pain may be aggravated by running on hard surfaces, uneven ground, or uphill.

Nonathletes with insertional Achilles tendinopathy are typically sedentary, overweight, and older than age 45 years. Women are more commonly affected than men. Pain in these patients appears to be associated with degenerative changes, rather than related to overuse. Their pain initially occurs intermittently but may become constant and chronic.

Biomechanical malalignment, including excessive pronation and cavus foot, has also been discussed as a cause. As a result of the specific insertional site medially and across the ankle and subtalar joint, runners who overpronate place unbalanced loads and torque on the Achilles tendon. These unbalanced loads make the Achilles tendon particularly susceptible to injury. Cavus feet have a decreased ability to absorb shock, which increases the stresses on the Achilles tendon.

Physical Examination

Physical examination will typically be normal unless an associated inflamed retrocalcaneal bursa or a posterolateral bony ridge is noted. In patients with advanced degenerative insertional Achilles tendinosis, tenderness

and prominence is localized to the Achilles tendon insertion posteriorly or posterolaterally (**Figure 1**). A bony prominence may or may not be present. Crepitus on palpation and generalized erythema also might be observed. Evaluations of range of motion may reveal decreased ankle dorsiflexion secondary to a tight heel cord. This pain may be exacerbated by active or passive forced dorsiflexion.

Differential Diagnosis

- Trauma (particularly a direct blow)
- Chronic shoe heel counter pressure
- Retrocalcaneal bursitis
- Insertional enthesopathy
- Seronegative spondyloarthropathies
  - Ankylosing spondylitis
  - Reiter's syndrome
  - Psoriatic arthropathy
  - Crohn's disease and ulcerative colitis
- Gout
- Sarcoidosis
- Diffuse idiopathic skeletal hyperostosis
- Prominent lateral calcaneal ridge (pump bump)

One or more of the authors or the departments with which they are affiliated have received something of value from a commercial or other party related directly or indirectly to the subject of this chapter.

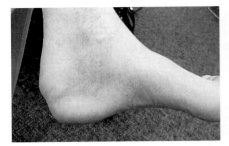

Figure 1 Prominence along the posterior aspect of the Achilles tendon insertion.

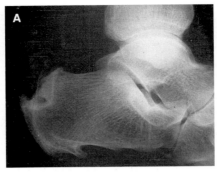

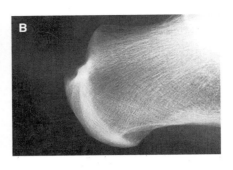

Figure 2 **A,** Lateral view of a degenerative calcific Achilles tendon. Note the prominent spur along the posterior calcaneus. **B,** Lateral view of the calcaneus showing a small calcific spur on the insertional site of the Achilles tendon.

- Insertional Achilles tendinitis
  - Degenerative-calcific
  - Overuse
  - Acute traumatic rupture (partial or complete)

Additional Work-up

The Achilles tendon can be imaged radiographically and with MRI. A lateral radiograph is often useful and may demonstrate a calcific spur along the posterior tuberosity (**Figure 2**). This spur may not be present in younger patients or early in the course of the disease. This spur, although intimately associated with the tendon, is not typically associated with the actual insertion of the Achilles tendon on the calcaneus. The Achilles tendon is in continuity with the posterior calcaneal insertional site more distal to the spur. A lateral radiograph will also allow visualization of Haglund's deformity, which is a prominent posterior and superior process on the calcaneus. On a lateral radiograph, a line can be drawn along the posterior border from the anterior tuberosity to the posterior tuberosity. A parallel line can then be drawn from the posterior superior articular facet to the posterior calcaneus. It is purported that any calcaneal process above this superior line is abnormal.

MRI allows detection of internal pathology of the tendon and inflammatory changes surrounding the tendon in the paratenon. In addition, MRI may be useful in the evaluation of the tendon in patients who may be candidates for surgical intervention. However, most injuries or diseases of the Achilles tendon can be diagnosed with physical examination alone, and the use of sophisticated imaging techniques is not required.

———————■

■ The Solutions

Treatment Options and Rationale
NONSURGICAL INTERVENTIONS

Nonsurgical modalities will be successful in more than 95% of patients with insertional Achilles tendinitis caused by overuse. Interventions should consist of initial rest or modified activity. Athletes may need to decrease their mileage and avoid running on hills or hard surfaces. Some athletes may begin cross-training to help maintain their level of fitness. Patients should apply ice to the tendon after activity and use nonsteroidal anti-inflammatory drugs as recommended by their physician. Shoe modification may consist of a heel lift and a soft counter or backless shoe. In the event that a biomechanical malalignment is identified, the use of a semirigid orthosis should be attempted. A soft posterior heel pad may also assist in padding and redistributing pressure along the posterior heel. Physical therapy and additional gentle stretching exercises can be initiated. Patients who are recalcitrant to these initial steps may require cast or walker boot immobilization for 4 to 6 weeks.

In our experience, the older (ie, 40s and older) sedentary population represents a degenerative problem that rarely becomes asymptomatic with nonsurgical care. In this patient population, nonsurgical management is usually successful less than half the time; surgical intervention is generally needed sooner. Despite this impression, a trial of nonsurgical care should be attempted. The use of corticosteroid injections is not indicated.

SURGICAL INTERVENTIONS

Central, isolated lateral or medial, combined medial and lateral, and J or hockey-stick incisions have been advocated to address maximal pathology and pain. The goal of surgery is to decompress bony impingement in the posterior heel and should consist of aggressive débridement of degenerated or calcified Achilles tendon, excision of the retrocalcaneal bursa, and removal of the superolateral ridge or Haglund's deformity and any insertional ridge on the posterior heel. Loss of integrity of the Achilles tendon necessitates augmentation with suture anchors and/or tendon graft. The risk of avulsion after partial excision of the

Achilles tendon and Haglund's deformity was found by one author to be minimized if the excision is performed from superior to inferior and less than 50% of the tendon is débrided. Significant defects may require augmentation with the flexor hallucis longus (FHL) tendon. Postoperatively, the patient is placed in a non–weight-bearing splint in resting equinus for 2 weeks. The patient is then placed into a walker boot with a heel lift 2 weeks postoperatively. Active range-of-motion exercises and weight bearing with gradual reduction of the heel lift are initiated at 4 weeks postoperatively until 8 weeks. The patient is then allowed to begin physical therapy for strengthening and stretching. The period of immobilization is extended for patients who underwent FHL tendon transfer. Patients should be advised that the recovery period is prolonged and may extend to 6 to 9 months postoperatively before the desired pain relief and level of activity can be achieved.

Author's Preferred Treatment and Rationale

Nonsurgical modalities should be continued for at least 6 months in nonathletic individuals. In the athletic population, modified training regimens with concomitant physical therapy and orthotics are aggressively implemented. We do not advocate aggressive stretching of the Achilles tendon because stretching may actually exacerbate the condition in most patients. We also are inclined to apply a weight-bearing cast for 4 weeks to allow complete rest of the Achilles tendon insertion. The athlete is allowed to exercise on a stationary bicycle or an elliptical training machine in the interim. Anecdotally, we have observed more than 90% improvement with this short period of immobilization and the gradual resumption of activity in patients with nondegenerative changes.

We also have found that nonsurgical measures are less effective in sedentary patients with advanced degenerative changes. The use of a soft heel pad, orthotic devices, and heel lifts are attempted. Physical therapy is not commonly used in this group as it appears to exacerbate symptoms. These patients may continue to have pain even with immobilization of the Achilles tendon. In addition, the chronic and constant nature of their pain typically necessitates early surgical intervention.

For the operation, the patient is placed in a prone position, and a thigh tourniquet is applied. A lateral incision is used almost exclusively unless an FHL graft is planned. The Achilles tendon is subperiosteally elevated lateral to medial and proximal to distal as far as needed to expose the calcific insertional ridge. A cuff of calcaneal periosteum is elevated to facilitate later repair. Degenerative and calcified tendon is aggressively débrided to healthy Achilles tendon. Bony decompression with a sagittal saw follows. The plane of the osteotomy is just anterior to the superior posterior calcaneal process and just distal to the calcific ridge, if present. If the insertional ridge is not present, then the osteotomy is taken to a point just proximal to the Achilles insertion. Aggressive bony decompression cannot be overemphasized. An intraoperative

fluoroscopic lateral view of the heel is used in all patients to confirm adequate bony decompression and to confirm complete excision of calcification within the Achilles tendon. All sharp medial and lateral edges are smoothed with a rasp and rongeur. The Achilles tendon repair is often augmented with suture anchors that help to secure the tendon to the bone edge, as well as to allow early motion (**Figure 3**).

If the preoperative evaluation reveals significant attenuation of the Achilles tendon that will require a graft, we prefer the medial-based, hockey-stick incision. This allows decompression of the Achilles tendon and retrocalcaneal space and harvest of the FHL tendon through a single incision. The FHL is harvested through this incision at the ankle. A biotenodesis screw is used to secure the tendon to the calcaneus and allows harvest of a shorter portion of the FHL tendon than would be required to secure the FHL tendon back onto itself. The FHL tendon transfer not only provides added tendon volume and muscle strength but also provides vascularity to the remaining Achilles tendon.

Patients must be advised that recovery time may be considerable, usually up to 8 to 10 months, to achieve the maximum improvement in symptoms and complete satisfaction with the surgical intervention.

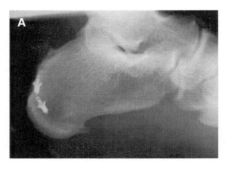 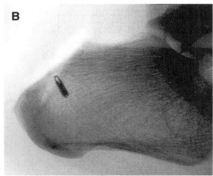

Figure 3 Lateral view of the patient in Figure 2, after surgical decompression of the posterior lateral spur (**A**) and augmentation of the Achilles tendon insertion with a suture anchor (**B**).

Management of Complications

Complications related to impaired wound healing and skin breakdown are common but usually superficial. A short period of dressing changes and immobilization may be required to address these complications. Injuries to the sural nerve or calcaneal branches have also been reported, but numbness around the incision is more common. This numbness, however, rarely causes long-term functional sequelae. Postoperative avulsion of the Achilles tendon has also been reported and is most often related to a fall or unexpected load within the first 8 to 12 weeks after surgery. Recurrent discomfort and pain has also been a difficult complication. Evaluation should begin by determining if the completed bony resection was adequate. If the bony resection was inadequate, MRI may be warranted to identify possible if degenerative tendon. In patients with a failed bony or soft-tissue decompression, a more aggressive procedure with a FHL transfer or augmentation of the Achilles tendon may be required. In addition, late reappearance of symptoms might indicate a recurrence of an insertional ridge or calcification within the tendon. The return of symptoms does not always, however, correlate with radiographic evidence of calcification and may simply represent progression of degenerative disease.

The author wishes to acknowledge the contribution of Simon Lee, MD, in the creation of this chapter.

References

Gerken AP, McGarvey WC, Baxter DE: Insertional Achilles tendonitis. *Foot Ankle Clin* 1996;2:237-246.

Kolodziej P, Glisson RR, Nunley JA: Risk of avulsion of the Achilles tendon after partial excision for treatment of insertional tendonitis and Haglund's deformity: A biomechanical study. *Foot Ankle Int* 1999;20:433-437.

Myerson MS, McGarvey WC: Disorders of the Achilles tendon insertion and Achilles tendinitis. *Instr Course Lect* 1999;48:211-218.

Watson AD, Anderson RB, Davis WH: Comparison of results of retrocalcaneal decompression for retrocalcaneal bursitis and insertional tendinosis with calcific spur. *Foot Ankle Int* 2000;21:638-642.

Coding

ICD-9 CODES

726.71   Achilles tendinitis

727.06   Tenosynovitis—ankle

CPT CODES

27650   Repair, primary, open or percutaneous, ruptured Achilles tendon

27652   Repair, primary, open or percutaneous, ruptured Achilles tendon with graft

28118   Ostectomy of calcaneus

Anterior Impingement of the Ankle

James W. Stone, MD

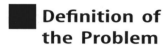 **Definition of the Problem**

Patient Presentation

The diagnosis of an impingement lesion of the ankle, particularly soft-tissue impingement, can be difficult because of the nonspecific nature of the presenting signs and symptoms. The presenting symptom may be pain, instability, locking, swelling, or a combination thereof. These symptoms usually occur after a traumatic event, but they may occur after a relatively minor recurrent injury or no injury at all. Impingement lesions usually cause well-localized pain, most commonly anterolateral, occasionally medial, but rarely posterior. Patients with rheumatoid arthritis, pigmented villonodular synovitis, and synovial chondromatosis may have poorly localized discomfort. Locking can be caused by physical impingement of the soft tissue or bony abnormality within the joint. Although the patient may have joint instability with episodes of giving way and frequent sprains, objective evidence of instability, such as pathologic joint opening on stress radiographs, is not usually present. Soft-tissue impingement lesions generally cause pain with activity (rather than pain with resting pain) and interfere with sports activity. Bony impingement lesions may cause pain only at end range of motion of the affected joint, and patients may actually report significantly limited joint motion.

Physical Examination

A careful physical examination is necessary to detect signs of soft-tissue or bony impingement and to rule out other causes of ankle pain, which are listed in the differential diagnosis. The physical signs of impingement lesions are nonspecific. Lateral impingement lesions typically cause localized tenderness over the anterolateral joint line and lateral gutter. Discomfort may be elicited by compression of the distal tibia and fibula in situations where syndesmotic injury has caused the soft-tissue impingement lesion to develop. The rarer instances of medial joint impingement result in localized medial joint line tenderness. Bony impingement lesions are associated with localized tenderness over the osteophyte prominence and may also be associated with swelling, evidence of generalized synovitis, and limited joint range of motion.

Differential Diagnosis

- Joint instability (lateral ligament injury, syndesmosis injury)
- Sinus tarsi syndrome or other subtalar disorder
- Tendinitis
- Osteochondral lesion of the talar dome
- Loose body
- Rheumatoid arthritis
- Pigmented villonodular synovitis
- Crystalline synovitis
- Synovial chondromatosis

Additional Work-up

Plain radiographs including AP, lateral, and mortise views are routinely obtained. Soft-tissue impingement lesions cannot be seen on plain radiographs, but bony impingement lesions can be seen. The amount of abnormal bone anterior to the tibia can be estimated by measuring the angle formed by tangents to the talar neck and anterior tibia (**Figure 1**). This angle is greater than 60° in the normal ankle. It has been shown that the size of the anteromedial osteophyte can be underestimated on a standard lateral radiograph. Therefore, a specific oblique view with the ankle rotated externally 30° and the x-ray tube tilted 45° craniocaudad is recommended for adequate evaluation of this lesion.

Lateral and anterior stress radiographs can be useful in evaluating the possible contribution of lateral ligament laxity. CT can be used preoperatively to identify the precise size and location of osteophytes so that the ex-

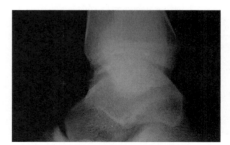

Figure 1 Preoperative lateral radiograph demonstrating an anterior tibial osteophyte in a 23-year-old man with anterior ankle pain and limited ankle dorsiflexion.

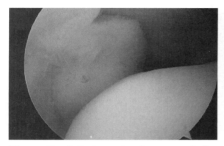

Figure 2 Soft-tissue impingement lesion in the lateral gutter as seen with the arthroscope in the anteromedial portal.

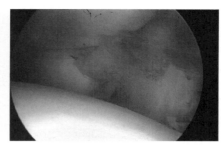

Figure 3 Anteroinferior tibiofibular ligament as seen with the arthroscope in the anteromedial portal.

tent of bone to be removed surgically can be estimated. However, CT is not necessary, especially as the surgeon's experience in arthroscopic evaluation and treatment grows. MRI has been shown in some studies to be capable of defining soft-tissue lesions of the ankle. However, the value of this study depends both on the quality of the scan itself and the capabilities of the radiologist interpreting the study. MRI is very useful in evaluating other soft-tissue and bony lesions of the ankle and may be used to rule out other causes of ankle disability.

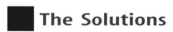

■ The Solutions

Treatment Options and Rationale

When the work-up for ankle pain has led to the likely diagnosis of soft-tissue impingement lesion, options for nonsurgical and surgical treatment are considered. If the symptoms have been present for only a short time or if only a short time has elapsed since the inciting injury, then a period of nonsurgical treatment is appropriate. Nonsurgical measures to be considered include rest, nonsteroidal anti-inflammatory medication, physical therapy, orthotics, and corticosteroid injection. Arthroscopic evaluation is

appropriate when nonsurgical means have failed to restore joint function.

Author's Preferred Treatment and Rationale

Both soft-tissue and bony impingement lesions in the ankle joint are best approached arthroscopically. Arthroscopy has several advantages over traditional open surgery. Arthroscopy is minimally invasive, requiring only two or three small incisions, and arthroscopic surgery can be performed on an outpatient basis with low risk of complications. The joint pathology can be addressed without stimulating even more extensive scar tissue as occurs with an open approach to the joint. Most important, proper use of the arthroscope allows a more complete evaluation of the entire joint, which is not possible with visualization obtained from limited open approaches.

The patient is positioned supine on the operating table while under general or spinal anesthesia. The ipsilateral hip and knee are flexed and supported by a padded leg holder, allowing the foot and ankle to hang freely in a plantigrade position. After sterile skin preparation and draping, a commercially noninvasive ankle distractor is applied to the midfoot and hindfoot, and distraction force is applied.

Small joint arthroscopes (2.7-mm diameter) facilitate joint entry and minimize the risk of iatrogenic articular cartilage injury. The routine working portals are anteromedial and anterolateral, with a posterolateral portal placed for

fluid inflow or instrumentation. The first step is a thorough, organized evaluation of the entire joint. The technique is detailed in numerous publications.

Soft-tissue impingement lesions are most commonly found in the lateral gutter, the anterolateral corner, and the intra-articular portion of the syndesmosis (**Figure 2**). Visualization is best with the arthroscope positioned in the anteromedial portal and the instruments in the anterolateral portal. A combination of basket forceps and shavers is used for complete resection of the abnormal tissue. Firm masses of tissue can be ablated using the bipolar cautery, which is also helpful in achieving hemostasis if bleeding is encountered.

Medial soft-tissue lesions are approached with the arthroscope in the anterolateral position and the instruments in the anteromedial position. Impingement of the inferior slip of the anterior inferior tibiofibular ligament (Bassett's ligament) on the underlying talus can occur. It should be noted that the ligament is a normal structure visible in every normal ankle (**Figure 3**). Before concluding that the ligament is responsible for pathologic impingement, some supporting evidence, such as localized synovitis in proximity, thickening of the ligament, or adjacent talar chondromalacia, should exist. An abnormal Bassett's ligament may be resected arthroscopically. Removal of the visible intra-articular portion of the ligament has no adverse effect on syndesmosis stability.

In rare instances, posterior impingement, usually involving the posterior syndesmotic ligaments, the posteroinferior tibiofibular ligament, and the tibial slip, can occur. The arthroscopic ankle surgeon must become facile in achieving posterior visualization, either with anterior approaches using both 30° and 70° arthroscopes or by using the posterolateral portal to view the posterior compartment.

Most bony impingements by osteophytes are anterior in location and

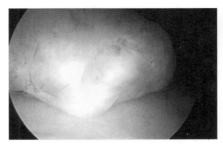

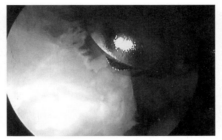

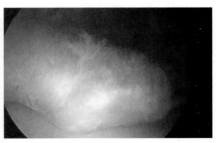

Figure 4 Intraoperative photograph of anterior osteophyte in the patient shown in Figure 1. The arthroscope is in the anteromedial portal.

Figure 5 The small joint shaver is used to strip the anterior soft tissues off the outer surface of the osteophyte so that the extent of the lesion can be clearly delineated.

Figure 6 The osteophyte is exposed before excision.

are readily approached arthroscopically (**Figure 4**). Joint distraction may not be required to address anterior osteophytes, and visualization may be enhanced by dorsiflexion of the ankle during the procedure, which allows the anterior capsule to be distended away from the osteophyte. Soft tissue and capsule adherent to the outer surface of the osteophyte must be stripped using a shaver or the bipolar cautery (**Figure 5**). After completely exposing the bone lesion, it may be removed with a round burr, osteotome, or pituitary rongeur (**Figure 6**). The lesions frequently extend medially onto the anterior surface of the medial malleolus, and this area must be included in the resection. A thorough inspection of the entire area must be performed to confirm complete resection (**Figure 7**). If there is any question as to the completeness of the resection, then an intraoperative radiograph should be obtained (**Figure 8**).

After removing the tibial osteophyte, the talar neck must be inspected for a "kissing lesion." Preoperative radiographs should alert the surgeon to the presence of a talar neck osteophyte, which should be resected in a manner similar to the tibial osteophyte to ensure complete removal of the impinging lesion.

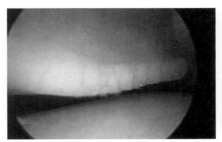

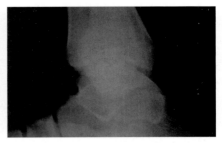

Figure 7 Arthroscopic view of the anterior joint after complete excision of the osteophyte.

Figure 8 Postoperative lateral radiograph of the ankle confirming complete excision of the osteophyte.

Management of Complications

Complications are rare after ankle arthroscopy. The incidence of complications related to bleeding, infection, or deep vein thrombosis are low with this minimally invasive surgical technique.

The most common complication in ankle arthroscopy is neurovascular injury directly related to the portals themselves. Using proper technique to create the portal, specifically ensuring that the incision includes only the skin, spreading the subcutaneous tissues with a blunt hemostat, and piercing the capsule with a blunt trochar, will minimize the risk of neurologic injury.

Portals should be made large enough to allow easy passage of the instruments into the joint to minimize soft-tissue injury from repeated instrument passes and thus decrease wound healing problems, including sinus tract formation. I have seen no problems directly related to the use of noninvasive joint distraction.

Incomplete resection of an osteophyte is a potential complication that can be prevented by thorough analysis of preoperative radiographic studies, which typically provide a good indication of the amount of resection necessary to achieve decompression of the joint. Intraoperative radiographs are another means of assuring adequate resection of the spur.

References

Bassett FG, Gates HS, Billys JB, et al: Talar impingement by the anteroinferior tibiofibular ligament: A cause of chronic pain in the ankle after inversion sprain. *J Bone Joint Surg Am* 1990;72:55-59.

DeBernardino TM, Arciero RA, Taylor DC: Arthroscopic treatment of soft-tissue impingement of the ankle in athletes. *Arthroscopy* 1997;13:492-498.

Ferkel RD, Karzel RP, Del Pizzo W, Friedman MJ, Fischer SP: Arthroscopic treatment of anterolateral impingement of the ankle. *Am J Sports Med* 1991;19:440-446.

Liu SH, Raskin A, Osti L, Baker CL, Jacobson K, Finerman G: Arthroscopic treatment of anterolateral ankle impingement. *Arthroscopy* 1994;10:215-218.

Tol JL, Verheyen CP, van Dijk CN: Arthroscopic treatment of anterior impingement in the ankle: A prospective study with a five- to eight-year follow-up. *J Bone Joint Surg Br* 2001;83:9-13.

Coding

ICD-9 CODE
718.07 Articular cartilage disorder, ankle and foot

CPT CODES
29897 Arthroscopy, ankle (tibiotalar and fibulotalar joints), surgical; debridement, limited

29898 Arthroscopy, ankle (tibiotalar and fibulotalar joints); surgical; debridement, extensive

■ Definition of the Problem

Patient Presentation

Many toenail problems initially present as trivial annoyances best handled by personal hygiene, over-the-counter products, or minimal physician intervention. However, a distinct subset of complex toenail maladies can cause severe pain and result in lifestyle changes; these problems require skilled evaluation and management.

Ingrown toenail is a painful condition caused by penetration of the nail into the lateral nail fold. Soft-tissue inflammation, aggravated by shoe wear, leads to a cycle of inflammation, erythema, infection, and purulent drainage. This condition is very common in adolescents (**Figure 1**). Pain at one or both of the great toenail folds, swelling, erythema, and purulent drainage are common on presentation. The adjacent skin may be heaped up and overlap the nail. Excess tissue and nail penetration may both be present.

Subugual hematoma is a painful condition resulting from direct trauma, usually a crush injury, causing bleeding in the enclosed space between the nail bed and nail plate (**Figure 2**). The pain is usually out of proportion to the seemingly minor presentation, and the patient is miserable. The great toenail is affected most often.

Black toenail (jogger's toe, ten-

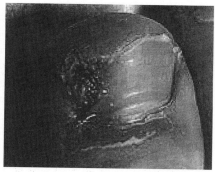

Figure 1 Ingrown toenail in which friable soft tissue is heaped up over the side of the nail. (Reproduced with permission from Coughlin M, Mann R: Toe nail abnormalities, in *Surgery of the Foot and Ankle,* ed. 7. St. Louis, MO, Mosby, 1999, Vol 2, pp 1033-1070.)

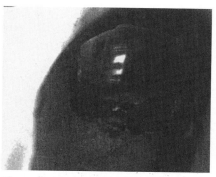

Figure 2 An acute blood clot causes pressure pain under the nail bed (subungual hematoma). (Reproduced with permission from Coughlin M, Mann R: Toe nail abnormalities, in *Surgery of the Foot and Ankle,* ed. 7. St. Louis, MO, Mosby, 1999, Vol 2, pp 1033-1070.)

nis toe) is chronic repetitive subungual bleeding that gives the nail a black appearance (**Figure 3**). It is caused by repeated stops and starts, running down hill, or in a runner who has an extensor deformity of the great toe in which the nail plate repeatedly impinges on the distal dorsal lining of the shoe. There will be single or multiple areas of subungual black discoloration. If the trauma is recent, the toe will be quite painful, and the distal phalanx and nail bed will be warm.

A partially or completely delaminated nail plate continues to grow but has lost contact and lies free at some point distal to the cuticle (**Figure 4**). Partial (onycholysis) or complete delamination (onychomadesis) of the nail can occur as a result of subungual bleeding, crush trauma, and seronegative or fungal disease. This condition appears to be more common in

women. Patients report that it catches on socks, is difficult to cut, and is painful from shoe wear.

A clubnail is characterized by pain in the distal toe and by surrounding soft tissue that hooks upward. An irregular, poorly attached nail stump may be present. A thickened, yellow nail with a progressive build-up of subungual debris is typical of fungal infection (onychomycosis) (**Figure 5**).

Physical Examination

Careful inspection of an irregular toenail may help identify an underlying disease process, such as a first sign of tumor, seronegative disease, metabolic problem, or immunosuppression. Circulation of the foot with an ingrown toenail should be assessed as

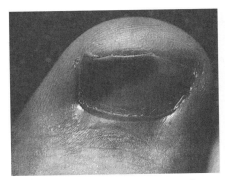

Figure 3 Black toenail, characterized as an old blood clot under the nail. (Reproduced with permission from Coughlin M, Mann R: Toe nail abnormalities, in *Surgery of the Foot and Ankle,* ed. 7. St. Louis, MO, Mosby, 1999, Vol 2, pp 1033-1070.)

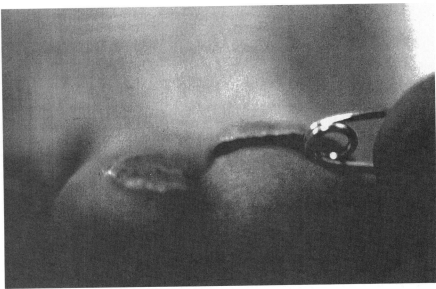

Figure 4 Delaminated nail in which the nail bed is attached only at the base. (Reproduced with permission from Coughlin M, Mann R: Toe nail abnormalities, in *Surgery of the Foot and Ankle,* ed. 7. St. Louis, MO, Mosby, 1999, Vol 2, pp 1033-1070.)

should signs of increasing infection, such as proximal streaking, local abscess, and adenopathy.

The entire distal phalanx of a toe with a subungual hematoma is affected. Any palpation increases pressure on the nail bed and increases pain. The material under the nail plate must be identified as blood, not pus. A radiograph must be obtained to rule out an underlying fracture.

A patient with black toenail should be carefully followed to ensure that the condition resolves with nail growth and is not an underlying tumor. A radiograph should be obtained to rule out a fracture or distal phalanx deformity.

Laceration of the toenail complex is an obvious injury, but careful inspection after adequate irrigation is necessary to evaluate the injury and/or avulsion of the nail bed and germinal matrix. The delaminated toenail is easily lifted up during physical examination.

The nail plate is critical to maintaining the smooth, low, rigid profile of the great toe. During gait, as the foot moves into toe-off, considerable upward pressure (floor force) is exerted on the distal tuft. The great toenail counteracts this pressure. In clubnail, loss of the nail plate (from disease, avulsion, or trauma) results in

upward deformation of the distal soft tissue of the toe, interfering with nail plate regrowth. During the prolonged period of nail regeneration, this irregular tissue acts as an obstacle to nail growth, and the nail plate may bunch up, or in worse situations, actually grow into the toe.

Fungal infections of the toenails are extremely common, affecting around 15% to 20% of the general population and over 50% of those older than age 70 years. The warm, moist environment inside the shoe leads to tissue maceration and nail penetration by the causative organism. *Trichophyton mentagrophytis* and *T rubrum* cause most of the most common distal subungual infections. Trauma, diabetes, aging, and immunosuppression increase rates of infection. Smoking and peripheral vascular disease are predictors of this disease.

Differential Diagnosis

Ingrown Toenail
- Improper cutting of nails
- Incurved nail impinging on the skin
- Subungual exostosis or tumor

- Paronychia
- Fungal infection
- Subungual hematoma
- Trauma with unrecognized open or closed fracture under the nail bed

Subungual Hematoma
- Infection
- Fracture

Black Toenail
- Fracture
- Subungual exostosis
- Malignant melanoma

Delaminated Toenail
- Trauma
- Drug reactions
- Thyroid disease
- Bacterial and fungal infections
- Psoriasis

Clubnail
- Trauma
- Fungal or bacterial infection
- Congenital deformity

Additional Work-up

Further work-up should include careful assessment of the circulation if the pulses are suspect, culture of any purulence, and radiographs to rule out local tumor, foreign body, or bone infection. A metabolic evaluation should be considered because a toenail infection may be the first sign of diabetes or other diseases of immunosuppression. If anything other than trauma is suspected, then work-up for an underlying disease or infection is indicated.

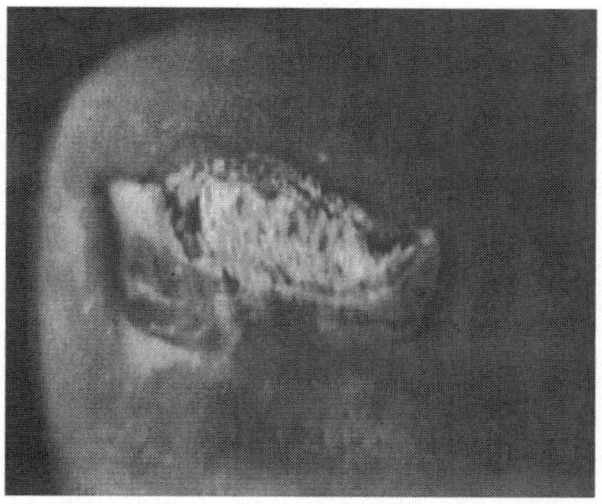

——————■

■ The Solutions

Treatment Options and Rationale

An understanding of the normal anatomy and characteristics of the toenail is essential for treatment (**Figure 6**). The hard keratin of the toenail provides stability and protection to the toe tip along with adding sensation. The close proximity of the nail to the distal phalanx is of concern because surgery may adversely affect normal nail growth.

The nail root is located beneath the proximal nail fold. Nail growth originates from the germinal matrix, which extends from the lunula to the proximal nail root (approximately 5 to 6 mm from the cuticle). This onychogenic germinal tissue actually extends lateral to the visible nail at the proximal nail fold. In addition, nail germination may occur from the hyponychium and lateral nail groove, making these areas potential sources of recurrent nail formation after matrix excision. The growing nail overlies and is attached to the nail bed. Distally the nail bed becomes the hyponychium. At that point the nail detaches and is now called the free edge. The nail folds protect the lateral edges of the nail, which lie in the nail groove.

Normal toenail growth occurs at 0.03 to 0.05 mm a day; nails take between 9 and 18 months to fully regrow after avulsion, which is approximately half the rate of finger nails. Nail

Figure 5 Crumbling fungal nail. (Reproduced with permission from Coughlin M, Mann R: Toe nail abnormalities, in *Surgery of the Foot and Ankle,* ed. 7. St. Louis, MO, Mosby, 1999, Vol 2, pp 1033-1070.)

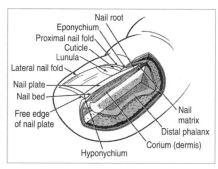

Figure 6 Longitudinal section of the distal end of a toe showing the components of the nail unit. (Reproduced with permission from Coughlin M, Mann R: Toe nail abnormalities, in *Surgery of the Foot and Ankle,* ed. 7. St. Louis, MO, Mosby, 1999, Vol 2, pp 1033-1070.)

growth peaks in adolescence and then decreases with aging. Nails grow faster in men than women and faster in pregnancy, in warmer climates, in patients with psoriasis, and in the dominant leg. Nail growth slows with immobilization, paralysis, decreased circulation, malnutrition, infection, and chemotherapy.

INGROWN TOENAIL

Initial treatment of an ingrown toenail involves soaks to reduce inflammation, application of desiccating agents (eg, alcohol or gentian violet), removal of the offending piece of nail, use of capacious shoes, and, perhaps, the use of a cotton wisp to elevate the free edge as it grows out. Often the tissue appears inflamed and possibly infected, but the routine use of antibiotics is not recommended except in patients who are immunocompromised, vascularly impaired, or in whom the cellulitis extends proximal to the hallux interphalangeal joint. With failure of nonsurgical care, surgical decompression is essential.

In adolescents the principal problem may be hypertrophy of one or both nail folds combined with pressure from shoe wear to cause suppuration and infection. Although local steroid cream may abate the problem,

plastic decompression of the nail fold works well.

After placing the affected toe under a digital block and using a 0.25-in Penrose drain as a tourniquet, an incision is made from the end of the toe to 5 mm proximal to the nail fold. An ellipse of skin, subcutaneous tissue, and extra fat 3 mm wide by 1 cm long is removed. The wound is then closed with No. 3-0 nylon sutures.

Any adjacent offending piece of nail is removed. When the sutures are removed at 3 weeks, the affected nail groove has been drawn away from the nail. This procedure can be done on both sides of the great toenail simultaneously.

When the toenail has grown distally and buried itself into the soft tissue of the toe tip, complete nail ablation is tempting; the unfortunate consequence is the development of a clubnail. Plastic decompression of the front of the toe with the same technique as described for the nail fold can be successful. With this procedure a wedge of soft tissue is removed so that the distal soft-tissue hump is brought below the leading edge of the nail. The sutures are removed at 3 weeks, and follow-up examinations are needed until the free edge grows over the soft tissue (**Figure 7**).

Partial and complete ablation, when done under a digital block and

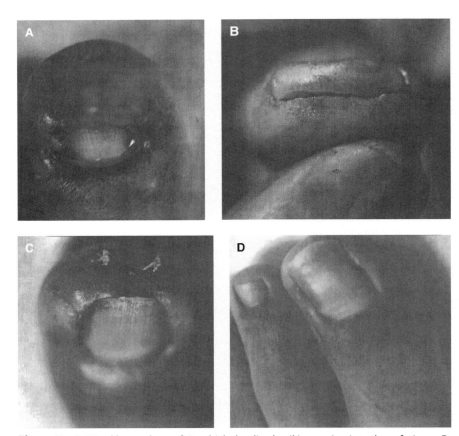

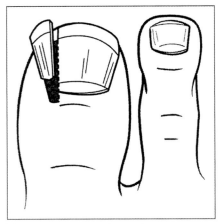

Figure 8 Winograd partial matrisectomy. Shaded area shows resection of matrix and nail bed. (Reproduced with permission from Coughlin M, Mann R: Toe nail abnormalities, in *Surgery of the Foot and Ankle,* ed. 7. St. Louis, MO, Mosby, 1999, Vol 2, pp 1033-1070.)

Figure 7 **A,** Distal heaped up tuft in which the distal nail is growing into the soft tissue. **B,** Distal soft tissue removed. **C,** Nail growing 3 weeks later. **D,** Healed nail at 6 months. (Reproduced with permission from Coughlin M, Mann R: Toe nail abnormalities, in *Surgery of the Foot and Ankle,* ed. 7. St. Louis, MO, Mosby, 1999, Vol 2, pp 1033-1070.)

with a Penrose drain tourniquet, offer the advantages of speed, rapid healing, and minimal pain. Ablation is especially effective for decompressing acute infection. The nail bed reepithelializes in 2 to 3 weeks, and the patient can wear shoes again. The problem lies in the high rate (40% to 70%) of recurrence. When the entire nail is ablated, regrowth may take 9 to 12 months, increasing the risk for club-nail formation.

For intractable ingrown toenail or a severe senile incurved nail, partial or complete toenail ablation is indicated. Partial nail ablation is performed once the infection has abated. After application of a digital block, perioperative antibiotics, and Penrose drain tourniquet, the affected outer 0.125-in border of the nail is split dis-tal to proximal with a nail splitter. An oblique incision is made in the corner of the proximal nail fold to expose the germinal matrix and lateral nail recess.

The attached pearly white germinal matrix is removed. Care must be taken to remove it from the underlying distal phalanx, the cuticle, and the lateral nail fold. The nail bed underlying the involved piece of nail is then removed using a Winograd procedure (**Figure 8**). The nail bed is maintained in the Heifetz modification (ie, keeping the nail bed following nail removal).

Sutures are placed to reapproximate the wound edges, and a compression dressing is applied. The dressing is changed at 24 to 48 hours. Nonabsorbable sutures are removed at 2 weeks. This procedure can be done on both sides of the great toe in a single sitting.

Complete ablation of the great toenail is done in a similar manner. The entire nail is grasped with a hemostat and elevated off the underlying nail bed with a freer elevator. An oblique incision is made at the medial and lateral nail folds; the nail is then pulled distally and avulsed. The cuticle, germinal matrix, eponychium, and proximal nail bed are excised. Care is taken to examine meticulously and to curet the lateral nail folds and the inferior portion of the proximo-dorsal area where residual germinal nail tissue may hide.

The wound is sutured with as little tension as possible, and a compression dressing is applied and changed at 24 to 48 hours. Nonabsorbable sutures are removed at 3 weeks. Regrowth of some nail plate may occur from residual germinal nail tissue but it is usually pain-free, and women desiring a more attractive foot frequently use polish on the area.

An average satisfaction rate of 80% to 85% is expected with partial nail ablation. Although some residual nail growth may occur in a rather high number of patients, most of it is asymptomatic. Results are similar for complete nail ablation. Epidermal inclusion cysts occur with some frequency after partial and complete nail ablation. Both respond well to excision.

Phenol and/or the use of a carbon dioxide laser are reported to be helpful as additional steps in ensuring nail removal. After partial or complete nail ablation, phenol (carbolic acid 88%) is placed on the germinal surfaces with cotton-tipped applicators. The adjacent soft tissues are protected with petrolatum jelly. After application the phenol is washed away with alcohol. Three separate 30 second applications are performed, and the wound is dressed. Dressings are changed daily until drainage has ceased. The phenol, which is contraindicated in the presence of vascular disease, may incite local inflammatory reaction with prolonged healing and drainage for many weeks.

The carbon dioxide laser is heralded as a cure for the postoperative recurrence of ingrown toenail. Partial nail and matrix excision followed by carbon dioxide laser treatment is associated with low recurrence.

With multiple symptomatic recurrences after repeated nail ablations, partial amputation of the distal tuft of the great toe along with all nail and germinal tissue (Syme or Thompson-Terwilliger procedure) is recommended. After application of digital block anesthesia, perioperative antibiotics, and a Penrose drain tourniquet, an elliptical incision is made to excise all of the nail fold, cuticle, proximal skin, nail bed, and germinal matrix (**Figure 9**, *A* and *B*). Half of the distal phalanx is excised, and the edges are smoothed and beveled with a rongeur. The longer plantar flap is then brought up over the end of the phalangeal bone and sutured to the proximal flap with nylon suture (**Figure 9**, *C*).

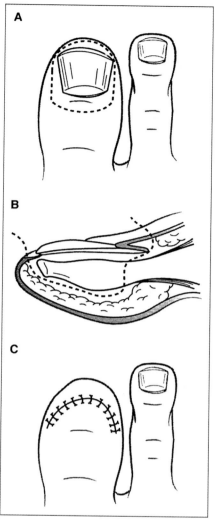

Figure 9 Nail ablation with partial removal of distal phalanx (Thompson-Termilliger procedure). (Reproduced with permission from Coughlin M, Mann R: Toe nail abnormalities, in *Surgery of the Foot and Ankle*, ed. 7. St. Louis, MO, Mosby, 1999, Vol 2, pp 1033-1070.)

A compression dressing is applied and changed at 24 to 48 hours. Weight bearing on the heel is permitted in a postoperative shoe, and sutures are removed at 3 weeks. The recurrence rate is very low, and a normal shoe can be worn.

SUBUNGUAL HEMATOMA

An acutely crushed, throbbing great toe with obvious subungual blood collection is a surgical emergency. Pressure is released and pain abated by evacuating the fluid through a hole made in the nail with a red-hot paper clip, nail drill, or portable cautery. The nail is left in place to prevent clubnail formation. This original nail may be lost as a new one grows in. If infection develops with purulent drainage the nail must be avulsed.

Most treated hematomas resolve without sequelae. However a crush injury can lead to subsequent subungual exostosis, clubnail, a thickened discolored nail, or one with pits and ridges.

BLACK TOENAIL

Chronic, painful blackened toenail is best managed with rest and warm soaks. The foot should be carefully examined to identify an extension deformity at the first metatarsophalangeal joint. The athletic shoes are inspected to assess whether the toe box is adequate for the excursion of the patient's great toe.

The patient should be advised that failure to treat this problem could lead to delamination and clubnail. Some individuals with chronic black toe may return several years later with such advanced changes that great toenail ablation may be the only curative modality.

DELAMINATED NAIL

If careful trimming and the application of topical antifungal agents are not helpful, complete ablation of the toenail is curative.

LACERATIONS

Lacerations of the nail bed or germinal matrix should be repaired when feasible to prevent an uneven scarred nail plate, which may entrap a growing nail. Repair may be impossible in the smaller nails.

The germinal matrix can be repaired after careful elevation of the proximal nail fold. Avulsed nail bed tissue should be replaced. Unfortunately, scarring and split nail deformity may still result despite an adequate repair.

FUNGAL INFECTIONS

Although fungal infections are quite common and cosmetically unappealing, they truly cause minimal disability. Frequent cutting, filing, and cleaning of the debris can allow proper shoe wear and save on destruction of expensive socks and hose. Severely thickened, unmanageable nails can be ablated. However the general population in the United States is excessively concerned about being disease-free and having normal looking nails.

Drug treatment is expensive, and many third-party payers will approve therapy only after positive cultures. The best choice of tissue for culturing is subungual debris (ie, nail scrapings) from the more proximal area. In an increasingly litigious society, the accuracy of the diagnosis should be confirmed before initiating treatment with potentially harmful drugs.

Griseofulvin, ketoconazole, and fluconazole still are included in many references as being effective for fungal nails. These drugs are obsolete, have many side effects, and are no longer used. Itraconazole (200 mg/day for 3 months) and terbinafine (250 mg/day for 3 months) are the two best drugs for current use, with terbinafine having a slight statistical edge. Pulsed dosing does not offer greater benefit than a continued dose.

Before prescribing these agents a frank discussion with the patient about possible side effects (liver, gas-

trointestinal, cardiovascular) and the odds of eventual cure is mandatory. Cures may not be noted until 3 to 4 months after drug cessation.

Patients are not only interested in a disease-free nail but also want a normal looking nail. Standard courses of terbinafine produced a disease-free normal nail in only 35% to 50% of patients, and intraconazole produced that effect in 25% to 40%.

Ciclopirox used as a gel or toe paint is safe. It causes only transient mild irritation, and when used for superficial mild disease with frequent filing, it can result in a 34% to 52% cure rate.

Author's Preferred Treatment and Rationale
INGROWN TOENAIL

With close attention to hygiene and nonsurgical care, a healthy, pain-free nail may result. However, given the slow rate of nail growth and average patient compliance, an unmonitored inflamed nail may get into serious trouble. Encouraging the patient to proceed in a timely manner with a nail problem that is obviously intractable can truly alter the patient's quality of life.

When there is hypertrophied soft tissue in an adolescent patient, I am quick to suggest soft-tissue decompression. It has low morbidity, heals quickly, and avoids further soft-tissue trauma. If there is associated incurving or ingrowing of the nail, I often perform decompression and partial nail ablation simultaneously.

Ablation has stood the test of

time. I think the key is to treat the ingrown nail as a serious problem, have excellent light, loupe magnification if necessary, and be meticulous about searching for the more obscure areas of germinal matrix deposition. I have seen no advantage to the addition of chemical cauterization. Laser ablation adds significant cost to the procedure without any perceived benefit. I have no experience with postoperative epidermal inclusion cysts.

I am often referred patients with recurrent problems despite multiple procedures. They are specifically sent for a terminal Syme procedure. However, I find that most can be helped with a meticulous repeated resection of the residual germinal nail tissue under loupe magnification. If that fails I will proceed with the Thompson-Terwilliger amputation.

FUNGAL INFECTIONS

I encourage good nail hygiene to help people easily fit into shoes and socks and try to downplay the cosmetic appearance of these usually pain-free, unsightly nails. If pushed, and there is minimal disease, I will prescribe ciclopirox 8% nail paint. Only after frank discussions and a positive nail culture will I prescribe oral terbinafine. Toenail ablation for a severely thickened nail is always an option.

Management of Complications
Complications from laceration repair are best handled by complete nail ablation.

References

Coughlin M: Toe nail abnormalities, in Coughlin M, Mann R (eds): *Surgery of the Foot and Ankle*, ed 7. St Louis, MO, Mosby, 1999, vol 2, pp 1033-1070.

Scher RK, Daniel CR: *Nails: Therapy, Diagnosis, Surgery*. Philadelphia, PA, WB Saunders, 1990.

Coding

ICD-9 CODES

110.1   Dermatophytosis of nail; Dermophytic onychia, Onychomycosis, Tinea unguium

681.10   Toe, cellulitis and abscess, unspecified

681.11   Onychia and paronychia of toe; Panaritium, Perionychia of toe

686.1   Pyogenic granuloma

686.9   Unspecified local infection of skin and subcutaneous tissue

703.0   Diseases of nail; Ingrowing nail, ingrowing nail with infection

703.8   Other specified diseases of nail; Dystrophia unguium, Hypertrophy of nail, Koilonychia, Leukonychia (punctata) (striata), Onychauxis, Onychogryposis, Onycholysis

703.9   Unspecified disease of nail

719.77   Other and unspecified orders of joint; Difficulty walking, ankle and foot

729.5   Other disorders of soft tissues; Pain in limb

757.5   Specified anomalies of nails; Anonychia, Congenital clubnail, koilonychia, leukonychia, onychauxis, pachyonychia

893.0   Open wound of toe(s): includes toenail; Without mention of complication

893.1   Open wound of toe(s): includes toenail; Complicated

924.3   Contusion of lower limb and of other unspecified sites; Toe, Toenail

928.3   Crushing injury of lower limb; Toe(s)

CPT CODES

11719   Trimming of nondystrophic nails, any number

11720   Debridement of nail(s) by any method(s); one to five

11721   Debridement of nail(s) by any method(s); six or more

11730   Avulsion of nail plate, partial or complete, simple; single

11732   Avulsion of nail plate, partial or complete, simple; each additional nail plate

11740   Evacuation of subungual hematoma

11750   Excision of nail and nail matrix, partial or complete (eg, ingrown or deformed nail) for permanent removal

11752   Excision of nail and nail matrix, partial or complete (eg, ingrown or deformed nail) for permanent removal; with amputation of tuft of distal phalanx

11755   Biopsy of nail unit, any methos (eg, plate, bed, matrix, hyponychium, proximal and lateral nail folds) (separate procedure)

11760   Repair of nail bed

11762   Reconstruction of nail bed with graft

11765   Wedge excision of skin of nail fold (eg, for ingrown toenail)

Stress Fractures of the Medial Malleolus

John A. Bergfeld, MD

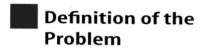 Definition of the Problem

Patient Presentation

Stress fractures of the medial malleolus are relatively rare, representing fewer than 10% of all stress fractures of the foot and ankle. They are becoming more common, however, as more people engage in vigorous exercise and competitive sports even into older age. A detailed history and a high level of suspicion are essential for recognition of a medial malleolar stress fracture. Presenting symptoms usually include pain during activities and tenderness over the medial malleolus that are present before an acute traumatic episode. Often the patient has aching or soreness over the medial aspect of the ankle for weeks or months before an acute episode of pain that significantly limits activity. Although a twisting injury may appear to have precipitated the pain, patients with stress fractures of the medial malleolus will have had soreness and pain over the medial aspect of the ankle before the acute injury. In runners, the pain may not start until part way into the run, and this early signal is often ignored. Patients may report a change in the type of athletic shoes worn or in the surface on which their sports are performed (eg, a change from grass to hard court for a tennis player). Medial malleolar stress fractures are most common in patients between the ages of 20 and 40 years and occur almost exclusively in athletes involved in sports that involve a significant amount of running and jumping.

A detailed patient history should elicit information about previous stress fractures, changes in shoes, any history of high arches, and the type and intensity of athletic activities. Additional predisposing factors that should be noted include osteoporosis, tobacco use, significant alcohol intake, hyperthyroidism, and anorexia nervosa—all of which are known to make bone more susceptible to stress fractures. In women, dietary history and irregularities in the menstrual cycle should be noted. A period of temporary inactivity with a return to vigorous activity also can predispose an individual to this injury.

Physical Examination

The entire foot and ankle should be carefully examined with the patient both standing and sitting. An evaluation of the hindfoot is important to determine if there is any hindfoot varus that might increase the forces placed on the medial malleolus. Although swelling is typically minimal with this injury, it usually is noticeable over the medial ankle when compared with the uninvolved contralateral ankle. Swelling and pain on both the lateral and medial aspects of the ankle are more likely to be produced by a rotational injury (ligament sprain) than by an isolated medial injury, such as a stress fracture of the medial malleolus. A thorough evaluation of the integrity of the posterior tibial tendon is important. To rule out posterior tibial tendinitis, palpation should detect an intact posterior tibial tendon, and the patient should be able to perform a single heel rise and have good plantar flexion and inversion strength against resistance. Finally, pain with posterior tibial tendinitis will be palpable on the tendon rather than on the bony medial malleolus. Evaluation of a patient's shoes is also important because excessive wear of the lateral aspect of the shoe indicates a significant varus deformity that increases stress over the medial ankle. Tibiotalar and subtalar joint ranges of motion are normal in a patient with a medial malleolar stress fracture.

Radiographs should be obtained even though reports suggest that initial radiographs reveal medial malleolar stress fractures in fewer than 50% of patients in whom the diagnosis is ultimately made. Radiographs may show a fissure line, with or without sclerosis, extending vertically or obliquely upward at the junction of the medial malleolus and the tibial plafond (**Figure 1**). Most medial malleolar stress fractures are in the posteromedial concave side of the tibia.

Differential Diagnosis
- Posterior tibial tendinitis
- Deltoid ligament sprain
- Ankle arthritis
- Tarsal tunnel syndrome
- Benign bone tumor
- Malignant bone tumor

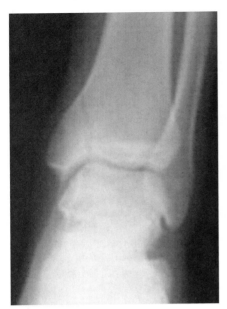

Figure 1 AP radiograph showing typical appearance of a medial malleolar stress fracture.

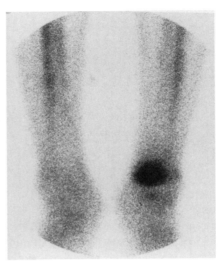

Figure 2 Positive bone scan for a medial malleolar stress fracture (right) compared with the contralateral normal ankle (left).

Additional Work-up

If initial radiographs are negative, as they often are with this injury, additional diagnostic imaging is necessary. A three-phase bone scan has traditionally been used (**Figure 2**), but MRI is currently the definitive imaging technique for diagnosis of a medial malleolar stress fracture. When used in the diagnosis of stress fractures, MRI is more sensitive than radiography and at least as sensitive as and more specific than bone scanning. Although CT provides excellent bony detail, MRI also provides valuable information about the surrounding ligaments, the posteromedial tendons, the articular cartilage, and the underlying bone of the ankle joint. On T2-weighted MRI scans, these fractures are seen as bands of low signal intensity surrounded by areas of high signal intensity produced by hemorrhage or edema. Once the diagnosis is established with MRI, CT can be obtained to provide better bony detail. On CT scans, a well-circumscribed, small, lytic lesion often can be seen in addition to the fracture line. This lesion

is believed to be the result of an earlier microfracture with subsequent reabsorption.

The Solutions

Treatment Options and Rationale

The bony changes associated with stress fractures are related to stress distribution in normal bone. Compression and tension forces are normally placed on any weight-bearing bone during physiologic loading. Bone has the ability to remodel in response to these forces, but this ability is limited by the physiologic tolerance of the bone structure, which is time, rate, and load dependent. When normal stresses are maintained within physiologic limits, remodeling occurs. However, when stresses exceed the physiologic limits of the bone, microfractures of the trabeculae occur and can propagate into a stress fracture. Healing of these fractures can occur only if the excessive stresses on the bone are decreased to a level within

the physiologic limits of the bone. Similar to anterior tibial and femoral neck stress fractures, the medial malleolar stress fracture is often caused by excessive tension forces and, therefore, is difficult to heal.

Two treatment options that reduce the stress forces in the medial malleolus to within its physiologic limits are casting and open reduction and internal fixation (ORIF). Because the normal internal rotation force of the talus is transmitted to the medial malleolus, casting that decreases this rotational force decreases stress on the medial malleolus. With dorsiflexion of the ankle, the wider anterior aspect of the talus fills the mortise and places stress on the medial malleolus. Casting decreases dorsiflexion and reduces this stress on the medial malleolus.

Casting or bracing that reduces stress on the medial malleolus will allow normal physiologic bone remodeling to heal the fracture. When treated with a casting program, patients with medial malleolar stress fractures are reported to be able to return to activities in an average of 6 weeks. The average time for complete healing of medial malleolar stress fractures treated with casting has been reported to be 6.7 months. A short leg cast or a removable walking boot can be used to immobilize the ankle, usually for 6 weeks, after which time the patient is gradually weaned from the cast or boot into an ankle-stirrup brace, and activity is gradually increased. Full activity is not allowed until the patient is free of symptoms. Once the stress fracture has healed, any predisposing factors elicited in the history should be altered. Alteration may require a change in the patient's training program, diet, or orthotic management of an ankle deformity.

The other treatment option for medial malleolar stress fractures is ORIF, which is reported to allow a faster return to activity (4.5 weeks) than immobilization (6 weeks) and faster healing of the stress fracture

(4.2 months compared with 6.7 months after casting). ORIF is performed through a small incision over the medial malleolus, with limited dissection to protect the blood supply to the medial malleolus. Screws are placed perpendicular to the fracture line to stabilize the fracture fragments and decrease motion at the fracture site, allowing the bone to undergo normal remodeling to heal the fracture.

Authors' Preferred Treatment and Rationale

Most medial malleolar stress fractures occur in athletes who return to the same activity that originally created the stress fracture. We favor ORIF in this group of patients, especially elite athletes. In our experience, surgical treatment of these injuries reduces the tension forces, allows more rapid rehabilitation and earlier return to full activity, and has a higher rate of fracture healing than nonsurgical treatment.

In nonathletes, a nonsurgical treatment program of casting with weight bearing as tolerated may be appropriate. We initially place this type of patient in a short leg weight-bearing cast for 3 weeks. Then a removable boot is placed for another 3 weeks, during which time range-of-motion exercises of the ankle are done. At 6 weeks, an ankle-stirrup brace is fitted, and clinical symptoms are monitored. Once symptoms are completely resolved, return to full activity is allowed. If pain recurs with return to full activity, we perform ORIF rather than continuing immobilization.

For ORIF of a medial malleolar stress fracture, the patient is placed supine on the operating table, and a limited incision is made medially. Because this most commonly is an oblique fracture rather than a vertically oriented fracture, we place two screws parallel to the joint line and a third screw obliquely from the tip of the medial malleolus up into the tibia (**Fig-**

ure 3). We believe this provides excellent fracture stabilization, which decreases stress along the fracture line and allows the normal remodeling process to heal the fracture. We prefer fully threaded solid cortical screws placed in a lag fashion. Depending on the size of the fracture fragment and the size of the individual, we use either 3.5- or 4.5-mm screws. Postoperatively, the patient is placed in a short leg splint for 1 week and is not allowed to bear weight. Then a removable walking boot is fitted, weight bearing is allowed as tolerated, and exercises to enhance ankle range of motion are initiated. The boot is removed at night during sleeping. At 3 weeks, strengthening exercises of the ankle are initiated. At 6 weeks, the boot is replaced by a stirrup brace, and activities are increased. When the patient is symptom-free, full activity is allowed. Any predisposing factors elicited in

the history are treated before the patient returns to full activity.

Management of Complications

The two most common complications after surgical treatment of medial malleolar stress fracture are painful hardware over the medial ankle and fracture nonunion. In a patient with a very thin ankle, it is important to countersink the screws to prevent the hardware from being prominent. When the hardware is prominent, padding around the screw heads decreases the pressure over the screws. If pain persists despite these conservative measures, screw removal can be considered, although we prefer not to remove the screws for at least 1 year after surgery. In an elite athlete, we try not to remove the hardware until his or her athletic career has ended.

Nonunion of a medial malleolar stress fracture is best treated surgi-

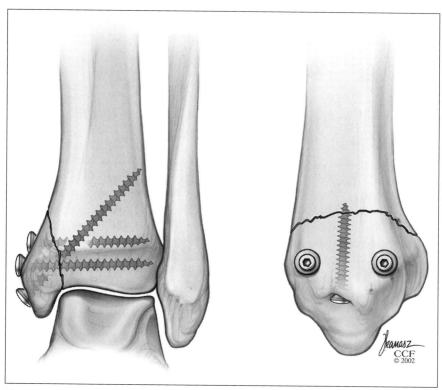

Figure 3 Mortise and lateral views of our preferred surgical fixation technique for medial malleolar stress fractures. (Reproduced with permission from the Cleveland Clinic Foundation)

cally. This requires a larger medial approach with exposure of the fracture site to remove any fibrous tissue that has developed. Both surfaces of the fracture are drilled with a 0.045-in Kirschner wire to stimulate vascular channels. We also pack the site with autogenous bone graft obtained from the calcaneus or from the iliac crest. If the fragment is large enough, repeat interfragmentary lag screws can be placed, or a medial buttress plate can be incorporated into the construct to decrease the stresses over the fracture site. We also use an external electrical or ultrasound bone stimulation device to aid healing of the fracture. A short leg non–weight-bearing cast is worn for 3 weeks, followed by a short leg weight-bearing cast for another 3 weeks, and then a removable cast boot with weight bearing as tolerated for another 3 weeks. At 9 weeks after surgery, the patient is weaned out of the cast boot and into a stirrup brace. Return to activity is not allowed for at least 3 months after surgery, and unrestricted activity is not allowed until the patient is pain-free.

The author wishes to acknowledge the contribution of Brian Donley, MD, in the creation of this chapter.

References

Korpelainen R, Orava S, Karpakka J, Siira P, Hulkko A: Risk factors for recurrent stress fractures in athletes. *Am J Sports Med* 2001;29:304-310.

Orava S, Karpakka J, Taimela S, Hulkko A, Permi J, Kujala U: Stress fractures of the medial malloelus. *J Bone Joint Surg Am* 1995;77:362-365.

Schils JP, Andrish JT, Piraino DW, Belhobek GH, Richmond BJ, Bergfeld JA: Medial malleolus stress fractures in seven patients: Review of the clinical and imaging features. *Radiology* 1992;185:219-221.

Shabat S, Sampson KB, Mann G, et al: Stress fractures of the medial malleolus: Review of the literature and report of a 15-year-old elite gymnast. *Foot Ankle Int* 2002;23:647-650.

Shelbourne KD, Fisher DA, Rettig AC, McCarroll JR: Stress fractures of the medial malleolus. *Am J Sports Med* 1988;16:60-63.

Coding

ICD-9 CODE
824.0   Fracture of ankle, Medial malleolus, closed

CPT CODE
27766   Open treatment of medial malleolus fracture, with or without internal or external fixation

CPT copyright © 2003 by the American Medical Association. All Rights Reserved.

Metatarsal Stress Fractures

Robert S. Adelaar, MD

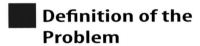

Definition of the Problem

Patient Presentation

Dull, aching pain in the forefoot is typical on presentation. Frequently the patient can walk but not run because of pain. Occasionally there is redness and swelling on the dorsum of the foot that can mimic cellulitis. The patient cannot continue the activity that caused the stress fracture. The length and geometry of the second metatarsal head, biomechanical problems, overuse fatigue, and metabolic factors can result in pathologic stress loading, leading to fatigue and possibly nonunions.

NORMAL ANATOMY AND PHYSIOLOGY

The second and third metatarsals usually are the longest and the most rigid in normal gait. The rigidity results from the metatarsocuneiform proximal articulation with its keystone architectural restraint. The attachments of the second metatarsal to the three cuneiforms provide cantilever force effect with normal weight bearing. Weight bearing puts a dorsiflexion stress on the head of the second metatarsal, which normally is countered by the plantar flexor muscles. The biomechanical vectors of dorsiflexion secondary to weight bearing and the opposed plantar muscle vectors are important in determining ultimate force distribution to the second metatarsal. The length of the second meta-

tarsal and the rigidity of its base normally create high stresses throughout the metatarsal area. The concentration of stress depends on the activity and position of the limb at contact.

The normal biomechanical anatomy of the foot, with proper support and no contributing abnormalities in alignment of the lower extremity, will respond to the stress related to the activity, duration, and position of the limb during stress concentration. For instance, in marathon running, men have a higher incidence of tibial and fibular stress fractures compared with women, who have a higher incidence of foot and ankle stress fractures. Variations in running mechanism and bone density would contribute to different locations of stress.

The bone density of the metatarsal also will affect its ability to withstand stresses. Insufficiency fractures occur in bones with altered biomechanical stability. Differences in bone density cause differences in the pattern of limb injury. The density of bone can be changed by variations of the menstrual cycle and whether a woman is taking birth control pills or hormonal replacement and by periods of altered weight bearing, such as cast immobilization, bed rest, or space exploration. Cadaver experiments have shown that metatarsal strength and bone density rather than geometry constitute the major factors in determining load to failure.

The blood supply of the second

metatarsal also affects the ability of the bone to withstand stress and repair itself in case of fracture. The blood supply is rich in the proximal and distal metaphyseal areas and least in the diaphyseal portion of the metatarsal. Usually a single nutrient artery enters the shaft of the metatarsal at the metaphyseal-diaphyseal junction. This is important because surgical procedures or fractures in the diaphyseal area are more difficult to heal than those in the metaphyseal area and often can interfere with this nutrient artery. Stress fractures in the metaphyseal area usually can be treated successfully by nonsurgical means. The diaphyseal stress injuries result in more nonunions and often need electrical augmentation or surgical treatment. Although it has not been demonstrated, I believe that osteonecrosis of the metatarsal head is related to a series of stress fractures that have healed, with sclerosis and eventual decreased blood supply into the metatarsal head area.

ABNORMAL ANATOMY

Abnormal anatomy will affect the amount and distribution of stress to the foot and ankle. Body weight, limb length, gastrocnemius-soleus weakness or contracture, lack of ankle dorsiflexion, hindfoot malalignment, hyperpronation, cavovarus alignment, forefoot metatarsal adduction deformity, forefoot malrotation or malalignment, decreased great toe motion, and toe deformities are all abnormal anatomic factors that can adversely affect stress on the metatarsals. Inability to dorsiflex the ankle secondary to contracture or exostosis increases the forces on the forefoot. Spasticity or Achilles tendon contracture also increases these forces. The cavovarus foot normally has decreased pronation and, therefore, transmits more stress to the forefoot metatarsals. The hyperpronated flatfoot increases stress to the medial portion of the forefoot. If there is an accompanying hallux valgus deformity with pronation, the first metatarsal complex cannot absorb its normal stress and has to transfer that stress to the other metatarsals. The second metatarsal is principally affected by this transfer. Hallux rigidus or operations that decrease motion of the first metatarsophalangeal (MTP) joint increase stress transfer to the second MTP joints. Forefoot contractures will alter the normal metatarsal stress distribution. An example is metatarsus adductus, which will load the fourth and fifth metatarsals. Abnormalities of the toes such as a clawtoe deformity cause hyperextension deformity at the MTP joint, thus increasing the stresses to the metatarsal head.

Conditions in which there is less stress on the first MTP complex, such as dorsiflexion deformity and hyperpronation with sesamoid rotation, will transfer stress to the lateral toes, particularly the second metatarsal. Surgi-

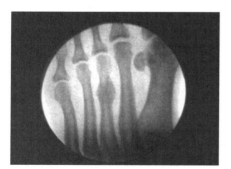

Figure 1 A 30-year-old female runner with a 4-month history of foot pain; notice the massive callus around the third metatarsal stress fracture.

cal procedures can also vary the motion of the first MTP joint. For reconstruction in hallux valgus, altered motion or pain and swelling in the first MTP joint will increase stress on the other metatarsals.

Physical Examination

When a patient is suspected of having a stress fracture, the physical examination is usually quite straightforward. Often, pain on palpation over the metatarsal area where the stress fracture is located differentiates it from problems in the metatarsal head or base articulations. There can be swelling and some change of coloration if there has been recent acute activity or bleeding into the tissue, but this is not common. Attention to abnormalities in limb length, rotation, muscle tone, and, in particular, tightness at the gastrocnemius-soleus complex is important. Abnormalities of foot contour, such as a flatfoot with increased pronation and a cavovarus foot with decreased pronation, transmit different stresses to different regions of the forefoot. Motion of the first metatarsal is also important because in conditions in which there is rigidity of the first MTP complex there are transfer stresses over to the lateral side as the patient tries to avoid bearing full weight on the first metatarsal. Deformities of the toes, such as claw toe deformities in which there is a hyperextension deformity at the MTP joint, increase stresses on the metatarsal. The pulses should be checked to ensure that there is adequate circulation, and sensory function should be checked to make sure there is no neurotrophic problem.

Differential Diagnosis
- Synovitis of the MTP joint
- Fibular collateral instability
- Claw toe deformities
- Digital nerve entrapment
- Metatarsal plantar keratosis

Additional Work-up

Routine radiologic views of the forefoot, including obliques views, will be positive in stress fractures only after the body has reacted to stress by forming callus or a fracture line (**Figure 1**). These usually are seen late in the disorder and cannot be relied on for an accurate early diagnosis. A bone scan is positive after a week and can serve as a screen to show intense bony activity but does not distinguish between high stress reactions, hyperemia, and fatigue fractures. MRI is the most accurate assessment of the type of stress in the metatarsal if it is obtained after the inflammatory focus has developed. MRI can be used to detect different edema patterns, which can give prognostic value as to length of pain. Patterns associated with linear fractures are usually the shortest as far as symptom complex duration is concerned.

———————————————◼

◼ The Solutions

Treatment Options and Rationale
Activity modification is the first treatment of an acute stress fracture, if it is possible to define the activity that caused the stress fracture such as a prolonged running program or a period with more intense activity than the individual had been accustomed to. In addition, some type of containment program, depending on the degree of swelling and tenderness in the fracture, should be used. If the patient has significant tenderness and swelling, then a short leg cast or walker boot would be appropriate for the first month. If radiographs do not show any sclerosis and very early fluffy callus after the first month, then a rocker-bottom shoe with activity modification would be appropriate. It usually takes 6 to 8 weeks to heal a fresh stress fracture.

If anatomic abnormalities are factors in the stress fracture, then treatment, such as an orthotic for passively correctable deformities, should be directed at the abnormal areas. Fixed deformities, such as varus hindfeet, first MTP arthritis, or hyperpronation, may need to be addressed surgically if the abnormal stress persists. The gastrocnemius-soleus complex is important, and stretching exercises should be done, but selective release eventually may be needed. Decreased dorsiflexion of the ankle is much more difficult to treat if it is secondary to degenerative arthritis. If there are large tibial and talar exostoses and the capsular contractures will allow increased motion, then range of motion may be improved by débriding the tibial exostosis. Orthotic devices have been shown in some studies to effectively reduce stress on the metatarsal.

Author's Preferred Treatment and Rationale

All of the treatments described herein, whether for the stress fractures themselves or for possible complications of treatment, are my preferred treatments.

Management of Complications

DELAYED UNION

Delayed union in the diaphysis of the second metatarsal is common but unusual in the proximal or distal metaphyseal areas where the blood supply is better. External bone stimulation with magnetic coils or ultrasound can be used, in addition to containment in a walker boot, until healing is complete. Abnormal anatomic factors should also be addressed as a potential cause of delayed healing and increased stress. Pa-

tient habits such as smoking are also factors in delayed healing.

NONUNION

Nonunions usually are stable and fibrous, occur in the diaphyseal portion of the second metatarsal, and are accompanied by callus and sclerosis. The blood supply to the area usually is decreased by multiple healing attempts with sclerosis of the medullary canal and is difficult to increase.

Reaming the medullary canal of the sclerotic diaphyseal shaft with a series of Kirschner wires or drills will improve the blood supply. While reaming, I lengthen the extensors and release the dorsal capsule at the distal MTP joint to allow hyperflexion. This technique allows the orthopaedic surgeon to acutely flex the proximal phalanx and enter the metatarsal head with a Kirschner wire and then to ream under fluoroscopy until a channel is created. As in other diaphyseal bones, only the outer third of the cortex of the second metatarsal is supplied by the periosteal blood supply. Because the blood supply of the diaphyseal shaft is primarily endosteal, it needs to be reestablished by reaming out sclerotic bone so new capillary buds can form.

Another approach for more severe fractures is open plating and resection of the nonunion accompanied by a dorsiflexion osteotomy to change the stress on the metatarsal head. An autogenous bone graft, usually from the pretibial or calcaneal area, is used if needed. I do not use synthetic bone; I usually use autologous cancellous bone. Dorsal plate fixation with compression to neutralize the dorsiflexion forces is my goal (**Figure 2**). I usually

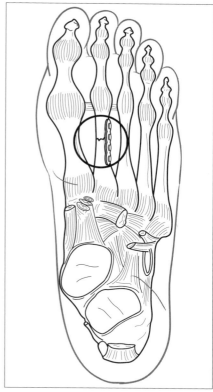

Figure 2 Nonunion of stress fracture of the second metatarsal treated with reaming of the canal with a 0.62-in Kirschner wire or cannulated drill (2.0) and a four-hole dorsal compression plate.

use a 2.4 dynamic compression plating system with six cortices above and below the area of concern. If the sclerotic area needs to be removed and the diaphyseal shaft reamed, an autogenous graft that can be taken with a saw from the pretibial area can be used with plating. The open approach is not often needed, and I must admit that I very rarely need to use this technique.

References

Kaufman KR, Brodine SK, Shaffer RA, Johnson CW, Collison TR: The effect of foot structure and range of motion on musculoskeletal overuse injuries. *Am J Sports Med* 1999;27:585-593.

Korpelainen R, Drava S, Karpekko J, Siira P, Hulkko A: Risk factors for recurrent stress fractures in athletes. *Am J Sports Med* 2001;29:304-310.

Muehleman C, Lidtke R, Berzins A, Becker JH, Shott S, Sumner DR: Contributions of bone density and geometry to the strength of the human second metatarsal. *Bone* 2000;27:709-714.

Oleson CV, Busconi BD, Baran DT: Bone density in competitive figure skaters. *Arch Phys Med Rehabil* 2002;83:122-128.

Warren MP, Brooks-Gunn J, Fox RP, Holderness CC, Hyde EP, Hamilton WG: Osteopenia in exercise-associated amenorrhea using ballet dancers as a model: A longitudinal study. *J Clin Endocrinol Metab* 2002;87:3162-3168.

Zanetti M, Steiner CL, Seifert B, Hodler J: Clinical outcome of edema-like bone marrow abnormalities of the foot. *Radiology* 2002;222:184-188.

Coding

ICD-9 CODES

733.81   Malunion of fracture

733.82   Nonunion of fracture

733.94   Stress fracture of the metatarsals

CPT CODES

20900   Bone graft, any donor area; minor or small (eg, dowel or button)

28320   Repair, nonunion or malunion; tarsal bones

28322   Repair nonunion or malunion; metatarsal, metatarsal with or without bone graft (includes obtaining graft)

28485   Open treatment of metatarsal fracture, with or without internal or external fixation, each

Jones Fracture of the Fifth Metatarsal

James A. Nunley, MD

■ Definition of the Problem

Patient Presentation

The typical patient is an athlete who sustained an acute injury and presents with pain along the lateral side of the foot. Stress Jones fractures also generally occur in the athlete and usually have a prodrome of some lateral aching pain while playing sports. The patient usually will have symptoms only with athletic activity and can walk with a normal gait.

The Jones fracture is a transverse or oblique fracture of the fifth metatarsal that occurs at the metaphyseal-diaphyseal junction and does not extend distal to the 4-5 intermetatarsal articulations. Unlike fifth metatarsal diaphyseal stress fractures, which result from repetitive loading above the fatigued strength of bone, a true Jones fracture is an acute injury resulting from direct or indirect trauma, with no history of prodomes. The exact mechanism of injury is uncertain, but it is thought to involve the rapid application of vertical and mediolateral forces to the fifth metatarsal, commonly with a plantar flexed ankle, while a large adduction force acts on the forefoot. Because abduction-adduction motion is very limited at the fifth tarsometatarsal joint, forced adduction can result in a fracture between the shaft and the immobile metatarsal base in the region bounded by the insertion of the peroneus brevis and tertius.

Physical Examination

Physical examination usually shows minimal swelling and no ecchymosis, but there will be tenderness over the base of the fifth metatarsal. There generally is minimal pain with eversion of the foot. AP, lateral, and oblique radiographs usually show the fracture. It is important when viewing the radiographs to avoid confusing a Jones fracture with other fractures that occur at the base of the fifth metatarsal, such as the avulsion fracture, which is a fracture of the tuberosity and does not involve the 4-5 intermetatarsal joint, or a more distal fracture in the diaphyseal region, which is usually a stress fracture (**Figure 1**).

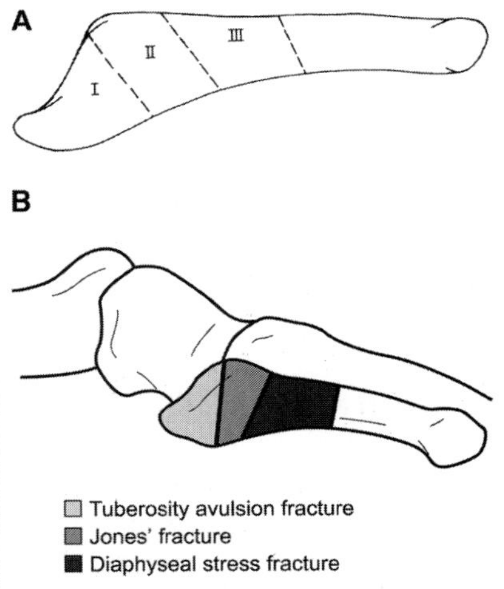

It is important in the physical examination of any patient presenting with either an acute Jones fracture or stress Jones fracture to assess for knee varus, hindfoot varus, or a plantar flexed first metatarsal. All of these conditions are capable of producing a varus force on the hindfoot, which can lead to failure in the treatment of this fifth metatarsal fracture unless the varus force is addressed simultaneously.

Differential Diagnosis

- Avulsion fracture of the fifth metatarsal
- Avulsion fracture of the beak of the calcaneus

Additional Work-Up

Additional work-up is rarely ever warranted, because the diagnosis is obvious from plain radiographs. It is, however, imperative to search either radiographically or with a thorough physical examination to assess for varus of the ankle, hindfoot, or forefoot.

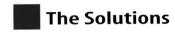

Figure 1 **A,** I, Tuberosity avulsion fracture; II, Zone of metaphyseal-diaphyseal junction; III, Shaft stress fracture zone. (Reproduced from Dameron TB: Fractures of the proximal fifth metatarsal: Selecting the best treatment option. *J Am Acad Orthop Surg* 1995;3: 110-114.) **B,** Fracture zones for proximal fifth metatarsal fractures. (Reproduced with permission from Lawrence SJ, Botte M: Jones' fractures and related fractures of the proximal fifth metatarsal. *Foot Ankle* 1993;14:360.)

Tuberosity avulsion fracture
Jones' fracture
Diaphyseal stress fracture

■ The Solutions

Treatment Options And Rationale

In 1927 Carp reported on 21 fractures of the base of the fifth metatarsal and

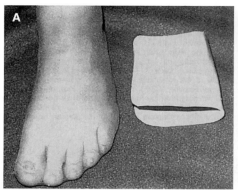 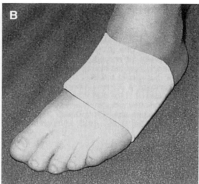

Figure 2 A, AP view of a functional brace for proximal fifth metatarsal fractures. The brace gains purchase on the metatarsals (including the fifth metatarsal head) distally, allowing full metatarsophalangeal motion in all toes. **B,** Dorsolateral view of a functional brace in place. (Reproduced from Dameron TB: Fractures of the proximal fifth metatarsal: Selecting the best treatment option. *J Am Acad Orthop Surg* 1995;3:110-114.)

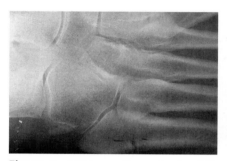 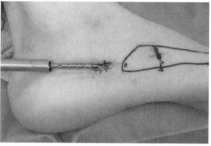

Figure 3 Oblique radiograph of a fifth metatarsal Jones fracture. Note the fracture line beginning on the lateral cortex and propagating to the 4-5 intermetatarsal articulation. (Reproduced with permission from Nunley JA: Jones fracture technique. *Tech Foot Ankle Surg* 2002;1:131-137.)

Figure 4 A cannulated drill is passed over the guide pin to ream the medullary canal. Notice that the soft-tissue protector has been withdrawn so that the drill may be visualized, but during the surgical procedure it is important to keep the drill guide down to the base of the bone so as not to injure the sural nerve or peroneal tendons. (Reproduced with permission from Nunley JA: Jones fracture technique. *Tech Foot Ankle Surg* 2002;1:131-137.)

Currently, the orthopaedist must decide between surgical or nonsurgical management. If the patient is willing to undergo nonsurgical treatment, that is, to wear a non–weight-bearing cast for 6 to 8 weeks or until fracture union, then there is anywhere from a 70% to a 90% chance that the fracture will heal. Dameron has introduced the concept of a molded orthotic (**Figure 2**) to suspend the fifth metatarsal, but there have been no series to report the results of this treatment. The final option is the surgical management that would involve the insertion of some type of an intramedullary screw or sliding onlay bone graft. Electrical stimulation has been reported to be successful for the treatment of delayed unions and nonunions but is not usually recommended for the primary fracture.

Author's Preferred Treatment and Rationale

I prefer surgical treatment of all acute Jones fractures and for all stress Jones fractures. I believe that the risk of surgery is minimal, the rehabilitation is greatly enhanced, and union generally is ensured. It is critically important that the surgical procedure be performed in an accurate anatomic fashion. I believe that the use of a noncannulated screw is extremely important because cannulated screws are not able to withstand repetitive stress. Nonunion has been reported in previous series when using a cannulated screw. It is also important that all the threads of the partially threaded screw cross the fracture site completely, but that the screw not be so long that it straightens the normally curved fifth metatarsal. Straightening the fifth metatarsal will cause lateral gapping and lead to delayed union or nonunion. I generally use either a 4.5- or 6.5-mm AO screw. The decision as to which screw to use is made at the time of surgery based on preoperative templating and the feeling the surgeon gets with the use of a bone tap during surgery.

The surgery is done percutane-

demonstrated a tendency toward delayed union, which he believed was related to poor blood supply of the fifth metatarsal. In 1975, Dameron reported on a large series of fractures of the fifth metatarsal, which included 100 patients with tuberosity avulsion fractures, but of his 20 proximal metaphyseal-diaphyseal fractures, 15 of which were treated conservatively, 12 showed union within 2 months to 1 year but 3 went on to nonunion, and ultimately 5 nonunions were treated with sliding bone grafts.

In 1983, DeLee took exception to the prevailing view, which was to treat all Jones fractures with a non–weight-bearing cast until union. He presented

the first primary surgical treatment of 10 athletes with fifth metatarsal stress fractures. All of the athletes were professional football players, and all of them were treated with percutaneous ASIF type 4.5 malleolar screws. Union was obtained in all the athletes at an average of 7.5 weeks, with all of them returning to their sport at an average of 8.5 weeks. Since then, numerous other techniques for surgical stabilization of Jones fractures have been presented. These include tension band wiring, minifragment screws, low profile plates, and cross pinning with Kirschner wires.

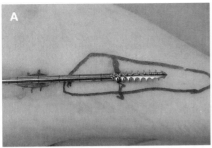
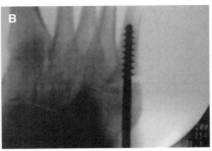
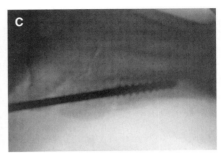

Figure 5   **A,** Tap overlying the fifth metatarsal demonstrating the length that the tap needs to go for all threads to cross the fracture site. **B,** Fluoroscan view demonstrating slight distraction of the fracture as the tap cuts threads distal to the fracture. **C,** Lateral view demonstrating how there is no penetration of the medial cortex. (Reproduced with permission from Nunley JA: Jones fracture technique. *Tech Foot Ankle Surg* 2002;1:131-137.)

ously, making a small 1-cm incision approximately 1 inch proximal to the base of the fifth metatarsal (**Figure 3**). The guide pin must be perfectly placed in the anteroposterior, lateral, and oblique planes within the center of the medullary canal of the fifth metatarsal. Any attempt to pass the cannulated drills and taps in which the guide pin has not been centered is likely to lead to penetration of the medial cortex or other fractures (**Figure 4**). Once the guide pin has been inserted, I overdrill with a 3.2-mm cannulated drill and withdraw both the guide pin and the drill. I next use the 4.5-mm tap and watch with the fluoroscope as I advance the tap, making sure that the threads on the tap completely cross the fracture site (**Figure 5**). If there is a good purchase by the tap in the distal metatarsal or if the distal metatarsal tends to rotate as the tap turns, this generally means that a 4.5-mm screw will provide adequate fixation. If

there is no purchase with the 4.5-mm tap, then I go up to a 6.5-mm screw.

I found that the 6.5-mm screw can be used in at least 80% of my patients. It is critically important to tap the entire distance the screw will be inserted; otherwise, the shaft will fracture as the screw is tightened down. Once the tap has been inserted completely in the distal metatarsal and channels cut into the diaphyseal medullary bone, an appropriately sized 6.5-mm screw is inserted (**Figure 6**). The wound is closed in routine fashion, and the patients are kept touch-down weight bearing in a splint for 2 weeks and then put in an orthotic as described by Dameron. I have the patients begin weight bearing between 2 and 4 weeks. Generally, the fractures are healed, and the patients have returned to normal activities between 6 and 8 weeks. In the athlete, to enhance early union, I use simultaneous electrical stimulation for 8 hours at night, and

I use ultrasonic stimulation for 20 minutes during the day.

Management of Complications

Complications occur for several reasons. The most common complication that I see is nonunion. Malunion has been extremely uncommon. Generally, a nonunion occurs with a cannulated screw. This type of screw can be extremely difficult to remove, especially if it is a titanium cannulated screw. I generally try to remove the screw and again perform the surgery percutaneously without taking down the fracture site. If it is not possible to remove the screw, a slot is made in the fifth metatarsal lateral border, the hardware is extracted, the nonunion site is freshened, and an onlay bone graft is performed. This graft may or may not be supplemented with a small fragment plate for further security.

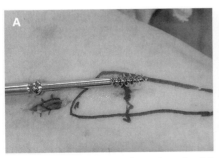
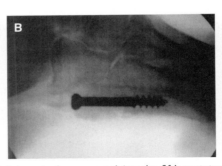
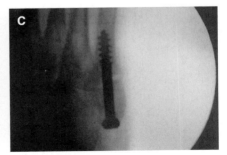

Figure 6   **A,** A 6.5-mm short-thread solid stainless steel screw overlying the fifth metatarsal will be inserted percutaneously. **B,** Lateral radiograph demonstrating excellent compression with all threads crossing the fracture. **C,** AP radiograph showing excellent purchase of the screw thread distal to the fracture without penetration of the medial cortex. (Reproduced with permission from Nunley JA: Jones fracture technique. *Tech Foot Ankle Surg* 2002;1:131-137.)

References

Dameron TB: Fractures of the proximal fifth metatarsal: Selecting the best treatment option. *J Am Acad Orthop Surg* 1995;3:110-114.

Glasgow MT, Naranja RJ, Glasgow SG, et al: Analysis of failed surgical management of fractures of the base of the fifth metatarsal distal to the tuberosity: The Jones fracture. *Foot Ankle Int* 1996;17:449-457.

Holmes GB Jr: Treatment of delayed unions and non-unions of the proximal fifth metatarsal with pulsed electromagnetic fields. *Foot Ankle Int* 1994;15:552-556.

Kelly IP, Glisson RR, Fink C, Easley ME, Nunley JA: Intramedullary screw fixation of Jones fractures. *Foot Ankle Int* 2001;22:585-589.

Nunley JA: Fractures of the base of the fifth metatarsal. *Orthop Clin North Am* 2001;32:171-180.

Nunley JA: Jones fracture technique. *Tech Foot Ankle Surg* 2002;1:131-137.

Rettig AC, Shelbourne KD, Wilckens J: The surgical treatment of symptomatic nonunions of the proximal (metaphyseal) fifth metatarsal in athletes. *Am J Sports Med* 1992;20:50-54.

Coding

ICD-9 CODE

825.25 Fracture of one or more tarsal and metatarsal bones. Fracture of other tarsal and metatarsal bones, closed, Metatarsal bone(s)

CPT CODE

28476 Percutaneous skeletal fixation of metatarsal fracture, with manipulation, each

CPT copyright © 2003 by the American Medical Association. All Rights Reserved.

Turf Toe

Robert B. Anderson, MD

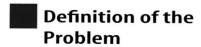

Definition of the Problem

Patient Presentation

The term turf toe was coined to describe hyperextension injuries of the hallux metatarsophalangeal (MTP) joint in athletes playing on artificial turf surfaces; however, there is no evidence to suggest that these injuries are more common on artificial turf than on natural grass fields. These injuries can lead to significant functional disability and may end an athletic career in sports in which toe push-off is important to performance.

The spectrum of turf toe injuries ranges from mild sprain of the MTP joint to complete rupture of the plantar plate with sesamoid retraction. Other than pain with activity, long-term sequelae include hallux rigidus, hallux valgus, and occasionally a cock-up deformity.

Presentation depends on the degree of injury and the time elapsed from the original injury. Turf toe constitutes a broad spectrum of injury with marked variability in the extent of soft-tissue involvement. Pain on weight bearing and difficulty with push-off are the most consistent markers of a significant injury. The classification of the turf toe injury was described in 1984. We have further developed this classification to include a gradation of injury based on signs and symptoms. **Table 1** shows a spectrum of injury that may extend to frank dislocation of the hallux MTP joint.

The primary mechanism of injury appears to be a hyperextension injury to the hallux MTP joint (**Figure 1**), which leads to varying degrees of injury to the plantar plate. There may be instances in which the base of the proximal phalanx impacts the metatarsal head, leading to a small osteochondral defect in this location. Often the athlete cannot recall the specific events of the incident; therefore, a review of the videotape, if available, may indicate the mechanism. Once the mechanism of injury is established, the physician can concentrate on determining the severity of the injury.

Physical Examination

Physical examination and suspicion of a turf toe injury are important to make this diagnosis in the athlete. The examination must start with a complete history of the events leading up to the injury. Observation of the foot should indicate the amount of swelling and the location of any ecchymosis. The hands-on examination of the foot includes palpation over the plantar capsular structures, the dorsal capsule, and the medial and lateral collateral ligaments. An attempt should be made to put the hallux MTP joint through a full range of motion. At the time of initial evaluation, range of motion may be difficult secondary to pain, and a digital block may aid in appropriately evaluating these injuries. The orthopaedist should look specifically for hypermobility with extension compared with the opposite foot (lack of a firm end point), mechanical block, or gross instability to a drawer (toe Lachman's) test (**Figure 2**). The presence of varus or valgus instability at the hallux MTP joint should also be assessed. Examination of the extensor and flexor tendons completes the physical examination of the foot.

In the event of late presentation, a cock-up posture to the hallux may be observed. This is caused by the lack of continuity of the flexor hallucis brevis (FHB) tendon and imbalance of the flexor hallucis longus (FHL) and extensor hallucis longus tendons. FHL tendon function may be weak or absent in these chronic injuries and may be accompanied by a flexion contracture of the hallux interphalangeal (IP) joint. Signs consistent with hallux rigidus may be present as well.

Differential Diagnosis

- Hyperextension injury of the MTP joint
- Hyperflexion injury of the MTP joint (sand toe)
- Sesamoiditis
- Sesamoid fracture
- Tendinitis
- Degenerative joint disease (hallux rigidus)
- Gouty arthropathy

Table 1   Classification of Acute Hallux MTP Joint Injuries

Type of Injury	Classification	Characteristics
Hyperextension (turf toe)	Grade 1—Stretching of the plantar complex	Localized tenderness, minimal swelling, no ecchymosis
	Grade 2—Partial tear	Diffuse tenderness, moderate swelling, ecchymosis, restricted movement with pain
	*Grade 3—Frank tear	Severe tenderness to palpation, marked swelling and ecchymosis; limited movement with pain; positive vertical Lachman's test, if pain allows
	Associated injuries	Medial or lateral injury; sesamoid fracture with bipartite diastasis; articular cartilage and subchondral bone bruise
Hyperflexion (sand toe)	Dislocation—Type I	Dislocation of the hallux with the sesamoids
		No disruption of the intersesamoid ligament Usually irreducible
	Type II II A	Associated disruption of intersesamoid ligament; usually reducible
	II B	Associated transverse fracture of one of the sesamoids; usually reducible
	II C	Complete disruption of intersesamoid ligament fracture of one of the sesamoids; usually reducible

*Grade 3 injuries may represent spontaneously reduced dislocations.

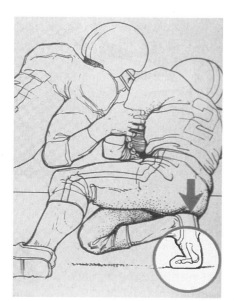

Figure 1   Turf toe is characterized by a dorsiflexion injury of the first MTP joint that damages the plantar structures. (Reproduced from Sullivan JA, Anderson SJ (eds): *Care of the Young Athlete* Rosemont, IL American Academy of Orthopaedic Surgeons, 2000, p 436.)

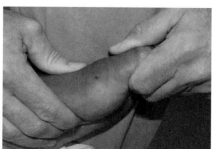

Figure 2   Lachman's test of the hallux MTP joint may indicate plantar plate injury.

Additional Work-up

LABORATORY STUDIES

Because most patients with turf toe injuries are athletes, laboratory work-up does not play a significant role in diagnosis or treatment. However, in the patient with presumed late sequelae of turf toe such as hallux rigidus, laboratory work-up may include studies to rule out other commonly seen causes such as gouty arthropathy. Laboratory studies for each patient must be appropriate to the presenting clinical picture.

IMAGING STUDIES

Following a thorough history and physical examination of the foot, radiographs should be obtained to further examine these hyperextension injuries. Bony abnormalities accompanying the soft-tissue injuries seen in these athletes can be seen on routine radiographs. These findings include capsular avulsions, sesamoid fractures, impaction fractures, diastasis of bipartite sesamoids, and proximal migration of the sesamoids.

Weight-bearing AP, lateral, and sesamoid axial views of both feet should be obtained. Comparison AP and lateral views often confirm the diagnosis. Proximal migration of the sesamoids typically is seen with complete rupture of the plantar complex. Evaluation of the radiographs should include comparing the distance from the distal pole of the sesamoids to the joint. The side-to-side difference should be less than 3.0 mm for the tibial sesamoid and less than 2.7 mm for the fibular sesamoid.

Dorsiflexion stress lateral views (with comparison views) may help delineate joint subluxation, sesamoid migration, or separation of a bipartite sesamoid or sesamoid fracture (**Figure 3**). As the proximal phalanx dorsiflexes, the distance to the distal pole of the tibial sesamoid should remain constant if the plantar ligamentous complex is intact. This distance should be compared with the distance on the uninjured side.

We believe that MRI best defines the soft-tissue injury and the presence of osseous and articular damage (**Figure 4**). MRI should be obtained in all patients in whom gross instability or asymmetric proximal migration of the sesamoids has been identified. T2-weighted and proton-density images should assist in decision making, as well as in grading the extent of the soft-tissue injury. In chronic injuries, the FHL should be closely assessed for longitudinal split tears or ruptures.

DIAGNOSTIC PROCEDURES
An arthrogram of the hallux MTP joint can reveal capsular injuries and assist in decision making but is not necessary given the availability of MRI. Although it is feasible, the joint rarely is anesthetized to examine for instability or to confirm the origin of pain.

The Solutions

Treatment Options and Rationale
NONSURGICAL TREATMENT
Nonsurgical treatment of all grades of turf toe injuries includes rest, ice,

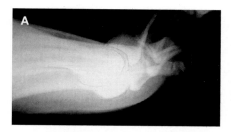
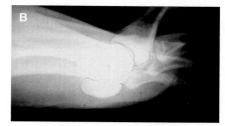

Figure 3 Dorsiflexion stress lateral radiographs of the uninjured (**A**) and injured (**B**) foot. Note the increased distance between the distal pole of the sesamoid and the base of the proximal phalanx. (Reproduced with permission from Watson TS, Anderson RB, Davis WH: Periarticular injuries to the hallux metatarsophalangeal joint in athletes. *Foot Ankle Clin* 2000;5:687-713.)

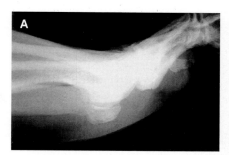
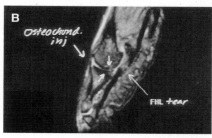

Figure 4 **A,** Lateral radiograph of a professional football wide receiver after sustaining a turf toe injury. Note the proximal migration of the sesamoids. **B,** Postinjury MRI scan defines associated injury patterns to bone and soft tissue. (Reproduced with permission from Watson TS, Anderson RB, Davis WH: Periarticular injuries to the hallux metatarsophalangeal joint in athletes. *Foot Ankle Clin* 2000;5:687-713.)

compression, and elevation (RICE). Principles that apply to most acute sprains of the musculoskeletal system apply to the hallux MTP joint as well. Once the injury is recognized, immediate application of ice with a compressive-type dressing may help reduce swelling. Adjunctive use of anti-inflammatory medication can also be helpful. Typically, a walker boot is applied for protective ambulation. In patients with significant soft-tissue injury or pain, a short leg cast with a toe spica extension in slight plantar flexion may be used (**Figure 5**). The patient's progress is closely monitored with return to activity based on symptoms and function. In returning to play, taping regimens provide compression while limiting movement at the MTP joint. A custom-made orthosis with a Morton's extension to limit hallux MTP motion can be placed in the shoe. The shoe can be modified by

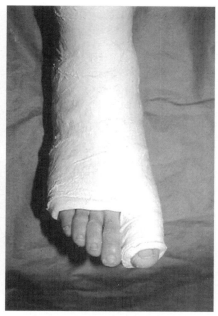

Figure 5 A short leg walking cast with toe spica extension in slight plantar flexion can be used in patients with significant soft-tissue injury or pain. (Reproduced with permission from Watson TS, Anderson RB, Davis WH: Periarticular injuries to the hallux metatarsophalangeal joint in athletes. *Foot Ankle Clin* 2000;5:687-713.)

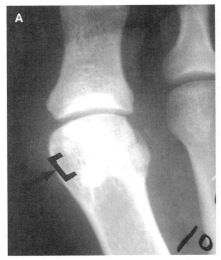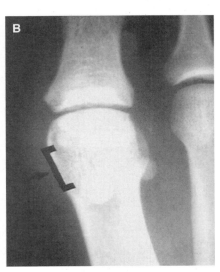

Figure 6 **A,** AP radiograph of a professional football player following a turf toe injury. Note the diastasis of the tibial sesamoid. **B,** AP radiograph 1 year later demonstrating progression of diastasis, which was associated with early clawing of the toe. (Reproduced with permission from Watson TS, Anderson RB, Davis WH: Periarticular injuries to the hallux metatarsophalangeal joint in athletes. *Foot Ankle Clin* 2000;5:687-713.)

placing an aluminum, steel, or carbon-fiber plate into the sole to further limit hallux MTP motion. Factory-made turf toe shoes are available and restrict forefoot bend. However, most running athletes are resistant to this modality because of a perceived loss of mobility. Cortisone and/or anesthetic injections are not advised in any injury to the hallux MTP joint, particularly when attempting to keep an athlete on the playing field. Injections create a neuropathic-like situation that may accelerate joint degeneration.

Most athletes with mild to moderate turf toe injuries return to sports with protection within 4 weeks. The more severe (grade 3) injuries may result in loss of playing time of at least 6 weeks, frequently requiring long-term immobilization and serial examinations. Return to play decisions are individualized because sprinters typically require more time to recover. In athletes with continued swelling and edema, modalities such as whirlpool and ultrasound with cold compression may be used as adjuncts to traditional therapy.

SURGICAL TREATMENT

There is a paucity of literature on the surgical management of hallux MTP joint injuries. This paucity stems from the general notion that surgery is rarely indicated in the treatment of this disorder. However, when nonsurgical treatment fails or an athlete is diagnosed with gross instability, the orthopaedist should be suspicious for pathology that necessitates surgical intervention. Indications for surgery include (1) a large capsular avulsion with an unstable joint, especially medial; (2) progressive diastasis of a bipartite sesamoid or sesamoid fracture; (3) retraction of sesamoids, single or both; (4) traumatic bunion and progressive hallux valgus; (5) a positive vertical Lachman's test; and (6) the presence of a loose body or chondral injury.

The surgical procedure chosen should address the specific pathology determined by diagnostic studies and physical examination. Our experience in the repair or reconstruction of hyperextension injuries has been derived from several athletes who sustained a turf toe and subsequently

were unable to perform at their preinjury levels. These athletes often reported pain with running activity and an inability to cut from side to side. Clinical findings included malalignment of the hallux, traumatic and progressive bunion deformity, clawing of the great toe, diminished flexor strength, generalized joint synovitis, and advanced degeneration of the joint. Radiographic analysis frequently showed proximal migration of one or both sesamoids and instances of progressive diastasis of bipartite sesamoids (**Figure 6**). MRI confirmed pathology through the plantar complex of this joint, frequently associated with injuries to the joint surface or FHL tendon. All instances of sesamoid migration associated with hyperextension injury have been associated with distal rupture and proximal migration despite the proximal capsular attachment to the metatarsal neck being weaker. It appears that the sesamoids rupture distally and migrate proximally because of the preservation of the flexor tendons, along with the abductor and adductor tendons, and their ability to retract.

Author's Preferred Treatment and Rationale
SURGICAL TREATMENT

The surgical incision used to access plantar injuries is longitudinal, placed medial or plantar medial, with the option to create a J-type incision by extending across the flexion crease at the base of the hallux. The latter is our preferred incision for more extensive injuries that often involve the proximal migration of both sesamoids (**Figure 7**).

Once the incision is made, it is imperative to identify and protect the plantar medial digital nerve. With the nerve mobilized and protected from excessive traction, the degree of injury to the plantar soft-tissue structures can be assessed.

If a simple plantar plate disruption with proximal retraction of the sesamoids has occurred, a primary repair is performed using nonabsorbable sutures. Plantar flexion at the hallux MTP joint assists in exposure. Repair of the soft tissues commences from lateral to medial across the plantar plate (**Figure 8**). If inadequate soft tissue is available distally, suture anchors are placed into the base of the proximal phalanx. If diastasis of the tibial sesamoid is involved, excision of the entire sesamoid with repair of the resultant soft-tissue defect typically is required. In the event of a small distal pole avulsion or diastasis, the distal pole is excised and soft tissues are repaired through drill holes in the remaining proximal pole. The soft-tissue repair of the plantar defect that follows tibial sesamoidectomy can be augmented with transfer of the abductor hallucis tendon (**Figure 9**). The transferred abductor tendon will function dynamically as a flexor tendon, as well as provide collagen for additional plantar restraint to dorsiflexion forces.

Occasionally, an athlete may present with late sequelae following an undiagnosed or untreated turf toe injury. These athletes typically report pain and weakness with push-off and difficulty running. Associated injuries can include dorsal chondral injury to the metatarsal head, synovitis, hallux rigidus, longitudinal splitting of the FHL, and clawing of the hallux with IP joint contracture (**Figure 10**). If the initial mechanism involved more of a straight medial stress, progressive hallux valgus deformity may be present.

The late reconstruction of a turf toe is substantially more difficult than a primary repair. Plantar soft-tissue reconstruction may require significant soft-tissue release with fasciotomies and fractional lengthening of the FHB and abductor hallucis tendon. Débridement of the hallux MTP joint with a dorsal cheilectomy is often nec-

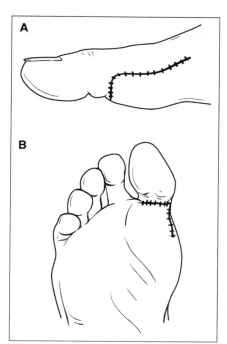

Figure 7 Plantar medial incision commonly used to correct turf toe injuries.

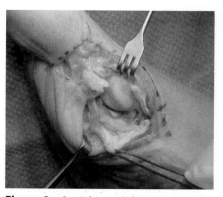

Figure 8 Straight medial incision used to address turf toe injury in a professional football player. Note plantar plate disruption. This was reefed to the proximal phalanx using nonabsorbable suture. The longitudinal split in the FHL tendon was repaired.

essary. In patients with a traumatic bunion, a modified McBride bunionectomy typically is used to allow release of the contracted lateral soft tissues with subsequent joint rebalancing.

For the athlete presenting with a claw toe or cock-up deformity of the hallux, decision making depends on

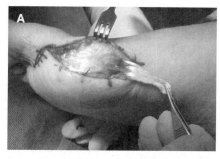

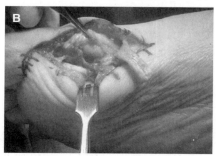

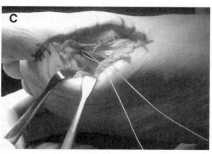

Figure 9 Technique of abductor hallucis tendon transfer for reconstruction of hallux MTP joint. **A,** Abductor hallucis tendon dissected from underlying capsule and immobilized proximally. **B,** Plantar defect following sesamoid excision. **C,** Transfer of the abductor hallucis tendon completed with attachment to the proximal phalanx. (Reproduced with permission from Watson TS, Anderson RB, Davis WH: Periarticular injuries to the hallux metatarsophalangeal joint in athletes. *Foot Ankle Clin* 2000;5:687-713.)

the flexibility of the joints. If the hallux IP and MTP joints are passively correctable to neutral, a flexor-to-extensor tendon transfer is performed. This transfer can be achieved either by splitting the flexor tendon and reapproximating dorsally into the extensor hood as described by Girdlestone-Taylor (**Figure 11**) or via a bone tunnel in the proximal phalanx. When the deformity involves a fixed contrac-

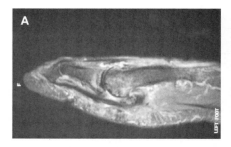

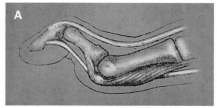

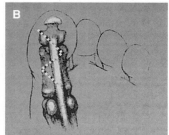

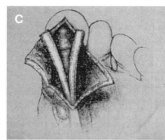

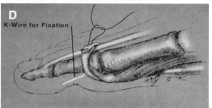

Figure 11 Technique for reconstruction of a claw toe deformity that is passively correctable. (Reproduced with permission from Watson TS, Anderson RB, Davis WH: Periarticular injuries to the hallux metatarsophalangeal joint in athletes. *Foot Ankle Clin* 2000;5:687-713.)

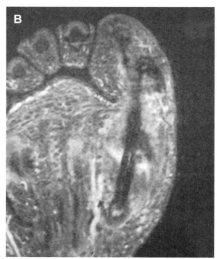

Figure 10 MRI scans of an athlete with a turf toe injury. **A,** Sagittal view shows plantar fluid underlying the MTP joint, consistent with a turf toe injury. **B,** Axial view shows associated injury with a longitudinal split of the FHL tendon.

ture of the IP joint, a hallux IP arthrodesis and a flexor-to-extensor tendon transfer as described above are recommended.

POSTOPERATIVE MANAGEMENT

The postoperative management of athletes is difficult because of the delicate balance between soft-tissue protection and early range of motion. First, it is important to avoid placing the hallux in more than 10° of plantar flexion, either through surgical reconstruction techniques or with postoperative external immobilization. Excessive plantar flexion may become fixed and difficult to compensate for in the running athlete. Our protocol includes external immobilization in approximately 5° to 10° of plantar flexion for 7 to 10 days. At that time, the athlete begins protective passive plantar flexion under the direct guidance of the athletic trainer or physical therapist. We avoid using active and passive dorsiflexion, as well as active plantar flexion. At rest, the toe is protected with a bunion splint using a plantar Velcro restraint and a removable posterior splint or cast boot. Non–weight-bearing ambulation is continued for 4 weeks. Then, range of motion of the hallux is gradually increased, and protected ambulation in a cast boot is introduced. At 2 months after surgery, the patient is placed into an accommodative athletic shoe with the protection of an insole plate that limits dorsiflexion. Active range of motion is instituted, and by 3 to 4 months after surgery, the patient is allowed to return to contact activity with the continued protection of taping techniques and shoe modifications.

The most difficult part of the treatment regimen is determining when an athlete will be able to return to play. We have found this depends on the athlete's position, level of discomfort, and healing potential. Once the athlete has maintained 50° to 60° of painless passive dorsiflexion of the hallux MTP joint, he or she usually is ready for a return to competition. The athlete is usually performing at a pre-injury level after approximately 6 to 12 months.

Management of Complications

Many of the complications associated with hyperextension injuries of the hallux MTP joint involve a delay in diagnosis. Potential complications following surgical repair of the plantar structures include injury to the plantar medial cutaneous nerve leading to a painful neuroma or paresthesia, hallux rigidus, loss of push-off strength, and failure of the repair. Joint stiffness with limited extension rarely occurs; however, a return to the operating room for a closed manipulation could be considered. The best treatment, however, is prevention with a well-guided physical therapy program and close follow-up by the orthopaedic surgeon. Progressive degeneration of the hallux MTP joint is likely over time, and the athlete needs to be advised about this probability even before beginning treatment.

———■

References

Anderson R: Turf toe injuries of the hallux metatarsophalangeal joint. *Tech Foot Ankle Surg* 2002;1:102-111.

Clanton TO, Ford JJ: Turf toe injury. *Clin Sports Med* 1994;13:731-741.

Clanton TO, Schon LC: Athletic injuries to the soft tissues of the foot and ankle, in Mann RA, Coughlin MJ (eds): *Surgery of the Foot and Ankle,* ed 6. St Louis, MO, Mosby, 1992, pp 1191-1200.

Rodeo SA, Warren RF, O'Brien SJ, Pavlov H, Barnes R, Hanks GA: Diastasis of bipartite sesamoids of the first metatarsophalangeal joint. *Foot Ankle* 1993;14:425-434.

Sammarco GJ: Turf toe. *Instr Course Lect* 1993;42:207-212.

Watson TS, Anderson RB, Davis WH: Periarticular injuries to the hallux metatarsophalangeal joint in athletes. *Foot Ankle Clin* 2000;5:687-713.

Coding

ICD-9 CODES

727.06   Tenosynovitis of foot and ankle

735.0   Hallux valgus (acquired)

735.2   Hallux rigidus

845.12   Sprain of MTP joint

905.4   Late effect of fracture of lower extremity

905.8   Late effect of tendon injury

CPT CODES

28220   Tenolysis, flexor, foot; single tendon

28240   Tenotomy, lengthening, or release, abductor hallucis muscle

28270   Capsulotomy; MTP joint with or without tenorrhaphy

28289   Hallux rigidus correction with cheilectomy

28292   Correction, hallux valgus; McBride type procedure

28294   Correction, hallux valgus (bunion) with or without sesamoidectomy; simple exostectomy (eg, Silver-type procedure) with tendon transplants (eg, Joplin-type procedure)

28315   Sesamoidectomy, first toe (separate procedure)

28899   Unlisted procedure, foot and toes

Stress Fracture of the Sesamoid

Judith F. Baumhauer, MD

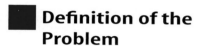

Definition of the Problem

Patient Presentation

The clinical presentation of sesamoid stress fracture is characterized by progressive prodromal symptoms of activity-related pain and swelling localized to the plantar aspect of the first metatarsal head. A detailed patient history is very important. Several factors have been found to increase the incidence of stress fractures, including participation in specific running and jumping sports such as cross-country running and dance that dynamically load the first metatarsal head. Changes in footwear with less shock-absorbing shoes or running shoes that have excessive wear predispose an individual to a stress fracture. In addition to questions concerning abrupt increases in training duration, the patient should be questioned about changes in training techniques or in the terrain in which the training occurs. The patient usually describes an insidious onset of discomfort and may report laterally based foot pain resulting from alterations in gait to avoid contact over the painful sesamoid. On rare occasions, neuritic symptoms or numbness may occur as the medial or lateral digital nerve is compressed by swelling and inflammation caused by the injury.

Physical Examination

Physical examination demonstrates point tenderness over the affected sesamoid. This tenderness is accentuated with dorsiflexion of the great toe as the affected sesamoid is placed in contact with the metatarsal head. The clinical appearance of the first ray can vary from focal plantar swelling to more generalized plantar and dorsal edema of the sesamoid and first metatarsophalangeal (MTP) joint. Active or passive first MTP joint dorsiflexion may be diminished secondary to pain. First MTP joint plantar flexion strength often is decreased. A positive Tinel's sign may be present along the medial or lateral plantar digital nerve adjacent to the injured sesamoid. The generalized foot architecture should be noted. A cavus foot has a plantar flexed first ray that increases axial load to the sesamoids. The tibial sesamoid is more commonly affected with sesamoid disease because it bears more weight during repetitive impact loading.

Oblique views of the foot are often the most helpful in evaluating the sesamoids (**Figure 1**). The lateral oblique view allows visualization of the fibular sesamoid, and the medial oblique view allows visualization of the tibial sesamoid. An AP view is also helpful; however, a standard lateral view of the foot usually is not useful. An axial view of the sesamoids should be obtained with any sesamoid pathology (**Figure 2**). These radiographic views may be normal initially; however, as bone resorption occurs adjacent to the fracture, the radiographs reveal the fracture line.

Differential Diagnosis

- Bipartite sesamoid
- Sesamoid-metatarsal arthrosis (osteochondritis)
- Osteonecrosis of the sesamoid
- Intractable plantar keratosis
- Synchondritis of the sesamoid
- Flexor hallucis longus tenosynovitis
- Infection of the sesamoid

Additional Work-up

If radiographs reveal no sesamoid pathology and the clinical suspicion is high, a technetium Tc 99m bone scan with pinhole collimation may be helpful. The sesamoid complex can be obscured on an AP bone scan when degenerative or posttraumatic articular changes of the first MTP joint are present. Therefore, a PA or oblique bone scan is more specific in distinguishing the sesamoid complex from articular disease of the first MTP joint. A marked difference in technetium Tc 99m uptake of the affected sesamoid is evident when compared with that of the unaffected foot (**Figure 3**).

MRI is helpful in delineating degenerative changes of the sesamoid-first metatarsal head articular cartilage, as well as confirming the diagnosis of a sesamoid stress fracture (**Figure 4**). Bone edema will be present at the region of the bone margins adjacent to the fracture. A bipartite sesamoid, which is an anatomic variant, will not display these

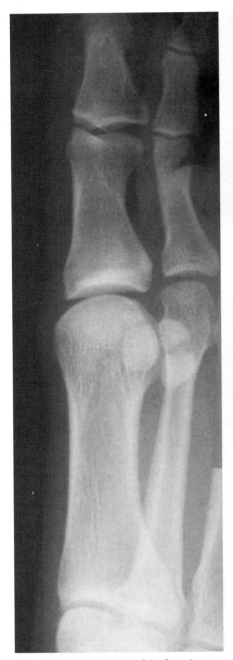

Figure 1 Oblique view of the foot demonstrating a transverse fracture of the lateral sesamoid.

bony changes. MRI is also helpful in ruling out osteonecrosis, flexor hallucis longus tenosynovitis, or infection.

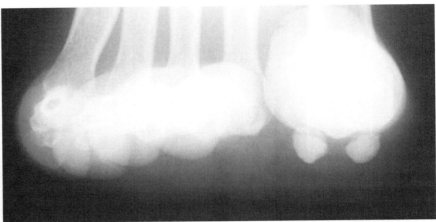

Figure 2 Axial view of the sesamoids demonstrating preservation of the sesamoid-metatarsal head articular surface.

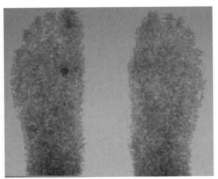

Figure 3 PA technetium Tc 99m bone scan demonstrating increased uptake of the lateral sesamoid of the left foot, consistent with a sesamoid fracture. The right foot uptake is normal.

The Solutions

Treatment Options and Rationale
Initial management of a sesamoid stress fracture consists of immobilization in a short leg non–weight-bearing cast that extends past the tips of the toes for 4 to 6 weeks. If the patient is asymptomatic after that time, an orthotic is fabricated to unweight the sesamoid through either posting proximal to the sesamoid or a U-shaped pad under the sesamoid. Any errors in training that may have precipitated the fracture are also corrected at this time. A slow, progressive return to physical activity is instituted.

If the patient's symptoms persist after casting, additional casting can be considered. However, because additional casting often is poorly tolerated, other options such as activity modification (training) and the use of a stiff-soled shoe, carbon footplate or Morton's extension orthosis, or foot taping and strapping should be considered. The taping, stiff shoe, or insole will limit first MTP joint motion, theoretically decreasing stress and strain of the sesamoid complex and providing additional protection to promote healing. An orthosis has the advantages of being moved from shoe to shoe and avoids the skin irritation that occurs with taping. Additionally, the orthosis can be posted proximal to the sesamoid or a relief can be used to aid in unweighting the sesamoid. Taping has traditionally been used during sports activities with no treatment rendered between games or practices. This type of intermittent treatment provides less protection to the injured sesamoid and is less desirable than shoe or insole modifications. These nonsurgical options should be tried for a minimum of 3 months before progressing to surgical intervention. Most recreational athletes will tolerate these modifications to shoe wear and activities, which result in slow, progressive improvement over 3 to 6 months. Competitive or professional athletes are

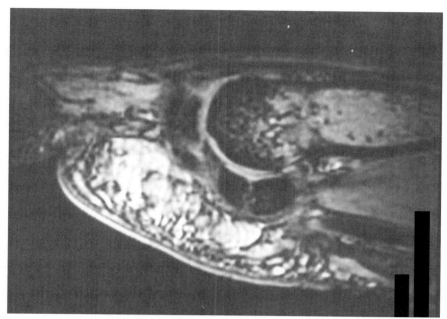

Figure 4 A lateral MRI of the great toe MTP joint. Note the prominent fracture line in the sesamoid with adjacent bone edema. The articular cartilage is well preserved, and there is no evidence of osteonecrosis.

more likely to opt for surgical intervention if initial casting is unsuccessful.

Surgical options include bone grafting or partial or complete excision of the sesamoid. Small case series have reported on the results of tibial sesamoid bone grafting. In the largest series of 21 patients, 90% of stress fractures healed in an average of 12 weeks. The only postoperative complication was medial plantar nerve paresthesias. Two patients who had a nonunion after bone grafting were noted to have instability of the bone fragments. The recommended indication for bone grafting is a persistent symptomatic sesamoid fracture following 6 months of nonsurgical management. The fracture characteristics amenable to bone grafting include well-aligned fragments without separation or instability. Fibular sesamoid bone grafting has not been reported.

Partial sesamoid resection has been reported in 14 patients with symptomatic multipartite and fractured sesamoids. No differences were found in the results between proximal or distal pole excisions. Results were good or excellent in 87% of patients, and no toe alignment deformities were encountered postoperatively.

Total sesamoid excision has been the most common surgical treatment of this problem. Although this surgery eliminates the painful sesamoid stress fracture, it results in decreased strength of the great toe, which obviously is less desirable in the athlete. Although varus and valgus drift of the great toe has been reported after sesamoid excision performed concurrently with a web space release for bunion correction, isolated removal of the sesamoid has not been shown to result in this complication.

Author's Preferred Treatment and Rationale

Initial management of a sesamoid stress fracture begins with a complete history of the patient's recreational and athletic activities over the last 6 months. Understanding the precipitating event(s) that led to the fracture is as important as healing the fracture to avoid recurrence. Treatment begins with short leg casting or bracing and no weight bearing for 4 to 6 weeks until the sesamoid is not ten-

der to palpation. Once the tenderness has resolved, a custom-molded total contact insert modified with a Morton's extension stiffener is used for an additional 8 to 12 weeks. Avoiding the suspected causative activity is recommended for an additional 8 weeks, with slow, progressive return to all activities thereafter while using an orthosis to modify sesamoid loading.

If the patient has continued pain after casting, MRI is ordered in preparation for surgical intervention. The fracture fragments are examined for arthrosis and/or osteonecrosis. A partial sesamoidectomy is performed with removal of the least involved or smallest pole of the sesamoid. Care is taken to close the defect in the flexor hallucis brevis that occurs with bone removal using a small bioabsorbable suture purse stitch. The patient is protected from weight bearing in a removable boot for 4 weeks. Early active and passive range-of-motion exercises are begun at the time of skin suture removal (2 weeks). Weight bearing in the boot is then allowed at 4 weeks postoperatively for 2 weeks. At 6 weeks, the patient weans into a sneaker and begins lower extremity strengthening and proprioception, with return to sports activities at 9 to 12 weeks.

Management of Complications

Injury to the tibial or fibular digital nerve branches can occur with sesamoid resection. The proper incision for a fibular sesamoidectomy is less than 2 mm from the lateral border of the bone to avoid nerve injury. The tibial sesamoid incision is placed on the inferior and medial aspect of the first metatarsal head, and the sesamoidectomy is performed through the joint. This technique makes injury to the tibial nerve branch less likely. Loss of great toe plantar flexion strength is minimized when the flexor hallucis brevis defect is closed.

■ References

Anderson RB, McBryde AM: Autogenous bone grafting of hallux sesamoid non-unions. *Foot Ankle Int* 1997;18:293-296.

Aper RL, Saltzman CL, Brown TD: The effect of hallux sesamoid excision on the flexor hallucis longus moment arm. *Clin Orthop* 1996;325:209-221.

Aper RL, Saltzman CL, Brown TD: The effect of hallux sesamoid resection on the effective moment of the flexor hallucis brevis. *Foot Ankle Int* 1994;15:462-470.

Van Hal MF, Keene JS, Lange TA, et al: Stress fractures of the great toe sesamoids. *Am J Sports Med* 1982;10:122-128.

■ Coding

ICD-9 CODE
733.99 Stress fracture of the metatarsals

CPT CODE
28315 Sesamoidectomy, first toe (separate procedure)

CPT copyright © 2003 by the American Medical Association. All Rights Reserved.

High Ankle Sprain-Syndesmosis Instability

Richard D. Ferkel, MD

▮ Definition of the Problem

Patient Presentation

The syndesmotic joint is stabilized by the anterior inferior tibiofibular ligament (AITFL), the interosseus ligaments, the posterior inferior tibiofibular ligament, and the transverse tibiofibular ligament, a distal and deep fascicle of the posterior inferior tibiofibular ligament. The interosseus membrane proximal to the syndesmotic joint provides additional stability to the joint (**Figure 1**). A high ankle sprain occurs when there is an injury to the distal syndesmotic joint as a result of disruption of the syndesmotic ligaments. A high ankle sprain usually occurs in younger patients as a result of an athletic injury. The most common mechanism of injury is a dorsiflexion of the ankle with a concurrent external rotation of the foot. A typical example of this type of injury occurs when a football player is tackled from behind as the athlete's foot is firmly planted on the ground at the instant the athlete has started moving toward the opposite side. Anterolateral ankle and lower leg pain and swelling develop immediately, typically accompanied by the inability to bear weight on the involved lower extremity.

The high ankle sprain with syndesmosis instability in the absence of periarticular fractures is a rare injury and commonly missed on initial examination. The pain and disability of a high ankle sprain lasts much longer than that of the usual lateral ankle sprain, particularly if proper treatment is not provided in a timely fashion.

Physical Examination

Early and accurate diagnosis of the high ankle sprain is the key to successful treatment. Once the diagnosis is established, patients, their families, coaches, and athletic trainers need to be educated with regard to this unique injury. The stability of the syndesmosis needs to be determined with available clinical and radiographic means.

There are several tests specific for the detection of the high ankle sprain. The palpation test (**Figure 2**) reveals localized tenderness at the anterior aspect of the syndesmotic joint, with or without concomitant tenderness, at the interosseous membrane more proximally in the leg when direct pressure is applied to this area. The squeeze test (**Figure 3**) is positive when compression of the midcalf produces pain in the area of the syndesmosis. The presence of pain is due to the abnormal movement of the distal fibula and tibia as a result of rupture of the syndesmotic ligaments. The external rotation test (**Figure 4**) is performed by applying gentle external rotation to the involved ankle and foot

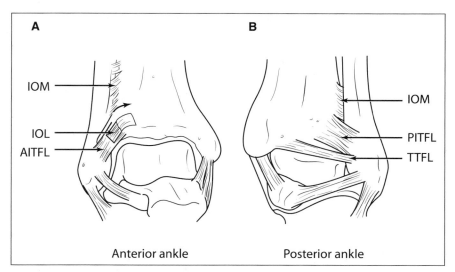

Figure 1 **A,** Anatomy of the anterior ankle, including the anterior inferior tibiofibular ligament (AITFL), interosseous ligament (IOL), interosseous membrane (IOM), anterior talofibular ligament, and calcaneofibular ligaments. **B,** Posterior view of the ankle, including the posterior inferior tibiofibular ligament (PITFL), transverse tibiofibular ligament (TTFL), and interosseous membrane (IOM).

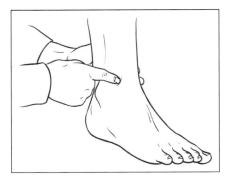

Figure 2 Palpation test for syndesmotic injury. It is important to differentiate pain in the syndesmosis from that in the lateral gutter and sinus tarsi. A separate, careful palpation should be made at each site.

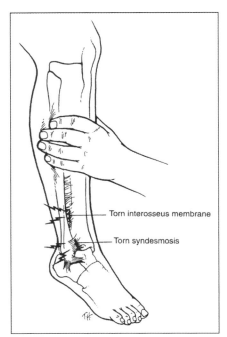

Figure 3 "Squeeze test" is used to diagnose injuries to the syndesmosis. It is positive when squeezing the fibula at the midcalf produces pain at the syndesmosis. (Reproduced with permission from Fu FH, Stone DA: *Sports Injuries: Mechanism, Prevention, Treatment.* Philadelphia, PA, Williams & Wilkins, 1994, p 986.)

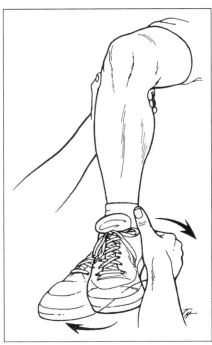

Figure 4 External rotation stress test produces significant pain in patients with syndesmosis sprains. It is positive when pain is produced at the syndesmosis with external rotation of the foot, while holding the leg stabilized with the knee flexed at 90°. This test can also be used to diagnose latent diastasis using stress radiography. (Reproduced with permission from Fu FH, Stone DA: *Sports Injuries: Mechanism, Prevention, Treatment.* Philadelphia, PA, Williams & Wilkins, 1994, p 986.)

while the knee is held to 90° of flexion. Exquisite tenderness at the syndesmosis confirms the injury. The modified external rotation test is very useful in the evaluation of a large and/or overweight patient with a suspected injury to the syndesmosis. This test is performed by having the patient stand on the affected foot and internally rotate the ipsilateral leg while a comparison is made to the contralateral lower extremity. The presence of tenderness at the affected ankle indicates a positive test.

A careful examination of the entire ankle, leg, and foot is necessary to rule out other associated injuries, including fractures and additional ligament tears.

Differential Diagnosis
- Ankle fracture-dislocation, including Maisonneuve fracture (Danis-Weber type C fracture)
- Syndesmotic ligament impingement
- Distal tibiofibular joint synovitis
- Distal tibiofibular joint arthritis
- Bone tumor at or near the syndesmosis, such as osteochondroma

Additional Work-up
AP, mortise, and lateral views of the injured ankle, and AP and lateral views of the ipsilateral leg are obtained during the initial examination of an injured ankle when syndesmosis instability is suspected. The tibiofibular clear space, the tibiofibular overlap, and the medial clear space are measured on the AP and mortise views (**Figure 5**). The tibiofibular clear space is the distance between the incisura fibularis of the posterior tibia and the medial border of the fibula, measured 1 cm proximal to the tibial plafond articular line on the AP and mortise views. The clear space is considered within normal limits when it is less than 6 mm. The tibiofibular overlap is the distance between the medial border of the fibula and the lateral border of the anterior tibia, measured 1 cm proximal to the tibial plafond articular line. At least 1 mm of overlap of the tibia and fibula on the AP and mortise views indicates a normal tibiofibular relationship. The medial clear space is the distance between the medial border of the talar dome and lateral border of the medial malleolus, measured 1 cm distal from the tibial plafond articular line. The medial clear space is considered normal when it is less than 4 mm. A detailed evaluation of tibiotalar joint congruity on the lateral view is important in the overall assessment of a syndesmosis injury. Anterior widening of the tibiotalar joint is consistent with syndesmotic injury. Comparison radiographs of the contralateral ankle should be obtained whenever necessary.

Definitive diagnosis of latent syndesmosis instability may not be possible without additional evaluations. An external rotation and abduction stress test of the ankle under general anesthesia and fluoroscopy will verify an unstable syndesmotic joint.

The use of ankle arthroscopy is extremely helpful in the assessment of dynamic syndesmotic instability and can be performed during the stress test of the ankle. Arthroscopy has the added benefit of simultaneous evaluation and treatment of intra-articular ankle lesions when they are present. In a study of patients with acute ankle fractures, ankle arthroscopy was 100% accurate in diagnosing syndesmosis disruption, but AP radiographs were only 48% accurate, and mortise views were only 64% accurate.

Bone scintigraphy using technetium Tc 99m pyrophosphate is sensitive for the detection of occult syndesmotic pathology. CT with bilateral comparison axial views is invaluable in confirming subtle widening of the syndesmotic joint when there is strong clinical evidence of syndesmosis instability in the presence of normal plain radiographs. In a similar manner, MRI scans comparing the injured and normal ankles are very useful in detection of ligament and cartilage abnormalities as well as joint incongruity of the syndesmotic and ankle articulations.

We consider a high ankle sprain acute when it has been present for less than 6 weeks and subacute when it has been present for more than 6 weeks. The sprain is chronic when it has been present for more than 3 months. A grading system for high ankle sprains is provided in **Table 1**. Most grade II

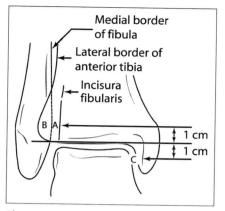

Figure 5 Normal radiographic relationships that are important in evaluation of the tibiofibular articulation. A= Tibiofibular clear space; B= Tibiofibular overlap; C= Medial clear space.

and all grade III acute high ankle sprains are associated with syndesmosis instability. Patients with these ankle sprains usually have much more ankle soft-tissue swelling, ecchymosis, and tenderness than those with a grade I injury.

Grade II ligament instability may be obscure on the initial evaluation. Additional radiographic studies including fluoroscopic stress examination of the ankle, CT and/or MRI are needed to confirm syndesmotic joint instability. Arthroscopy provides additional diagnostic and therapeutic options in the management of grade II ligament injury without overt diastasis.

A grade III high ankle sprain without periarticular fracture is a very

rare entity. Grade III injury represents a serious insult to the ankle and the ipsilateral lower extremity. The ankle is markedly unstable. This is usually the result of a high-energy axial loading of the ankle in dorsiflexion while the foot is forcefully externally rotated and abducted. There is marked pain and swelling of the ankle and the leg with frank diastasis of the syndesmosis and widening of the medial ankle mortise (**Figure 6**). A careful assessment of the local neurovascular structures and tendon integrity is critical in the initial evaluation of this type of injury.

The management of patients with subacute or chronic syndesmosis pain and instability is always a challenge. The goals of restoring and maintaining syndesmotic and tibiotalar joint congruity and stability have remained the same. The presence or absence of arthritis ultimately dictates the available treatment options and prognosis. Accurate diagnosis by using various clinical and diagnostic tools before the commencement of a definitive surgical procedure is essential. Groups who have separately studied syndesmotic injuries emphasize the importance of arthroscopy in the diagnosis and treatment of these injuries. Arthroscopy allows (1) direct palpation of the syndesmosis, (2) visual evaluation of the integrity of the anterior and posterior inferior tibiofibular ligaments, and (3) dynamic assessment of the tibiofibular joint.

Subacute or chronic ankle pain after injury may be caused by syndes-

Table 1 Grading System for High Ankle Sprains

Grade	Description	Joint Stability	Mechanism
I	Partial AITFL	Joint stable	Dorsiflexion (DF) ± external rotation (ER)
II	Partial or complete AITFL Partial interosseous ligament tear (IOL)	Joint either mildly or moderately unstable	DF + ER
III	Complete tear of syndesmotic ligaments + Deltoid ligament avulsion ± Interosseous membrane tear (IOM)	Joint markedly unstable	DF + ER ± abduction

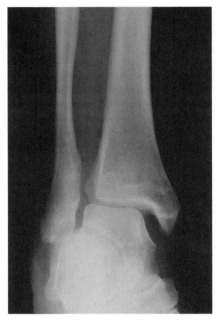

Figure 6 Frank diastasis of the syndesmosis and widening of the medial ankle mortise without a fracture.

motic ligament impingement. Synovitis and scar formation can occur in the areas of the anterior and/or posterior inferior tibiofibular ligaments, with subsequent soft-tissue impingement. Arthroscopic evaluation reveals injected, inflamed synovium surrounding the AITFL extending into the distal tibiofibular joint. In some patients, the synovitis may extend along the joint line all the way to the posterior inferior tibiofibular ligament. The occurrence of syndesmotic impingement with a separate distal fascicle of the AITFL has been reported.

The Solutions

Treatment Options and Rationale
NONSURGICAL TREATMENT OF GRADE I HIGH ANKLE SPRAINS
A patient with an acute grade I syndesmotic ligament injury has a stable ankle. Nevertheless, this type of injury needs to be treated early with a non–weight-bearing cast for 1 to 3 weeks until the acute ankle pain and swelling are resolved. This initial intervention is followed by protected weight bearing with a walker boot or lace-up ankle support. A comprehensive regimen of physical therapy to minimize late pain and disability is started as soon as the acute pain and swelling are resolved. Patients with grade I ligament injury usually return to their previous level of functional activities, including sports in 6 to 8 weeks. The individual is ready to return to sports when he or she can perform push-off and independent single-leg hop forward and lateral without ankle pain or weakness. Grade I syndesmosis sprains have been reported to result in poor outcomes at both 6 weeks and 6 months compared with other studied ankle injuries. This unexpected finding suggests that the extent of injury of grade I sprains is underestimated and that rehabilitation may be incomplete. Therefore, physicians and patients must be aware of the need to thoroughly complete the recommended course of treatment.

TREATMENT OF GRADE II HIGH ANKLE SPRAINS
Most grade II injuries are associated with syndesmosis instability. Percutaneous insertion of a transsyndesmotic screw is performed to provide syndesmosis stabilization once mechanical instability of the distal tibiofibular joint is established. Postoperatively, the patient is allowed early range of motion of the ankle without weight bearing for at least 6 to 8 weeks. Protected weight bearing with a walker boot may be initiated after 8 weeks in patients who are compliant with therapy. In general, the syndesmotic screw is removed approximately 3 months after its insertion. The ankle is protected with a lace-up ankle support while the patient undergoes aggressive physical therapy. Patients can transition to full weight bearing as tolerated.

We do not recommend nonsurgical treatment with non–weight-bearing cast immobilization alone as the treatment of choice for dynamic instability of the syndesmosis. Syndesmotic stabilization with internal fixation provides the distal tibiofibular joint with the optimal protection for healing while allowing functional rehabilitation. Satisfactory restoration of the stability and function of the syndesmosis in a timely fashion minimizes disability and recurrence of instability. Patients are usually able to resume participation in sporting activities in approximately 4 to 6 months.

TREATMENT OF GRADE III HIGH ANKLE SPRAINS
Closed and/or open anatomic reduction of the syndesmotic and tibiotalar joints is imperative for grade III high ankle sprains once acute swelling of the ankle and leg is managed. Initially, arthroscopy may be used to treat all intra-articular pathology. This includes débridement of both the syndesmotic and deltoid ligament tears, which will facilitate reduction of the joints. Medial ankle joint exploration is necessary when the anatomic reduction of the syndesmosis is not obtained. Occasionally, proximal fibular osteotomy is performed to correct plastic deformation of the distal fibula. The transsyndesmotic screw is inserted when anatomic reduction of the syndesmosis is achieved. Anatomic repair of the deltoid ligament and/or syndesmotic ligaments can be completed as necessary before skin closure. The ankle is immobilized in a short leg non–weight-bearing cast for 4 to 6 weeks. Non–weight-bearing ankle range of motion is started after 4 to 6 weeks of immobilization. Physical therapy and protected partial weight bearing in a walker boot is started after 8 to 10 weeks in a compliant patient but delayed until 12 weeks in a non-

compliant patient. The syndesmotic screw is removed 3 to 4 months after surgery. The patient continues to participate in a comprehensive physical therapy program until satisfactory functional recovery is achieved.

MANAGEMENT OF SUBACUTE OR CHRONIC SYNDESMOSIS PAIN AND INSTABILITY

Arthroscopic and occasionally open débridement of the syndesmotic and tibiotalar joints are invariably necessary before anatomic reduction is possible during late reconstruction. Syndesmotic ligaments are repaired through bone holes and/or with the use of suture anchors after the syndesmosis is reduced and stabilized. Autologous tissue, allograft, or synthetic ligament may be used to reconstruct deficient syndesmotic ligaments. An ideal choice of tendon graft is the long extensor tendon of the second and third toe. More than one transyndesmotic screw of a larger diameter (6.5 mm) is usually required to achieve rigid internal fixation of the syndesmosis to allow proper healing. Occasionally tibiofibular synostosis may be required to maintain reduction in late reconstruction of the syndesmosis. Autologous bone graft is harvested from either the distal medial tibia or the proximal tibial metaphysis and placed in the distal tibiofibular joint with internal fixation to promote synostosis. The stiffness produced by the synostosis (**Figure 7**) is usually well tolerated and compatible with high-level athletic performance.

ANKLE ARTHRODESIS OR TOTAL ANKLE ARTHROPLASTY

Ankle arthrodesis or total ankle arthroplasty becomes the treatment of choice when there is significant arthrosis of the tibiotalar joints.

FIXATION OF THE SYNDESMOSIS

Fixation of the syndesmosis continues to be controversial. Most surgeons, however, agree that one or

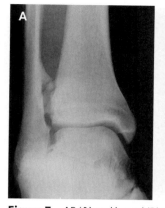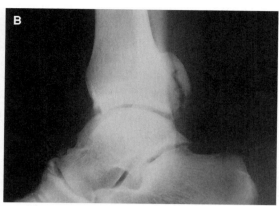

Figure 7 AP (**A**) and lateral (**B**) radiographs demonstrating calcification of the interosseous membrane with synostosis between the tibia and fibula. This professional football player initially had severe pain but once the synostosis matured, his pain disappeared and he was able to return to professional play.

two 3.5- or 4.5-mm fully threaded and tapped cortical screws engaging three or four cortices are adequate for the stabilization of the syndesmosis. In general, more and larger diameter (6.5-mm) screws are used for the following situations: (1) large or overweight patients, (2) noncompliant patients, (3) difficult reduction procedures, (4) late reconstruction procedures, (5) patients with suboptimal bone quality, and (6) patients with neuropathy. Occasionally, it is necessary to overdrill or lag the screws in difficult late reconstruction situations. Polylactide bioabsorbable screws are occasionally used in nonathletes who do not desire to have another procedure for screw removal or who are not expected to return for follow-up. A regular washer or a two-hole plate "washer" may be used on bones with suboptimal quality or in revision cases. A four-hole plate may be used in high-performance athletes, with syndesmotic screws inserted through the two central holes. The plate is left in place after the removal of the syndesmotic screws to avoid stress fracture of the fibula at the syndesmotic screw holes.

A recent study concluded that anatomic reduction of the syndesmosis may be performed in any po-

sition of ankle flexion without compromising ankle dorsiflexion. Further confirmation of this finding is necessary.

The syndesmosis is mobile as the fibula moves up and down, rotating and translating medially and laterally during ankle range of motion and weight-bearing activities. The stiffness of the fixation limits normal syndesmosis motion and function. Therefore, removal of the syndesmotic screw is recommended before the patient returns to full activities and unprotected weight bearing.

TREATMENT OF SYNDESMOTIC IMPINGEMENT

Treatment of syndesmotic impingement includes débridement of the torn syndesmotic ligaments anteriorly, centrally, and inferiorly, including the tibiofibular joint. If a separate fascicle of the AITFL is abrading against the lateral talar dome, it should be excised. From anatomic studies, we have observed that approximately 20% of the syndesmotic ligament is intra-articular. Therefore, complete removal of the intra-articular portion leaves approximately 80% of the ligament intact and does not predispose the patient to any iatrogenic instability.

Author's Preferred Treatment and Rationale

Arthroscopy is routinely used in the diagnosis and treatment of grade II and grade III injury, particularly when there is uncertainty regarding the syndesmosis instability. One percutaneous 4.5-mm fully threaded and tapped cortical screw engaging four cortices is used to stabilize the syndesmotic joint. Two screws are used in patients who are overweight and, occasionally, in those who are competitive athletes. A four-hole plate may be used in competitive athletes as described. We believe keeping the ankle in neutral dorsiflexion during the reduction and stabilization of syndesmosis avoids overtightening of this joint. The syndesmotic screw is routinely removed approximately 3 months after surgery, before the patient returns to full, unprotected weight bearing and athletic activities.

Aggressive surgical intervention for a grade III injury is performed as soon as the acute tissue swelling is under control. A Robert-Jones bulky dressing and a short leg non–weight-bearing cast in the immediate preoperative and postoperative period are effective in reducing swelling and providing immobilization of the severely injured lower extremity. The syndesmotic screw(s) may be left in place longer than 3 to 6 months if additional fixation time is deemed necessary to ensure proper healing.

We prefer arthroscopic evaluation and débridement of the ankle joint and percutaneous internal fixation of the syndesmosis as the initial treatment option in patients with subacute or chronic syndesmosis instability, provided closed reduction is satisfactory. We proceed with open débridement and reduction of the distal tibiofibular and tibiotalar joints if the closed reduction is unsuccessful. Internal fixation and ligament repair and/or reconstruction are performed as described. However, inserting two to three larger diameter screws through a plate is frequently necessary to achieve desired fixation for proper healing. Screws usually are not removed until 4 to 6 months after surgery. Screw removal may not be necessary in patients with a synostosis unless the patients are experiencing symptoms related to the hardware.

We advocate timely and aggressive physical therapy rehabilitation for all grades of high ankle sprain until full functional recovery of the involved lower extremity is accomplished.

Management of Complications

The patient with a grade III sprain needs to be informed of the potential for a compartment syndrome.

Problems commonly encountered postoperatively include ankle stiffness, longer than expected time lost from athletic participation, screw loosening, screw breakage, loss of reduction, stress fracture of the fibula, and arthrosis. Virtually all of these problems can be avoided or minimized if the clinician and the patient follow the described treatment guidelines and recommendations. Ankle arthrodesis or total ankle arthroplasty is indicated for patients with painful arthrosis.

The author would like to acknowledge Jiun-Rong Peng, MD, for contributing to this chapter.

References

Ferkel RD: *Arthroscopic Surgery: The Ankle and Foot.* Philadelphia, PA, Lippincott-Raven, 1996.

Ogilvie-Harris DJ, Reed SC: Disruption of the ankle syndesmosis: Diagnosis and treatment by arthroscopic surgery. *Arthroscopy* 1994;10:561-568.

Peng JR: Solving the dilemma of the high ankle sprain in the athlete. *Sports Med Arthrosc Rev* 2000;8:315-325.

Scranton PE Jr: Isolated syndesmotic injuries: Diastasis of the ankle in the athlete. *Tech Foot Ankle Surg* 2002;1:88-93.

Takao M, Ochi M, Naito K, et al: Arthroscopic diagnosis of tibiofibular syndesmosis disruption. *Arthroscopy* 2001;17:836-843.

Coding

ICD-9 CODES

845.0   Sprains and strains of ankle

845.03   Tibiofibular (ligament), distal

845.01   Deltoid (ligament), ankle

CPT CODES

27692   Repair, primary, disrupted ligament, ankle; collateral

27698   Repair, secondary, disrupted ligament, ankle, collateral

27829   Open treatment of distal tibiofibular joint (syndesmosis) disruption, with or without internal or external fixation

27842   Closed treatment of ankle dislocation; requiring anesthesia, with or without percutaneous skeletal fixation

27846   Open treatment of ankle dislocation, with or without percutaneous skeletal fixation; without repair or internal fixation

27848   Open treatment of ankle dislocation, with or without percutaneous skeletal fixation; with repair or internal or external fixation

29897   Arthroscopy, ankle (tibiotalar and fibulotalar joints), surgical debridement, limited

29898   Arthroscopy, ankle (tibiotalar and fibulotalar joints), surgical debridement, extensive

CPT copyright © 2003 by the American Medical Association. All Rights Reserved.

Midfoot Strain in the Athlete

James A. Nunley, MD

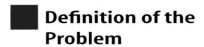

Definition of the Problem

Patient Presentation

Midfoot strains in the athlete represent a spectrum of injuries to the Lisfranc ligament complex that range from partial sprains with no displacements to complete tears with frank displacement. Complete injuries that result in wide diastasis between the first and second metatarsals may present with different patterns of tarsometatarsal displacement, and diagnosis usually is not difficult. Subtle midfoot sprains (diastasis of 1 to 5 mm between the first and second metatarsals) are difficult to diagnose and can be a cause of significant long-term disability and frustration for the athlete, but even more difficult to recognize is a partial capsular tear with no diastasis. This injury can result in an inability to play sports at an elite level for many months.

Although sprains of the midfoot are not common in the general population, certain athletes experience a much higher rate of injury. Typically the athletic injury occurs with an axially loaded plantar flexed foot. The athlete will frequently feel a popping or tearing sensation. Ecchymosis is unusual. There may be mild swelling. Usually the athlete is able to continue to practice or play, but the following day pain limits activity. Tenderness may be very mild as may be swelling. Usually the athletic trainer will have applied ice, and this may very well help to keep the swelling and tenderness to a minimum.

Midfoot sprains are the second most common athletic injury after metatarsophalangeal joint injuries that occur in football players, especially offensive linemen. This injury typically is caused by a low-velocity indirect force, and most athletes can describe an axial longitudinal force applied to the plantar flexed foot with some element of rotation. There has been no specific classification system to guide the investigation and management of these injuries. However, classification schemes for traumatic Lisfranc injuries that occur because of high-velocity traumatic injuries have been well described. I described a classification scheme and a treatment regime for the athletic midfoot sprain.

In this classification scheme, stage I injury is a sprain to the Lisfranc ligament with no diastasis or arch height loss, but increased uptake on bone scintigraphy (**Figure 1**). Stage II sprains have a 1-2 intermetatarsal diastasis of between 1 and 5 mm resulting from a failure of the Lisfranc ligament. There is no arch height loss. Stage III sprains display 1-2 intermetatarsal diastasis and loss of arch height as represented by a decrease in the distance between the plantar aspect of the fifth metatarsal and the plantar aspect of the medial cuneiform on an erect lateral radiograph.

Physical Examination

It is imperative that the athletic trainer, as well as the sports medicine physician or any treating physician,

has a high index of suspicion because if this diagnosis is not sought after it frequently will be missed. The physical findings will be subtle, and in the mildest case the athlete will be able to walk without a limp but will not be able to run and participate at an elite level without pain. The earlier the diagnosis can be established, the quicker a treatment regime can be organized.

Differential Diagnosis
- Contusion of the foot
- Avulsion of the peroneus tertius

Additional Work-up

In addition to a high index of suspicion, radiographic examination is critical. The most common mistake that I see is that radiographs are not weight bearing. It is essential to have standard weight-bearing AP and lateral radiographs of both feet (**Figure 2**). These radiographs allow for comparison of the space between the first and second metatarsals. If the radiographs are completely normal and the index of suspicion is high, I recommend radionuclide imaging (**Figure 3**). In my experience, this test has been 100% reliable in both specificity and sensitivity. There have been no patients in my personal series in which a bone scan has failed to identify the involved injury. Although some will argue that MRI investigation can yield similar results, in my personal series MRI has been unable

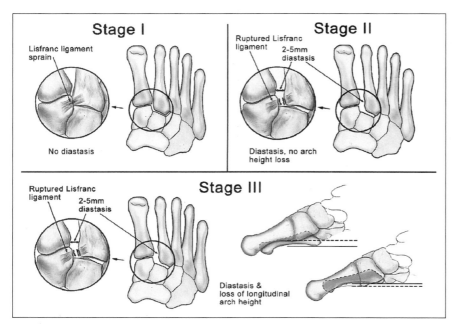

Figure 1 Midfoot sprain classification system. Stage I is a sprain to the Lisfranc ligament with no diastasis or arch height loss seen on radiographs but increased uptake on bone scintigraphy. Stage II sprains have a first to second intermetatarsal diastasis of 1 to 5 mm because of failure of the Lisfranc ligament but no loss of arch height. Stage III sprains display first to second intermetatarsal diastasis and loss of arch height, as represented by a decrease or inversion of the distance between the plantar aspect of the fifth metatarsal bone and the plantar aspect of the medial cuneiform bone on an erect lateral radiograph. (Reproduced with permission from Nunley JA, Vertullo CJ: Classification, investigation, and management of midfoot sprains: Lisfranc injuries in the athlete. *Am J Sports Med* 2002;30:871-878.)

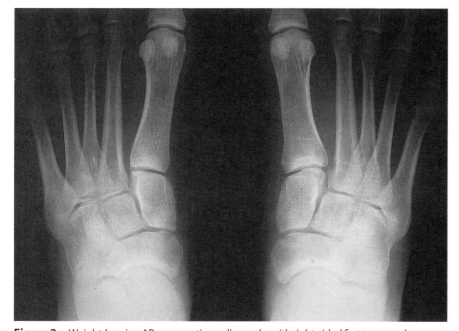

Figure 2 Weight-bearing AP comparative radiographs with right-sided first to second metatarsal bone diastasis caused by lateral displacement and failure of the second tarsometatarsal joint (B2 pattern). Note the ossification in the diastasis secondary to late diagnosis and treatment. (Reproduced with permission from Nunley JA, Vertullo CJ: Classification, investigation, and management of midfoot sprains: Lisfranc injuries in the athlete. *Am J Sports Med* 2002;30:871-878.)

to show this injury as often as the bone scan.

The sequence of capsular ligamentous disruption in a Lisfranc fracture-dislocation has been described; however, the pathoanatomy of these isolated subtle athletic injuries has not been fully investigated. My hypothesis is that stage I injury represents a dorsal capsular tear and sprain without elongation of the Lisfranc ligament. Because of the low energy imparted in this injury, the Lisfranc complex is stable and shows a normal appearance on weight-bearing radiographs. However, a bone scan will show increased uptake indicating where the injury occurred.

The stage II injury represents a greater force with elongation or disruption of the Lisfranc ligament but the plantar capsular structures remain intact. The weight-bearing radiograph may show diastasis but there will not be collapse of the longitudinal arch. Stage II injuries with B1 displacement undergo failure of the capsular ligamentous structures of the medial cuneiform and Lisfranc ligament that allows a medial deviation of the first ray. Stage II injuries with B2 displacement patterns undergo failure of the capsular ligamentous structure of the second metatarsocuneiform joint and the Lisfranc ligament, leading to the lateral displacement of the second metatarsal and diastasis. In stage III injuries, a significant force is applied to the midfoot that causes disruption of the dorsal capsule, Lisfranc ligament, and plantar capsular ligamentous structures of multiple metatarsal joints, and that may produce bony fracture.

In my series of patients with this injury, 50% of the patients with diastasis of the 1-2 metatarsal had normal non–weight-bearing radiographs. Failure to obtain weight-bearing radiographs would have resulted in misdiagnosing a subtle tarsometatarsal dislocation. Although some authors have advocated the use of stress radiographs under fluoroscopy with anesthesia, the single patient in my series who underwent stress

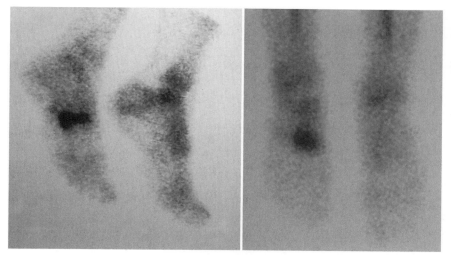

Figure 3 Diagnostic AP and lateral delayed bone scans with increased uptake at the second tarsometatarsal joint. (Reproduced with permission from Nunley JA, Vertullo CJ: Classification, investigation, and management of midfoot sprains: Lisfranc injuries in the athlete. *Am J Sports Med* 2002;30:871-878.)

radiographs displayed no diastasis until weight-bearing radiographs were obtained and a bone scan confirmed the injury. If the patient is unable to stand for a weight-bearing radiograph because of pain, another consideration is to obtain the radiograph with the patient under ankle-block anesthesia. Nevertheless, bone scintigraphy seems to be totally accurate.

━━━━━━━━■

The Solutions

Treatment Options and Rationale

The management of stable nondisplaced sprains in the athlete is not controversial; these athletes respond successfully to nonsurgical management with appropriate orthoses and rehabilitation. The management of midfoot sprain with a subtle diastasis is controversial. A subtle diastasis sprain represents a true Lisfranc injury, and the treatment differs from anatomic reduction to acceptance of the injury in the athlete.

Meyer and associates reported on 22 athletes with midfoot sprain who were treated nonsurgically; three patients had diastasis of the 1-2 metatarsal. Two of their three patients initially were misdiagnosed as having nondisplaced sprains, and the third had nonsurgical management despite a diastasis. This athlete experienced a recurring midfoot sprain with return to activity. Hence, 33% of their patients with diastasis that were treated nonsurgically continued to have pain.

Shapiro and associates have reported on nine athletes with stage II diastasis of between 2 and 5 mm. One athlete with 5 mm of diastasis was treated with open reduction internal fixation while the other eight athletes with 2 to 3 mm of diastasis had an excellent outcome at an average of 34 months, with an average time until return to sport of 4 months. In my series, two patients with similar diastasis were unable to play their respective sport at 4 and 10 months after similar nonsurgical treatment. Only after a late open reduction internal fixation were both patients able to return to sport. In my series, return to sport averaged 14.4 weeks. This timing is im-

portant for athletic trainers and coaches to understand. Midfoot strain is not a benign injury and even with proper treatment will result in significant morbidity.

Author's Preferred Treatment and Rationale

Patients with nondisplaced injury (stage I) are treated in a non–weight-bearing, well-molded fiberglass cast for 6 weeks. If the patient is pain-free on cast removal, a custom-molded orthosis that supports the medial longitudinal arch is prescribed, and the patient undergoes a sport-specific gradual return to function. If the patient is still symptomatic after cast removal, a weight-bearing ankle-foot orthosis is prescribed for an additional 4 weeks.

Patients with stage II and stage III injuries undergo closed or open reduction and internal fixation with partially threaded 4.5-mm cannulated screws (**Figure 4**). Closed reduction is possible in most patients, especially with stage II injury. Under adequate regional anesthetic control and fluoroscopic visualization, a large bone tenaculum forceps is percutaneously placed around the second metatarsal and the medial cuneiform. Under fluoroscopy the physician can watch the reduction as the tenaculum is closed. If this treatment is successful and the tarsometatarsal joint is completely closed, a percutaneously inserted guide wire for a 4.5-mm partially threaded cancellous screw is placed from the medial cuneiform through the second metatarsal to the outermost cortex of the second metatarsal. After appropriate measurement of the length, as well as drilling and tapping, a partially threaded 4.5-mm screw is inserted from medial to lateral. Stage II injuries have been subdivided into B1 and B2, in which a B1 injury has partial incongruity with medial dislocation of the medial ray or first metatarsal. This injury requires a second screw, which is inserted from

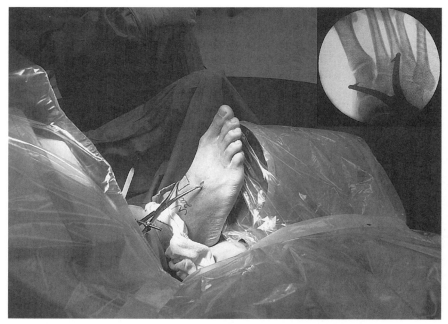

Figure 4 Percutaneous fluoroscope-guided reduction of the diastasis undertaken with a large bone tenaculum. The inset fluoroscopic image shows the reduction before cannulated screw fixation. (Reproduced with permission from Nunley JA, Vertullo CJ: Classification, investigation, and management of midfoot sprains: Lisfranc injuries in the athlete. *Am J Sports Med* 2002;30:871-878.)

the medial cuneiform into the intermediate cuneiform. B2 injuries are partial incongruity with lateral dislocation of the second metatarsal and are treated with a single percutaneous screw from the medial cuneiform to the base of the second metatarsal.

If closed treatment fails to obtain a perfect anatomic reduction or if the patient presents late, then open reduction with removal of fibrous scar tissue and closure of the diastasis followed by screw fixation is undertaken.

After surgery, patients do not weight bear for 8 weeks. Toe touch is initiated at 8 weeks, progressing to full weight bearing by week 12. Once full weight bearing has been accomplished, the patient is fit with a custom shoe orthosis to maintain the medial arch and is returned to sport-specific rehabilitation.

It is important during the immediate postoperative and the entire rehabilitative phase that the athletic trainer and/or physical therapist concentrate on motion of the flexor and extensor tendons to the great toe. In my experience, this has been an area where stiffness tends to occur and can lead to pain with great toe motion. This problem is easily solved with appropriate therapy but must be watched for carefully.

Screw removal occurs at 12 to 14 weeks in athletes weighing less than 200 lb. However, a minimum of 24 weeks before screw removal is recommended for those weighing more than 200 lb. Generally, screws are removed according to the specific athletic season, and it is not unusual for athletes to play for at least a year with the screw still in place while the arch is maintained by means of an arch support in the athletic shoe. The screw can be removed between training periods, depending on the sport.

Management of Complications

The only complications with which I am familiar are failure to recognize the injury and rediastasis once the screw has been removed. The former should be solved by paying attention to the procedure described in the previous section. If the latter occurs and the patient is symptomatic, a screw can be reinserted and left for a longer period of time; if the patient is asymptomatic, he or she can be treated with a foot orthosis inside the athletic shoe.

References

Clanton TO: Athletic injuries to the soft tissues of the foot and ankle, in Coughlin MJ, Mann RA: *Surgery of the Foot and Ankle,* ed 7. St. Louis, MO, Mosby, 1999, pp 1178.

Curtis MJ, Myerson M, Szura B: Tarsometatarsal joint injuries in the athlete. *Am J Sports Med* 1993;21:497-502.

Meyer SA, Callaghan JJ, Albright JP, et al: Midfoot sprains in collegiate football players. *Am J Sports Med* 1994;22:392-401.

Nunley JA, Vertullo CJ: Classification, investigation, and management of midfoot sprains: Lisfranc injuries in athletes. *Am J Sports Med* 2002;30:871-879.

Shapiro MS, Wascher DC, Finerman GA: Rupture of Lisfranc's ligament in athletes. *Am J Sports Med* 1994;22:687-691.

Coding

ICD-9 CODE

838.03 Closed dislocation, tarsometatarsal (joint)

CPT CODE

28606 Percutaneous skeletal fixation of tarsometatarsal joint dislocation, with manipulation

CPT copyright © 2003 by the American Medical Association. All Rights Reserved.

Salvage of Failed Heel Pain Surgery

Lew C. Schon, MD

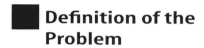

Definition of the Problem

Patient Presentation

Patients with pain after failed surgery for plantar fasciitis, heel spur syndrome, subcalcaneal bursitis, or first branch or lateral plantar nerve entrapment typically report symptoms that reflect a more neurologic process than did symptoms before surgery. Preoperative pain in the plantar medial aspect of the heel that was worse on rising in the morning may have become persistent unremitting neuralgia that is not affected by activity or posture. New symptoms often include burning, sharp, shooting, tingling, radiating, stabbing, and/or electric pain radiating from the heel into the foot and/or up the leg following the course of the tibial nerve. Pain intensity typically is unbearable and chronic from the moment of surgery. Foot cramping or spasms may occur. Patients may be unable to touch or put pressure on the medial and/or plantar-medial aspect of the heel, with abnormal gait resulting. Patients often experience a strange finding of exquisite hypersensitivity in a zone that is "numb." This phenomenon, called anesthesia doloroso, is indicative of severe nerve trauma and reflects deafferentation.

Patients whose preoperative symptoms were typical of an overuse condition (plantar fasciitis) may fare better with treatment of pain after failed surgery. Those whose preoperative symptoms were more neurologic, as in a direct impact from a fall, have a poorer prognosis. Overall, if overuse etiology is implicated in the original symptom, the prognosis is more predictable and favorable than with other more neurologic etiologies.

Physical Examination

On physical examination, patients who have failed to respond to surgery for plantar fasciitis exhibit an antalgic gait, avoiding weight bearing on the heel. Range of motion of the foot and ankle typically is unaffected. There may be decreased sensation along the course of the calcaneal nerve(s) or, less commonly, decreased sensation along the branches of the tibial nerve. Frequently, the incision(s) from previous surgery are exquisitely sensitive to touch. Percussion along the course of the tibial nerve elicits tingling, burning, or lancinating pain that travels along the course of the most affected nerve branch.

Patients may experience tenderness along the course of the nerves adjacent to the affected nerves, with pain typically noted along the sural nerve trunk, other branches of the tibial nerve, and the saphenous nerve. In patients who have had a tarsal tunnel release to alleviate heel pain, there may be pain with range of motion of the ankle. In these patients, a thickened scar with lack of normal tissue mobility is consistent with adhesions between the traumatized tissues and the nerve, a condition known as adhesive neuralgia or traction neuritis.

Signs of abnormal sudomotor or vasomotor activity such as edema, sweating, color change, and temperature change indicative of severe nerve trauma are often found and indicate complex regional pain syndrome (CRPS) type II. Spontaneous pain in the heel or along the distribution of the traumatized nerves that is not provoked by posture or activity can be a manifestation of ectopic nerve discharge or ectopic neuralgia. Pain experienced with positional changes or induced by activity or palpation is known as nociceptive neuralgia.

Differential Diagnosis

- Radiculopathy
- Systemic neuropathy
- Posterior tibial tendon rupture
- Rupture of accessory muscles in the distal medial ankle
- Space-occupying lesions, neurolemmomas, ganglions
- Subtalar arthritis
- Calcaneal stress fracture
- Subcalcaneal fat pad atrophy
- Rheumatologic disorders (seropositive and seronegative arthropathies and fibromyalgia)
- Plantar fascia rupture
- Tarsal coalition

Additional Work-up

Additional work-up includes radiographs to rule out bony lesions. A technetium Tc 99m bone scan may be helpful to rule out stress fractures or occult subtalar arthritis. MRI may show posterior tibialis tendon pathology that may have been previously unrecognized but

349

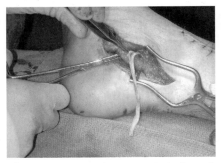

Figure 1 The saphenous vein is ligated, and the vein is harvested.

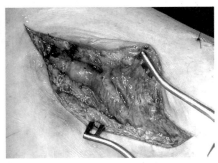

Figure 2 The nerve has been wrapped with the saphenous vein, which was split longitudinally and wrapped around the nerve in a spiral fashion.

led to an acquired flatfoot and resulting chronic heel pain. MRI may also show neurolemmomas or other space-occupying lesions. Electrodiagnostic studies are supportive but are most useful to exclude other neurologic conditions that may cause persistent pain, such as radiculopathy, neuropathy, or more proximal nerve lesion. Nerve studies may support the presence of two nerve problems or lesions, as seen in double-crush phenomenon. Local injections of nerves or joints with anesthetic agents can help to define the location of the pathology.

The Solutions

Treatment Options and Rationale
Mechanical or other conditions such as tumors that may cause problems should be evaluated. Patients are categorized as having stump neuroma, adhesive neuralgia, nociceptive neuralgia, ectopic neuralgia, or CRPS type II. Minimally invasive treatment should be initiated, first with topical medications and short leg bracing and then with transcutaneous electric nerve stimulation units, oral medications, focal injections of steroids, and pain management with a team approach that includes psychological and rehabilitation specialists. After this initial noninvasive treatment, minimally

invasive treatments may include sympathetic nerve blocks, intravenous regional blocks, or peripheral nerve blocks. Intravenous infusion with lidocaine may be considered and, if successful, can indicate a good response to oral mexiletine.

Surgical intervention is indicated for patients with focal pathology that has not responded to the noninvasive and minimally invasive treatment alternatives. Patients are indicated for surgery when they have clinical features of unaddressed pathologies, such as focal neuroma or adhesive neuralgia, or failed or incomplete proximal nerve release. In general, the more focal and nociceptive the syndrome, the better the anticipated results.

Surgical intervention includes neurolysis, revision nerve release with vein wrap, neuroma transection and stump burial, and implantable nerve stimulation. For patients with focal stump neuromas, a revision of the prior surgery with a more proximal extension of the nerve release is considered. The stump neuroma is identified and removed from the zone of previous surgery, cut more proximally, and buried into deep tissues away from any mechanical trauma. For patients with suspected nerve entrapment, a revision neurolysis or more proximal extension of the prior neurolysis is indicated. However, tibial nerve transection is not recommended because results of this

procedure have been poor at Union Memorial Hospital, Baltimore, Maryland.

For the patient with adhesive neuralgia from scarring of the tissue bed around the nerve, a revision nerve release in conjunction with a barrier procedure such as vein wrap may be considered. In this procedure, an incision is made through the previous scar, extending more proximally and distally, and the nerve is freed from surrounding dense scar tissue. The ipsilateral saphenous vein is exposed beginning at the ankle and extending to just below the knee. Care is taken to avoid the saphenous nerve during this procedure. The branches of the vein are ligated on both sides (vein and leg side), and the vein is harvested (**Figure 1**). The vein is then inflated with local anesthetic, which maintains the vein in a distended state. The vein is split longitudinally and wrapped around the nerve endothelial side down in a spiral fashion; care is taken not to wrap the vein too tightly to avoid additional constriction of the nerve (**Figure 2**). Postoperative immobilization is for 2 to 3 weeks, with a removable brace used to facilitate ambulation and function.

Peripheral nerve stimulation (PNS) is indicated for a patient with ectopic neuralgia if the patient has had previous nerve transection or a barrier procedure. PNS is indicated with involvement of a single nerve such as the tibial nerve or one of its branches. If multiple nerves are involved, spinal cord stimulation is preferred. For those patients failing all treatments, an intrathecal indwelling pain medication pump or limb ablation with transtibial amputation may be considered.

With any of these procedures, a 50% improvement can be expected in approximately 75% of patients when the specific clinical criteria for surgeries are met. Each of the procedures also carries the risk that the condition will become worse after surgery. Recovery from these procedures tends to be prolonged, with maximum improvement occurring 6 to 30 months after surgery.

Author's Preferred Treatment and Rationale

PNS can provide relief from chronic pain for many patients and should be considered despite the demanding procedure, high maintenance, and high complication rate. An ongoing prospective study at Union Memorial Hospital found that 32 of 37 patients were satisfied with the procedure, and 45% cited overall improvement, increased walking and sleeping ability, and improved work status.

The PNS apparatus (Medtronic, Minneapolis, MN) includes a pulse generator, electrodes embedded in a silicone sheath (lead), and a connecting wire. The tibial nerve is exposed proximal to the previous surgery with the patient under general anesthesia. The wound is injected with local anesthetic, avoiding the tibial nerve. The patient is removed from anesthesia, and the lead is placed on the nerve (**Figure 3**). The lead is connected to a temporary pulse generator and current is applied to identify the area that provides maximum comfort. This area usually corresponds with paresthesias along the course of the affected nerves. If the paresthesias are unpleasant or painful, a new location on the nerve is tested. If no comfortable stimulation can be achieved, the stimulation procedure is terminated. When the stimulation produces relief, the patient is mechanically tested with deep palpation or percussion of the zones of pain, including the zone of anesthesia doloroso, to ensure adequacy of pain coverage. Manipulation and joint mobilization should be performed to ensure that the effectiveness of the stimulation does not vary

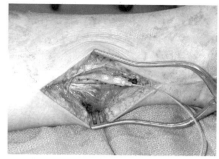

Figure 3 The lead is placed on the nerve. The location of the tibial nerve is shown.

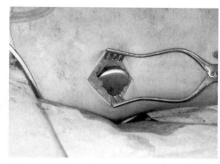

Figure 4 The pulse generator is inserted into a subcutaneous pocket in the medial thigh.

with changing tension or compression between the nerve and the electrodes.

Once the position of the leads is finalized, the leads are sutured to the epineurium. The patient is again tested for effectiveness of the stimulation. After final adjustments in lead placement are made, the patient is reanesthetized. A subcutaneous pocket is made in the medial thigh for insertion of the pulse generator (**Figure 4**). A tunneling rod is used to run the extension wire from the generator to the lead that houses the electrodes, avoiding mechanically vulnerable sites for all components. Placement of the generator in areas of fatty tissue along the posterior medial aspect of the leg, knee, or thigh is preferable. Patients are immobilized for 3 months postoperatively with a brace that can be removed for range-of-motion and strengthening exercises.

Management of Complications

Standard complications include wound problems, scar pain, stiffness, atrophy, and infection, especially if there is a history of infection. With implantable nerve stimulators, infection may occur in 5% to 7% of patients. A neurostimulator infection that is recognized early may be managed with intravenous anti-

biotics. Once there is evidence of purulence, some or all of the hardware must be removed. Patients may experience changes in the pattern of stimulation that often can be easily dealt with by external reprogramming of the implanted devices. Less frequently a fluid leak, which can result in altered or lost stimulation, may occur somewhere along the wires or lead. This problem correlates with specific electrical readings that can be made externally by means of interrogation between the external programmer and the internal implanted device. Revision of the hardware is warranted when a fluid leak causes loss of effective coverage. The leads may fatigue and break, an occurrence recognizable through external interrogation of the system, the lead may lose effective contact on the nerve, or the nerve may become less susceptible to the neurostimulation; these conditions may require revision of the lead. The implantable pulse generator is replaced after 1 to 3 years, depending on the intensity of the electrical stimulation required by the patient. The generator replacement is a simple procedure that can be performed with the patient under local anesthesia and with minimal recovery complications.

References

Schon LC, Anderson CD, Easley ME, et al: Surgical treatment of chronic lower extremity neuropathic pain. *Clin Orthop* 2001;389:156-164.

Schon LC, Baxter DE: Heel pain syndrome and entrapment neuropathies about the foot and ankle, in Gould JS (ed): *Operative Foot Surgery*. Philadelphia, PA, WB Saunders, 1994, pp 192-208.

Schon LC, Lam PW, Easley ME, et al: Complex salvage procedures for severe lower extremity nerve pain. *Clin Orthop* 2001;391:171-180.

Coding

ICD-9 CODES

337.22	Reflex sympathetic dystrophy of the lower limb
355.5	Tarsal tunnel syndrome
355.71	Causalgia of lower limb
355.8	Mononeuritis of lower limb, unspecified
355.9	Mononeuritis of unspecified site
729.2	Neuralgia, neuritis, and radiculitis, unspecified
928.21	Crushing injury of lower limb, ankle
959.7	Injury, knee, leg, ankle, and foot
997.61	Neuroma of amputation stump

CPT CODES

20926	Tissue grafts, other (eg, paratenon, fat, dermis)
28035	Release, tarsal tunnel (posterior tibial nerve decompression)
28899	Unlisted procedure
64575	Incision for implantation of neurostimulator electrodes; peripheral nerve (excludes sacral nerve)
64585	Revision or removal of peripheral neurostimulator electrodes
64590	Incision and subcutaneous placement of peripheral neurostimulator pulse generator or receiver, direct or inductive coupling
64595	Revision or removal of peripheral neurostimulator pulse generator or receiver
64704	Neuroplasty; nerve of hand or foot
64708	Neuroplasty, major peripheral nerve, arm or leg; other than specified
64782	Excision of neuroma; hand or foot, except digital nerve
64784	Excision of neuroma; major peripheral nerve, except sciatic
64787	Implantation of nerve end into bone or muscle (list separately in addition to neuroma excision)
95972	Complex brain, spinal cord, or peripheral (except cranial nerve) neurostimulator pulse generator/transmitter, with intraoperative or subsequent programming, first hour
95973	Complex brain, spinal cord, or peripheral (except cranial nerve) neurostimulator pulse generator/transmitter, with intraoperative or subsequent programming, each additional 30 minutes after first hour (List separately in addition to code for primary procedure)

SECTION 7
Trauma

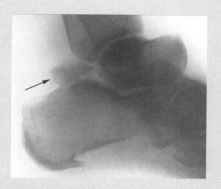

Roy W. Sanders, MD
Editor

Management of Postoperative Wound Complications

L. Scott Levin, MD, FACS

■ Definition of the Problem

Patient Presentation

The potential for postoperative wound complications in the foot and ankle may be even greater than for other regions because of the diminished amount of subcutaneous soft tissue and muscle in the foot and ankle and the dependent position of the extremity. Any excessive postoperative pain and swelling at the foot and ankle region should generate a high index of suspicion that there may be more serious postoperative complications, such as formation of sinus tract, skin slough, compartment syndrome, skin necrosis, or a deep infection.

Cellulitis is not uncommon after foot and ankle surgery. With a superficial infection, the skin is warm and erythematous. The area may be tender to palpation but is not fluctuant. In patients with deep infections, the skin may be warm, tender, swollen, and fluctuant. Joint infections may be manifested by increasing pain with joint motion, swelling, and drainage.

Physical Examination

Infections after foot and ankle surgery can have disastrous consequences. These are more common after open traumatic injuries than after elective surgical procedures because open traumatic injuries are contaminated with microorganisms that are on the skin or introduced at the time of injury. Furthermore, tissue destruction and devascularization may hinder the body's infection-fighting mechanisms.

A fracture blister is a delamination of the skin layers when the epidermis separates from the dermis. The inflammatory fluid that is contained within these blisters is sterile. If these blisters are unroofed, then the sealed environment is converted to the equivalent of a second-degree burn, and the dermis will reepithelialize. After sterility of the fracture blister is violated, a granulating wound can become colonized with bacteria. The dermis usually is intact unless the internal pressure from a hematoma or protruding bone fragment causes skin necrosis similar to a pressure sore. This necrosis can occur when there has been marked pressure on the blood supply to the skin for a prolonged period of time. When fracture blisters are removed from this type of skin contusion, the underlying dermis may appear dusky white or even dark black, indicating full-thickness soft-tissue necrosis. Soft-tissue reconstruction may be indicated if internal fixation is to be considered.

SOFT-TISSUE INFECTIONS

Infection is one of the most important factors contributing to nonunion, loss of function, and other complications after foot and ankle trauma. However, early recognition and aggressive treatment may limit the severity of the complication.

In cellulitis, leukocyte count and temperature may be elevated. The most common causative organisms are *Staphylococcus aureus* and *Streptococcus*. It is important to distinguish cellulitis from a deep infection associated with abscess formation. Patients who are immunocompromised are at a higher risk for a deep infection after surgery. Plain radiographs, MRI, and needle aspiration may be helpful in making the diagnosis.

A critical differential diagnosis is necrotizing fasciitis, characterized by rapidly progressive necrosis and edema of the subcutaneous fat and fascia progressing to septic shock, end organ failure, and amputation or death. The most common causative organism is *Streptococcus pyogenes*, but the infection may be caused by multiple organisms. Clinical signs of necrotizing fasciitis include tense edema and erythema that do not respond to antibiotics or elevation. Patients appear toxic and febrile. Crepitus may be palpable because of subcutaneous emphysema. The wound often appears unremarkable, even though the deep infection is intensive.

In cases of necrotizing fasciitis, the relatively unremarkable appearance of the extremity may be misleading and may contribute to a delay in diagnosis, resulting in increased morbidity and potential mortality. Liquefactive necrosis of the fat and superficial fascia leads to the characteristic appearance of grayish, watery, and foul-smelling fluid often referred to as "dishwater pus." The necrotic fascia present at the time of surgical exploration is pathognomonic of necrotizing fasciitis.

JOINT INFECTION
The patient may have fever, leukocytosis, and an elevated erythrocyte sedimentation rate. Plain radiographs, MRI, and needle aspiration can be helpful in making the diagnosis. Existing joint implants may be associated with infections.

OSTEOMYELITIS
Bone infections after foot and ankle surgery can be difficult to diagnose and treat, especially following surgery on the calcaneus. Fever, local pain, edema, exudative drainage, and elevated leukocyte count and erythrocyte sedimentation rate are typical findings but in some cases may be absent. Radiographic changes may include a rounded lucent area surrounded by sclerotic bone, with nearby cortical or periosteal thickening. MRI and indium In 111 labeled leukocyte scintigraphy may be helpful in defining the extent of the infection. Definitive diagnosis is made by bone biopsy and culture.

DEHISCENCE
Wound dehiscence may occur after foot and ankle surgery, even in the absence of infection. Causative factors include poor nutritional status, postoperative swelling, and a history of smoking. The dehisced wound may become infected.

Differential Diagnosis
- Soft-tissue necrosis
- Fracture blister
- Dehiscence
- Superficial infection/cellulitis
- Deep infection
- Abscess
- Osteomyelitis
- Necrotizing fasciitis
- Gas gangrene

Additional Work-up
None

The Solutions

Treatment Options and Rationale
Performing an open reduction through unstable skin may cause postoperative swelling, inability to close the wound, or breakdown of skin edges resulting in exposure of bone and hardware. Whether or not to operate through areas of fracture blisters is controversial. When surgery is delayed for 7 to 10 days to allow blisters to resolve before proceeding with surgery, the hematoma that accumulates after an acute fracture may permeate the tissues and cause fibrosis and a "woody" consistency. If the fracture blister ruptures, turbid fluid accumulates under the collapsed epidermal layer, and colonized bacteria from

Table 1 Débridement Guidelines

Structure	Procedure
Skin, subcutis	Sharp knife dissection to bleeding dermis. Trim edges 1 to 2 mm to create a clean wound edge. Cut fat back to healthy fat. Punctate bleeding and minimal hemosiderin staining.
Fascia	May be débrided sharply and should be removed if not vascularized. Fascia has a network of vessels that can be seen with loupe magnification. Low threshold to open and extensively explore compartment.
Muscle	Débride to contractile muscle (ie, pink and bleeding from cut myosomes).
Bone	Fragments devoid of soft-tissue attachments should be removed.
Nerve	Be aware of cutaneous nerves; they may cause painful neuromas. Epineurium can be removed if contaminated fascicles remain. If the nerve is not vascularized, it can be salvaged provided it does not desiccate and wound closure is achieved early.
Vessels	Remove perforated, thrombosed segments. Identify main vascular trunks. If not intact and if there is no flow, segmental vascular débridement is done. Ligate major and clip minor vessels. Identify, mark, and protect viable major vessels that can be used for vascular access during immediate or delayed free tissue transfer.
Pulsatile irrigation	Caveat: avoid implosion of foreign material, hydrodissection of tissue planes, and insufflation of tissues.
Deflate tourniquet	Evaluate structures for bleeding.

(Reproduced with permission from Germann G, Sherman R, Levin LS: *Decision Making in Reconstructive Surgery*. New York, NY, Springer-Verlag, 1999.)

the skin may cause an infection. Surgery under these circumstances may be associated with a greater risk of deep infection and wound slough. Therefore, it may be safer to operate through an unruptured fracture blister, perform the appropriate internal fixation and wound closure, and subsequently treat the blister bed as a burn. With this approach, the dermis may seal, and the wound may epithelialize using silver sulfadiazine cream as skin therapy.

SOFT-TISSUE INFECTION

Five to 7 days of treatment with oral antibiotic agents such as dicloxacillin, cephalexin, or clindamycin often is sufficient for cellulitis. Soaks, splinting, elevation, and intravenous antibiotics may be required. Surgical débridement and broad-spectrum antibiotic therapy are the initial treatment of deep infection with abscess formation. Once the infecting microorganism is identified from cultures, the antibiotic is changed accordingly.

The technique for surgical drainage is based on obtaining adequate decompression of infected compartments. Multiple incisions may be

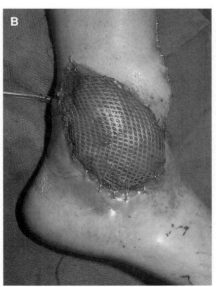

Figure 1 Tibia after bone débridement with punctate bleeding from healthy bone (paprika sign).

required to débride deep infections of the foot. Extensive irrigation and débridement often is required to remove infected tissue adequately, and multiple procedures may be necessary to eradicate the infected debris. Placing drains and packing open wounds may allow ongoing drainage while the wound begins to heal.

Treatment of necrotizing fasciitis includes immediate radical débridement well beyond the margins of the cellulitis until healthy muscle and fascia can be seen. Early surgical débridement is the key for successful treatment. Repeated débridement is warranted at 12- to 24-hour intervals until the infection is controlled. A combination of intravenous broad-spectrum antibiotics, such as a cephalosporin against *Staphylococcus* and *Streptococcus*, penicillin against anaerobes, and gentamicin against gram-negative organisms, is recommended. The patient may deteriorate rapidly, and early amputation may be necessary to control a rapidly progressing infection.

JOINT INFECTION

Joint infection is promptly treated with irrigation, débridement, and intravenous antibiotics. Severe joint space infections may cause marked fibrosis, chondrolysis, and destructive arthritis. The joint wound and capsule are left open, and drains are used. Postoperative irrigating systems are no longer used. The prognosis depends on duration of the infection before treatment, the causative organism (gram-negative infections are worse than gram-positive infections), preexisting joint disease, host immunocompetence, and the specific joint involved. Treatment of a joint implant infection includes implant removal and intravenous antibiotic therapy for

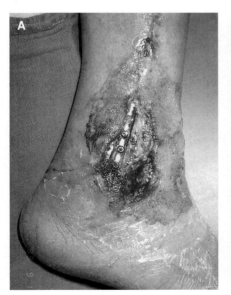
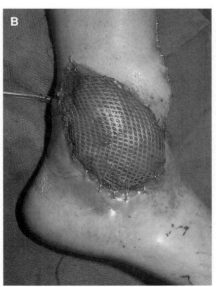
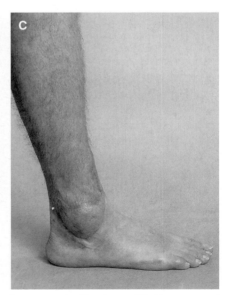

Figure 2   A, Exposed implant at the lateral malleolus. **B,** Immediate postoperative result after removal of implants, débridement, and coverage with a free rectus abdominis flap and skin graft. **C,** Result 1 year after surgery.

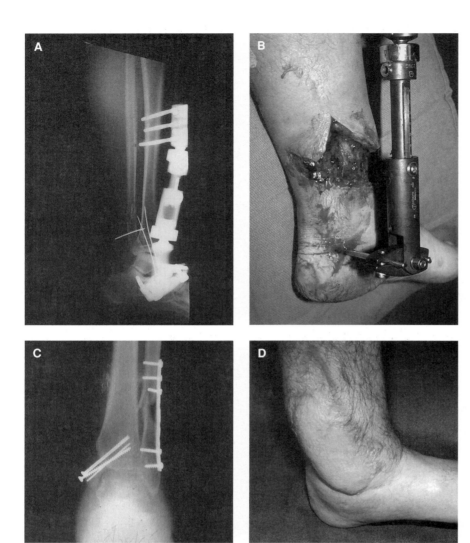

Figure 3   Radiograph (**A**) and clinical photograph (**B**) of a type IIIB open fracture that initially was treated with débridement, percutaneous pins, and external fixation. The inadequate fixation was revised 5 days after the injury using plates and screws. At the same time, the soft-tissue defect was covered with a free gracilis flap. Radiographic (**C**) and clinical (**D**) appearance 1 year after surgery.

6 weeks. After eradication of the infection, arthrodesis may be performed.

OSTEOMYELITIS

Chronic osteomyelitis may be characterized by a chronic wound that has remained arrested in one of the stages of wound healing. The goal of treatment is to convert this chronic wound into an acute wound so that it can progress through the normal phases of wound healing. The factors necessary for adequate healing include adequate

blood flow to the area, control of the infection, and correction of medical and nutritional abnormalities.

Palpable pulses do not always signify sufficient arterial tissue inflow. If the flow is questionable, a formal noninvasive vascular evaluation including toe pressures may be performed. An ankle-brachial index of less than 0.45 or a toe pressure of less than 40 mm Hg is considered a risk factor for poor wound healing. If the flow is insufficient, débridement may

be limited until the limb has been revascularized. Venous congestion and lymphedema are managed with elevation, compression, stockings, and pneumatic pumps.

Osteomyelitis may be addressed with surgical débridement to excise all nonviable tissue until the wound surfaces consist of normal, healthy tissue. Intraoperative assessment is used to guide the débridement of skin, subcutaneous tissue, fascia, muscle, tendons, nerves, and vessels (**Table 1**). For bone débridement, evaluation of sequestrum and necrotic segments of cortical bone may be guided by both preoperative CT scans or tomograms and intraoperative appearance. All areas devoid of vascularity are resected, and cortical bone stripped from the periosteum is débrided. Bone is débrided until punctate bleeding from the cortical bone is encountered, indicating bone viability (**Figure 1**). After débridement, treatment includes soft-tissue coverage, reduction of dead space, antibiotic beads, fracture stabilization, and delayed bone grafting, if necessary.

Osteomyelitis that develops in conjunction with internal fixation or exposed hardware is characterized by the presence of microorganisms in the glycocalyx (**Figure 2**). The glycocalyx is a biofilm or slime that adheres to metal, dead bone, and tissue, protecting bacteria from antibiotics and host-defense mechanisms. Therefore, metallic implants are removed when possible. However, stable implant retention may be beneficial to minimize the potential for edema and soft-tissue trauma associated with motion at the fracture site. In the presence of acute infections, after open reduction and internal fixation, the implant often remains stable and may be left in place until the fracture unites. If the fracture is not united and the hardware is not providing stability, the hardware is removed and the fracture stabilized with an external fixator. If the internal fixation device is stabilizing a nonunited

Table 2 Treatment Algorithm for the Management of Soft-Tissue Problems Associated With Calcaneal Fractures

Type	Description*	Treatment
Type I	Closed fracture treated with ORIF, unable to close skin	Porcine grafts, skin grafts: split or meshed
Type II	Closed fracture treated with ORIF, wound breakdown	Local flaps (medialis pedis, dorsalis pedis abductor hallucis fasciocutaneous, myocutaneous, peroneal flap, anterior tibial fasciocutaneous, flexor hallucis brevis)
Type III	Traumatic large soft-tissue loss with adequate bone stock	Local flaps Free flaps Skin (radialis, lateral arm, scapular/parascapular flap) Muscle (rectus abdominis, gracilis flap)
Type IV	Traumatic loss of bone and soft tissue	Free iliac crest bone graft and skin flap
Type V	Calcaneal osteomyelitis	Local muscle flap Free muscle flap (rectus abdominis, gracilis flap) Amputation
Type VI	Unstable heel pad	Custom orthotic, custom shoe Free skin flap (innervated radialis, lateral arm flap)

*ORIF, open reduction and internal fixation
(Adapted with permission from Levin LS, Nunley JA: The management of soft-tissue problems associated with calcaneal fractures. *Clin Orthop* 1993;290:151-156.)

articular fracture, it is usually left in place. For infected nonunions, the internal fixation device is removed, and the fracture may be stabilized with an external fixator. The historic practice of making relaxing incisions to pull the skin together with retention sutures is strongly discouraged because the results are unpredictable and failure may be more difficult to salvage.

Soft-tissue closure is addressed according to the level of complexity required from the simplest procedure (primary closure) to skin grafting, lo-cal flaps, regional flaps, and free tissue transfer. However, primary closure or skin grafting for treatment of osteomyelitis rarely is feasible, and distally based flaps such as the sural flap are usually too small and may not help to eliminate dead space. Therefore, free tissue transfer may be required in the foot and ankle region. Free flap coverage within 1 week after trauma generates the most favorable results (**Figure 3**). Chronic wounds may be covered with a free flap immediately after they are transformed to healthy, acute wounds.

The free tissue transfer may be tailored to the requirements of the recipient site, and flap selection may vary by region. For the ankle and dorsum of the foot, thin and pliable soft-tissue coverage is provided by fasciocutaneous flaps such as the lateral arm flap, radial forearm flap, and scapular or parascapular flap. We believe the radial forearm flap is the most desirable plantar resurfacing for the heel (**Table 2**), particularly if the flap is innervated (**Figure 4**). Muscle flaps are preferred on exposed bone, in

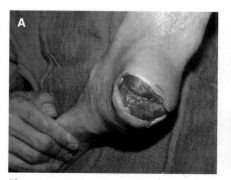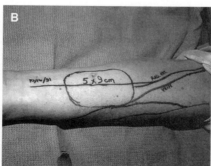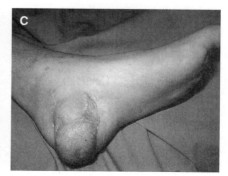

Figure 4 **A,** Chronic heel wound resulting from calcaneal osteomyelitis (type V, Table 2). **B,** Flap design before harvesting the radial forearm flap. **C,** Appearance 1 year after transfer of a free radial forearm flap.

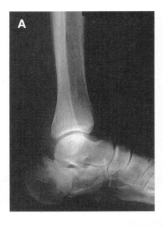

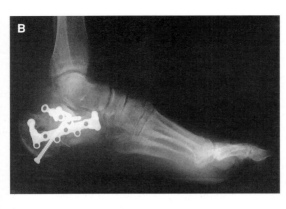

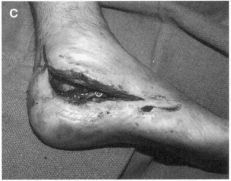

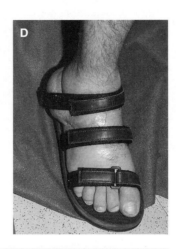

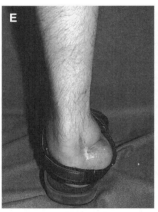

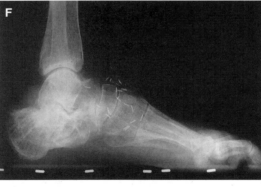

Figure 5 **A,** Intra-articular calcaneal fracture. **B,** Improved bony alignment after open reduction and internal fixation with plates and screws. **C,** Exposed hardware following skin slough after surgery (type V, Table 2). Clinical (**D** and **E**) and radiographic (**F**) results after removal of hardware and transfer of a free serratus flap.

nonunion, usually is postponed for 6 to 8 weeks after flap coverage.

After free tissue transfer, the interface between the flap and the surrounding tissue must be healed before any type of weight bearing is allowed, usually a minimum of 4 to 6 weeks after surgery. This is particularly important for the plantar surface of the foot, such as the heel, instep, and forefoot. Furthermore, elevation of the foot and ankle for 2 to 3 weeks is important for healing of venous and lymphatic channels. After 2 weeks, patients are encouraged to place the lower extremity in a dependent position for brief periods of progressively increased duration.

Skin grafts should be totally epithelialized and the dermal elements hypertrophied before weight bearing; this usually requires 6 weeks. Skin grafts should be kept moist with emollients and water-based creams to prevent dessication and fissuring, which may cause localized infection and breakdown of the skin graft over the muscle.

After the flaps are fully healed, patients often will benefit from a customized shoe with an orthotic insert, custom molded to accommodate height and shape changes from free tissue transfer. The shoe may be modified with a double-upright brace to stabilize the foot in the varus-valgus plane and a rocker bottom. Chronic edema is managed with a custom-measured support stocking.

Author's Preferred Treatment and Rationale

We have described our preferences to the various conditions in the previous section.

Management of Complications

The entire chapter covers this topic.

The author wishes to acknowledge the contribution of Christoph Heitmann, MD, in the creation of this chapter.

——————————■

large cavitary defects, and in the reconstruction of the entire plantar surface of the foot. The most frequently harvested muscles include the rectus abdominis, gracilis, and serratus anterior (**Figure 5**). The muscle flaps are covered with a skin graft. These flaps may resist shear forces and become fibrotic with time. If the muscle flaps do not fill the existing dead space, antibiotic spacers may be useful. Bone grafting, if required for bone defects or

References

Attinger CE, Bulan E, Blume PA: Surgical debridement: The key to successful wound healing and reconstruction. *Clin Podiatr Med Surg* 2000;17:599-630.

Donley BG, Philbin T, Tomford JW, Sferra JJ: Foot and ankle infections after surgery. *Clin Orthop* 2001;391:162-170.

Hallock GG: Utility of both muscle and fascia flaps in severe lower extremity trauma. *J Trauma* 2000;48:913-917.

Levin LS, Nunley JA: The management of soft-tissue problems associated with calcaneal fractures. *Clin Orthop* 1993;290:151-156.

Patzakis MJ: Management of acute and chronic osteomyelitis, in Chapman MW (ed): *Chapman's Orthopaedic Surgery*, ed 3. Philadelphia, PA, Lippincott Williams and Wilkins, 2001, pp 3533-3560.

Coding

ICD-9 CODES

457.2   Lymphangitis (chronic) (subacute)

682.7   Other cellulitis and abscess; foot, except toes

730   Osteomyelitis, periostitis, and other infections involving bone

CPT CODES

11043   Debridement; skin, subcutaneous tissue, and muscle

11044   Debridement; skin, subcutaneous tissue, muscle, and bone

15756   Free muscle or myocutaneous flap with microvascular anastomosis

15757   Free skin flap with anastomosis

28899   Unlisted procedure, foot or toes

Pilon Fractures

Paul T. Fortin, MD

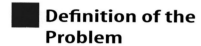

Definition of the Problem

Patient Presentation

Pilon fractures may be caused either by a serious traumatic event that is associated with multiple injuries or by rotational injuries. Specific knowledge of the mechanism of injury is an important aspect of the assessment of pilon fractures. High-energy injuries such as motor vehicle accidents, falls from heights, and industrial accidents must be differentiated from low-energy, torsional injuries. The likelihood of postoperative complications including wound healing problems and long-term sequelae, such as posttraumatic arthrosis, is directly related to the energy of the injury. High-energy injuries are more likely to be associated with complications. Injuries that involve significant axial loading are typically associated with implosion of the articular surface. The position of the foot at the time of impact will determine whether the injury occurs in the anterior, posterior, or central portion of the plafond. In addition to the compressive load, shearing or tensile forces can lead to marked disruption of the bone and gross instability at the level of the metaphysis.

Physical Examination

A systematic assessment of the neck, back, and other extremities is neces-

sary to rule out associated injuries, especially in patients who sustained a high-energy trauma. Some of these patients may be sent to referral centers several hours or days after the injury. This delay can lead to considerable swelling, and the soft tissue may be compromised. The integrity of the skin and degree of injury to the soft tissues is an extremely important part of the assessment. A disruption of skin integrity with open fractures usually occurs at the level of the medial metaphyseal-diaphyseal junction where the spike of the tibial shaft extrudes. Closed fractures with significant displacement can cause tenting of the thin medial soft-tissue envelope, creating an impending open fracture. This necessitates prompt reduction and provisional immobilization. Fracture blisters can occur several hours after the injury and reflect the severity of the soft-tissue injury. Blood-filled fracture blisters should be differentiated from those filled with clear fluid because blood-filled blisters represent a full-thickness epidermal injury. The size and position of these blisters should be considered when planning definitive treatment. The Tscherne classification system differentiates high-grade and low-grade injuries to the soft tissue in patients with closed fractures. Factors associated with more severe injuries to the soft tissue include direct trauma, blistering, compartment syndrome, muscle damage, and compromise of the neurovas-

cular system. Serial physical examinations are necessary in patients who have high-energy injuries because of the risk of compartment syndrome. The clinician should also be aware of any comorbid factors such as a history of diabetes mellitus, tobacco use, neuropathy, peripheral vascular disease, and advanced age that may affect the patient or affect the proposed treatment plan.

Differential Diagnosis

- Trimalleolar ankle fracture with large posterior plafond fragment
- Supination-adduction ankle fracture with marginal impaction of plafond

Additional Work-up

Radiographic evaluation should include AP, lateral, and mortise views of the ankle as well as full-length views of the tibia when there is diaphyseal extension of the fracture. Three anatomic zones to be considered in the decision-making process are the articular surface, the metaphysis, and the fibula. Traction radiographs can be very helpful to define the pattern of the fracture (**Figure 1**). This is most commonly done after provisional stabilization with an external fixator. Occasionally, a radiograph of the opposite ankle can be useful for comparison and preoperative planning. CT is essential for the preoperative work-up. Compared with plain radiographs, CT scans more accu-

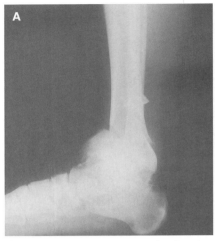

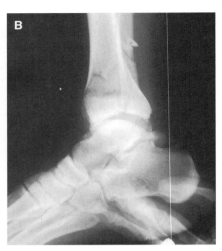

Figure 1 **A,** Lateral radiograph of a pilon fracture. **B,** After longitudinal traction was applied, the fracture pattern was better defined.

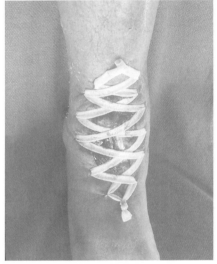

Figure 2 Attempted surgical treatment of a pilon fracture 2 days after injury resulting in an inability to close the wound; ultimately, flap coverage was required.

rately define the position and displacement of the fragments, amount of comminution, and any impaction of the articular surface. A CT scan often helps to define the most appropriate surgical approach based on the location of the major fracture lines. As with plain radiographs, the CT scan is often more informative after the fixator has been placed and there is distraction of the fragments. The AO/

ASIF classification system of distal tibial fractures is relatively simple and generally accepted.

The Solutions

Treatment Options and Rationale

One of the most important issues regarding treatment of pilon fractures is the decision to render definitive treatment. If a surgeon has limited experience treating pilon fractures or limited support from services such as plastic surgery, provisional stabilization and transfer to a tertiary care center is advisable. Poorly executed attempts at definitive fixation can result in disastrous bone and soft-tissue complications that are very difficult to salvage (**Figure 2**).

Indications for surgical intervention include significant articular incongruity (> 2 mm), axial malalignment, and open fractures. Most of these fractures are best treated with surgical intervention to restore joint congruity and limb alignment. Cast immobilization may be the best treatment option for nondisplaced frac-

tures or fractures in patients with significant comorbid factors.

The timing of a definitive fixation is crucial. Particularly with high-energy fractures, a lengthy delay of tibial fixation is often necessary. Until recently, many surgeons suggested operating immediately (within 6 hours) after injury or after a delay of only 5 to 7 days. Soft-tissue swelling peaks approximately 5 to 7 days after injury, and delaying definitive fixation for 2 to 3 weeks is often necessary to avoid soft-tissue complications. Fracture blisters should be healed and the skin should wrinkle before definitive fixation of the tibia is performed. In the acute setting, the fracture should be provisionally stabilized. This is typically done with a simple spanning external fixator placed in distraction. This approach has several advantages in that immediate ligamentotaxis helps to reduce the fracture fragments, decreases dead space and hemorrhage, and lessens the amount of ongoing insult to the soft tissue. Stabilization of the fracture also limits the amount of manipulation and stripping necessary at the time of definitive fixation. Often only the large impacted articular segments need direct manipulation. Spanning external fixation can be done in conjunction with open reduction of the fibula. The indications for fibular plating are somewhat controversial. Plating the fibula potentially contributes to provisional stability and restoration of limb alignment. It demands, however, that the fibular reduction be anatomic. Plating the fibula in a malrotated or shortened position will likely prevent anatomic reduction of the tibia because of the attachments of the anterolateral tibial articular fragment to the fibula (**Figure 3**). In patients with high-energy injuries, the fibula is commonly markedly comminuted; thus, restoration of proper fibular length and rotation can be difficult.

Methods of definitive fixation are numerous and involve either plat-

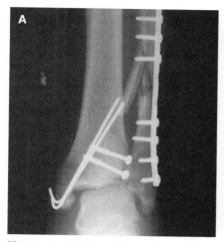

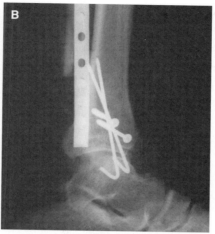

Figure 3 AP (**A**) and lateral (**B**) radiographs showing inadequate restoration of fibular length, precluding anatomic reduction of the tibial articular surface, resulting in a malunion.

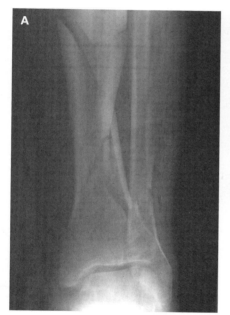

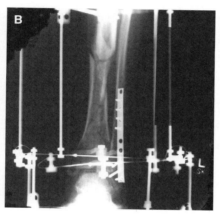

Figure 4 **A,** Distal tibia fracture with significant diaphyseal comminution. **B,** Small pin/wire external fixator used for stabilization.

ing or a combination of external fixation with minimal internal fixation. The method used for a particular fracture is selected based on fracture type, soft-tissue status, and surgeon preference.

EXTERNAL FIXATION WITH MINIMAL INTERNAL FIXATION

External fixation with minimal internal fixation is a popular means of treating pilon fractures. It has the advantage of limiting the dissection of soft tissue and diminishing the risk of wound problems. CT is used to identify the primary fracture lines, and incisions are made directly over the fracture after indirect reduction with ligamentotaxis. Because of the difficulties in manipulating multiple articular fragments through a limited incision, this technique can result in a less than anatomic reduction of the articular surface. Relative indications for this technique include fractures with large articular fragments, severe metaphyseal comminution, open fractures, and situations in which soft tissues are not amenable to an extensile exposure. Articulated fixators that span the ankle joint are popular because they are relatively easy to apply. It may take months for the metaphyseal component of the fracture to heal before the fixator can be removed. Therefore, stiffness of the ankle and subtalar joint may result. Small pin fixators that do not cross the ankle joint are an alternative if the articular fragments are sufficiently large to ensure stable fixation of the distal portion of the construct.

PLATING METHODS

Plating methods have evolved from the use of large bulky implants that require extensile exposure to the use of lower profile implants. Percutaneous plating techniques can help to minimize dissection of soft tissue and limit wound problems. The basic AO tenets proposed by Ruedi and Allgower are still useful: (1) restoration of fibular length, (2) articular reconstruction, (3) bone grafting the tibial metaphysis, and (4) medial or anterior buttress plating to stabilize the metaphysis. The standard pilon incision is one fingerbreadth lateral to the tibial crest and proceeds along the course of the tibialis anterior tendon. Dissection is performed just medial to the tibialis anterior tendon taking care to leave the tendon and paratenon intact. A full-thickness flap is elevated off the anterior tibia in an extraperiosteal fashion in an attempt to leave periosteal attachments intact. Because of intact tibia-fibula ligamentous attachments, the anterolateral joint fragment often acts as a reference point to which the remainder of the articular surface can be reconstructed provided that the fibular length and rotation have been adequately restored. The anteromedial fragment can be hinged open to expose any centrally depressed fragments. Any subarticular voids that exist after restoration of the

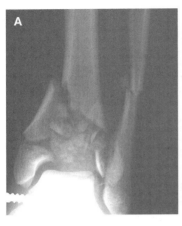
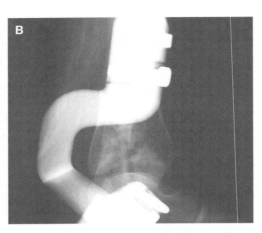
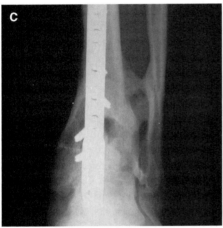
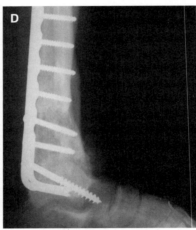

Figure 5 Tibial plafond fracture with severe comminution and irreparable articular surface (**A** and **B**) treated with primary fusion (**C** and **D**).

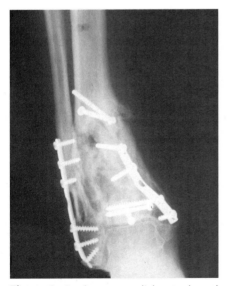

Figure 6 Inadequate medial metaphyseal fixation leading to varus malunion.

This technique, however, is associated with fewer anatomic reductions and a higher incidence of osteoarthrosis. Immediate open reduction and plating is associated with an unacceptably high rate of wound problems and subsequent deep infection. Results from a series of staged treatment of tibial plafond fractures suggest that these fractures can be safely managed with open reduction and plating if tibial fixation is sufficiently delayed. Tibial fixation was delayed an average of 2 to 3 weeks in these series. Deep infection due to wound problems occurred in up to 3% of patients with closed fractures. Long-term follow-up of surgically treated tibial plafond fractures suggests that osteoarthrosis will develop in most patients even when the joint surface has been reduced anatomically. Patient satisfaction and functional outcome, however, do not necessarily correlate with the radiographic severity of osteoarthrosis.

Author's Preferred Treatment and Rationale

For most tibial plafond fractures, staged reconstruction is an effective method of treatment. Application of a simple spanning external fixator and simultaneous plating of the fibula are performed in the acute setting. The incision is typically made on the posterolateral border of the fibula to ensure an adequate skin bridge between the anterior and lateral incisions. Extreme care is taken to ensure that fibular length and rotation are properly restored. External fixator pins must be placed away from the proposed incision(s) for tibial fixation. CT after fixator placement is typically helpful to confirm the position and orientation of the fragments once they have been provisionally reduced with ligamentotaxis. The information obtained from imaging studies serves as the basis for a well-designed preoperative plan. A delay in fixation of the tibia of 2 weeks or more is not uncommon depending on the status of the soft tissues.

joint surface should be bone grafted. Finally, the metaphyseal component of the fracture is neutralized with a medial and/or anterior plate.

CONCLUSIONS

Advances in surgical techniques and appropriate timing of procedures have significantly improved the results of surgical management of tibial plafond fractures. Currently published data are inadequate to make valid comparisons of the two most commonly used methods, external fixation with limited internal fixation and staged open reduction and plate fixation. A spanning external fixator and limited internal fixation minimizes wound problems and results in acceptable functional outcome for most patients.

A standard anteromedial pilon incision is used if there is significant residual displacement of the articular segments following placement of the external fixator that necessitates an extensile exposure. Distraction across the joint facilitates visualization of the articular surface. The joint is reconstructed working from posterior to anterior and lateral to medial. Fragments are provisionally fixed with Kirschner wires. Bioabsorbable pins or small diameter screws are sometimes helpful to address small intercalary articular fragments. Small fragment cortical lag screws are used for larger articular fragments. A low profile or precontoured neutralization or buttress plate is used on the anterior and/or medial surface depending on the fracture pattern. If the fracture fragments are large and not markedly displaced or impacted, smaller incisions made directly over the fracture lines and percutaneous reduction with the aid of fluoroscopy may be used to reconstruct the joint surface. The metaphyseal component of the fracture can then be stabilized by placement of a percutaneous precontoured plate that is placed in a subcutaneous tunnel on the medial face of the tibia. This procedure avoids undermining of the tenuous skin over the subcutaneous portion of the tibia.

Open fractures are treated in much the same manner. After adequate irrigation and débridement, large articular pieces of the plafond may be fixed provisionally in the acute setting with lag screws, provided further soft-tissue dissection and insult to the soft tissue is not required to accomplish the fixation. A spanning external fixator is placed, and definitive fixation is performed after coverage of the soft tissue. In patients with soft tissues that are persistently in poor condition or who have severe metaphyseal comminution, a small pin circular fixator may be used as a definitive means of treatment (**Figure 4**).

In the rare instance that the ar-

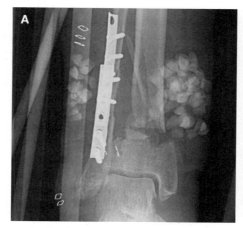
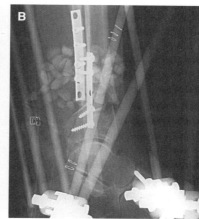
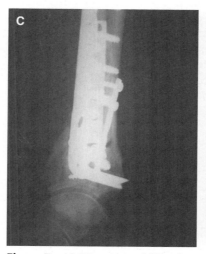
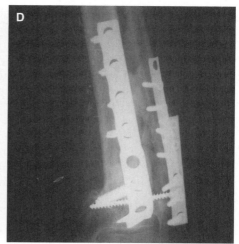

Figure 7 AP (**A**) and lateral (**B**) radiographs of an open tibial plafond fracture with severe metaphyseal comminution treated initially with an articulated fixator. Delayed union of the metaphyseal component necessitated a second procedure. AP (**C**) and lateral (**D**) radiographs following posterior plating and bone grafting.

ticular surface is irreparable because of severe comminution, consideration is given to primary arthrodesis (**Figure 5**). This can be done through a posterolateral approach in the subacute period once all swelling has subsided and healing has occurred.

Management of Complications

Wound problems are the most frequent complication following pilon fractures. Fortunately, most of these are superficial skin sloughs that can be managed effectively with oral antibiotics, local wound care, and delaying ankle motion. Proper timing of the surgical procedures, limited exposure,

low-profile implants, and skillful surgical technique are factors that can help minimize disastrous deep wound infection. With contemporary techniques of staged fixation, the reported incidence of deep wound infection is estimated to range from 0% to 6%. Deep infection necessitates wide débridement, long-term antibiotics, soft-tissue coverage, and secondary skeletal reconstruction in some patients. Cavitary bone defects may be amenable to simple bone graft techniques. Large segmental defects can be extremely difficult to manage and may require bone transport to salvage the limb. Amputation may be necessary in patients who have an uncontrollable infection, large skeletal and/or soft-tissue defects, or in patients with co-morbid factors that preclude limb salvage.

Articular malunion is the result of inadequate reduction and is very difficult to manage. Depending on the degree of joint incongruity, ankle fusion may be the only alternative when inaccurate reduction leads to advanced posttraumatic arthritis. Large articular pieces left unreduced resulting in malunion can occasionally be treated with intra-articular osteotomy and restoration of the joint surface if detected before the development of significant arthritis or ankylosis of the joint.

Inadequate medial metaphyseal fixation can result in extra-articular malunion as the distal tibia collapses into varus (**Figure 6**). A supramalleolar osteotomy may be required to restore axial alignment to the extremity and prevent accelerated wear of the tibiotalar joint.

Inadequate restoration of fibular length can also lead to an extra-articular malunion and may prevent reduction of the tibial articular surface (**Figure 3**).

Nonunions typically occur at the metaphyseal-diaphyseal junction and can be the result of traumatic devascularization of the fracture fragments, soft-tissue stripping at the time of surgery, and inadequate stabilization of the metaphyseal component of the fracture. Failure of the metaphysis to heal is sometimes encountered with the articulated fixator that spans the ankle joint if the fixator has reached its limit because of pin loosening and/or infection. This failure to heal necessitates another procedure such as bone grafting and plating to heal the tibia (**Figure 7**).

The development of tibiotalar arthrosis is a factor of the energy of the injury, the amount of joint comminution leading to cartilage necrosis, and the quality of the reduction. Ulti-

mately, functional outcome is closely related to the accuracy of the reduction. An anatomic reduction, however, does not prevent tibiotalar arthrosis. Long-term follow-up studies suggest that posttraumatic arthrosis occurs in more than half of all patients who sustain a pilon fracture despite an anatomic reduction. The development of posttraumatic arthritis presumably reflects the impaction injury to the articular surface leading to irreparable damage to the cartilage. Loss of ankle motion is a common consequence of tibial plafond fractures. Rigid fixation that allows early ankle motion can help limit this loss of motion. External fixators that span the ankle and/or subtalar joint are associated with greater loss of motion of both of these joints.

The author wishes to acknowledge the contribution of Greg Nowinski, MD, in the creation of this chapter.

References

Etter C, Ganz R: Long-term results of tibia plafond fractures treated with open reduction internal fixation. *Arch Orthop Trauma Surg* 1991;110:277-283.

Patterson MJ, Cole JD: Two-staged delayed open reduction and internal fixation of severe pilon fractures. *J Orthop Trauma* 1999;13:85-91.

Ruedi T: Fractures of the lower end of the tibia into the ankle joint. Results 9 years after open reduction and internal fixation. *Injury* 1973;5:130-140.

Sirkin M, Sanders R, Dipasquale T, Herscovici D: A staged protocol for soft tissue management in the treatment of complex pilon fractures. *J Orthop Trauma* 1999;13:78-84.

Coding

ICD-9 CODES

823.20   Fracture of tibia and fibular, shaft, closed tibia alone

823.22   Shaft, closed, fibula with tibia

823.30   Shaft, open, tibia alone

823.31   Shaft, open, fibula with tibia

823.80   Unspecified part, closed tibia alone

823.90   Unspecified part, open, tibia alone

CPT CODES

27824   Closed treatment of fracture of weight bearing articular portion of distal tibia with or without anesthesia; without manipulation

27825   Closed treatment of fracture of weight bearing articular portion of distal tibia with skeletal traction and/or requiring manipulation

27826   Open treatment of fracture of weight bearing articular portion of distal tibia with internal or external fixation; fibula alone

27827   Open treatment of fracture of weight bearing articular portion of distal tibia with internal or external fixation; tibia only

27828   Open treatment of fracture of weight bearing articular portion of distal tibia with internal or external fixation; both tibia and fibula

Malunion of Ankle Fracture and Chronic Syndesmotic Instability

David B. Thordarson, MD

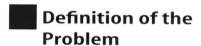 Definition of the Problem

Patient Presentation

All patients with an ankle fracture malunion or chronic syndesmotic instability have a history of previous trauma. Perhaps the most important historic information will be their prior treatment of the given problem. Most patients will fall into one of two categories: failed nonsurgical or failed surgical treatment.

All details from previous operations including timing of surgery, type of fixation, bone quality, and intraoperative difficulties are important. The patient's age is also a consideration but perhaps is not as important as previous treatment. Older patients (age 65 years or older) with an asymptomatic ankle who will be placing less stress on their ankle may not require surgical reconstruction. Younger patients (age 40 years or younger) with any significant degree of talar displacement will require surgical reconstruction to minimize the altered joint biomechanics and contact stresses. The degree and location of pain should be noted when questioning the patient; however, factors related to pain will not likely influence decisions regarding reconstruction of malunited fractures. Other potentially pertinent information includes complications from previous surgical treatment such as infection or wound healing problems.

Physical Examination

Physical examination should include a standard evaluation of the ankle, including range of motion, because significant stiffness preoperatively bodes poorly for postoperative range of motion. The location of previous scars and any distal sensory deficits should be recorded.

In patients with malunion of an ankle fracture, medial-lateral stress testing (Cotton test) can be performed to identify any gross medial-lateral instability. This test is somewhat subjective, but it can provide useful information about the degree of widening of the syndesmosis. In patients with syndesmotic instability, pain with external rotation stress at the ankle and tenderness of the syndesmosis and deltoid ligament should be noted.

Standard radiographic assessment should include three weight-bearing radiographs (AP, lateral, and mortise views) of the ankle. In patients with ankle fracture malunion, comparison views of the opposite ankle should be obtained to measure the degree of displacement. The degree of displacement can be determined by measuring the medial clear space, the tibiofibular clear space, and the talocrural angle. Although the tibiofibular clear space has been used to determine the degree of lateral displacement of the talus, I rely more on the medial clear space because it is the easiest to view and the most reproducible on a mortise radiograph.

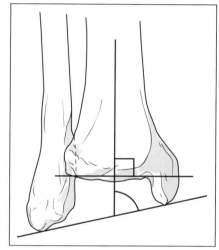

Figure 1 The talocrural angle is used to evaluate fibular shortening compared with the contralateral, normal side. (Adapted with permission from Rolfe B, Nordt W, Sallis JG, Distefano M: Assessing fibular length using bimalleolar angular measurements. *Foot Ankle* 1989;10:106.)

The talocrural angle can be quite helpful in determining the degree of fibular shortening (**Figure 1**). External rotation deformity can be difficult to discern on plain radiographs. Some lateral impaction of the plafond might be observed in patients with shortening of the fibula, in addition to lateral shift of the talus, and this impaction may require surgical attention.

Differential Diagnosis
- None for ankle fracture malunion
- Chronic ligamentous pain without instability for syndesmotic injuries

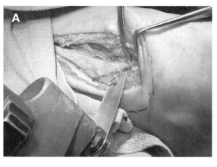
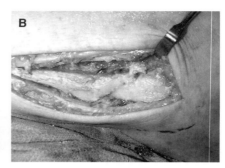
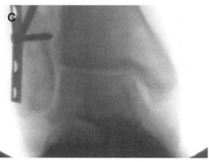
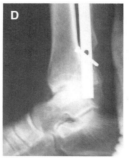

Figure 2 **A,** Intraoperative photograph showing the oblique osteotomy of a malunited supination-external rotation ankle fracture. **B,** Subsequent translation of the osteotomy with approximately 5 mm of lengthening. **C,** Intraoperative mortise image with reduced medial clear space and talocrural angle. **D,** Postoperative lateral view demonstrating lengthening through osteotomy and hardware.

Additional Work-up

In patients with syndesmotic instability, external rotation stress views of the ankle can be obtained to look for medial clear space widening. In patients with an ankle fracture malunion, on occasion, CT just proximal and through the ankle joint can be helpful to identify an external rotation component to the malunion deformity.

■ The Solutions

Treatment Options and Rationale
ANKLE FRACTURE MALUNION

The most important factor in selecting the treatment of an ankle fracture malunion is the severity of persistent displacement in the context of the pa-

tient's age. Most ankle fracture malunions will cause some degree of pain, although on occasion patients will have little or no pain at the time of surgical intervention. In younger patients (age 40 years or younger), however, any significant degree of displacement will lead to significant changes in contact stresses and thus eventual degenerative changes. Biomechanical studies have demonstrated that persistent lateral shift of the talus, shortening of the fibula, and to a lesser extent, external rotation, all lead to increased contact stresses in the ankle joint. In a young patient, this can be anticipated to lead to degenerative changes over time. Patients who have lateral shift of the talus with shortening and impaction of the lateral plafond are at high risk for rapidly developing arthritic changes. If a young or middle-aged patient (approximately age 40 years or less) has any combination of 2 mm of lateral

shift of the talus, 2 mm of shortening of the fibula, or 5° of external rotation of the distal fibular fragment, I believe that surgical reconstruction is indicated. There is no nonsurgical treatment of this problem except palliative bracing, but this will not improve the abnormal contact stresses.

Ankle malunions will generally fall into one of two anatomic types: (1) residual of supination-external rotation injuries with a malunited long oblique fracture at or near the level of the syndesmosis, or (2) pronation-external rotation deformities that have a malunion at a variable level proximal to the ankle joint. In both scenarios, it is easiest to reconstruct the malunion by essentially recreating the initial fracture deformity.

Supination-external rotation fracture malunions are best treated by attempting to recreate the plane of the initial fracture in the distal fibula (**Figure 2**). The external rotation deformity can be corrected by taking additional bone off the lateral aspect of the osteotomy such that the external rotation corrects when the osteotomy is fixated. Lengthening of this osteotomy is performed by sliding along the obliquity of this osteotomy, as is the lateral translation (**Figure 2**, *B*). Fixation usually includes some type of small fragment plate and screws placed laterally and shaped to fit the sometimes unusual contour of the lateral fibula after this corrective osteotomy. In general, up to 5 mm of lengthening can be achieved without having to use a push-pull screw. A lag screw should be placed across the osteotomy before applying the plate.

Pronation-external rotation malunions are best treated by recreating the fracture transversely through the fibula and proximal to the syndesmosis (**Figure 3**). With significant shortening, which is frequently a significant component of this deformity, significant mobilization of the distal fragment, including disruption of the intraosseous ligaments and mem-

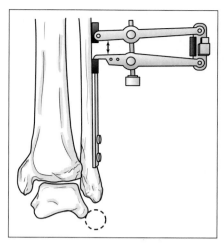

Figure 3 A push-pull screw is placed proximal to the plate to allow for distraction of the ankle to reestablish appropriate length. (Adapted with permission from Marti RK, Besselaar FP, Raaymakers E: Malunion, in Ruedi TP, Murphy WM (eds): *AO Principles of Fracture Management*. New York, NY, Thieme, 2000, p 793).

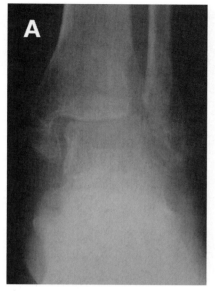

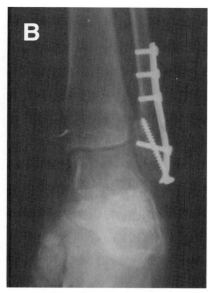

Figure 4 **A,** Preoperative AP view demonstrating malunited supination-external rotation bimalleolar ankle fracture. **B,** Postoperative AP view demonstrating plating with reduction obtained through the malunion site in the fibula. Attempts at reduction of the medial malleolus led to fragmentation with subsequent excision with suture anchor present in medial malleolar remnant used to repair deltoid ligament.

brane up to the osteotomy, is usually necessary to allow the distal translation of this fragment. While mobilizing the distal fibular fragment, it is frequently necessary to débride all of the fibrous tissue and ligamentous remnants in the interosseous area using a small curved rongeur. I find that it is usually easiest to secure a small fragment plate with screws to the distal fragment and distract this by placing a push-pull screw proximally and using either a distractor or a lamina spreader between the push-pull screw and the proximal edge of the plate to reestablish normal length. Intraoperative radiographs can be very important to assess the talocrural angle to confirm that the necessary amount of intraoperative lengthening has been obtained. Syndesmotic screws can help to reduce any lateral translation of the distal fibular fragment. If necessary, despite being contrary to conventional surgical wisdom, a syndesmotic lag screw can be placed if difficulty is encountered when reducing the lateral translation.

In both supination- and pronation-external rotation malunions with any degree of lateral talar shift, a separate arthrotomy directly overlying the medial gutter of the ankle is needed to permit débridement of the deltoid ligament remnants, which frequently prevent closure of the medial clear space. In addition, after the lateral malleolar fragment has been reduced intraoperatively, the reduction of the talus can be assessed through this medial arthrotomy both visually and by palpation with a Freer elevator. After intraoperative fixation, AP, lateral, and mortise radiographs or fluoroscopic images should be obtained to assess the degree of correction (**Figure 4**).

SYNDESMOTIC INSTABILITY AND PAIN

Patients with syndesmotic instability may have pain in the syndesmosis that is diffuse throughout the ankle or localized over the deltoid ligament. If preoperative external rotation stress radiographs demonstrate persistent instability, débridement of the syndesmosis and placement of syndesmotic fixation is indicated. I prefer making a

small incision laterally just along the anterior edge of the fibula at the level of the syndesmosis to allow direct access to the syndesmosis for débridement with a rongeur. After completely débriding the syndesmosis interosseous ligament, two syndesmotic screws can be placed to maintain this reduction. In cases of Maisonneuve malunion, it may be necessary to perform a fibular lengthening osteotomy in addition to débriding and reducing the syndesmosis. Assessment of the talocrural angle in preoperative comparison views of the opposite ankle can show fibular shortening.

Syndesmotic fixation choices include 3.5- or 4.5-mm fully threaded cortical screws placed through three or four cortices. Stainless steel screws have typically been used for this fixation. There are proponents for each of these options for syndesmotic fixation. Syndesmotic screws placed through all four cortices provide greater stability but do not allow toggling of the screw in the tibia and will, in theory, lead to a higher rate of screw breakage. Larger 4.5-mm screws are obviously stronger than 3.5-mm screws and are less likely to break but more likely to lead to a stress fracture through the syndesmotic screw hole in the fibula. One of the most common clinical scenarios for chronic syndesmotic instability is redisplacement of the syndesmosis after removal of syndesmotic screws. For this reason, I do not remove syndesmotic screws before 3 months and usually not until 6 months after surgery if stainless steel screws have been used.

Recent studies have shown the success of bioabsorbable screws for fixation of the syndesmosis. Fully threaded 4.5-mm polylactide screws (Bionx; Blue Bell, PA) have been successful for this indication and do not require removal (**Figure 5**).

Author's Preferred Treatment and Rationale

ANKLE FRACTURE MALUNION

I treat supination-external rotation fracture malunions by attempting to reestablish the initial oblique distal fibular fracture as described in the previous section. Frequently, there is a great deal of difficulty in translating the fracture fragment both distally and medially. A medial arthrotomy overlying the anterior aspect of the joint should be performed to débride any ligamentous and fibrous debris in the medial gutter that may be blocking reduction. In such scenarios, significant stripping of the syndesmotic ligament and everything except the anterior talofibular, calcaneofibular, and posterior talofibular ligaments is performed to increase the mobilization of the distal fibular fragment. Direct visualization of the talar reduction through the medial arthrotomy can be helpful in these situations. On occasion, a syndesmotic screw may help to maintain the reduction, even in a supination–external rotation fracture pattern.

In pronation-external rotation fractures, I typically prefer to make the osteotomy through the original

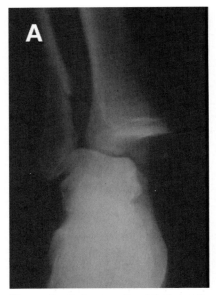
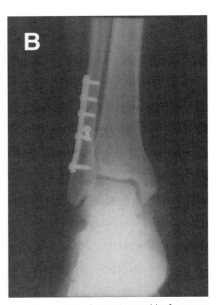

Figure 5 **A,** Preoperative AP view following pronation-external rotation ankle fracture-dislocation with obvious severe syndesmotic disruption. **B,** Postoperative AP view demonstrating anatomic reduction of the fibula. Note the empty screw hole with visible screw track where a bioabsorbable, radiolucent screw has been placed, maintaining the syndesmotic reduction.

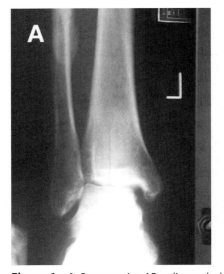
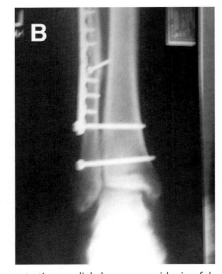

Figure 6 **A,** Preoperative AP radiograph demonstrating medial clear space widening following pronation-external rotation malunion. **B,** Postoperative AP radiograph demonstrating reduction of the medial clear space.

fracture plane. However, if it is very proximal to the ankle joint, the osteotomy can be performed 3 to 5 cm above the level of the ankle joint to minimize the disruption of ligaments. In general, a seven- or eight-hole plate is used as three screws through six cortices are secured through the plate

below the osteotomy before translating the fragment distally using a push-pull screw. Once the fracture is reduced, the proximal screws are placed, and interpositional bone graft is placed in the fracture gap. If the amount of translation performed is minimal (less than 5 mm), I use a tre-

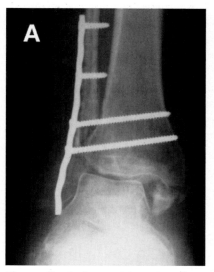
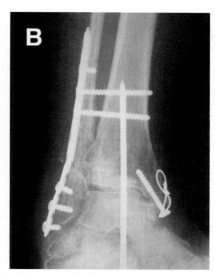

Figure 7 **A,** Preoperative AP radiograph following two failed open reduction and internal fixation procedures for bimalleolar ankle fracture. Six months following injury, the patient has markedly osteopenic bone. **B,** Postoperative AP radiograph demonstrating tension band wiring of the medial malleolus as a result of marked osteopenia and a large, smooth Steinmann pin placed across the ankle joint to stabilize the ankle at the time of surgery. Lateral fixation had bone grafting of a significant gap at the osteotomy site caused by previous marked shortening of the lateral malleolar fragment.

phine of bone graft from the calcaneus to fill the osteotomy gap. For situations with more than approximately 5 mm of translation, I use two or more trephines of bone graft from the iliac crest to fill the osteotomy gap. An additional hole distally in the plate is used for syndesmotic fixation in these patients (**Figure 6**). Frequently, the syndesmotic screw in these complex malunions is placed in a lag fashion to help force the lateral fibular fragment medially in patients who have significant lateral displacement. If a nonunion of the medial malleolus is present, it should also be reduced and fixed. With a fragment smaller than 1 cm, a tension band technique can be helpful to prevent fragmentation of the malleolar fragment when inserting hardware. On occasion, the fragment will be too small or comminuted and will require excision.

SYNDESMOTIC INSTABILITY
My preferred treatment of syndesmotic instability is predicated on proper diag-

nosis of the condition. If the patient has demonstrable instability with widening of the medial clear space on external rotation stress views, then débridement of the syndesmosis and internal fixation are necessary. A lateral incision along the anterior aspect of the fibula is made, and the syndesmosis is débrided completely with a small, curved rongeur to permit an anatomic reduction and induce a healing response. If the patient has persistent medial clear space widening, then a medial arthrotomy of the ankle joint will be necessary to remove any scarred, infolded deltoid ligament remnants from the ankle fracture malunion. For syndesmotic instability, I prefer using fully threaded 4.5-mm polylactide, bioabsorbable screws. Either one or two screws can be used, depending on the degree of instability.

In patients with a malunited Maisonneuve, I débride the syndesmosis and medial ankle gutter in a similar manner. In these situations, a large tenaculum is placed across the syndesmosis and used to compress it

maximally with the ankle in neutral flexion. A fully threaded 4.5-mm stainless steel cortical screw may be necessary for maximal strength of fixation. If there is still difficulty in reducing the syndesmosis, it can sometimes be fully reduced by placing the syndesmotic screw in a lag fashion by overdrilling the fibula, despite this technique being contrary to AO principles. If the syndesmosis still cannot be reduced, it most likely will be secondary to a malunion of the fibula. Presumably, patients will have preoperative AP and mortise radiographs that demonstrate a normal fibular length when compared with the contralateral side. If the fibula is shortened or has an external rotation deformity, then an osteotomy should be performed as outlined above.

On occasion, a patient will have a persistently symptomatic syndesmosis despite a lack of evidence of instability. An injection of lidocaine can be administered under fluoroscopic control as a diagnostic tool to confirm that the pain is emanating from the syndesmosis. A small amount of a corticosteroid can also be administered to try to achieve long-lasting pain relief. If a patient has only transient pain relief with an injection of a corticosteroid, then arthroscopic débridement of the syndesmosis may be necessary.

Management of Complications
The most common complication leading to failure of either of these procedures is persistent malunion. These problems need to be treated based on their etiology. On occasion, malunion is a result of failure of fixation because of hardware failure, lack of adequate intraoperative correction, or loss of screw fixation. Occasionally, there is a gradual loss of reduction as a patient begins bearing weight. In patients with failed fixation who have marked osteopenia, I will, on rare occasion during a revision operation, place a large Steinmann pin inferiorly from the calcaneus through the talus and

into the distal tibial plafond to maintain the reduction. This procedure will cause a small amount of articular cartilage damage and lead to some additional joint stiffness (**Figure 7**). However, in patients with severe osteopenia, this may be the only way possible to maintain a reduction. Simply sliding the new plate along the fibula and placing the screws in bone that has not previously had screws inserted is a possibility for some patients. Sometimes cancellous screws will provide greater purchase in osteopenic bone than cortical screws.

Patients with persistent pain and no demonstrated instability after syndesmotic instability surgery deserve a course of nonsurgical treatment, including therapy, bracing, and injections before any surgical treatment. In these patients, CT or MRI through the syndesmosis can be helpful to identify any pathology of bony or soft tissue.

Wound complications and/or infections should be managed with aggressive débridement and appropriate antibiotic therapy. Nonunion of an osteotomy requires takedown of the nonunion and bone grafting with either local bone graft from the calcaneus or graft from the hip. With each subsequent failed procedure, a longer period of protected immobilization is necessary.

References

Thordarson DB, Motamed S, Hedman T, Ebramzadeh E, Bakshian S: The effect of fibular malreduction on contact pressures in an ankle fracture malunion model. *J Bone Joint Surg Am* 1997;79:1809-1815.

Thordarson DB, Samuelson M, Shepherd LE, Merkle PF, Lee J: Bioabsorbable versus stainless steel screw fixation of the syndesmosis in pronation-lateral rotation ankle fractures: A prospective randomized trial. *Foot Ankle Int* 2001;22:335-338.

Weber BG, Simpson LA: Corrective lengthening osteotomy of the fibula. *Clin Orthop* 1985;199:61-67.

Yablon IG, Leach RE: Reconstruction of malunited fractures of the lateral malleolus. *J Bone Joint Surg Am* 1989;71:521-527.

Yablon IG, Heller FG, Shouse L: The key role of the lateral malleolus in displaced fractures of the ankle. *J Bone Joint Surg Am* 1977;59:169-173.

Coding

ICD-9 CODES

733.81   Malunion of fracture

733.82   Nonunion of fracture

845.03   Sprains and strains, Tibiofibular (ligament), distal

CPT CODES

27792   Open treatment of distal fibular fracture (lateral malleolus), with or without internal or external fixation

27814   Open treatment of bimalleolar ankle fracture, with or without internal or external fixation

27822   Open treatment of trimalleolar ankle fracture with or without internal or external fixation, medial and/or lateral malleolus; without fixation of posterior lip

27829   Open treatment of distal tibiofibular joint (syndesmosis) disruption, with or without internal or external fixation

Malunion of Ankle Fractures

Donald R. Bohay, MD

■ Definition of the Problem

Patient Presentation

Patients who have a malunion of an ankle fracture invariably present with pain that is usually poorly localized and accompanied by activity-related swelling that worsens as the day progresses. With increasing pain, patients tend to limit their physical activities, including the amount of time spent walking. Some patients may note a sensation of instability resulting from loss of normal ligamentous or bony support to the ankle joint.

Physical Examination

The physical examination begins with an evaluation of the patient's gait, alignment, and range of motion. An antalgic gait is usually evident, with a decrease in ankle range of motion, especially dorsiflexion. Walking on the toes is often painful. Although significant malalignment or joint instability may be evident on physical examination, alignment frequently appears to be normal. Instability is often subtle and may be difficult to detect by physical examination alone. The determination of ligamentous instability should include tests for lateral, medial, posterior, and syndesmotic instability. Lateral ligamentous instability can be evaluated by performing anterior drawer and inversion talar tilt stress tests to assess the integrity of the anterior talofibular ligament and calcaneofibular ligaments. The eversion talar tilt stress test is useful in the determination of deltoid ligament instability. Abduction external rotation stress testing is used to evaluate syndesmotic instability or lateral talar shifting. A palpable clunk noted on abduction external rotation stress indicates shifting of the talus as it abuts against the adjacent lateral malleolus. A clunk may also be evident on adduction stress testing as the subluxated talus reduces against the adjacent medial malleolus. When in doubt, stress radiographs with comparisons to the contralateral ankle should be obtained.

Radiographs should include AP, mortise, and lateral views of the affected ankle and comparison views of the contralateral ankle. When an articular step-off is suspected, oblique views are helpful to better visualize the entire joint surface. CT can be helpful in preoperative decision making and in planning surgical procedures. When ordered, CT should always be obtained in two planes with fine cuts of 1 to 2 mm.

An AP radiograph is useful in evaluating syndesmotic widening by measuring the tibiofibular overlap and the tibiofibular clear space. The tibiofibular overlap is defined as the overlap between the anterolateral tibial prominence and the medial border of the fibula. The tibiofibular clear space measures the distance between the lateral border of the posterior tibial malleolus and the medial border of the fibula at a distance 1 cm proximal to the tibiotalar joint (**Figure 1**, *A*). Tibiofibular overlap values less than 10 mm are considered abnormal, and tibiofibular clear space measurements greater than 5 mm are abnormal. A mortise view is useful in measuring the medial tibiotalar clear space, which should be equal to the joint space of the plafond and no more than 4 mm (**Figure 1**, *B*). Shenton's line of the ankle is also assessed, which is the contour of dense cortical bone across the distal tibia and over the syndesmotic space to the fibula, where a small bony spike is seen (**Figure 1**, *C*). The talocrural angle and talofibular arcuate line are measured on the mortise view and are useful in determining fibular length. The talocrural angle (normally 83° or within 2 mm of the opposite ankle) is the angle formed by drawing a line that connects the tips of the medial and lateral malleoli with a line perpendicular to the tibial articular surface (**Figure 1**, *D*). The arcuate line is normally an unbroken circle that connects the lateral talar articular surface and the inferior recess in the distal fibula that houses the peroneal tendons (**Figure 1**, *C*). Alterations in fibular length will lead to changes in these measurements compared with normal or compared with the opposite ankle.

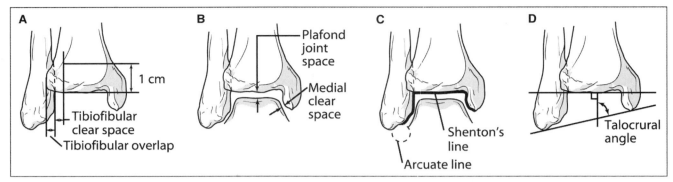

Figure 1 Radiographic measurements of a normal ankle. **A,** AP view. Tibiofibular overlap and tibiofibular clear space should be greater than 10 mm and less than 6 mm, respectively. **B,** Mortise view. The medial clear space should be symmetric to the remaining joint space and less than 4 mm. **C,** Mortise view. Shenton's line and the talofibular arcuate line should be unbroken. **D,** The talocrural angle should be 83° ± 2° and within 2° of the opposite ankle.

Differential Diagnosis
- Nonunion
- Neuropathic joint
- Infection
- Reflex sympathetic dystrophy or neuropathic pain

Additional Work-up
When contemplating reconstruction of a malunited ankle fracture, laboratory tests such as a complete blood cell count with differential, erythrocyte sedimentation rate, and C-reactive protein might be considered. Scintigraphic or MRI studies should be considered if there is a history of or concern about an infectious process. Nerve conduction velocity studies can be performed if neuropathy is suspected, and a vascular work-up might be completed if peripheral vascular disease is suspected based on the clinical examination. Appropriate medical consultation and work-up should be pursued when necessary to ensure that the patient is a sound candidate for surgical treatment.

The Solutions

Treatment Options and Rationale
In the past, patients with malunited ankle fractures were followed until symptoms become intolerable, at which point arthrodesis would be performed. In the past 2 decades, there has been renewed interest in early restoration of anatomic osseous and articular alignment and stability in patients with a malunited ankle fracture. This renewed interest has corresponded with an increased understanding of the natural history of these malunited fractures and the likelihood of the development of arthritis. Favorable results have been reported for clinical studies of malunited fibula fractures treated with osteotomy and realignment. The indications for reconstruction of malunited fibula fractures have been expanded as a result of these data.

Recent biomechanical studies have enhanced understanding of the changes in tibiotalar contact stresses associated with malunited fractures. Changes in tibiotalar contact stresses and contact surface area are now known to occur with fibular shortening or translation of as little as 2 mm and with external rotation of as little as 5°. These increases in contact stresses can occur even in the absence of any shift in the talus. The fact that symptomatic fibular malunions can occur despite evident talar instability would support the notion that isolated fibular displacement can alter tibiotalar joint mechanics.

Two distinct types of ankle malunions have been identified. (1) Overt malunions are those in which talar displacement or tilt is obvious on standard radiographs. (2) Occult malunions are those in which no discernable talar displacement or radiographic abnormality is evident on casual inspection of radiographs. On closer inspection, subtle degrees of fibular shortening or malrotation that corresponded with poor clinical results were observed. These abnormalities ultimately require realignment osteotomy to achieve satisfactory outcomes.

The most common cause of malunions around the ankle is inadequate reduction or fixation of AO type B or C ankle fractures. Often the fibula heals in a shortened, translated, or externally rotated position, resulting in a deformity that adversely affects the distal tibiofibular, talofibular, and tibiotalar articulations. When the fibula shortens, the normal buttressing effect of the lateral malleolus is lost, and the talus may shift or rotate laterally. When left alone, lateral plafond impaction with premature wear of the lateral aspect of the joint results in a valgus deformity. If the fibula has been reduced but the syndesmosis has been inadequately stabilized, the syndesmosis may widen, again leading to lateral talar subluxation and premature wear (**Figure 2**). Biomechanical studies indicate that

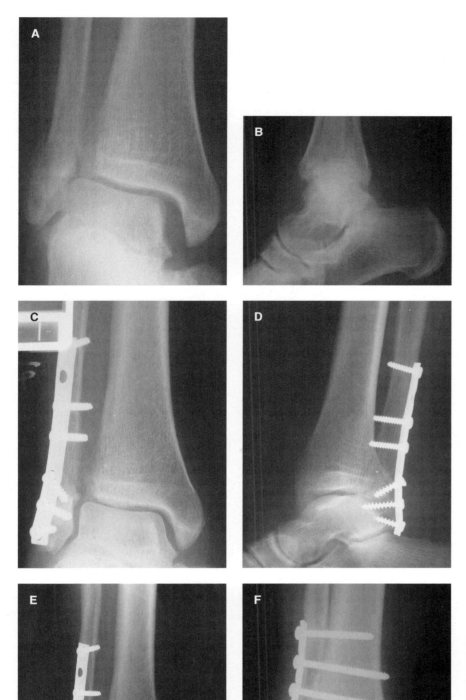

Figure 2 AP **(A)** and lateral **(B)** radiographs of a 62-year-old woman with type I diabetes mellitus who sustained a Weber B fibula fracture treated by open reduction and internal fixation. Postoperative mortise **(C)** and lateral **(D)** radiographs show a well-reduced medial clear space. Six months later, syndesmotic widening is noted on abduction stress angle radiograph **(E)**. Note the laterally subluxated talus, widened tibiofibular clear space, and decreased tibiofibular overlap. **F,** Mortise radiograph obtained after open reduction and internal fixation of the syndesmosis and medial ankle débridement. Multiple syndesmotic screws were used to stabilize syndesmosis. The patient had an excellent clinical result at 1-year follow-up.

contact surface area is decreased, and contact stresses on the lateral aspect of the tibiotalar joint are increased under such scenarios, which likely accelerate lateral plafond impaction and cartilaginous wear. Reconstructive osteotomy restores normal anatomy, and joint mechanics help reverse adverse changes in contact pressure and contact surface area associated with malreduction.

Extension deformities of the fibula can also be seen in AO type C ankle fractures or following treatment of pilon injuries associated with a fracture of the fibular shaft (**Figure 3**). These deformities usually are a result of poor initial reduction, which can easily be compromised by extensive cortical comminution. The deformity is exaggerated at the level of the talofibular articulation and leads to anterior translation of the lateral malleolus. This alters the relationship of the syndesmosis and talofibular articulation, leading to lateral ankle pain. This altered relationship may also contribute to anterior talar translation, commonly observed after certain anterior pilon fractures.

Malunited medial and posterior malleolar fractures are much less common. Very little information regarding posterior malleolar malunions has been published. Because the posterior malleolar fragment often indirectly reduces when the fibular fracture is reduced, residual displacement of the posterior malleolus should lead to an evaluation of fibular malreduction. Posterior malleolar fragments that are less than 25% of the total surface area of the joint are not associated with posterior instability, and reconstruction of smaller malunited fragments should be performed only if the fragment causes significant pain relating to an articular step-off. Posterior tibiotalar instability resulting in malunion of larger fragments will lead to rapid joint destruction and is a direct indication for reconstructive osteotomy if

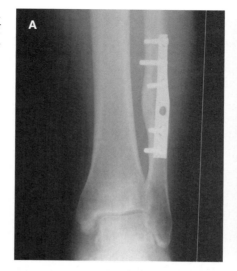
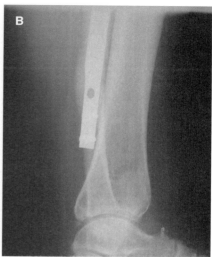
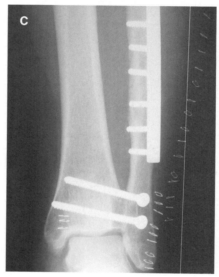
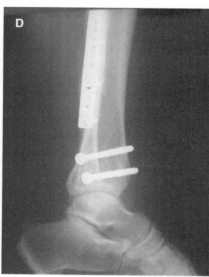

Figure 3 Postoperative AP (**A**) and lateral (**B**) radiographs of 42-year-old woman with a Weber C ankle fracture and malunited fibular fracture resulting from poor initial reduction show an extension deformity of the fibula. The patient reported lateral ankle pain on presentation. AP (**C**) and lateral (**D**) radiographs after syndesmosis revision with fibular osteotomy and open reduction and internal fixation. The patient had complete pain relief and an excellent clinical result.

irreversible changes in the joint have not already been demonstrated.

Malunited medial malleolar fractures most frequently occur following nonsurgical treatment of unstable or displaced ankle fractures. Because of the difficulty in maintaining alignment with immobilization alone, unstable ankle fractures are generally treated surgically. Certain fracture patterns are associated with a higher

incidence of malreduction, even with surgical treatment. Supination adduction injuries of the ankle are associated with an oblique or vertical medial malleolar fracture and may have medial articular impaction at the medial plafond. They can easily be malreduced with open reduction and internal fixation if care is not taken to place lag screws perpendicular to the fracture line and/or reduce the impacted

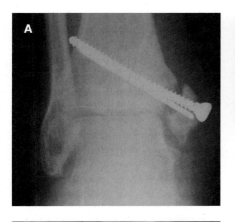
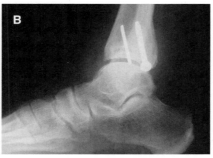
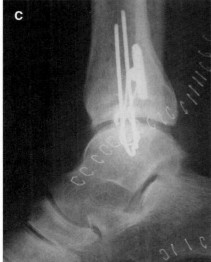
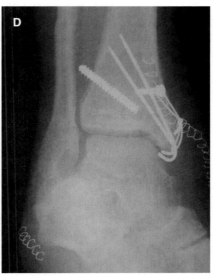

Figure 4 AP **(A)** and lateral **(B)** radiographs of a 32-year-old man with ankle pain following open reduction and internal fixation of a medial malleolus fracture show malunited/nonunited fracture. Lateral **(C)** and mortise **(D)** views obtained after revision with open reduction and internal fixation and bone grafting. Note that anatomic alignment was restored, and the patient had a pain-free clinical result.

injury. Certainly, the sooner the reconstruction is performed, the more likely that primary fracture lines can be identified to facilitate reduction and the less likely that severe fibrosis or irreversible articular changes will occur. The decision for early intervention should be made after careful assessment and clinical judgment of the likelihood for significant improvement of symptoms and the prevention of progressive wear.

Author's Preferred Treatment and Rationale
FIBULAR MALUNIONS

Characterizing fibular malunions as occult or overt malunions is helpful in planning surgical treatment. An occult malunion has no lateral talar shift or talar tilt and is associated with an isolated fibular deformity. If treated early, the primary fracture line can be identified and mobilized, and all intervening callus and fibrous tissue can be removed. Fibrosis will be particularly evident in the anterior syndesmotic area and will need to be resected to allow proper reduction of the syndesmotic joint. The distal fragment needs to be mobilized distally and internally rotated in external rotation type injuries, which are the most common types encountered. This procedure requires some syndesmotic release in addition to resection of syndesmotic scar tissue. Once that has been accomplished, the distraction can be performed by using a laminar spreader or bone distracter.

Visualizing the talofibular articulation and syndesmosis by maintaining an anterior dissection helps to facilitate the reduction. Once achieved, the reduction is provisionally held with Kirschner wires placed transversely from the fibula into the tibia and talus. The reduction is then confirmed with radiography, with attention to restoration of the tibiofibular clear space, medial clear space, tibiofibular overlap, talocrural angle, and arcuate line. Once a satisfactory

component (**Figure 4**). Standard placement of lag screws from inferomedial to superolateral should be avoided because it leads to translational forces that tend to displace the medial malleolar fracture superiorly, resulting in an articular step-off. Any discussion of the treatment of ankle malunions should, therefore, include prevention of malunions through primary anatomic reduction and rigid stabilization of the injured components that lead to joint incongruity or instability. A complete synopsis of this topic is beyond the scope of this discussion.

The decision to intervene with a reconstructive procedure can be difficult, particularly if the patient has very few symptoms. Often the bone quality will be poor as a result of disuse osteopenia, and fibrosis and scars may jeopardize placement of the incision. The best time to intervene has not been clearly defined. Reconstructions delayed for up to 3 years after initial fracture management may produce satisfactory functional results if significant arthritic wear of the joint is not evident. Most untreated instances of significant malalignment, however, progress to arthritis within 1 year of reduction is confirmed, the fibula is stabilized with a 1/3 tubular plate along the posterolateral or lateral surface. If the primary fracture line was reestablished, supplemental bone grafting typically is not needed. When a transverse osteotomy is performed, the gap resulting from the fibular lengthening should be filled with autogenous bone graft. Corticocancellous graft is recommended for defects of 1 cm or more, but smaller defects can be filled with cancellous graft obtained from the ipsilateral proximal tibia.

Because of the soft-tissue mobilization in the syndesmosis, a transsyndesmotic screw is used to stabilize the distal tibia to the distal fibula if the syndesmosis has been rendered unstable. This screw is placed through the plate and across four cortices, in nonlag fashion, after the syndesmotic reduction is obtained. The screw is held with a large bone clamp placed across the distal tibia and fibula. In overt malunions, the talus must first be reduced under the tibia to reduce the fibula appropriately; this procedure may require resection of scar tissue in the medial joint space or osteotomy of a malunited medial malleolar fracture. Once the medial clear space is reduced and the talus is positioned appropriately, the fibula is reduced and stabilized in the same manner as in occult fibular malunions. Postoperatively, patients are placed into a bulky compressive splint until the incisions are dry and the swelling has subsided, usually for 10 to 12 days. Patients are then maintained in a removable cast boot to allow for early range-of-motion exercises. Weight-bearing activities can be performed, as tolerated, once bony union is obtained, which usually occurs within 6 weeks after surgery.

MEDIAL MALLEOLAR MALUNIONS

The approaches to treatment of medial malleolar malunions are based on the same principles as for treatment of lateral malleolar malunions. The goal should be anatomic restoration of the joint surface. Bone quality often can be poor as a result of disuse, and adjustments in fixation may be needed if standard lag screw fixation is inadequate. A tension band construct, medial spring plate, or buttress plate are alternative fixation solutions. Large malunited fragments should be osteotomized and reduced using direct visualization into the joint with an anteromedial arthrotomy. If the fragment is small and below the joint line, consideration should be made for fragment excision with deltoid reattachment, which does not adversely affect the result. Postoperative rehabilitation is similar to that after treatment of fibular nonunions.

POSTERIOR MALLEOLAR MALUNION AND NONUNION

Posterior malleolar malunion and nonunion of up to 20% of the articular surface should be treated with open reduction and internal fixation in symptomatic patients when there is little evidence of arthritis and when the fragment is significantly displaced and/or associated with joint instability. In the absence of instability, treatment decisions should be based on the likelihood that restoration of articular congruity will reduce pain. These injuries are often associated with a malreduced fibula, which should also be addressed by the treatment plan. Exposure of the posterior malleolus in the face of fibular malunion can be facilitated by transfibular osteotomy with reflection of the fibula from proximal to distal on an intact collateral ligament hinge. This requires complete release of the syndesmotic ligaments and allows for thorough débridement of the syndesmotic space. The posterior malleolus can be addressed readily through this exposure, with direct reduction of the tibial articular surface and lag screw or buttress plate fixation.

Once open reduction and internal fixation of the posterior malleolar fragment is completed, the fibula can be reduced and stabilized with a 1/3 tubular plate incorporating one or more transsyndesmotic screws. This exposure allows direct visualization of the tibial articular surface, the syndesmosis, and the lateral talus.

In the absence of any fibular malalignment, the posterior malleolus can be exposed through a posterolateral approach. If the primary fracture line can be identified, it should be taken down and all intervening callus and fibrous tissue removed to allow reduction. If no fracture line is visible, the malunion is osteotomized under fluoroscopic guidance. In this situation, an indirect reduction of the joint surface is performed. Intraoperative imaging should be used to confirm the reduction before the definitive fixation is placed. Oblique radiographs may allow better visualization of the posterior malleolar reduction than standard radiographs. Postoperative management is similar to that described previously for other surgical interventions.

Management of Complications

Complications after reconstructive procedures for malunited ankle fractures are similar in scope to those seen following any fracture surgery. Such complications might include infection, wound healing problems, nerve injury, nonunion, stiffness, and persistent pain. Wound healing becomes more problematic in patients who have extensive scar formation or adherent surgical scars. Surgical planning should include a careful assessment of where surgical incisions should be made and full-thickness soft-tissue flaps should be developed down to bone. If wound healing is impaired, prompt treatment with débridement and soft-tissue coverage procedures are paramount to a satisfactory outcome. Joint stiffness can be minimized by early joint mobilization in the postoperative period and judicious use of physiotherapy. Rigid fixation should be achieved to allow for early mobilization. Not all patients will be pain-free at the conclusion of treatment, and the patient should be advised about this in advance. Most patients, however, benefit in terms of relief of symptoms and preservation of joint function when the procedure is performed in appropriate candidates. Clinical experience and judgment regarding the surgical skills required must take precedence over technological advances. An arthrodesis should be considered when reconstruction is not feasible or does not achieve the desired results.

The author wishes to acknowledge the contribution of John G. Anderson, MD, in the creation of this chapter.

References

Miller SD: Late reconstruction after failed treatment for ankle fractures. *Orthop Clin North Am* 1995;26:363-373.

Thordarson DB, Motamed S, Hedman T, Ebramzadeh E, Bakshian S: The effect of fibular malreduction on contact pressures in an ankle fracture malunion model. *J Bone Joint Surg Am* 1997;79:1809-1815.

Weber D, Friederich NF, Muller W: Lengthening osteotomy of the fibula for post-traumatic malunion: Indications, technique and results. *Int Orthop* 1998;22:149-152.

Wyss C, Zollinger H: The causes of subsequent arthrodesis of the ankle joint. *Acta Orthop Belg* 1991; 57(suppl 1):22-27.

Yablon IG: Treatment of ankle malunion. *Instr Course Lect* 1984;33:118-123.

Yablon IG, Heller FG, Shouse L: The key role of the lateral malleolus in displaced fractures of the ankle. *J Bone Joint Surg Am* 1977;59:169-173.

Coding

ICD-9 CODES

733.81   Malunion of fracture

733.82   Nonunion of fracture

CPT CODES

20900   Bone graft, any donor area; minor or small (eg, dowel or button)

20902   Bone graft, any donor area; major or large

27625   Arthrotomy, ankle, with synovectomy

27705   Osteotomy; tibia

27707   Osteotomy; fibula

27829   Open treatment of distal tibiofibular joint (syndesmosis) disruption, with or without internmal or external fixation

Occult Fractures About the Subtalar Joint

Michael P. Clare, MD

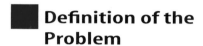

Definition of the Problem

Patient Presentation

Patients with fractures of the lateral process of the talus typically present with a clinical picture identical to that of a lateral ankle sprain and commonly are misdiagnosed as having simple ankle sprains. Misdiagnosis of these fractures, commonly known as the snowboarder's fracture, can eventually result in significant arthrosis involving both the ankle and subtalar joints.

Patients who have fractures of the anterior process of the calcaneus present with pain and swelling directly over the calcaneocuboid joint, located roughly at a point equidistant from the tip of the lateral malleolus to the base of the fifth metatarsal. These fractures occur either as avulsion fractures following an inversion injury or, less commonly, as compression fractures in higher energy abduction injuries to the foot.

Patients with fractures of the posterior process of the talus typically describe a sudden injury and have pain and swelling in the posterior ankle on presentation. These fractures can involve either tubercle (or both) and are considered intra-articular fractures because the entire inferior surface is in continuity with the posterior articular surface of the subtalar joint. These fractures occur either as an avulsion fracture following a hyperdorsiflexion injury or as a

compression or impingement fracture resulting from a forced plantar flexion injury.

Patients with fractures of the medial process or sustentaculum typically have pain and swelling in the medial hindfoot distal to the medial malleolus.

Physical Examination

The mechanism of injury in fractures of the lateral process of the talus is classically described as acute dorsiflexion and inversion of the hindfoot, transmitting shear stresses from the calcaneus to the lateral process of the talus; other possible mechanisms include dorsiflexion and external rotation injuries in snowboarders and stress fractures in athletes. Patients typically exhibit swelling and ecchymosis about the lateral hindfoot and sinus tarsi area and have tenderness to palpation just anterior and inferior to the tip of the lateral malleolus. These fractures typically occur in isolation but also can occur with higher energy trauma, such as talar neck fractures, supination-adduction type ankle fractures, subtalar dislocations, and avulsion fractures of the distal fibula. Routine AP, lateral, and mortise views of the ankle should be obtained, and because the diagnosis often is missed on routine radiographs of the ankle, a high index of suspicion must be maintained.

The avulsion fracture of the anterior process of the calcaneus occurs as a result of forced inversion

and plantar flexion, which increases tension within the bifurcate ligament. The fragment is typically small with minimal intra-articular involvement, and the fracture may occur alone or in conjunction with other intra-articular fractures to the calcaneus. The compression fracture occurs as a result of a forceful abduction injury with compression of the calcaneocuboid joint surfaces. The fragment can vary in size but is larger with more articular involvement; it often displaces superiorly and posteriorly, resulting in joint incongruity. Patients exhibit tenderness to palpation in the sinus tarsi, particularly overlying the calcaneocuboid joint. Passive motion to the subtalar joint is markedly decreased. Standard radiographs of the foot and ankle should be obtained to rule out the presence of other injuries, particularly when there are compression-type injuries.

Patients with lateral tubercle fractures have tenderness to palpation just anterior and lateral to the Achilles tendon and exhibit crepitus with plantar flexion of the foot and tenderness with passive motion of the flexus hallucis longus (FHL) tendon. All of these symptoms are included in the so-called os trigonum syndrome. Standard radiographs of the ankle and foot should be obtained initially to rule out the presence of other injuries.

Medial tubercle fractures are much less common and occur as a

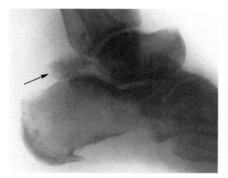

Figure 1 Lateral radiograph of a subtalar dislocation associated with a posterior process of the talus fracture (arrow).

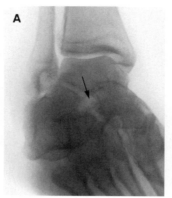
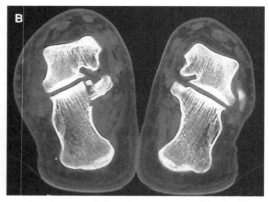

Figure 2 **A,** Bröden view of a sustentaculum fracture of the calcaneus (arrow). **B,** Semicoronal CT scan of a sustentaculum fracture of the calcaneus.

result of a dorsiflexion and pronation injury, causing avulsion of the posterior deltoid ligament. These fractures also can occur in the presence of a medial subtalar dislocation. Patients exhibit tenderness and a firm mass behind the medial malleolus, usually with some loss of the normal posteromedial contour. Standard radiographs of the ankle and foot should be obtained.

Fractures involving the entire posterior process are exceedingly rare and are difficult to visualize on plain radiography. These fractures are also common in the presence of a subtalar dislocation (**Figure 1**).

Sustentaculum fractures occur as a result of axial load and inversion of the hindfoot. The mechanism for medial process fractures is believed to be a shearing force, such as the force from an axial load, producing a vertical fracture line. Patients with these fractures exhibit tenderness to palpation along the medial hindfoot and with passive FHL motion, particularly with sustentaculum fractures. Standard axial, lateral, and Bröden views of the calcaneus should be obtained.

Differential Diagnosis

- Lateral ankle sprain (anterior talofibular or calcaneofibular ligaments)

- Avulsion fracture or other subtle fracture of the lateral malleolus
- Acute tear or other injury to the peroneal tendons
- Fifth metatarsal fracture
- Os trigonum injury; trigonal process (fused os trigonum) fracture
- Acute tear or other injury to the FHL or flexor digitorum longus tendons
- Plantar fascia rupture
- Stress fracture of the calcaneus

Additional Work-up

A fracture of the lateral process of the talus is best visualized on a mortise or modified internal rotation mortise view (20° to 25° of internal rotation), which puts the lateral process of the talus on direct profile in the frontal plane. Alternatively, an AP radiograph that demonstrates both the lateral talar process and the subtalar joint can be obtained with the ankle in 45° of internal rotation and 30° of plantar flexion. CT allows assessment of the size of the fragment, the degree of articular involvement, the comminution of the fragments, and the extent of displacement, all of which are critical factors in decision making.

Although often subtle, a fracture of the anterior process of the calcaneus is best visualized on an oblique view of the foot and must be

distinguished from a calcaneus secondarium, a rare accessory ossicle with a rounded, smooth contour usually lying adjacent to the anterior process. CT evaluation may be beneficial in delineating the size and displacement of the fracture.

Lateral tubercle fractures are best visualized on the lateral view of the ankle and must be distinguished from an os trigonum, a variable accessory ossicle with a rounded, smooth contour lying adjacent to the lateral tubercle. Medial tubercle fractures are often difficult to visualize; the fragment is usually medial and dorsal relative to the remainder of the talus. A bone scan may be useful in distinguishing an acute fracture from an asymptomatic os trigonum. CT is beneficial in delineating the size and displacement of the fracture, particularly in medial tubercle fractures and fractures involving the entire posterior process, and it always should be obtained following reduction of a subtalar dislocation.

The fracture line for fractures of the medial process and sustentaculum of the calcaneus can be visualized on plain radiographs. However, CT can be obtained if concerns exist as to extension of the fracture line into the articular surface of the middle or posterior facets (**Figure 2**).

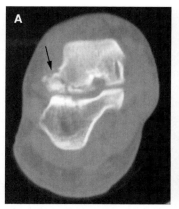
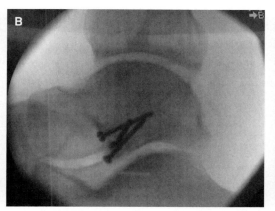
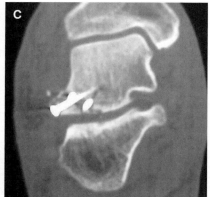

Figure 3 **A,** Semicoronal CT scan of a lateral process of the talus fracture. Note the large fragment (arrow) and surrounding comminution. **B,** Lateral radiograph following ORIF of the lateral talar process with minifragment screw fixation. **C,** Semicoronal postoperative CT scan. Note fixation of the large fragment and near complete preservation of the articular surface.

The Solutions

Treatment Options and Rationale

Critical factors in determining appropriate treatment of a fracture of the lateral process of the talus include the size of the fragment, the amount of comminution, and the degree of displacement. Intuitively, the larger the fragment, the higher the likelihood of articular involvement and the more aggressive the treatment required. Displaced fractures often fail to adequately heal, whereas malunited fractures may lead to persistent symptoms and posttraumatic subtalar arthritis. Nondisplaced fractures may be treated nonsurgically with cast immobilization and restricted weight bearing for 4 to 6 weeks. Displaced (> 2 mm) fractures with single large fragments can be treated by closed reduction and casting or by open reduction and internal fixation (ORIF), whereas fractures with smaller or comminuted fragments may require primary excision.

Treatment of a fracture of the anterior process of the calcaneus is based on the size and the extent of displacement of the fragment. Poor results and long-term disability may occur if the fracture is unrecognized and inadequately treated. Small, nondisplaced

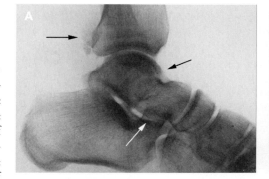
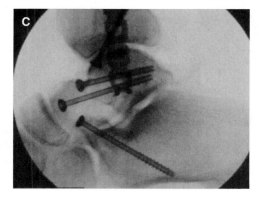
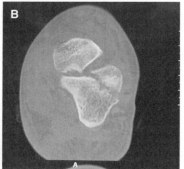

Figure 4 **A,** Lateral radiograph of an anterior process of the calcaneus fracture. Note the size and displacement of the fragment (white arrow). Note also the talar neck and distal fibula fractures (black arrows). **B,** Semicoronal CT scan of displaced anterior process of the calcaneus fracture. **C,** Lateral radiograph following ORIF of the anterior calcaneal process with small fragment screw fixation.

fragments involving less than 20% to 25% of the articular surface may be treated nonsurgically with cast or boot immobilization and restricted weight bearing for 4 to 6 weeks. There is some controversy as to the size of the fragment requiring surgical treatment; however, the extent of articular involvement usually increases with increasing size of the fragment. In com-

pression-type injuries with larger, displaced fragments, ORIF may be required to restore joint congruity.

Lateral tubercle fractures are usually nondisplaced or minimally displaced and can be managed nonsurgically with immobilization in a walking cast or boot in 15° of equinus for 4 to 6 weeks. Displaced medial tubercle fractures are usually larger than expected, and the FHL tendon may interpose in the area and block reduction. Smaller fragments can be managed nonsurgically with boot immobilization for 6 weeks. Larger fragments may require ORIF, particularly if there is significant involvement of the ankle or subtalar joint.

Fractures involving the entire posterior process typically include fragments involving a significant proportion of the articular surface of the subtalar and ankle joints. Because this fracture is essentially a two-joint injury, surgical management often is required.

Nondisplaced sustentaculum tali fractures can be managed nonsurgically with boot immobilization and restricted weight bearing. Larger, displaced sustentaculum fractures may require closed reduction and casting or ORIF. Medial calcaneal process fractures can be managed nonsurgi-

cally with boot immobilization while allowing the patient to bear weight to tolerance.

Author's Preferred Treatment and Rationale

I routinely order CT to better define the fracture pattern in fractures of the lateral process of the talus (**Figure 3**, *A*). I prefer to treat truly nondisplaced fractures with boot immobilization and restricted weight bearing for 6 weeks. I believe, however, that displaced intra-articular fractures cannot be anatomically reduced and reliably maintained through closed methods. Because these fractures are essentially two-joint injuries, I treat displaced fractures with ORIF if at all possible, using small and minifragment screws (**Figure 3**, *B*). Such fractures can be exposed through an Ollier-type approach, which should allow adequate visualization of the fragments. I excise any comminuted fragments too small

to be adequately fixed while attempting to stabilize and preserve as much of the articular surface as possible (**Figure 3**, *C*). I use a controlled ankle motion (CAM) boot postoperatively so that early motion can be instituted while maintaining weight-bearing restrictions for 6 weeks. I allow patients undergoing primary excision of all fragments to bear weight in a CAM boot after incision healing.

Because fractures of the anterior process of the calcaneus often are missed, a high index of suspicion must be maintained. If the fragment is not well visualized on plain radiographs, I use CT to better define the fracture pattern (**Figure 4**, *A* and *B*). I treat small nondisplaced fractures with minimal articular involvement with boot immobilization and weight-bearing restrictions for 4 to 6 weeks. I treat larger displaced fractures involving more than 25% of the articular surface with ORIF through an abbrevi-

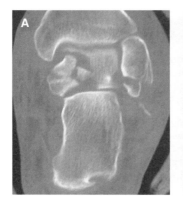

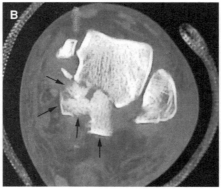

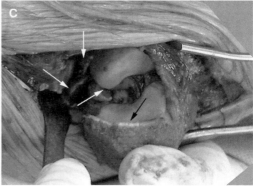

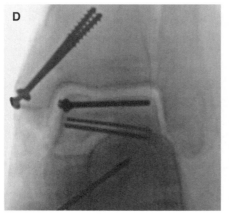

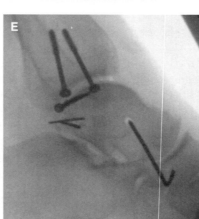

Figure 5 **A,** Semicoronal CT scan of a fracture involving the entire posterior process of the talus. Note the multiple displaced fragments. **B,** Axial CT scan of a fracture involving the entire posterior process of the talus. Note the multiple displaced fragments (arrows). **C,** Intraoperative view of a fracture involving the entire posterior process of the talus (white arrows). The fracture was exposed through a medial malleolar osteotomy (black arrow). Mortise (**D**) and lateral (**E**) radiographs following ORIF of the posterior process of the talus using minifragment screws. The inferior fragments required Kirschner wire fixation because they were too small to withstand screws.

ated Ollier-type approach using mini- or small fragment screws (**Figure 4**, *C*). Compression-type fractures may require stabilization with a small, cervical H-plate to buttress the fragment and maintain joint reduction. I use a CAM boot in patients postoperatively to allow early motion activities while maintaining restricted weight bearing for 4 to 6 weeks.

I routinely use CT to delineate the fracture patterns of both lateral and medial tubercle fractures and, especially, of fractures involving the entire posterior process (**Figure 5**, *A* and *B*). I treat truly nondisplaced lateral tubercle fractures with cast immobilization and restricted weight bearing for 6 weeks. I manage lateral tubercle fractures that are progressing to symptomatic nonunion with boot immobilization for 6 weeks and, if symptoms persist, with delayed excision through a posterolateral approach, followed by aggressive postoperative physical therapy.

Larger displaced fractures, especially those of the medial tubercle or entire posterior process and involving significant portions of articular surface, cannot be reduced reliably and held anatomically by closed methods. I prefer treating these displaced fractures with ORIF, if at all possible, using minifragment screws because these fractures are essentially two-joint injuries. Exposure of medial tubercle or entire posterior process fractures may require a medial malleolar osteotomy for sufficient visualization (**Figure 5**, *C*). I usually excise any comminuted fragments too small to be adequately fixed while attempting to preserve as much of the articular surface as possible, particularly in the subtalar joint (**Figure 5**, *D* and *E*). I use a CAM boot postoperatively so that early motion can be instituted while maintaining weight-bearing restrictions for 6 weeks.

I usually use CT for sustentaculum fractures to better delineate the fracture fragment. I treat nondisplaced sustentaculum fractures with boot im-

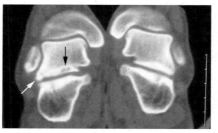

Figure 6 Semicoronal CT scan of posttraumatic subtalar arthritis from an unrecognized, untreated fracture of the lateral process of the talus (white arrow). Note formation of a subchondral cyst (black arrow).

mobilization and restricted weight bearing for 6 weeks. I prefer to treat larger displaced fragments with ORIF through a medial approach using small and minifragment screws. I use boot immobilization postoperatively to allow early motion activities while restricting weight bearing for 6 weeks. I manage medial process fractures with boot immobilization for 6 weeks, allowing the patient to bear weight to tolerance.

Management of Complications

Chronic fractures of the lateral process of the talus caused by a missed or delayed diagnosis will often result in a nonunion or delayed union and subsequent subtalar or talofibular arthritis (**Figure 6**). CT evaluation should be obtained to identify loose fragments and to assay the extent of articular involvement and arthritic changes. If it is recognized early, excision of a persistent loose fragment may prevent more significant posttraumatic arthritis. The results of excision, however, are somewhat unpredictable, and patients may ultimately require a subtalar arthrodesis. Patients with loose fragments in the presence of significant subtalar arthritis are best managed with an arthrodesis (**Figure 7**). Differential injections can be used to determine the extent of joint involvement in patients with arthritis in both the subtalar and talofibular joints; the subtalar joint is typically more symptomatic in these instances.

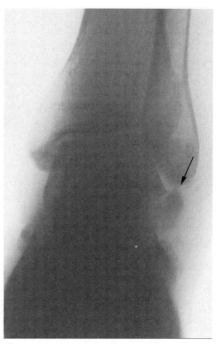

Figure 7 AP radiograph of an acute lateral talar process fracture. Note the size and displacement of the fragment (arrow). The fracture was missed originally and resulted in posttraumatic subtalar arthritis.

Unrecognized anterior process fractures may result in a nonunion that, if asymptomatic, can be treated with simple observation. Patients with symptomatic nonunions can be treated initially with immobilization and corticosteroid injections; if symptoms persist, CT should be obtained. Fragments involving less than 25% of the articular surface can be excised. ORIF may be considered for larger fragments, provided the remaining articular surface is well preserved. Arthrodesis should be considered if there is significant posttraumatic arthritis.

Patients with symptomatic lateral tubercle nonunions will have pain with extreme plantar flexion and diminished range of motion in the ankle or subtalar joints. In these patients, delayed primary excision of the fragment may relieve the pain and restore range of motion. Untreated or nonunited medial tubercle fractures may cause tarsal tunnel-like symptoms that should be relieved by release of the overlying retinaculum and/or excision of the fragment. Patients developing significant posttraumatic arthritis, especially in the subtalar joint, can be managed with arthrodesis.

Sustentaculum fractures may result in triggering or impingement of the FHL, which may ultimately require tenolysis or decompression. Displaced fractures may result in a nonunion that, if small, can be treated with simple excision. Larger fragments may require ORIF. Medial process fractures may result in persistent plantar medial pain or bony prominence that can be treated by local modalities and shoe modifications.

————————■

■ References

Boon AJ, Smith J, Zobitz ME, Amrani KM: Snowboarder's talus fracture: Mechanism of injury. *Am J Sports Med* 2001;29:333-338.

Degan TJ, Morrey BF, Braun DP: Surgical excision for anterior process fractures of the calcaneus. *J Bone Joint Surg Am* 1982;64:519-524.

Ebraheim NA, Skie MC, Podeszwa DA, Jackson WT: Evaluation of process fractures of the talus using computed tomography. *J Orthop Trauma* 1994;8:332-337.

Fitzgibbons TC, McMullen ST, Mormino MA: Fractures of the calcaneus, in Rockwood CA (ed): *Fractures in Adults*, ed 5. Philadelphia, PA, Lippincott, 2001, pp 2133-2179.

Veazey BL, Heckman JD, Galindo MJ, McGanity PLJ: Excision of ununited fractures of the posterior process of the talus: A treatment for chronic posterior ankle pain. *Foot Ankle* 1992;13:453-457.

Coding

ICD-9 CODES

716.17   Other and unspecified arthropathies, Traumatic arthropathy, ankle and foot

718.17   Loose body in joint, ankle and foot

825.0   Fracture of one or more tarsal and metatarsal bones, Fracture of calcaneus, closed

825.21   Fracture of one or more tarsal and metatarsal bones, Fracture of other tarsal and metatarsal bones, closed, Astragalus

825.31   Fracture of one or more tarsal and metatarsal bones, Fracture of other tarsal and metatarsal bones, open, Astragalus

905.4   Late effects of musculoskeletal and connective tissue injuries, Late effect of fracture of lower extremities

CPT CODES

27620   Arthrotomy, ankle, with joint exploration, with or without biopsy, with or without removal of loose or foreign body

27870   Arthrodesis, ankle, open

28120   Partial excision (craterization, saucerization, sequestrectomy, or diaphysectomy) bone (eg, osteomyelitis or bossing); talus or calcaneus

28400   Closed treatment of calcaneal fracture; without manipulation

28415   Open treatment of calcaneal fracture, with or without internal or external fixation

28430   Closed treatment of talus fracture; without manipulation

28435   Closed treatment of talus fracture; with manipulation

28445   Open treatment of talus fracture, with or without internal or external fixation

28715   Arthrodesis; triple

28725   Arthrodesis; subtalar

28740   Arthrodesis, midtarsal or tarsometatarsal, single joint

Calcaneal Fracture—Primary Arthrodesis

Adolph S. Flemister, Jr, MD

■ Definition of the Problem

Patient Presentation

Intra-articular calcaneal fractures most commonly occur in industrial workers who fall from a height or in individuals involved in high-energy motor vehicle accidents. Patients have moderate to severe pain and swelling localized to the hindfoot. Bilateral fractures are common as are other foot and ankle, lower extremity, and spinal fractures. In cases of traumatic injury, some patients may have multiple injuries that are so severely painful that they may not initially report significant foot pain.

Physical Examination

In general, the hindfoot will be severely swollen, tender, and ecchymotic. Blistering is common and may develop within a few hours after injury. Open fractures usually are associated with a medial wound. A thorough physical examination is necessary to identify any associated injuries, specifically examination of both lower extremities and the thoracolumbar spine.

For patients who present with severe pain and paresthesias, compartment pressures should be measured to rule out compartment syndrome. Several portable pressure monitors are commercially available. Compartment pressures of 30 mm Hg or greater are considered an indication for fasciotomy.

Differential Diagnosis

- Isolated intra-articular calcaneal fracture
- Associated lower extremity fracture
- Associated spinal fracture
- Compartment syndrome

Additional Work-up

AP and lateral views of the foot and calcaneal axial views should be obtained in patients suspected of having a calcaneal fracture. The lateral view will indicate the extent of the injury to the posterior facet and the calcaneocuboid joint (**Figure 1**). Injuries to the talus or talonavicular joint are also best viewed on a lateral view. The AP view helps to further evaluate the calcaneocuboid joint injury and any disruption at the talonavicular joint. An axial radiograph of the heel reveals the increased width and angulation of the calcaneal tuberosity. Patients who present with symptoms at the thoracolumbar spine must also be evaluated with the appropriate radiographs of the spine.

If plain radiographs reveal an intra-articular calcaneal fracture, two-dimensional CT should be ordered. Transverse images provide information regarding injury to the calcaneocuboid joint, the width of the tuberosity, the amount of posterior facet depression, and the extent of injury to the sustentaculum. Coronal cuts are useful for evaluation of the widening and comminution of the lateral wall, as well as the angulation and displacement of the tuberosity fragment. Most importantly, these coronal cuts allow evaluation of the comminution of the posterior facet (**Figure 2**). With this information, fractures can be classified according to the system of Sanders, which is prognostic for outcomes after surgical treatment of fractures. In this system, type I fractures are non-displaced; type II have two posterior facet fragments; type III have three posterior facet fragments; and type IV

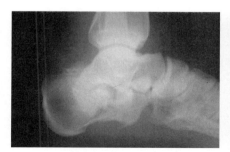

Figure 1 Lateral radiograph showing a calcaneal fracture.

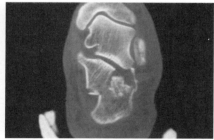

Figure 2 Coronal CT scan showing posterior facet comminution.

have four or more fragments. These fractures are further categorized by the location of the fracture lines along the posterior facet.

———————————■

■ The Solutions

Treatment Options and Rationale

There is no consensus regarding the best treatment of displaced intra-articular calcaneal fractures. In particular, the management of Sanders type IV fractures is controversial. Good and excellent results are often achieved with surgical treatment of type II and type III fractures. However, satisfactory results following open reduction and internal fixation (ORIF) of type IV fractures have been reported in only a small percentage of patients. These poor outcomes are most often associated with an inadequate reduction of the posterior facet.

Nonsurgical treatment consists of short-term immobilization in a bulky Jones-type dressing. Once patients are comfortable, they can be switched to a removable cast boot and range-of-motion exercises can be started. Non–weight-bearing status is required for about 3 months. This treatment approach avoids the complications associated with surgery, but leaves the patient with an incongruent and malaligned subtalar joint, a shortened and widened heel, and peroneal tendon and calcaneofibular impingement. Severe subtalar arthritis will develop in most patients, accompanied by varying degrees of chronic pain and loss of function.

Salvage of calcaneal malunions can be difficult. Exostectomy of the prominent lateral wall relieves calcaneofibular impingement. An in situ subtalar arthodesis will address subtalar arthritis. If anterior ankle impinge-

ment is present, however, a bone block arthrodesis is required. The latter is a particularly difficult procedure that involves placing a wedge of bone in the posterior facet in an effort to restore calcaneal height and talar inclination. Compared with in situ subtalar arthrodeses, bone block arthrodeses are associated with higher rates of complications, specifically wound problems, nonunion, and malunion. Varus malunions of the tuberosity are addressed with osteotomies.

ORIF is performed to anatomically restore the height, width, and alignment of the calcaneus. Most importantly, an anatomic reduction of the posterior facet must be achieved. Numerous methods have been described to achieve these goals with overall good clinical results obtained for Sanders type II and type III fractures. However, satisfactory results following surgical treatment of Sanders type IV fractures are less common. Most of these poor results correlate with an inability to achieve an adequate reduction of the posterior facet. Primary arthrodesis combined with ORIF is recommended for these fractures. The initial open reduction restores the calcaneal height and width, and the fusion avoids the late sequela of posttraumatic arthritis. In this scenario, patients have one operation and one recovery period; as a result, a more rapid return to function is possible.

Author's Preferred Treatment and Rationale

ORIF with primary arthrodesis is recommended for all Sanders type IV fractures. Patients with acute injury are placed into a bulky Jones-type dressing with a posterior mold. If no other injuries are present, most patients can be discharged to home with oral analgesics. Some patients may require an overnight hospital stay for pain control. Surgery should be sufficiently delayed to allow for the resolution of soft-tissue edema and the re-

turn of skin wrinkles but should be performed within 21 days of injury. Approximately 3 weeks after injury, mobilization of fracture fragments becomes significantly more difficult.

All patients are given appropriate antibiotic therapy preoperatively. Patients undergoing unilateral fusions are placed in the lateral decubitus position on a radiolucent table. If bilateral procedures are planned, patients are placed in a prone position to allow lateral access to both feet. Tourniquet control is used throughout the procedure. The calcaneus is approached laterally through an L-shaped extensile incision, and full-thickness flaps are maintained to avoid late wound necrosis. Kirschner wires (K-wires) are placed into the fibula, talar neck, and cuboid to act as retractors and to avoid excessive manual retraction. The lateral wall fragments are identified and lifted away from the calcaneal body to expose the buried articular fragments. These fragments are elevated and aligned with the sustentacular fragments and temporarily held with K-wires. The tuberosity is then reduced under the sustentaculum. Aligning the anterior corner of the most lateral posterior facet fragment with the posterior corner of the anterior calcaneal fragment restores the angle of Gissane. Lateral, axial, and Broden views are then obtained fluoroscopically.

In patients with Sanders type IV fractures, an adequate reduction of the posterior facet cannot be obtained and the decision is made to perform a subtalar arthrodesis. The K-wires holding the posterior facet are replaced with small fragment screws, and a lateral buttress plate is used to maintain the alignment of the calcaneal body. The remaining cartilage on the calcaneus and talus is completely denuded. Either autogenous bone graft or some form of allograft material should be used to supplement the fusion. One or two large, partially threaded cannulated screws (at least 6.5 mm) are then placed from the calcaneal tuberosity

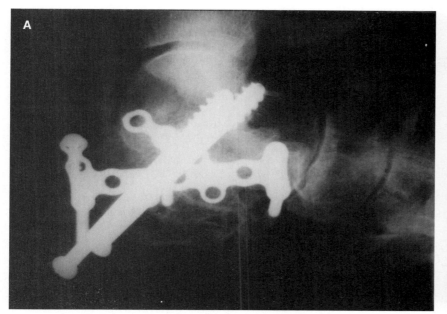

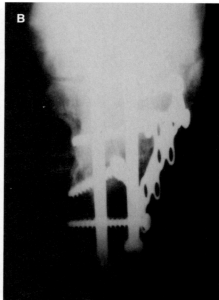

Figure 3   Lateral **(A)** and axial **(B)** radiographs showing arthrodesis.

across the subtalar joint (**Figure 3**). Care should be taken not to overly compress the joint as this can lead to some loss of height. Frequently, screws from either the plate or posterior facet may need to be removed to allow passage of the subtalar screws. Final positioning of the hardware and alignment of the fracture should be checked with fluoroscopy before closure.

Postoperatively, the patient is placed in a below-knee posterior splint. The wound is checked after 1 week, and sutures are kept in place until the wound has completely healed, which is usually at approximately 3 weeks. Immobilization in a non–weight-bearing short leg cast is continued for 10 to 12 weeks. Progressive weight bearing and physical therapy are then initiated.

Management of Complications

Wound healing problems, nonunion, malunion, sural neuritis, and hardware irritation are potential complications following primary arthrodesis of intra-articular calcaneal fractures. Of these complications, wound dehis-

cence is the most common. Most often this occurs at the apex of the incision and is noticed shortly after suture removal. If the wound does not appear infected, the cast can be windowed and local wound care performed. Oral antibiotics should be administered if cellulitis or superficial infection is suspected. Patients who have deep infections require multiple débridements and intravenous antibiotics. Every attempt should be made to retain the hardware until adequate bony healing has occurred. If there is a persistent infection, however, early removal of hardware may be required, followed by application of an external fixator across the subtalar joint. Patients who have a deep infection that requires multiple débridements may need require a free tissue transfer.

Sural neuritis or neuromas are uncommon if an extensile lateral approach is used because the nerve is protected in the anterior flap. If there is injury to the nerve, transsection of the nerve proximally and burial of the stump in muscle are required. Lateral plate irritation or discomfort over the tuberosity screw head may occur.

Hardware removal should be delayed until the calcaneal fracture has healed and the subtalar joint fused.

Varus malunion of the hindfoot is the most common malalignment problem following primary arthrodesis. Initially, this can be managed with a lateral heel wedge placed either in the shoe or on the sole, depending on the amount of correction required. Because this is a fixed deformity, symptoms may persist, in which case a corrective osteotomy is required. Nonunion of the fractured calcaneus is extremely rare, but nonunion of the attempted subtalar arthrodesis is more common. If nonunion is suspected, CT will often be helpful to make a definitive diagnosis. In patients who have a nonunion, I usually try some form of bone stimulator in an effort to avoid revision. If treatment with a bone stimulator is unsuccessful, then débridement of the nonunion and bone grafting are required. Two large cannulated screws are then placed across the subtalar joint.

References

Buch BB, Myerson MS, Miller SD: Primary subtalar arthodesis for treatment of comminuted calcaneal fractures. *Foot Ankle Int* 1996;17:61-70.

Flemister AS, Infante AF, Sanders R, Walling AK: Subtalar arthrodesis for complications of intra-articular calcaneal fractures. *Foot Ankle Int* 2000;21:392-399.

Huefner T, Thermann H, Geerling J, Pape HC, Pohlemann T: Primary subtalar arthodesis of calcaneal fractures. *Foot Ankle Int* 2001;22:9-13.

Sanders R: Displaced intra-articular fractures of the calcaneus. *J Bone Joint Surg Am* 2000;82:225-250.

Sanders RW, Fortin P, Dipasquale T, Walling AK: Operative treatment of 120 displaced intra-articular calcaneal fractures: Results using a prognostic computed tomography scan classification. *Clin Orthop* 1993;290:87-95.

Coding

ICD-9 CODES

825.0   Fracture of one or more tarsal and metatarsal bones, Fracture of calcaneus, closed

825.1   Fracture of one or more tarsal and metatarsal bones, Fracture of calcaneus, open

CPT CODES

28415   Open treatment calcaneal fracture

28420   Open treatment with autograft

28725   Subtalar arthrodesis

CPT copyright © 2003 by the American Medical Association. All Rights Reserved.

Missed Lisfranc Injury

Robert B. Anderson, MD

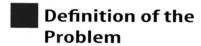

Definition of the Problem

Patient Presentation

Approximately 20% of Lisfranc injuries are missed at the time of the initial examination. Because a large number of these midfoot injuries are purely ligamentous, clinicians should have a strong suspicion of Lisfranc injuries when evaluating patients with midfoot injuries. In our experience, recreational athletes may have a Lisfranc injury if they have sustained a twisting injury to the foot, have radiographs that are interpreted as "negative," and are subsequently diagnosed with a midfoot sprain. All age groups are susceptible to this potential problem. Therefore, it is mandatory to look for subtle signs and symptoms of Lisfranc injuries in patients with chronic midfoot pain, regardless of its etiology. Patients may have a history of difficulty with weight bearing, possibly associated with diffuse pain and swelling.

Physical Examination

A thorough physical examination begins with an evaluation of gait to determine whether the gait is antalgic. An examination of stance may detect asymmetries, including loss of arch height, an abducted posture to the foot, and a dorsomedial midfoot prominence. Any areas of localized tenderness should be identified while the patient is seated. Frequently, this

tenderness will be in the region of the Lisfranc ligament. Pain may be reproduced with manipulation of the midfoot joints, particularly pronation-abduction and supination-adduction. Because these injuries may not be confined to the tarsometatarsal joint, proximal and distal joints must also be carefully evaluated. A vascular examination should be performed, and the function of the deep peroneal nerve to the first web space might also be assessed.

Weight-bearing AP, lateral, and oblique radiographs should be obtained because spontaneous reduction may occur after a ligamentous injury (**Figures 1** and **2**). Radiographs of a normal foot should show the following: (1) a consistent relationship between the medial margin of the middle cuneiform and the medial aspect of the second metatarsal; (2) an unbroken line between the medial base of the fourth metatarsal and the medial margin of the cuboid on an oblique view; and (3) an unbroken line between the dorsum of the first and second metatarsals and their corresponding cuneiforms on a lateral view. Any disruption of these relationships suggests a Lisfranc injury. In addition, flattening of the arch suggests a midfoot injury.

The radiographs should be assessed for subtle associated findings, such as compression fractures of the cuboid, second metatarsal base fracture, a "fleck sign" representing a small avulsion fracture of the base of the second metatarsal, lesser metatar-

sophalangeal joint dislocations, metatarsal head and neck fractures, and intercuneiform diastasis. When in doubt, radiographs of the contralateral foot, obtained while the patient is standing, can be used for comparison.

Differential Diagnosis
- Stable midfoot sprain
- Unstable Lisfranc injury
- Degenerative joint disease of the midfoot
- Inflammatory arthropathy of the midfoot (pseudogout)
- Posterior tibial tendon dysfunction

Additional Work-up
Weight-bearing radiographs, preferably in which the patient is standing on one leg, are usually adequate to elicit joint diastasis. In general, formal stress testing is not necessary if the patient can bear full weight on the involved limb. If the patient is not weight bearing, formal stress testing can be performed with fluoroscopic imaging.

A fluoroscopic examination may be useful if stress radiographs are unobtainable, but the mainstay of evaluation with imaging techniques should be radiographs. Adequate anesthesia must be used with fluoroscopic imaging. The patient's limbs should be maneuvered to elicit joint diastasis with pronation-abduction and supination-adduction.

Two-dimensional CT can help assess fracture patterns and plantar comminution. Also, a coronal (or splay) reconstruction of the midfoot transformed

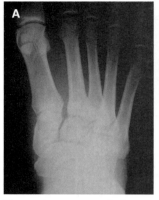
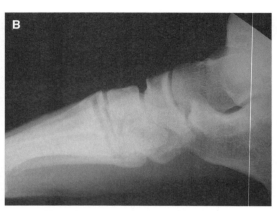

Figure 1   Non–weight-bearing AP (**A**) and lateral (**B**) radiographs of the right foot in a 39-year-old man who sustained a twisting injury approximately 1 week before presentation. Note the slight diastasis between the first and second metatarsal bases, as well as slight dorsal subluxation of the second metatarsal base. No obvious fractures are noted.

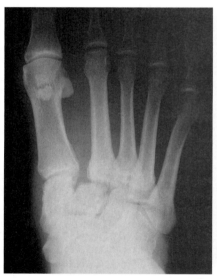

Figure 2   Weight-bearing AP radiograph of the right foot in the same patient demonstrates markedly increased diastasis between the first and second metatarsal bases, along with significant lateral translation of the second metatarsal. Also note the subtle diastasis of the medial and middle cuneiform interspace. Again, no fractures are identified. These findings are consistent with an unstable, ligamentous Lisfranc injury.

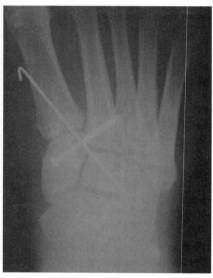

Figure 3   The same patient after open reduction and internal fixation. Note the reduction of the second metatarsal base with a home run screw in place, as well as closure of the first and second metatarsals and intercuneiform diastasis.

from a mortise configuration to a flattened plane may be useful. This allows a detailed, simultaneous examination of all of the tarsometatarsal joints.

Bone scans may be useful for patients who have persistent pain but no radiographic evidence of midfoot instability.

MRI may be useful to assess purely ligamentous injuries, synovitis, and subtle osteochondral injuries. With improvements in availability and quality, MRI may replace bone scanning as the imaging technique of choice in patients who have chronic pain but normal radiographs.

———————▶■

The Solutions

Treatment Options and Rationale

Persistent malalignment of the Lisfranc joint complex greatly increases the risk of late degenerative changes and deformity; therefore, the goals of treatment are to obtain and maintain anatomic reduction. Any amount of displacement in a healthy, active patient warrants surgical reduction and fixation. In the past, closed reduction and percutaneous pin fixation have been advocated for the treatment of minimally displaced injuries. In recent years, there has been a trend to perform open reduction for Lisfranc injuries that require surgical stabilization. Open reduction allows direct visualization of the fracture fragments and facilitates the removal of interposed soft tissue and debris. Whether to use screws or percutaneous pins for fixation remains a point of controversy. The current trend is to use screws for the first through third tarsometatarsal joints, including a "home run" screw from the medial cuneiform through the base of the second metatarsal (**Figure 3**). The rationale is that ligamentous injuries may take 3 to 6 months to heal, which is longer than the life span of a simple pin. The most commonly used screws are 3.5- or 4.5-mm AO cortical screws. For the fourth and fifth tarsometatarsal joints, buttressing in the form of percutaneous 0.062-in Kirschner wires (K-wires) usually will be sufficient.

The surgical procedure is usually followed by a 4- to 6-week period of non–weight-bearing immobilization, and subsequently a 4- to 6-week period of protected weight bearing in a cast or boot. With regard to hardware, there has been a trend toward leaving screws in place for a minimum of 3 months, or indefinitely if patients are asymptomatic.

Author's Preferred Treatment and Rationale

TIMING OF TREATMENT

When feasible, we perform surgery on these patients on initial presentation, before swelling becomes significant. In the acute setting, we attempt surgery as soon as swelling allows. We do not hesitate, however, to wait up to 3 weeks to allow swelling to resolve and soft tissues to consolidate. For missed Lisfranc injuries, there is an ongoing debate regarding when it is too late to attempt primary reduction and fixation. Unfortunately, there are no published data to support a specific recommendation regarding the optimal timing of this treatment. We attempt open reduction and internal fixation (ORIF) up to 12 weeks from the time of injury, assuming there is no significant chondral damage that might require a primary fusion. It is reasonable to treat minimally displaced injuries presenting after 3 months symptomatically and follow the patient's clinical progress, with the knowledge that realignment arthrodesis is always an option and has no time constraints.

SURGICAL TECHNIQUE FOR REDUCTION AND FIXATION

For ORIF, a linear dorsal skin incision is fashioned over the interval between the first and second metatarsal bases, extending proximally to the naviculocuneiform joint when intercuneiform instability is encountered. The reduction and fixation proceeds from medial to lateral.

All unstable joints must be identified and débrided of interposed tissue. Areas of chondral injury are assessed and documented. The neurovascular bundle lying over the Lisfranc ligament is identified, mobilized, and protected throughout the procedure.

The first tarsometatarsal joint is reduced and pinned temporarily. The second metatarsal base is reduced with a tenaculum and pinned in the "home run" fashion, which is medial cuneiform to the base of the second

metatarsal. This step is critical because the second metatarsal base is the keystone of the midfoot. We often use a guide wire from a cannulated screw system so that a cannulated drill may be used to ensure precise placement in the second metatarsal base.

Any intercuneiform diastasis is reduced with a tenaculum and secured with a K-wire placed perpendicular to the joint itself. The third tarsometatarsal joint is reduced and pinned if necessary.

The fourth and fifth tarsometatarsal joints are usually anatomically aligned at this point in the procedure, and a 0.062-in K-wire is percutaneously placed from the fifth metatarsal base into the midfoot to act as a buttress. If these joints require reduction, however, a second dorsal incision is made in line with the fourth metatarsal. The fourth and fifth tarsometatarsal joints are reduced and secured with one or two 0.062-in K-wire(s).

Screws are then placed to secure the first to third tarsometatarsal joints, as well as the intercuneiform joint, in a manner similar to that used for the placement of K-wires. We prefer to use a 3.5-mm cortical screw and avoid the lag technique. A 4.5-mm screw may be required for procedures in large or obese patients. Cannulated screws (4.0 to 4.5 mm) may be used for the home run screw.

We have been using bioabsorbable screws (3.5 and 4.0 mm) in our patients who are not competitive athletes. The use of these screws obviates the need for future screw removal, which offers a clear advantage. Strength characteristics of the absorbable screws remain in question. For that reason, we do not typically use them in high-demand patients or those requiring early or aggressive rehabilitation, as is required for competitive athletes.

POSTOPERATIVE CARE AFTER REDUCTION AND FIXATION

For nonathletes, postoperative care typically involves 6 weeks in a non–

weight-bearing cast, followed by removal of the percutaneous pins. The patient is then kept in a walking cast or cast boot for another 4 to 6 weeks. After cast removal, accommodative shoes with a longitudinal arch support are used.

For competitive athletes, a non–weight-bearing splint is used for 2 weeks, followed by use of a removable boot (still non–weight-bearing) for another 4 weeks to allow for the initiation of gentle range-of-motion exercises in a pool. The patient is then allowed to bear weight in a boot for another 6 weeks, and rehabilitation is continued. At 16 weeks, the patient is allowed to return to competitive play with appropriate protection. A longitudinal arch support with turf toe plate is used for at least 6 months.

One question frequently asked following ORIF of Lisfranc injuries is whether the hardware needs to be removed. For nonathletes, we typically leave all screws in unless the patient is symptomatic. For competitive athletes, we usually remove all screws across the tarsometatarsal joints at 6 months postoperatively. Intercuneiform screws are left in permanently. After the removal of hardware, the patient is restricted from contact sports for 8 weeks.

SURGICAL TECHNIQUES FOR POSTTRAUMATIC ARTHRITIS

For the first through third tarsometatarsal joints, as well as the intercuneiform joints, definitive treatment of posttraumatic arthritis involves fusion of the joints responsible for the patient's symptoms. The affected joints are identified by differential injection. For most patients, in situ fusion is involved; however, for patients who have significant deformity, corrective arthrodesis may be performed. When performing a fusion, it is essential to recreate the talo-first metatarsal line, as well as reduce the second tarsometatarsal joint (the keystone) in both the anteroposterior and lateral planes. Our typical sequence of reduc-

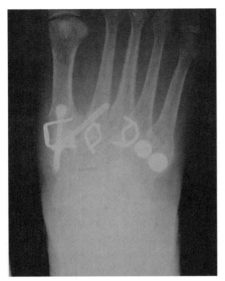

Figure 4 AP radiograph showing an example of a midfoot arthrodesis. Note the use of ceramic sphere spacers for the fourth and fifth tarsometatarsal joints.

tion and fixation for fusion is similar to that used for ORIF of acute injuries. One primary difference is the use of an additional screw to secure the first tarsometatarsal joint, as well as lag technique and liberal use of bone graft or bone graft substitutes. More recently, we have used dorsal compression staples to augment fixation of the first through third tarsometatarsal joints.

Arthritis of the fourth and fifth tarsometatarsal joints is rarely symptomatic, and the rule of thumb is to avoid fusion of these joints if at all possible. If painful arthritis of the fourth and fifth tarsometatarsal joints is associated with an abduction deformity and medial column arthritis, a realignment fusion of the medial column should be considered first, as this will often unload the lateral column. If there is isolated and/or persistent pain associated with the fourth and fifth tarsometatarsal joints, as documented by differential injection, tendon interposition arthroplasty may be performed using the peroneus tertius. This is performed through a separate dorsolateral approach, avoiding branches of the superficial peroneal and sural nerves. Recently, we have also performed arthroplasty of these joints with ceramic spheres (**Figure 4**). This procedure is currently an off-label use for these implants, as they were originally indicated for carpometacarpal arthroplasty. We have observed early clinical success with this technique; however, additional follow-up and more long-term data are needed.

Management of Complications

The most common late complication of Lisfranc injuries is posttraumatic arthritis. Although ORIF of unstable injuries can reduce this risk, the risk can never be completely eliminated. It is important to remember that radiographic evidence of degenerative change does not always correlate with symptoms. Treatment of posttraumatic arthritis, therefore, should involve only those patients who are symptomatic. The temptation to treat the radiographic evidence should be avoided. Furthermore, in those patients who are symptomatic, it is important to identify the specific joints responsible for the patient's symptoms. We have found differential joint blocks performed by a radiologist under fluoroscopic guidance to be quite useful. A mixture of a long-acting anesthetic and a steroid preparation is used. The patient is then asked to keep a diary of his or her pain. A helpful adjunct to injection of medications is the use of a longitudinal arch support and stiff-soled shoes, with or without a rocker bottom.

The author wishes to acknowledge the contribution of William C. James, III, MD, in the creation of this chapter.

————————■

References

Horton GA, Olney BW: Deformity correction and arthrodesis of the midfoot with a medial plate. *Foot Ankle* 1993;14:493-499.

Johnson JE, Johnson KA: Dowel arthrodesis for degenerative arthritis of the tarsometatarsal (Lisfranc) joints. *Foot Ankle* 1986;6:243-253.

Mann RA, Prieskorn D, Sobel M: Mid-tarsal and tarsometatarsal arthrodesis for primary degenerative osteoarthrosis or osteoarthrosis after trauma. *J Bone Joint Surg Am* 1996;78:1376-1385.

Myerson MS, Fisher RT, Burgess AR, Kenzora JE: Fracture dislocations of the tarsometatarsal joints: End results correlated with pathology and treatment. *Foot Ankle* 1986;6:225-242.

Sangeorzan BJ, Veith RG, Hansen ST Jr: Salvage of Lisfranc's tarsometatarsal joint by arthrodesis. *Foot Ankle* 1990;10:193-200.

Coding

ICD-9 CODES

715.97   Osteoarthrosis, unspecified whether generalized or localized, ankle and foot

825.25   Fracture of other metatarsal bones, closed

838.03   Dislocation of tarsometatarsal joint, closed

CPT CODES

28615   Open treatment of tarsometatarsal joint dislocation, with or without internal or external fixation

28730   Arthrodesis, midtarsal or tarsometatarsal, multiple or transverse

28740   Arthrodesis, midtarsal or tarsometatarsal, single joint

SECTION 8
Diabetic Foot

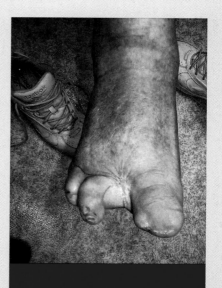

Elly Trepman, MD
Editor

Reconstruction of Acute Midfoot Charcot Arthropathy

Elly Trepman, MD

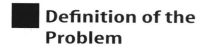

Definition of the Problem

Patient Presentation

Charcot neuropathy of the foot and ankle is a neuropathic syndrome most commonly observed in patients with diabetes mellitus, leprosy, and alcoholic neuropathy. The patient presents with a history of swelling and erythema. Sensory neuropathy is present, and the patient may have neuropathic symptoms including paresthesias, dysesthesias, and a history of painless wounds. Approximately half the patients report no pain because of the sensory neuropathy, but the other half report neuropathic pain or pain that may be disproportionately less than might be expected for the skeletal trauma present.

A history of trauma may be absent or vague. The absence of normal protective sensation may cause progressive aggravation of repetitive microtrauma. Furthermore arteriovenous shunting and hyperemia may cause osteopenia that may make the bones and joints more susceptible to injury. This combination of factors may cause progressive and extensive fracture-dislocation. The midfoot, including the tarsometatarsal (TMT) and midtarsal joints, is involved most commonly. Limited ankle dorsiflexion from contracture of the gastrocnemius-soleus complex may contribute to increased midfoot stresses and contribute to breakdown of this region.

The patient may or may not have noticed a change in the shape of the foot, which may be masked by swelling. Fracture-dislocation of the TMT joints may result in widening of the midfoot, collapse of the longitudinal arch, and a rocker-bottom foot with forefoot abduction. The patient may have difficulty fitting shoes on the rocker-bottom foot. The bony prominences and increased pressures on the skin may cause ulcers that may become infected, placing the foot at risk for abscess, osteomyelitis, and amputation.

The symptoms often are present for many months, and the patient may give a history of several previous medical evaluations and treatment of misdiagnosed conditions such as infection, gout, or rheumatoid arthritis.

Physical Examination

The patient may have a swollen and erythematous foot that is warmer to touch than the opposite foot. Some patients examined early in the process may have no deformity, or early deformity may be masked by marked swelling. Once deformity develops, there may be widening of the midfoot and presence of bony prominences with pressure signs such as local erythema or an ulcer. The location of the bony prominences may be varied; however, a common pattern includes prominences at the plantar midfoot and medial TMT region. If the arch has collapsed, the patient may have marked forefoot abduction associated with ulcers at the medial forefoot (**Figure 1**).

Bilateral involvement, either synchronous or later, may occur in approximately 30% of patients.

Sensory neuropathy is confirmed by lack of sensitivity to the 5.07 Semmes-Weinstein monofilament. Signs of motor neuropathy include contractures such as claw toes or a tight heel cord. Signs of autonomic neuropathy include dry scaly skin that may crack and become inflamed or infected.

Initial radiographs may be negative for bone or joint involvement, leaving soft-tissue swelling as the only finding. However, closer inspection or follow-up radiographs may reveal subtle fragmentation and subluxation or diastasis at the midtarsal or TMT joints. When progressive instability occurs, radiographs may show either complete dislocation with no fracture or extensive fracture-dislocation with bony fragmentation. There may be widening of the midfoot with medial dislocation of the first cuneiform or first metatarsal bone, forefoot abduction at the TMT joints, or plantar dislocation of the cuneiforms or cuboid. If the foot is left unreduced, radiographs in later stages may show progressive bony consolidation with residual deformity. Management of the chronic midfoot Charcot foot is discussed in chapter 64.

Differential Diagnosis

- Traumatic fracture
- Infection
- Rheumatoid arthritis

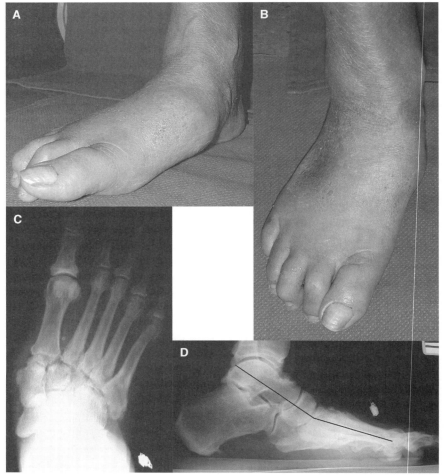

Figure 1 A 67-year-old man with a 20-year history of diabetes and previous right femoropopliteal bypass vascular graft and a right posterolateral heel ulcer that healed with dressings. After shoveling in the garden using the right foot to push the shovel down, he noted collapse of the right foot with associated pain and swelling. At the resulting plantar medial midfoot bony prominence, a noninfected, superficial, 1.5-cm diameter ulcer developed but healed with 3 weeks of total contact casting. Pulses were intact. Clinical photographs (**A** and **B**) show deformity of the right foot with forefoot abduction, plantar medial midfoot prominence, and collapse of the arch. Radiographs showed Lisfranc Charcot fracture-dislocation with forefoot abduction (**C**) and collapse of the arch with plantar flexion of the talus relative to the metatarsals (**D**).

- Gout
- Peripheral vascular disease

Additional Work-up

The differential diagnosis of the swollen, erythematous, warm foot in the neuropathic patient includes Charcot arthropathy and infection. The absence of any history of ulcer is evidence against deep infection. Although hematogenous infection may occur, the most common cause of infection in the neuropathic foot is direct bacterial invasion from a wound. Elevation of the foot may help distinguish between the two diagnoses; the erythema of the hyperemic Charcot foot may decrease with elevation but the erythema of cellulitis may persist despite elevation. In this setting, it is not uncommon for the medical service to specifically request that the orthopaedic surgeon perform a bone biopsy and deep culture. However, if there is no history of ulcer, a biopsy may subject the acutely inflamed Charcot foot to an iatrogenic infection and probably should be deferred.

A negative technetium Tc 99m bone scan may exclude the diagnosis of Charcot arthropathy, but a positive bone scan may be indicative of either Charcot arthropathy or deep infection. Additional imaging studies, such as bone scans with indium or gallium or MRI with gadolinium enhancement, may or may not be helpful diagnostically.

An acute Charcot arthropathy and deep infection may coexist in the same foot, especially in the presence of an ulcer. If an ulcer is present, a biopsy may be helpful. If the diagnosis is unclear from clinical and radiographic evaluation, a period of strict bed rest and mild elevation and splinting may improve the clinical signs of the Charcot foot. Empiric antibiotics may be considered but may be stopped if clinical improvement occurs. If there is no clinical improvement, especially if the patient has signs and symptoms of an infection (fever, chills, and leukocytosis), then a biopsy may be advised.

■

The Solutions

Treatment Options and Rationale

The goals of treatment include resolution of the Charcot process with a stable foot that may be fitted with functional footwear, including shoes and orthoses, for activities of daily living. Historically, treatment of acute Charcot arthropathy (stage 1) consisted of protective immobilization; however, sometimes the instability is so severe that the foot cannot be controlled with a cast. Early surgical stabilization is indicated if there is displacement and ulceration; the development of an ulcer at this stage indicates that the risk of recurrent ulceration is high even if the ulcer can successfully be treated nonsurgically. Other factors that may contribute to failure of nonsurgical treatment, such as obesity or a funnel-shaped leg, are indications for surgical stabilization of the acute Charcot foot.

If an ulcer is present, it is preferable, if possible, to defer Charcot reconstruction until the ulcer is healed by means of off-loading (total contact casting or prefabricated bracing) and surgical débridement. An ulcer that has not healed may increase the potential risk of postoperative infection from bacterial colonization of the ulcer. However, gross instability may prevent ulcer healing in some patients. Surgical stabilization of the Charcot foot with external or internal fixation and management of the ulcer with appropriate irrigation, débridement, and antibiotic coverage may be justified in these patients. An infected ulcer is a contraindication to open reduction and internal fixation, but stability of the bones and soft tissues may be achieved in this setting with an external fixator.

The goals of surgical reconstruction include realignment or reduction of the fracture-dislocation and arthrodesis with the foot in a neutral-plantigrade position. These goals may be achieved with open reduction and internal fixation. If extensive bony destruction, fragmentation, and collapse have occurred, then bony excision may be required to enable reduction without residual bony prominences. For midfoot Charcot arthropathy, this reduction may require excision of bone from the metatarsal bases, cuneiforms, or cuboid. Correction of alignment in midfoot Charcot arthropathy when the arch has collapsed and the forefoot is in abduction includes restoration of the arch and neutral forefoot position. Internal fixation may be

achieved with plate screw constructs or multiple screws.

In the patient with diabetic neuropathy, the risks of surgery may include an increased risk of infection, wound dehiscence, hardware failure, and nonunion. However, if an ulcer has already occurred, a foot with severe rocker-bottom or forefoot abduction deformity that is treated nonsurgically and allowed to heal in the displaced position may be at even greater risk for recurrent ulceration leading to deep infection or amputation. Therefore, surgery is justified if the risks of nonsurgical treatment are potentially greater than the risks of surgery. Furthermore, reconstructive surgery in the chronic stage (Eichenholtz stage III) may be more technically challenging than in the acute stage (Eichenholtz stage I) because osteotomy may be required after consolidation of the Charcot process. When surgery can be performed in the acute stage (Eichenholtz stage I) with close patient monitoring, antibiotic coverage, adequate arterial supply, reasonable patient compliance, and frequent wound inspection, the risks of a limb-threatening infection or wound problems from surgical treatment may be less than the risk of a limb-threatening infected ulcer developing in a nonreduced foot. This relative risk of surgical versus nonsurgical treatment is discussed with the patient and documented in the medical record.

For acute Charcot arthropathy (Eichenholtz stage I), the patient is maintained at bed rest (no weight bearing), and surgery is deferred until swelling, erythema, and increased warmth are improved.

SURGICAL APPROACH
The medial aspect of the Lisfranc region is exposed through a medial incision centered at the plantar palpated border of the first metatarsocuneiform joint. This incision usually extends from the plantar aspect of the midshaft of the first metatarsal to the plan-

tar aspect of the navicular bone and is curved convex plantar because of the rocker-bottom deformity. The subluxated first metatarsocuneiform joint is exposed. The risk of a painful neuroma of the medial plantar nerve is rare in the patient with neuropathy.

The second and third metatarsocuneiform joints and the first-second and second-third intercuneiform joints are exposed through a dorsal longitudinal incision while taking care to avoid injury to the dorsalis pedis artery.

CORRECTION OF ALIGNMENT AND PREPARATION OF ARTHRODESIS
The exposed articular surfaces of the metatarsocuneiform and intercuneiform joints are débrided of residual articular cartilage and fibrous tissue using curets and rongeurs. The joint surfaces are further prepared for arthrodesis by "fish scaling" the surfaces with an osteotome and making multiple small drill holes to increase surface area and promote vascularity. An Achilles tendon lengthening is done if the foot and ankle are not easily dorsiflexed beyond neutral.

The joints are reduced to as close to anatomic alignment as possible. Reduction usually involves manipulating the forefoot out of abduction and dorsiflexion. In the acute Charcot foot (Eichenholtz stage I), osteotomy usually is not required. A small amount of residual malalignment or displacement at the joints may contribute to marked residual deformity at the distal aspect of the forefoot. Therefore, the overall alignment of the forefoot relative to the hindfoot is evaluated intraoperatively to improve the potential for correct alignment after reduction. If soft-tissue structures or bony deformity blocks reduction, the joint is débrided until reduction can be achieved. This reduction may appear less anatomic than reduction of an acute nonneuropathic Lisfranc fracture-dislocation because of the bony fragmentation that may be present in the neuropathic foot. However, if the

overall alignment of the foot is restored, a stable arthrodesis without
bony prominences may be achieved.

Provisional fixation may be accomplished with Kirschner wires. With
the foot and ankle held in neutral position, the metatarsal heads are palpated
to confirm that they lie in a smooth
plane. Residual excessive dorsiflexion
or overcorrection into excessive plantar
flexion is avoided because it may cause
increased localized pressure and ulceration at a prominent metatarsal head.

FIXATION

Plate fixation may be achieved along the
plantar or plantar medial aspect of the
first metatarsocuneiform joint region
with a small fragment one third tubular
plate, stacked one third tubular plates, a
dynamic compression plate (DCP), or a
limited contact DCP (LC-DCP; Synthes,
Paoli, PA). In this location, the plate
may serve as a tension band plate in addition to providing fixation and compression. Small fragment screws may be
used, or large fragment (4.5-mm)
screws may be used with the one third
tubular plate for improved screw purchase. If additional stability is required,
the plate may be extended as needed to
bones such as the navicular bone that
are not necessarily included in the fusion. Additional screws, including
metatarsocuneiform screws and intercuneiform screws, are used as needed
for fixation. Alternate fixation methods
may include screws alone or external
fixation. Satisfactory alignment and
fixation are corroborated clinically and
fluoroscopically.

Cancellous bone graft is taken from
the distal tibial metaphyseal region
through a 2- × 1-cm cortical window
made with a microsagittal saw. The cortical fragment is replaced after the cancellous bone is removed, enabling cortical
healing to minimize the risk of tibial fracture through a cortical stress riser.

POSTOPERATIVE CARE

The foot and ankle are immobilized in
a well-padded plaster U-splint with

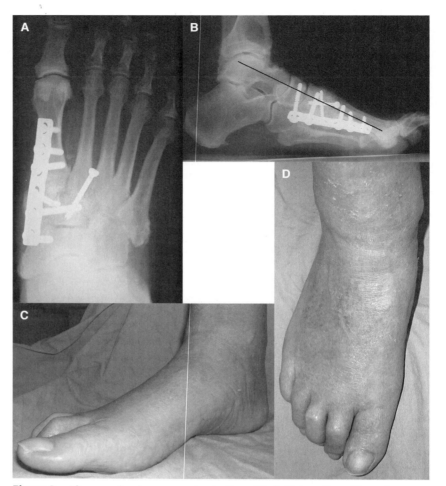

Figure 2 After vascular clearance and reduction of the initial swelling with casting, open
reduction and arthrodesis of the first, second, and third TMT joints and first-second and
second-third intercuneiform joints was performed with distal tibial cancellous bone graft.
AP (**A**) and lateral (**B**) radiographs show fixation with a small fragment LC-DCP from the
navicular to the first metatarsal and an additional 4.5-mm cannulated screw at the second
metatarsocuneiform joint. No Achilles tendon lengthening was done. The patient progressed to touchdown weight bearing in a total contact cast at 4 months after surgery,
partial weight bearing in a removable walker boot fitted with a custom Plastazote insole at
6 months, full weight bearing in the boot at 7 months, and weight bearing in an ankle-foot
orthosis with a full-length rocker-bottom shoe at 9 months postoperatively. Clinical photographs (**C** and **D**) obtained 17 months after surgery, show that the foot remained stable
with maintenance of correction of the forefoot position, TMT alignment, and plantar arch.

plantar plate and abdominal pads at
the malleoli and heel to protect
against ulceration. The splint is replaced on the first or second postoperative day and weekly thereafter until
the surgical wounds are healed. The
sutures remain in place for 3 to 4
weeks. The patient is not allowed to
bear weight for 3 to 6 months, depending on resolution of postoperative swelling, erythema, and progres-

sion of bony consolidation on
radiographs. Subsequently, orthoses
are provided and weight bearing is
progressed.

Author's Preferred Treatment
and Rationale

The procedure is done with the patient under general or spinal anesthesia. In most instances, a thigh tourniquet is used with a pressure of

275 mm Hg. Prior to inflation of the tourniquet, the dorsalis pedis pulse is palpated and marked with a marking pen, and the accurate location of the second-third intermetatarsal longitudinal incision is identified, using fluoroscopic guidance and a metal instrument outside the foot, and marked. This marking is helpful because if the incision is misplaced several millimeters, exposure of the joints and surgical fixation may be more difficult.

The fixation I prefer consists of two stacked small fragment one third tubular plates with large fragment (4.5-mm) screws. The small fragment DCP or LC-DCP (**Figure 2**) is stronger than the stacked one third tubular plates but is more difficult to contour, may be used only with small fragment (3.5-mm) screws, and may be too bulky and prominent. The bone stock is usually poor, and the large fragment (4.5-mm) screws used with the stacked one third tubular plates provide better screw purchase than small fragment (3.5-mm) screws.

Before provisional and definitive fixation, the foot and ankle are held in neutral position and one index finger is held across the plantar metatarsal head region to confirm planar alignment of the sesamoid-lesser metatarsal head region without bony prominence. Care is taken to reduce the forefoot out of dorsiflexion and abduction. The foot and ankle are inspected from all angles, including dorsal, plantar, medial, lateral, anterior, and posterior views, and security of fixation is assessed with mechanical examination and AP, oblique, and lateral fluoroscopic radiographs.

The patient is not allowed to bear weight for 6 months after surgery. If there is adequate consolidation of the arthrodesis, weight bearing is advanced in a prefabricated non-hinged removable walker boot fitted with a custom, heat-molded, full-length soft Plastazote insole (Zotefoams, Inc, Walton, KY). When the patient is fully ambulatory, a Plastazote-lined, custom ankle-foot orthosis (AFO) or custom molded leather ankle brace with built-in plastic AFO is fabricated, and shoes are modified with a rigid rocker-bottom sole and a custom, heat-molded, soft Plastazote insole. Follow-up is continued at 3 to 6 month intervals. If the foot remains stable after 1 year of full weight bearing, the AFO is tapered but the rigid rocker-bottom sole and soft insole are continued indefinitely.

Management of Complications

General risks of surgery include anesthetic problems, infection, wound dehiscence, neurovascular injury, and thrombophlebitis. Infection is managed with wound culture, débridement as needed, and antibiotics. Infections may be polymicrobial, and consultation from a specialist in infectious diseases may be helpful. Wound drainage or dehiscence is treated using half-strength povidone-iodine dressings and oral antibiotics, with weekly wound checks until dehiscence is resolved. If surgery is done in the setting of an unhealed ulcer, antibiotics are used prophylactically, and the patient may be maintained on oral empiric antibiotics until all wounds are completely healed; however, this treatment is controversial and may be associated with the risk of developing resistant organisms.

Risk of nonunion may be decreased with discontinuation of smoking before surgery, use of rigid fixation, and cancellous bone grafting. Asymptomatic, stable nonunion may be managed with protective orthoses and rocker-bottom shoes. Revision arthrodesis may be indicated for unstable nonunions, as evidenced by progressive deformity or ulceration. Hardware failure may occur even if consolidation of the fusion is successful; if there are signs of inflammation or hardware prominence, hardware removal may be indicated.

References

Johnson JE: Operative treatment of neuropathic arthropathy of the foot and ankle. *J Bone Joint Surg Am* 1998;80:1700-1709.

O'Malley DF, Conti SF: Results of distal tibial bone grafting in hindfoot arthrodeses. *Foot Ankle Int* 1996;17:374-377.

Pinzur MS: Benchmark analysis of diabetic patients with neuropathic (Charcot) foot deformity. *Foot Ankle Int* 1999;20:564-567.

Schon LC, Easley ME, Weinfeld SB: Charcot neuroarthropathy of the foot and ankle. *Clin Orthop* 1998;349:116-131.

Simon SR, Tejwani SG, Wilson DL, Santner TJ, Denniston NL: Arthrodesis as an early alternative to nonoperative management of Charcot arthropathy of the diabetic foot. *J Bone Joint Surg Am* 2001;82:939-950.

Trepman E, Nihal A, Pinzur MS: Charcot neuroarthropathy of the foot and ankle. *Foot Ankle Int*, in press.

Coding

ICD-9 CODES

250.6   Diabetes with neurological manifestations

707.1   Ulcer of lower limbs, except decubitus

713.5   Charcot's arthropathy associated with other disorders classified elsewhere

727.81   Other disorders of synovium, tendon, and bursa, Contracture of tendon (sheath); short Achilles tendon (acquired)

733.82   Malunion and nonunion of fracture; nonunion of fracture

825.35   Fracture of one or more tarsal and metatarsal bones, open

CPT CODES

20902   Bone graft, any donor area; major or large

27685   Lengthening or shortening of tendon, leg or ankle; single tendon (separate procedure)

28730   Arthrodesis, midtarsal or tarsometatarsal, multiple or transverse

28740   Arthrodesis, midtarsal or tarsometatarsal, single joint

Chronic Midfoot Charcot Rocker-Bottom Reconstruction

Lew C. Schon, MD

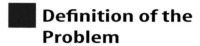

Definition of the Problem

Patient Presentation

Patients with a chronic midfoot Charcot rocker-bottom foot present with a history of an acute Charcot episode including a hot, swollen, erythematous foot (Eichenholtz stage I). Some patients do not recall an antecedent initiating event. The original manifestation may have been undiagnosed or misdiagnosed as an infection. After a period of casting, bracing, and not bearing weight, there is a decrease in swelling, warmth, and erythema indicative of a healing Charcot foot (Eichenholtz stage II). Ultimately the patient presents with a deformed foot that has minimal swelling, erythema, and warmth, consistent with the final stage of the Charcot process (Eichenholtz stage III).

Patients range in age from approximately 30 years to older than 70 years. Both sexes are equally affected. All patients have a history of neuropathy with diminished tactile sensation and often have proprioceptive derangements such as wide-based gait and tendency to fall. In my practice, more than 60% of these patients have diabetes mellitus. Of all patients, 15% to 20% have idiopathic neuropathy; the remaining patients have abnormal sensation secondary to hereditary sensory motor neuropathy, congenital insensitivity to pain, syringomyelia, rheumatologic disorders, alcoholism, infection, or posttraumatic neuropathy.

Approximately 30% of patients in my practice have bilateral involvement. Although classically Charcot neuroarthropathy results in a painless deformity, 30% to 40% of patients may have pain as a presenting symptom. However, the pain is much less than expected given the clinical and radiographic findings.

Physical Examination

A Charcot classification system categorizes chronic Charcot midfoot rocker-bottom deformity based on anatomic location (type) and degree of deformity (stage). Identifying the location helps in understanding the clinical features, such as where the bony prominences are likely to occur. Determining the type also helps identify what surgical correction is needed. The stage or severity helps identify the progression of disease. A stage A foot rarely requires surgical intervention, whereas a stage C foot often requires either extremely aggressive nonsurgical treatment that will be fraught with complications or surgery. The risks for ulceration and osteomyelitis are also greater in stage C.

Type I deformity occurs at the metatarsocuneiform joints and is characterized by a medial plantar prominence and often abduction at the midfoot level (**Figure 1**). A type II deformity occurs at the naviculocuneiform joints and is characterized by a plantar lateral prominence under the fourth and fifth metatar-

socuboid joints. This foot is abducted in 50% of patients and adducted in the other 50% of patients. The type III deformity occurs at the naviculum with fragmentation and/or osteonecrosis of this bone. This deformity is characterized by adduction, supination of the foot, and a plantar lateral prominence under the cuboid as a result of medial column shortening relative to the lateral column. A type IV deformity occurs at the transverse tarsal joints and is characterized by prominence under the calcaneocuboid joint and/or the talonavicular joint.

In stage A, the arch is low but not flat. In stage B, the midfoot is in the same plane as the metatarsal and calcaneus, and in stage C, the midfoot is below the plane of the metatarsals and calcaneus (**Figure 2**).

With increasing severity of the deformity, an ulcer or osteomyelitis is more likely to develop at the bony prominence. Ulcers should be probed to determine ulcer depth and to investigate possible occult deep space infection. If the probe touches bone, osteomyelitis is usually present. Although, in general, the chronic Charcot foot is minimally swollen, hot, and erythematous, occasionally an acute Charcot episode indicates additional deterioration of the foot with reactivation of the Charcot process.

Pulses are examined to determine whether vascular status is compromised to any extent that may re-

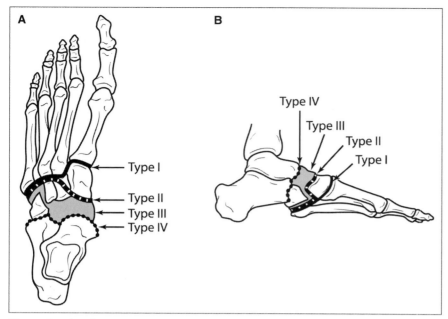

Figure 1 Classification of chronic Charcot rocker-bottom deformities. AP (**A**) and lateral (**B**) views. (Reproduced with permission from Schon LC, Weinfeld SB, Horton GA, Resch S: Radiographic and clinical classification of acquired midtarsus deformities. *Foot Ankle Int* 1998;19: 394-404.)

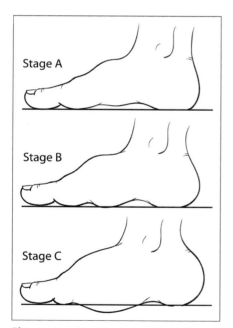

Figure 2 Classification of staging of chronic Charcot rocker-bottom deformities. (Reproduced with permission from Schon LC, Weinfeld SB, Horton GA, Resch S: Radiographic and clinical classification of acquired midtarsus deformities. *Foot Ankle Int* 1998;19: 394-404.)

quire vascular surgical intervention before orthopaedic treatment. If there is any question about the quality of the pulses or if the patient has any history of vascular pathology, I obtain arterial Doppler tests with toe pressures. An ankle-brachial index of 50% or higher indicates good vascularity for healing. The inability to feel a monofilament of 10 g is typically encountered in these patients.

Differential Diagnosis

- Soft-tissue infection (cellulitis or abscess)
- Osteomyelitis
- Septic joint space infection
- Arthritis or arthropathy (osteonecrosis, fracture, tendon rupture)
- Rheumatologic disorders (rheumatoid arthritis, gout)

Additional Work-up

Radiographs may indicate hypertrophic aggressive or destructive arthropathy. Varying degrees of bone fragmen-tation, zones of osteolysis, periosteal bone growth, and sclerosis may be observed, depending on the stage of the disease. Radiographs may reveal evidence of concomitant arthritis, osteonecrosis, fracture, dislocation, or subluxation. A technetium Tc 99m bone scan may have increased uptake in patients with a Charcot foot or in those with an infection. Scans using indium In 111-labeled leukocytes may be active in patients with an acute Charcot foot but are rarely active in patients who have a chronic Charcot foot. MRI may help to identify deep space infections, abscesses, and septic joints. However, marrow space edema, bone and joint destruction, and soft-tissue edema can be evident on MRI in patients with either Charcot arthropathy or osteomyelitis. Some have recommended gadolinium-enhanced MRI to distinguish a Charcot foot from an infected foot, although I have not found this to be helpful. Therefore, the differential diagnosis would rely on the physical examination and other imaging studies.

The Solutions

Treatment Options and Rationale

Most chronic midfoot rocker-bottom deformities can be managed nonsurgically, including bracing, custom-molded or accommodative shoes, foot orthoses, and intermittent callus or ulcer débridement. An acute-on-chronic process should be addressed with off-loading and total contact casting or Charcot bracing.

An arthrodesis of the Charcot midfoot or hindfoot is indicated when there is an unstable deformity, recurrent ulceration, persistent osteomyelitis, or a deformity that cannot be braced. At times, a limited ostectomy can be performed before an arthrodesis. Occasionally when the foot is intrinsically stable, an ostectomy may be sufficient for treatment and thus more aggressive osteotomy or fusion might not be required.

Patients with severe Charcot rocker-bottom deformity (stage C) with a complete reversal of the arch have a high risk of instability, recurrent ulceration, and persistent osteomyelitis. When the deformity occurs through dislocated joints without fractures, the foot is even more unstable and is less likely to consolidate. In these patients, arthrodesis with stabilization of the medial and lateral columns of the foot may be indicated.

Recently, better results have been obtained using more extensive hardware configurations and prolonged postoperative immobilization. Two advances that improve correction and increase the rigidity of fixation are the closing wedge osteotomy-arthrodesis and plantar plate fixation.

In severe type I or type II deformities, a typical correction is to perform a transpedal plantar-based wedge osteotomy and fusion through a medial and lateral approach. The wedge in type I deformity includes the metatarsocuneiform joints. In type II deformities, the wedge includes the naviculocuneiform joints and the 4-5 metatarsocuboid joints. The bones are then stabilized using a plantar-medial plate and either a dorsolateral or a plantar-lateral plate. With osteomyelitis, an external fixator is used for stability. The gastrocnemius and soleus

are lengthened to correct the equinus hindfoot deformity.

Type III and type IV midfoot deformities, both of which involve the calcaneocuboid joint, may require correction by a triple arthrodesis. Stabilization of the calcaneocuboid component of the triple fusion may be achieved with the use of a single long axial screw driven from the calcaneal tuberosity into the cuboid. When the rigid deformity is more severe, a wedge osteotomy and arthrodesis may be indicated. Modification of the surgery includes adjustments for the apex of the deformity and the plane of correction. Lengthening of the gastrocnemius and soleus is necessary to correct the equinus hindfoot deformity.

Midfoot and hindfoot fusions for Charcot deformities involve technically demanding surgical intervention as well as time-consuming and labor-intensive postoperative care. However, limbs that were marginally salvageable with high maintenance requirements before surgical intervention appear to be much more functional with lower maintenance requirements after surgery.

Author's Preferred Treatment and Rationale

For reconstruction of a chronic Charcot rocker-bottom foot, a closing wedge osteotomy, arthrodesis, and a plantar plating procedure are performed. A dorsal opening wedge osteotomy with structural bone graft interposition should be avoided in

patients with a chronic Charcot rocker-bottom foot.

A very high degree of intraoperative and postoperative vigilance is necessary to avoid complications. Reduction should achieve a properly configured plantigrade foot with restoration of an arch and even weight distribution of the metatarsals and calcaneus. Fixation must be rigid with mechanically sound constructs that can withstand acute and cyclic loading.

An extensile exposure is used for the transpedal osteotomy and arthrodesis. A curvilinear incision is made along the medial aspect of the foot with the inferior aspect of the incision sweeping in the plantar direction at the apex of the deformity (**Figure 3**, *A*). Full-thickness skin flaps are preserved, and the deep dissection proceeds to the fascia of the abductor hallucis muscle (**Figure 3**, *B*). The muscle belly is retracted in the plantar direction to identify the first metatarsal, medial cuneiform, medial talus, and/or naviculum as needed (**Figure 3**, *C*). The periosteum is incised longitudinally along the junction of the medial and plantar aspects of the medial ray using electrocautery. The deep fascial edge of the abductor hallucis is retracted in the plantar direction, and the plantar limb of the dissection is continued beneath the medial column (staying directly on the bone) using an electrocautery blade to minimize bleeding. A sharp periosteal elevator is then used to continue the dissection across the plantar

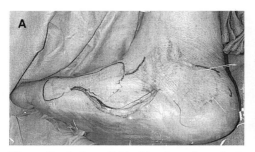 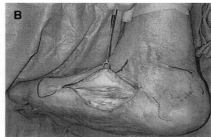 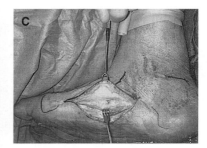

Figure 3 **A,** A medial incision is made at the junction of the plantar and medial margins of the midfoot. **B,** Full-thickness skin flaps are preserved as deep dissection proceeds to the fascia of the abductor hallucis muscle. **C,** The muscle is retracted down in the plantar direction.

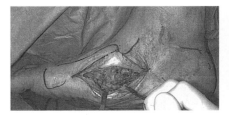

Figure 4 Subperiosteal dissection is done at the plantar base of the planned wedge.

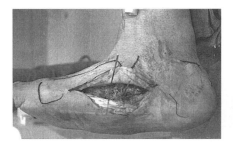

Figure 5 Converging guide wires mark the edges of the wedge for the midfoot osteotomy.

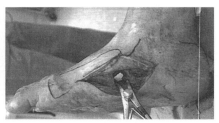

Figure 6 Transpedal osteotomy-arthrodesis is performed. A plantar-based closing wedge is created. The osteotomy traverses the deformed arthritic joints from medial to lateral through all bones. A lamina spreader is used to ensure that there are no obstructions and the surfaces are flat.

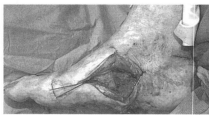

Figure 7 Transpedal closing wedge. The osteotomy-arthrodesis is reduced and held with guide wires.

aspect of the foot (**Figure 4**). Typically, the apex of the deformity will be at the joints, and thus the deformed joint surfaces are resected in the wedges. Care is taken to avoid dissection in the intermetatarsal area between the bases of any of the metatarsals where communicating arteries are vulnerable. A dorsal periosteal-capsular sleeve is developed to create a cuff of tissue for later closure. The insertions of the anterior and posterior tibial tendons may be identified and preserved as part of the thick dorsal sleeve, but complete detachment is avoided. At times, especially in the presence of a severe abduction deformity (in which a large medial-based closing wedge osteotomy is required), it is advisable to lift a sliver of the medial aspect of the cuneiform while leaving the insertion of the tendon intact. When treating a foot that has both an abduction deformity and a rocker-bottom deformity, the wedge is trapezoidal. If the foot has a rocker-bottom deformity without adduction or abduction, the wedge is triangular.

Correction of the rocker-bottom deformity is achieved by a coronal plane midfoot osteotomy and arthrodesis with wedge resection. The osteotomy and arthrodesis should be planned to cross the apex of the deformity and the associated joints affected by the disease process. The wedge is usually biplanar. A medially or laterally based triangular wedge is used to correct an abducted or adducted rocker-bottom deformity, respectively. The edges of the wedge are first marked by two converging guide pins inserted into the bone (**Figure 5**). The ends of the pins should meet at the outer cortex of the relevant bone in the lateral column (for a medial-based closing wedge) or medial column (for a lateral-based closing wedge). The final position of the pins is confirmed by fluoroscopy with both AP and lateral views. Two osteotomy cuts are then made with a sagittal saw along the inner borders of the converging guide pins. The saw blade is rotated slightly away from the vertical plane into an oblique position so that more bone

will be resected plantarly than dorsally. The resulting cross-section of the wedge (as viewed from the medial aspect of the foot) should be trapezoidal with a plantar base. The resected wedge of bone and any remaining bone fragments are identified and removed. The degree of the wedge correction reflects the degree of the deformity. For example, with a 30° lateral talo-first metatarsal angle, the angle at the apex is approximately 30°. Generally, the size of the wedge at its base ranges from 1 to 2.5 cm (**Figure 6**).

Reduction of the midfoot is achieved by reapproximating the bone edges in a closing-wedge fashion until stable bone-to-bone contact is achieved. This maneuver should correct both the abduction deformity of the forefoot and the rocker-bottom deformity of the midfoot. The reduction is assessed both clinically and with fluoroscopy. Fine adjustments can be made by resecting more bone if necessary. Any pronation or supination component of the forefoot deformity can be corrected by rotating the forefoot in relation to the midfoot through the osteotomy site. As soon as the optimal alignment has been achieved, the reduction is temporarily held by guide wires, and multiple 4.0-, 4.5-, or 5.0-mm cannulated screws are used for fixation (**Figure 7**). If the bone quality is poor, the screws may be extended across primarily uninvolved joints to gain better fixation of the osteoporotic bone. The lateral column may be reinforced with a long 6.5-mm axial screw driven from the posterior calcaneal tuberosity into the cuboid and sometimes extending into the base of the fourth metatarsal. Applying a plantar plate can provide additional stabilization of both columns. I typically use four- to six-hole one third tubular plates. Proper positioning of the hardware is confirmed with fluoroscopy (**Figure 8**). Postoperatively, the foot is immobilized in a non–weight-bearing cast for 3 months

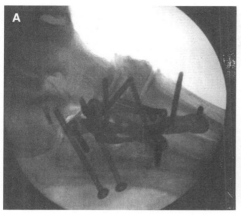

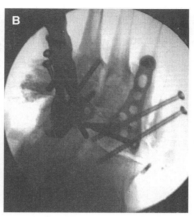

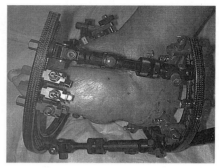

Figure 8   Lateral (**A**) and AP (**B**) fluoroscopic views demonstrate a plantarly applied medial plate stabilizing the medial column and a dorsally applied lateral plate stabilizing the fourth and fifth metatarsocuboid arthrodesis.

Figure 9   An external fixator maintains the reduction of the osteotomy-arthrodesis in a patient treated for osteomyelitis and open ulcer.

followed by bracing. Radiographs are obtained to monitor healing. After the foot is judged to be stable, braces and orthotics replace the cast.

No hardware is used where there is an active ulcer or osteomyelitis at the time of surgery. An external fixator is used for stabilization in these situations (**Figure 9**). The frame is constructed with multiple thin transfixing wires placed through the metatarsals, attached to a ring, and then tensioned. The hindfoot is similarly transfixed with pins in a plane perpendicular to the longitudinal axis of the calcaneus. The two rings are then compressed to maintain the reduction. Percutaneous Kirschner wires crossing the fusion site are helpful in maintaining the correct alignment. The external fixator is often removed by 3 to 5 months. The patient does not bear weight for at least 3 months; protected and progressive weight bearing in a cast or brace follows for the next 3 to 12 months.

Lengthening of the gastrocnemius and soleus muscles is usually required. A triple-cut Hoke-style distal lengthening can be supplemented by a midleg gastrocnemius and soleus lengthening using the Strayer technique. Deep posterior ankle capsular release is rarely required.

Management of Complications

After correction, redundant soft tissues often resemble the initial deformity. With time, progressive weight bearing, and more physiologic stresses, these tissues may remodel. Additional surgical reconstruction is not necessary for this condition provided that bone configuration is appropriate.

Broken hardware may need to be removed if the hardware is prominent. Broken hardware often means that the foot is not adequately healed and indicates the need to curtail weight bearing and increase immobilization. Alternatively, a broken screw may result from normal movement in unfused joints that have been transfixed by hardware to achieve additional stability during healing. In this scenario, hardware failure is expected and does not necessarily indicate loss of fixation at the site of the osteotomy or fusion.

The Charcot process may become activated during the healing process and is heralded by increased swelling, warmth, or erythema or by radiographic evidence of adjacent joint involvement. In roughly 10% of patients, the Charcot process extends to the talus or the forefoot. The acute process is controlled by immobilization with no weight bearing. In a few instances, osteonecrosis of the talus may occur. This osteonecrosis may

not always be controllable with nonsurgical management because the talus dissolution may result in ankle instability and uncontrollable deformity. In these patients, the fusion may be extended proximally by tibiocalcaneonavicular arthrodesis.

Superficial infection is managed with oral or intravenous antibiotics and immobilization with no weight bearing. Pin tract infections often require débridement and, rarely, the insertion of new wires. A deep infection is rare but requires aggressive repetitive débridement and treatment with antibiotics. The hardware may be left intact if it is still providing stability. If the hardware has failed or if the infection is uncontrollable, the hardware must be removed and an external fixator applied.

Incomplete or delayed unions are treated by a prolonged period of immobilization without weight bearing and the use of external or internal electric bone stimulation. Bone grafting or revision fixation is rarely needed. Surgery to stabilize the medial or lateral column may help complete the healing process and facilitate union in some patients. Revision surgery with or without revision wedge resection or treatment of other symptomatic joints may be necessary in patients in whom nonunion or malunion results in a foot that cannot be fit with braces and shoes.

References

Schon LC, Easley ME, Cohen I, Lam PWC, Badekas A, Anderson CD: The acquired midtarsus deformity classification system: Interobserver reliability and intraobserver reproducibility. *Foot Ankle Int* 2002;23:30-36.

Schon LC, Easley ME, Weinfeld SB: Charcot neuroarthropathy of the foot and ankle. *Clin Orthop* 1998;349:116-131.

Schon LC, Weinfeld SB, Horton GA, Resch S: Radiographic and clinical classification of acquired midtarsus deformities. *Foot Ankle Int* 1998;19:394-404.

Coding

ICD-9 CODES

707.15 Ulcer of other part of foot

715.37 Osteoarthrosis, localized, not specified whether primary or secondary, ankle and foot

730.07 Acute osteomyelitis, ankle and foot

733.81 Malunion of fracture

733.82 Nonunion of fracture

736.70 Unspecified deformity of ankle and foot, acquired

736.71 Acquired equinovarus deformity

838.02 Closed dislocation, midtarsal (joint)

CPT CODES

20692 Application of a multiplane (pins or wires in more than one plane), unilateral, external fixation system (eg, Ilizarov, Monticelli type)

20974 Electrical stimulation to aid bone healing; noninvasive (nonoperative)

20975 Electrical stimulation to aid bone healing; invasive (operative)

27606 Tenotomy, percutaneous, Achilles tendon (separate procedure); general anesthesia

27687 Gastrocnemius recession (eg, Strayer procedure)

28262 Capsulotomy, midfoot; extensive, including posterior talotibial capsulotomy and tendon(s) lengthening (eg, resistant clubfoot deformity)

28320 Repair, nonunion or malunion; tarsal bones

28715 Arthrodesis; triple

28735 Arthrodesis; with osteotomy (eg, flatfoot correction)

CPT copyright © 2003 by the American Medical Association. All Rights Reserved.

Ankle and Hindfoot Charcot Arthropathy

Timothy R. Daniels, MD, FRCSC

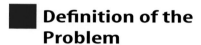

Definition of the Problem

Patient Presentation

Patients with Charcot arthropathy have a warm, swollen erythematous foot with varying degrees of deformity and instability on presentation. Most commonly they will have had diabetes mellitus for more than 10 years but, occasionally, a Charcot event is the first indication of diabetes. The type of diabetes has a marginal effect on the incidence of Charcot arthropathy; patients with type I diabetes mellitus have only a slightly higher preponderance toward a Charcot event. The rate of collapse and the degree of deformity are variable. Patients are at greatest risk during the initial stage (fragmentation stage).

Charcot collapse of the ankle and hindfoot can be the result of repetitive trauma or an acute event such as a sprain or a fracture. Most diabetic patients with Charcot arthropathy have bounding pulses on presentation and capillary blood flow in the foot that is up to five times the normal rate. The diabetic neuropathy can cause autonomic dysfunction leading to increased blood flow and arteriovenous shunting in the extremities, resulting in bone resorption. The sensory neuropathy decreases the patient's ability to recognize harmful external forces to the foot. The peripheral motor neuropathy is characterized by a large pattern of muscle weakness leading to structural deformities such as claw toes (intrinsic muscle weakness), cavus foot (overpull of the strong invertors of the foot), and equinus contractures at the ankle (overpull of the strong gastrocnemius-soleus complex). These structural deformities lead to increased weight distribution through the forefoot and midfoot, causing elevated shear forces at the midtarsal joints and the plantar skin beneath the metatarsal heads or bony prominences. This Charcot collapse of the foot and ankle often occurs at the joints. The frequency of Charcot involvement of the subtalar joint complex is 30% to 35%, and the incidence at the ankle joint is 5% to 10%.

Physical Examination

The lower extremities are evaluated for skeletal deformity, extent of soft-tissue contractures, vascular sufficiency, integrity of the soft tissues (depth of the ulcer if present), and the stage of the deformity. Collapse at the ankle joint or through the subtalar joint complex can present as either a hindfoot valgus or varus deformity; the direction of the deformity may be influenced by the premorbid position of the hindfoot. Varied patterns of skeletal deformity can occur when both the ankle joint and the subtalar joint complex are involved.

Although the etiology of a neuropathic ulcer is multifactorial, the extent and location of the deformity and associated pressure primarily determine the absence or presence of ulceration. If the ankle joint collapses into varus, the patient often has ulceration over the tip of the fibula or plantar to the fifth metatarsal tuberosity. Valgus collapse may be associated with ulcerations at the medial malleolus, at the navicular tuberosity, or beneath the medial cuneiform. Ulceration through the calcaneal fat pad is unusual, but if it is present, the patient should be evaluated for vascular insufficiency and/or osteomyelitis of the calcaneus.

Careful assessment of hindfoot and forefoot motion may determine the degree of instability and identify areas of the foot at high risk for ulceration. Significant motion within the Charcot joint complex suggests that stability has not been restored; this places the foot and ankle at substantial risk of further collapse. The unstable deformities are difficult to stabilize with a brace because hypermobility may result in increased shear forces between the orthosis and bony prominences, resulting in ulceration. Decreased joint motion in the foot has also been identified as a risk factor for ulceration resulting from increased plantar pressures that occur during the steady state of walking, especially through the forefoot. An equinus contracture of the ankle substantially increases the risk of forefoot ulceration and must be addressed if surgical correction of the Charcot deformity is being considered. Functional shortening of the gastrocnemius-soleus complex can be difficult to assess in the presence of a hindfoot deformity; however, a contracted gastrocnemius-

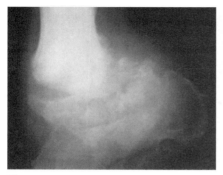

Figure 1 Lateral radiograph of a hindfoot that has undergone Charcot collapse with a hypertrophic response. Large shelf osteophytes extend anteriorly and posteriorly in an attempt to stabilize the collapsed joint complex.

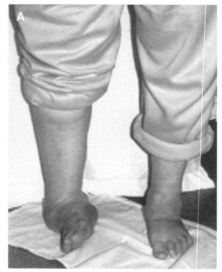

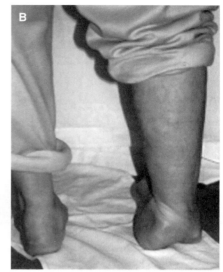

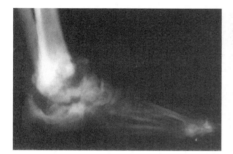

Figure 2 Lateral radiograph of a hindfoot that has undergone Charcot collapse with an atrophic response. Note the bone resorption at the anterior aspect of the tibia, the talar neck and body, and the calcaneal posterior facet.

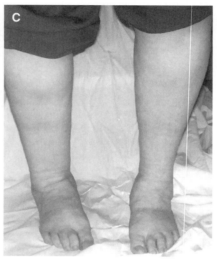

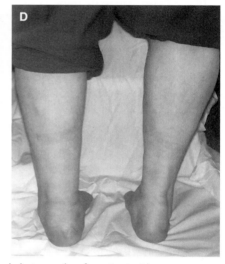

Figure 3 Anterior (**A**) and posterior (**B**) clinical photographs of a patient with a severe varus deformity of the ankle-hindfoot complex and ulceration over the tip of the fibula. The deformity was corrected with a talectomy and tibiocalcaneal arthrodesis. Anterior (**C**) and posterior (**D**) appearance of the lower extremity at 5 years after surgery. This patient had a Charcot arthropathy of the opposite side. She was managing at home with bilateral nonarticulating ankle-foot orthoses.

soleus complex can act as a major deforming force and compromise the surgical correction.

Inadequate blood flow to the extremity with Charcot arthropathy is unusual. Occasionally, patients have a remote history of Charcot collapse followed by vascular insufficiency and ulceration. It is, therefore, important to confirm that pulses are palpable. Additional vascular studies are rarely necessary in patients with acute collapse but may be indicated if pulses are difficult to palpate.

The integrity of the soft tissues requires close evaluation, particularly those surrounding any bony prominences. Débridement of callus is es-

sential to exclude the presence of an underlying ulcer and to decrease the cutaneous pressure over the bony prominence. If an ulcer is present, devitalized tissue should be débrided to decrease bacterial contamination and to create a fresh wound, which has a greater tendency to heal. Accurately documenting the size and depth of an ulcer is also important in the development of a treatment protocol. Ulcers

that extend to joints, bone, or ligaments usually require thorough débridement. If the ulcer probes to a hard bony surface with no overlying bursa, an associated osteomyelitis should be assumed until proven otherwise. Plain radiographs, CT, MRI, and nuclear medicine studies can help determine if the bone is infected; however, intraoperative biopsy of the involved bone is definitive.

Occasionally patients have a draining ulcer, excessive swelling, and moderate erythema. Clinically, it may be difficult to determine if the swelling and erythema are a result of the Charcot process or a spreading cellulitis. The typical constitutional signs and symptoms of infection are not reliable because they can be absent in patients with diabetes. A useful clinical test is to elevate the affected leg above the patient's heart for 15 minutes. The swelling will noticeably decrease if it is a result of the Charcot process. If an active infection is present, the leg will remain tensely swollen and erythematous.

The primary purpose of radiography is to identify the anatomic area involved in the Charcot collapse, to define the deformity, and to assess bone quality and quantity, especially before surgical correction and stabilization. Plain radiographs should include weight-bearing AP and lateral views of both feet and ankles. CT is an excellent method of assessing bone stock. The Charcot process is often hypertrophic on radiographs, characterized by the formation of large shelf osteophytes in a frustrated attempt to stabilize the injured and unstable joint complex (**Figure 1**). Less commonly, an atrophic Charcot process evolves, leading to resorption of entire bones such as the talus or navicular (**Figure 2**). The amount of bone available will, in part, determine the complexity of the surgical procedure, the type of fixation that can be used, and the necessity for bone graft.

In the Charcot foot, the process of osseous collapse and fragmentation can result in a disruption of the blood supply to the involved bones, resulting in the development of avascular fragments of bone and/or osteonecrosis of entire bones such as the talus. CT is a useful tool with which to quantitate the amount of bone fragmentation and collapse. This information may be useful in determining whether the talus should be incorporated into the fusion mass or a talectomy is required.

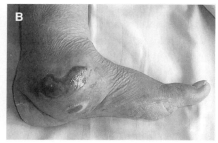
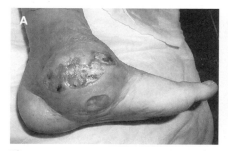

Figure 4 **A,** Acute pes planus deformity caused by collapse through the subtalar and Chopart joints. The patient has an acutely swollen foot and a superficial ulcer over the prominent medial malleolus and talar head. **B,** The swelling and size of the ulcer have decreased substantially after 2 weeks of bed rest, local wound care, and elevation of the foot. The foot was surgically realigned at this stage.

Differential Diagnosis
- Peripheral neuropathy
- Cellulitis
- Osteomyelitis
- Gout

Additional Work-up
Multiple attempts at needle aspiration of the affected area in the emergency department can lead to contamination and subsequent cellulitis and/or osteomyelitis. Evaluation includes laboratory studies (white blood cell count, erythrocyte sedimentation rate, and C-reactive protein) and studies such as ultrasonography to rule out a deep abscess or fluid collection. If a fluid collection is identified, CT- or ultrasound-guided aspiration may be helpful.

The Solutions

Treatment Options and Rationale
Patients with diabetes and hindfoot Charcot collapse pose a challenging clinical scenario for several reasons. First, many of them have had poorly controlled diabetes for more than 10 years. As a consequence, they have end-stage organ disease of multiple systems with varying degrees of renal compro-

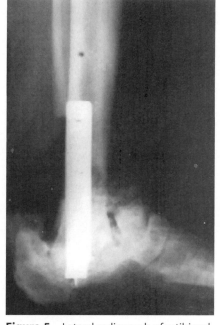

Figure 5 Lateral radiograph of a tibiocalcaneal arthrodesis with a blade plate obtained 1 year after surgery. The talus was fragmented and could not be incorporated into the fusion. The posterior portion of the posterior facet was excised to create a flat surface for apposition to the distal tibia. The navicular lies against the anterior aspect of the tibia. A stable and painless pseudarthrosis has developed.

mise, restricted vision, poor muscle function, difficulties with proprioception (poor balance), and compromised soft-tissue integrity. Second, the Charcot collapse often has resulted in major fragmentation and/or resorption of the hindfoot's osseous support. Limited bone stock confounds the orthopaedic surgeon's ability to adequately stabilize the hindfoot. Third, osteomyelitis is not uncommon and, once well established, is difficult to eradicate. These factors make it paramount that a multidisciplinary team properly prepares the patient for surgery and recovery.

The orthopaedic surgeon must emphasize to the patient that the goal of the surgery is to establish a properly aligned foot so that a brace can be worn and the foot remains ulcer-free. Surgical correction of a malaligned Charcot hindfoot is a difficult salvage procedure with the sole purpose of avoiding a below-knee amputation (**Figure 3**).

The timing of surgery depends on several variables such as the extent of deformity and instability, the presence of cellulitis and/or osteomyelitis, the status of the soft tissues, and the stage of presentation. Historically, surgical realignment of a deformed ex-

tremity was recommended when the Charcot process was consolidated (Eichenholtz stage III). However, delay is not always feasible or safe because Charcot collapse of the ankle and hindfoot can be a rapid and dramatic process, and a severe varus or valgus deformity of the hindfoot can evolve within days and progress even if the patient does not bear weight on the foot. Ulceration over the bony prominences may occur and can result from tension as the tissue is stretched over the bony prominence rather than from the direct pressure of weight bearing (**Figure 4**, *A*). Therefore, earlier stabilization may limit the destructive effects of instability on the soft tissues about the malleoli.

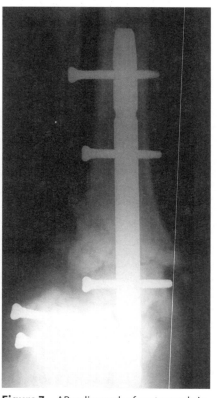

Figure 7 AP radiograph of a retrograde intramedullary reconstruction nail that has cut out of the calcaneus within 6 months after surgery. The bone stock and bone quality within the calcaneus was not sufficient. Some intramedullary nails allow for a locking screw in the sagittal plane of the calcaneus that may improve the distal stability of the fixation.

Author's Preferred Treatment and Rationale

Patients with severe, progressive deformities (Eichenholtz stage I) are admitted to the hospital for a 1- to 2-week period of bed rest, foot elevation, and ulcer care. Within days, the swelling and erythema of the surrounding soft tissues decrease. Once the erythema has resolved and there is a positive wrinkle test of the skin surrounding the ankle, surgical reconstruction may be performed (**Figure 4**, *B*). If the patient has a stable deformity or later stage disease and nonsurgical treatment has failed, then surgery is scheduled on an elective basis.

Preoperative antibiotics are administered; the type of medication depends on the culture results, the presence of osteomyelitis, and the state of the ulcer, if present. The surgical incision may need to be through or adjacent to a superficial ulcer because the ulcer might not heal until the deformity is corrected. The primary goals of surgery are to correct the deformity and maintain the correction with rigid internal and/or external fixation. The surgical approach for an unstable, deformed Charcot hindfoot differs from most elective procedures of the foot and ankle. Preservation of superficial sensory nerves or various muscle-tendon complexes is not required in the neuropathic foot. An extensile lateral approach to the hindfoot is used, and the peroneal tendons and the distal portion of the peroneal musculature may be excised, if necessary. If a posterior approach is required, the tendinous portion of the Achilles tendon may be excised. These muscles are no longer functional after the arthrodesis, and the decrease in soft-tissue bulk aids in relieving tension on the wounds after closure. When performing a lateral approach, the distal aspect of the calcaneus is routinely exposed without preserving the sural nerve. Pain or numbness/dysesthesia are uncommon in the neuropathic foot;

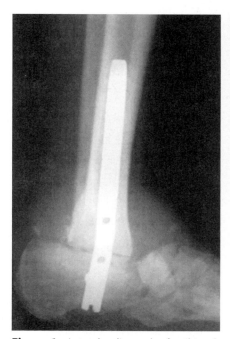

Figure 6 Lateral radiograph of a tibiocalcaneal arthrodesis using a retrograde intramedullary reconstruction nail obtained 4 years after surgery. Stable, painless tibiocalcaneal and tibionavicular pseudarthroses have developed.

however, proper exposure for insertion of the implant is essential.

The surgical approach to most Charcot ankle deformities consists of a lateral incision over the fibula and a medial incision starting just above the medial malleolus and extending along the medial border of the foot. Anterior or posterior incisions are used less frequently. The lateral approach is used to osteotomize the fibula and rotate it posteriorly to maintain the posterior soft-tissue attachments. A 1- to 2-cm section of the fibular diaphysis is removed to accommodate the shorten-ing that occurs after preparation of the joints or excision of the talus. The osteotomy of the fibula allows for adequate exposure of both the ankle and subtalar joints. Avascular fragments of bone, bursa, and fibrous tissues are excised. The soft-tissue attachments to the talus are evaluated. If the soft tissues surrounding the talar neck appear to be intact, then attempts are made to preserve the talus. However, it is not uncommon for the talus to be almost devoid of all soft-tissue attachments, and in some patients the entire talus extrudes from the wound once the lateral exposure is performed. In this circumstance, the talus is excised and either used as bone graft or discarded if associated with a deep ulcer or osteomyelitis. The cartilage of the joint surfaces is removed, and a high-speed burr with copious irrigation is used to expose fresh cancellous bone. If required, a medial approach is then used to excise the medial malleolus and prepare the talonavicular joint for arthrodesis.

If the talus is excised, a tibiocalcaneal arthrodesis is performed. In the deformed Charcot ankle, the calcaneus usually does not lie beneath the tibia; therefore, it is difficult to properly position the calcaneus in preparation for arthrodesis. Furthermore, application of internal fixation such as a lateral blade plate or screws may be difficult because of the step-off between the lateral border of the tibia and the lateral border of the calcaneus. The bony apposition between the tibia and the calcaneus may be improved by excising the posterior border of the posterior facet to create a flatter surface for coaptation with the tibia.

To obtain stabilization, a pediatric blade plate may be used (blade length, 30 or 40 mm; four- to six-hole plate). The distal fibula is excised to expose the lateral surface of the tibia. The blade portion of the plate is inserted in the posterior and lateral portion of the calcaneus, and the plate is secured to the lateral or posterolateral border of the tibia (**Figure 5**). The fixation can be augmented by one or two cannulated screws from the calcaneus into the anterior cortex of the tibia. After tibiocalcaneal fixation, the navicular is positioned anterior to the medial border of the tibia, and the tibionavicular gap is filled with bone graft and stabilized with 4.0 cannulated screws or fully threaded Kirschner wires. A stable pseudarthrosis often develops between the tibia and the navicular that does not require further intervention.

Other forms of internal fixation used include a retrograde intramedul-

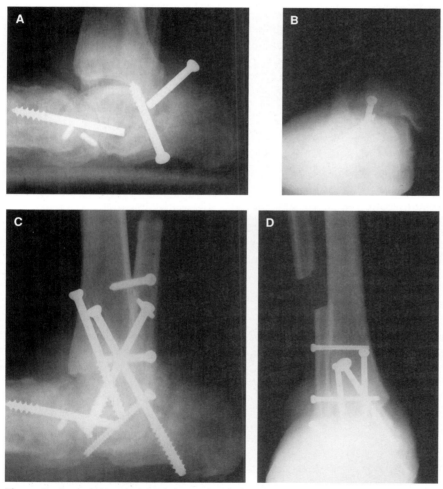

Figure 8   Lateral (**A**) and AP (**B**) radiographs of a failed triple arthrodesis for severe hindfoot Charcot collapse. The patient had a persistent flatfoot deformity and ulceration over the medial malleolus on presentation. Lateral (**C**) and AP (**D**) radiographs of salvage with tibiotalocalcaneal arthrodesis. The fibula was osteotomized and transferred distally to serve as a lateral stabilizer. Posterior soft-tissue attachments to the fibula were preserved to maintain blood supply.

lary reconstruction nail (**Figure 6**). With this method, the bone within the calcaneus can be deficient and cutting out of the nail may occur (**Figure 7**). The insertion site for the nail is in the anterior and medial aspect of the calcaneus near the middle facet. If the insertion site is too posterior and/or lateral, the hindfoot is translated in an anterior and/or medial direction as the nail is passed up through the medullary canal of the tibia. Retrograde nails are now available with calcaneal screw holes in the sagittal plane; their use improves the fixation distally. Retrograde nails are difficult to use in severe deformities because it may be difficult to position the calcaneus properly for nail insertion.

If the talus is preserved, a pantalar arthrodesis may be performed. This can be achieved with various forms of fixation devices; the preferred choice is cannulated 7.0- and 4.5-mm screws with preservation of the fibula. Postoperatively, the patients are placed in a removable below-knee brace for ulcer care. If the ulcer is deep, vacuum-assisted therapy may be instituted. The patient is advised to remain on non–weight-bearing status for a period of 8 to 12 weeks. Once the arthrodesis has matured and the swelling stabilized, the patient is fitted with a total contact ankle-foot orthosis.

Management of Complications

Salvage of failed fixation or failed arthrodesis of the Charcot hindfoot can be the result of an unstable pseudarthrosis and/or infection. It is imperative to identify the cause of failure because this will influence treatment options. If an infection is identified, it is unlikely to be eradicated while internal fixation devices are stabilizing the pseudarthrosis. In this circumstance, removal of hardware, placement of antibiotic impregnated methylmethacrylate or bone substitute, and stabilization with an external fixator is considered as an alternative to amputation.

In the absence of infection, salvage of failed fixation has a better prognosis. Salvage techniques may vary depending on bone stock and quality of the soft tissues (**Figure 8**).

References

Guyton GP, Saltzman CL: The diabetic foot: Basic mechanisms of disease. *Instr Course Lect* 2002;51:169-181.

Johnson JE: Operative treatment of neuropathic arthropathy of the foot and ankle. *J Bone Joint Surg Am* 1998;80:1700-1709.

Lin SS, Lee TH, Wapner KL: Plantar forefoot ulceration with equinus deformity of the ankle in diabetic patients: The effect of tendo-Achilles lengthening and total contact casting. *Orthopedics* 1996;19:465-475.

Pinzur MS, Kelikian A: Charcot ankle fusion with a retrograde locked intramedullary nail. *Foot Ankle Int* 1997;18:699-704.

Simon SR, Tejwani SG, Wilson DL, Santner TJ, Denniston NL: Arthrodesis as an early alternative to nonoperative management of Charcot arthropathy of the diabetic foot. *J Bone Joint Surg Am* 2001;82:939-950.

Coding

ICD-9 CODES

718.27   Pathological dislocation, ankle and foot

718.47   Contracture of joint, ankle and foot

719.77   Difficulty in walking, ankle and foot

733.16   Pathologic fracture of tibia or fibula

733.17   Pathologic fracture of ankle or foot

733.82   Nonunion of fracture

733.87   Malunion and nonunion of fracture, ankle and foot

733.93   Stress fracture of tibia or fibula

733.94   Stress fracture of the metatarsals

CPT CODES

27870   Arthrodesis, ankle, open

28705   Arthrodesis; pantalar

28715   Arthrodesis; triple

Ankle Fractures in Patients With Diabetes Mellitus

Michael S. Pinzur, MD

Definition of the Problem

Patient Presentation

To illustrate the problems considered in the evaluation and treatment of ankle fractures in patients with diabetes mellitus, four patients are presented who have had the disease for more than 10 years. The first patient is a 57-year-old man with type II diabetes mellitus who presented to the emergency department 1 day after sustaining a twisting injury to his ankle. He had minimal pain but decided to seek care because of the gross swelling. The second patient is a moderately obese 59-year-old patient with type I diabetes mellitus who had ankle discomfort and swelling after sustaining a twisting injury. The third patient is a 59-year-old man with type II diabetes mellitus who fell and was not able to bear weight on a painful, swollen ankle. The fourth patient, a woman with type I diabetes mellitus, noticed increased swelling and some discomfort following a misstep from a curb.

Physical Examination

All four patients had very swollen ankles on presentation with no breaks in the skin or signs of infection. However, a "simple" nondisplaced fracture in the foot or ankle of a patient with diabetes mellitus may be the first stage in a process that can lead to foot deformity, tissue breakdown, infection,

lower extremity amputation, and premature death. Of the more than 16 million people with diabetes mellitus in the United States, 25% have lost protective sensation as the result of peripheral neuropathy. This condition is considered a far more important risk factor for the development of diabetic foot ulcers, Charcot foot arthropathy, and lower extremity amputation than the presence of asymptomatic peripheral vascular disease. Examination of the four patients for peripheral neuropathy using a Semmes-Weinstein 5.07 (10 g)

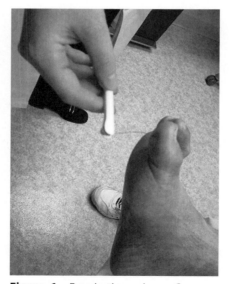

Figure 1 Examination using a Semmes-Weinstein 5.07 (10 g) monofilament. This nylon filament is one of a series of varied thickness filaments that can impart specific amounts of pressure to skin, depending on the thickness and stiffness. Ten grams of pressure applied to skin appears to be the threshold for detecting loss of protective sensation in individuals with peripheral neuropathy.

monofilament revealed that none was able to feel pressure (**Figure 1**).

How well each patient's blood glucose level was controlled, whether or not insulin was required to manage it, was determined by hemoglobin A_{1C} level studies. Vascular inflow was assessed by determining the strength of dorsalis pedis and posterior tibial pulses. All four patients had excellent vascular inflow with strong pulses and no signs of systemic infection, as measured by fever, chills, elevated white blood cell count, or increased insulin requirement.

Differential Diagnosis
- Acute Charcot arthropathy of the ankle
- Acute ankle fracture with loss of protective sensation

Additional Work-up

Metabolic associated forms of osteoporosis, combined with the loss of protective sensation, are likely responsible for the increased incidence of fracture in patients with diabetes mellitus. The peripheral neuropathy and altered balance increase with duration of the disease. The impaired granulocyte and immune function in this patient population adds to the staggering potential for morbidity following fracture. While there is no optimal way to clinically measure these functions, they have been shown with good scientific evidence.

■ The Solutions

Treatment Options and Rationale

In the examples presented, one patient healed uneventfully and two healed only after extensive surgery. The fourth required immediate ankle arthrodesis following her evaluation. Her process progressed during her initial treatment by her local physician. The reason for this diverse outcome is found in the initial differential diagnosis. Ankle fractures in patients with diabetes mellitus heal, albeit with an increased risk of morbidity. An ankle fracture that is actually the initial presentation of Charcot arthropathy is associated with more inherent risk and potential morbidity than the classic insidious presentation. This increase is a result of the biomechanical bending forces applied to the ankle compared with the plantigrade foot. Weight bearing in the ankle is applied through the tibia and accepted by the calcaneus, which is lateral to the weight-bearing axis, producing a bending moment. The plantigrade foot lies perpendicular to the weight-bearing line, so no bending moment is applied. Although the patient with a Charcot foot is almost always insensate to the Semmes-Weinstein 5.07 monofilament, the orthopaedic surgeon must remember that the insensate patient may also sustain a relatively low-energy fracture.

The fracture associated with the presentation of the first patient was actually the initial presentation of a Charcot ankle (**Figure 2**). The initial surgery achieved an anatomic reduction. The patient complied with the recommended treatment of non–weight-bearing immobilization until there was radiographic evidence of fracture union. Unfortunately, the hyperemia and bone resorption associated with the acute Charcot arthropathy process greatly decreased the screw-holding capacity of the bone and the reduction was lost. The joint was irreversibly damaged, requiring

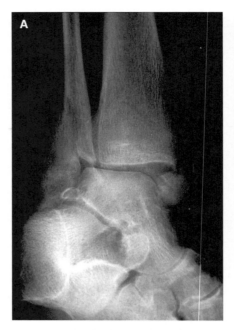
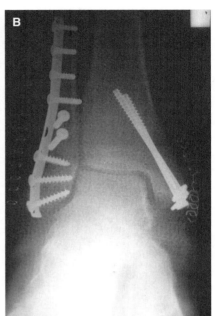
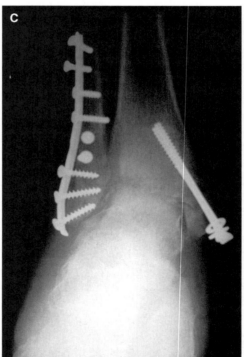
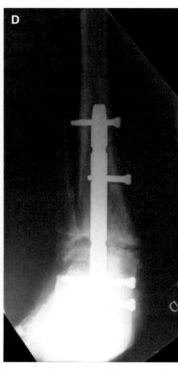

Figure 2 AP radiographs of a 57-year-old man with long-standing type II diabetes mellitus who presented to the emergency department 1 day after sustaining a twisting injury to his ankle. **A,** Initial radiograph. **B,** Immediately after surgery. **C,** Six weeks after surgery. The patient had been strictly compliant to a non–weight-bearing regimen. **D,** One year after successful tibiocalcaneal arthrodesis.

salvage with tibiocalcaneal arthrodesis.

The low-energy minimally displaced fracture that occurred in

the second patient was also an initial presentation of an acute Charcot arthropathy (**Figure 3**). Although the literature is consistent that a

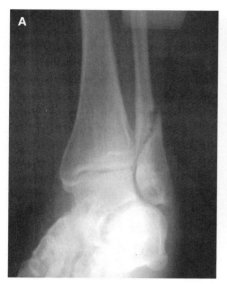
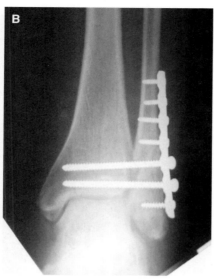

Figure 3 AP radiographs of a moderately obese 59-year-old patient with type I diabetes mellitus after a twisting injury to the ankle. **A,** After 12 weeks of immobilization in a short leg cast. The patient followed a non–weight-bearing regimen during this time. **B,** After open reduction and rigid internal fixation. Again, the patient attempted to not bear weight.

nondisplaced ankle fracture in an insensate ankle, whether it is in a patient with diabetes mellitus or with an acute Charcot ankle, should be managed with immobilization and avoidance of weight bearing, this approach is based on anecdotal information. The forces applied to the non–weight-bearing ankle may

preclude closed treatment. Rigid internal fixation in this scenerio may lessen the risk for the initial failure seen in the first patient.

The third patient had the most uneventful course (**Figure 4**). His history was consistent with a traumatic injury. Because his ankle was insensate, he was treated with open reduc-

tion and rigid internal fixation. He did not bear weight until there was radiographic evidence of fracture healing. He returned to work as a machine operator. When the fourth patient presented, her ankle was irreversibly damaged, and tibiocalcaneal arthrodesis was the only reasonable option (**Figure 5**). She initially presented to a local physician who treated her with a non–weight-bearing cast. The deformity developed during treatment, and the patient was referred to me. I advised immediate ankle arthrodesis.

When specialists who treat acute Charcot foot arthropathy were surveyed, most agreed on nonsurgical management, but one half allowed weight bearing with immobilization in a total contact cast. Patients with diabetes mellitus and an ankle fracture should be followed closely. The recent trend in the literature suggests early surgical stabilization, yet this recommendation is based on anecdotal experience from individuals in whom the fracture was located in the foot. The plantigrade foot is very amenable to stress neutralization with either a total contact cast or surgical stabilization. However, Charcot arthropathy occurs far less often in the ankle than the foot. Due to the offset stresses applied to the talus on the calcaneus, there are appreciable bending forces applied to the ankle. The addition of rotational stresses makes neutralization of the Charcot ankle with a cast very difficult.

Author's Preferred Treatment and Rationale

Although data collected through evidence-based medicine do not exist for treating Charcot arthropathy of the ankle, it appears very reasonable that early surgical intervention with a goal of achieving extremely rigid internal fixation may well be the conservative approach to a problem that otherwise has often resulted in transtibial amputation.

It is prudent to delay weight bearing until radiographic bony callus

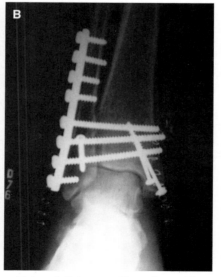

Figure 4 AP radiographs of a 59-year-old man with type II diabetes mellitus who could not bear weight on his ankle after a fall. **A,** Initial radiograph following the acute ankle injury. **B,** Nine months following open reduction and rigid internal fixation. The patient did not bear weight until there was radiographic evidence of fracture callus.

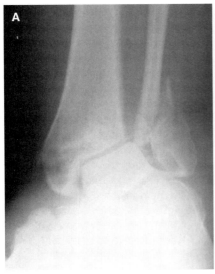
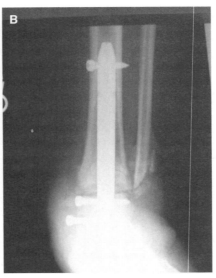

Figure 5 AP radiographs of a woman with type I diabetes who described discomfort and swelling after a misstep from a curb. She sustained a nondisplaced ankle fracture **A,** After 4 weeks of treatment in a short leg cast. She used a wheelchair and did not bear any weight; the cast was changed every week. **B,** At 3 months after surgery, just before she returned to her work as a teacher.

is observed. This non–weight-bearing period should be tempered with the potential for the development of osteopenia and the risk for insufficiency fracture. There have been anecdotal reports of the application of autograft or allograft augmentation and pulsed electromagnetic field or ultrasound therapy to this patient population. As yet, there is no laboratory or clinical evidence to support their application in this very complex high-risk patient population.

Management of Complications
Complications associated with ankle fractures in patients with diabetes mellitus have been discussed in the case studies in this chapter.

References

Brodsky JW: The diabetic foot, in Coughlin MJ, Mann RA (eds): *Surgery of the Foot and Ankle,* ed 7. St. Louis, MO, Mosby, 1999, pp 895-969.

Connolly JF, Csencsitz TA: Limb threatening neuropathic complications from ankle fractures in patients with diabetes. *Clin Orthop* 1998;348:212-219.

Early JS, Hansen ST: Surgical reconstruction of the diabetic foot. *Foot Ankle Int* 1996;17:325-330.

McCormack RG, Leith JM: Ankle fractures in diabetics. *J Bone Joint Surg Br* 1998;80:689-692.

Myerson MS, Henderson MR, Saxby T, Short KW: Management of midfoot diabetic neuroarthropathy. *Foot Ankle Int* 1994;15:233-241.

Pinzur MS: Charcot's foot. *Foot Ankle Clin* 2000;5:897-912.

Pinzur MS, Shields N, Trepman E, Dawson P, Evans A: Current practice patterns in the treatment of Charcot foot. *Foot Ankle Int* 2000;21:916-920.

Simon SR, Tejwani SG, Wilson DL, Santner TJ, Denniston NL: Arthrodesis as an early alternative to nonoperative management of Charcot arthropathy of the diabetic foot. *J Bone Joint Surg Am* 2000;82:939-950.

Coding

ICD-9 CODES

250.60 Diabetes mellitus, type II or unspecified type, not stated as uncontrolled, with neurologic manifestations

250.61 Diabetes mellitus, type I, not stated as uncontrolled, with neurologic manifestations

713.50 Arthropathy associated with type II diabetes mellitus, Charcot arthropathy

713.51 Arthropathy associated with type I diabetes mellitus, Charcot arthropathy

824.2 Fracture of ankle, lateral malleolus, closed

824.6 Fracture of ankle, trimalleolar, closed

CPT CODES

27822 Open treatment of trimalleolar ankle fracture, with or without internal or external fixation, medial and/or lateral malleolus; without fixation of posterior lip

28705 Arthrodesis; pantalar

CPT copyright © 2003 by the American Medical Association. All Rights Reserved.

Dilemmas in Lower Extremity Amputation

Michael S. Pinzur, MD

■ Definition of the Problem

Patient Presentation

The question of limb salvage versus amputation must be addressed in many clinical situations. In the patient with peripheral vascular disease, the benefits of vascular bypass surgery or angioplasty must be weighed against the associated potential morbidities. In complex mutilating limb injuries, will limb salvage serve the patient better than amputation and prosthetic limb fitting? Will limb salvage surgery for osteosarcoma provide a long-term result similar to amputation? In any clinical scenario in which limb preservation and amputation are options, four issues must be addressed before initiating treatment, regardless of the diagnosis.

1. Will limb salvage outperform amputation? A reasonable estimate must be made regarding the ultimate functional capacity of the preserved limb compared with amputation and prosthetic limb fitting.

2. What are realistic expectations associated with limb salvage? Not every patient receives the best possible outcome following surgery. Most receive an "average" result based on the condition and treating physician.

3. What are the costs associated with limb salvage? Costs go beyond financial considerations. Are there sufficient resources to accomplish limb salvage? If salvage takes a great deal of time, will the financial resources of the patient be exhausted? Will the psychological strain associated with disease damage the patient's relationships?

4. What are the risks? Can the patient medically tolerate multiple reconstructive surgeries? What about the potential for sepsis?

The judicious physician will address each of these issues before proceeding with treatment.

Physical Examination

The vascular status of the foot is assessed by examination of pulses, warmth, and capillary refill. Presence or absence of protective sensation is determined with the Semmes-Weinstein 10-g monofilament. The foot is examined to determine which parts must be removed to treat the disease and which parts can be salvaged. Alignment and deformity are assessed, including equinus, varus, and valgus deformity. The potential residual limb is considered with respect to function in standing and walking, including balance and fitting of shoes and orthoses. For example, if the medial three rays must be amputated because of gangrene in a diabetic neuropathic foot, the residual fourth and fifth rays may be susceptible to breakdown and may need to be included in the amputation.

Differential Diagnosis

- Diabetes mellitus (neuropathy, ulcer, infection, Charcot arthropathy, gangrene)
- Peripheral vascular disease
- Trauma (complex mutilating injury)
- Infection (necrotizing fasciitis, gas gangrene, abscess, osteomyelitis)
- Tumor
- Congenital anomaly
- Chronic pain

Additional Work-up

Plain radiographs of the foot and ankle, including weight-bearing views, are obtained to assess bony structure, alignment, and extent of involvement with the pathologic process such as infection or tumor. Further imaging studies such as CT, MRI, and nuclear medicine scans may be helpful in assessing the underlying condition and limits of the involved tissue. Infection is further evaluated with complete blood cell count, erythrocyte sedimentation rate, and C-reactive protein.

If vascular impairment is suspected, toe and ankle pressures are obtained. Toe pressure of less than 40 mm Hg is a prognostic indicator of poor healing potential. Vascular consultation including arteriography may clarify indications for vascular reconstruction.

———————————————■

■ The Solutions

Treatment Options and Rationale

Ernest Burgess taught that amputation surgery should be constructive sur-

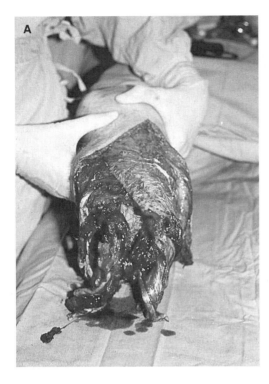

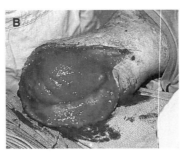

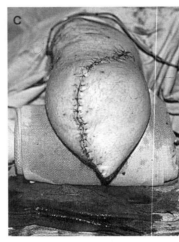

Figure 1 Open traumatic transtibial amputation. **A,** Surgical débridement of all infected nonviable tissue. **B,** A viable medial gastrocnemius muscle was used to construct a soft-tissue envelope to enclose the bone. **C,** When the wound was viable with no signs of infection, the skin was closed, leaving a residual limb with a soft-tissue envelope composed of mobile muscle and full-thickness skin. (Reproduced from Pinzur MS: Current concepts: Amputation surgery in peripheral vascular disease. *Instr Course Lect* 1997;46:501-509.)

gery, the first step in the rehabilitation of a patient with a nonfunctional limb. In the United States, approximately half of all lower extremity amputations (more than 50,000 a year) are performed on individuals with diabetes mellitus. Approximately 40% of amputations are for nondiabetic peripheral vascular disease, and 10% are for tumor, congenital anomalies, or other etiologies. The relatively small group of patients who undergo amputations as a result of trauma and congenitally associated conditions is actually the largest population of individuals receiving ongoing prosthetic care. These patients are generally young and have a long life expectancy,

whereas patients with diabetes mellitus and peripheral vascular disease have a significantly shorter life expectancy.

It is essential that outcome expectations be carefully factored into the decision-making process when lower extremity amputation surgery is contemplated. Staged surgeries, tissue expanders, and free tissue transfer techniques may be appropriate for the patient with a traumatic injury, in whom an optimal residual limb is crucial to long-term function. These same techniques may expose patients who have diabetes mellitus or lack of vascular function to too great a risk of morbidity or may consume too much

treatment time in patients with limited life expectancy and functional capacity.

The potential residual limb morbidity that occurs with immediate prosthetic fitting may not be justified in the traumatically injured patient who can better tolerate periods of limited activity, if this will improve the likelihood of a durable residual limb that will be essential to his or her long-term quality of life. In contrast, multiple limb salvage surgeries and prolonged perioperative periods in which weight bearing is avoided may lead to aerobic deconditioning and joint flexion contracture in elderly patients with diabetes mellitus, a group that has limited functional potential and a shorter life expectancy to benefit from this treatment. Although controversial, several authors have reported that immediate postoperative prosthetic fitting can be used in patients with diabetes mellitus, if carefully applied.

The benefits of amputation at the foot or ankle level are (1) normal weight-bearing tissues are retained, (2) there is little disability or increase in the metabolic cost of walking, (3) there is little risk for losing functional independence, (4) minimal physical therapy is required, and (5) patients rarely require hospitalization for rehabilitation.

SOFT-TISSUE MANAGEMENT IN TRAUMATIC AMPUTATION

Traumatic amputation should be considered a Gustilo-Anderson grade III injury. All nonviable tissue should be excised. The expected final level should not be made at the initial débridement. Guillotine transverse amputations should be avoided. Because there is usually an element of crush at the amputation level, the orthopaedic surgeon must consider that the amputation is being performed through the zone of injury. Constrictive dressings or skin traction only add trauma to the remaining tissue within the zone of injury. Tissue elas-

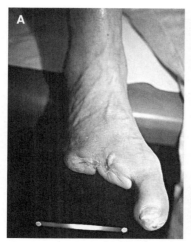 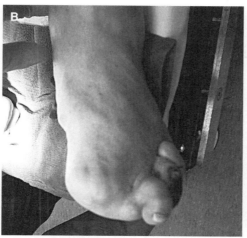

Figure 2 **A,** Amputation at the level of the proximal metaphysis of the hallux proximal phalanx retains essentially the same function without the risk of late ulceration from the difficult-to-accommodate hallux. **B,** In this case, amputation of the remaining toes is the treatment of choice, leaving a contour that is readily accommodated with standard therapeutic footwear.

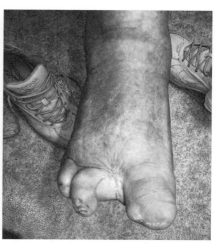

Figure 3 Disarticulation of the hallux at the interphalangeal joint and amputation of the second toe at the level of the proximal metaphysis was performed 1 year ago. The retained partial second toe prevents a late pathologic hallux valgus.

ticity will allow normal tissue tension to be reestablished following recovery from the crush injury. As with open fracture treatment, patients should return to the operating room every 48 to 72 hours for débridement until the tissues appear healthy. At the time of definitive wound closure, normal tissue tension and muscle unit lengths can be reestablished (**Figure 1**). Soft tissues should be handled carefully in patients with diabetes mellitus. Grasping the skin or applying tension to the soft-tissue envelope should be avoided as trauma or stretching can lead to failure of the soft-tissue envelope.

FOREFOOT AMPUTATION

Forefoot amputation produces little disability in patients with diabetes mellitus and patients who are dysvascular. Normal plantar weight-bearing tissue is retained. There is some decrease in walking stability as a result of the decreased size of the weight-bearing platform and the lessened lever arm available for push-off during the terminal stance phase of gait. Peripheral neuropathy leads to both loss of protective sensation and balance. Tissue failure occurs when stresses associated with increased direct pressure and shear overcome the ability of the tissues to accommodate these pathologic loads.

Considerable controversy is associated with first ray and hallux amputation. Every attempt should be made to retain the proximal metaphysis of the hallux proximal phalanx with the insertion of the flexor hallucis brevis. When this tendon insertion is lost, the sesamoids may migrate proximally and stability during terminal stance is diminished. The type of skin flap generally is dictated by the available viable soft tissue.

The contour of a retained residual partial foot is important. Prominent toes, especially in insensate feet, are susceptible to pressure ulcers (**Figure 2**). Disarticulation of the second toe provides an unopposed leverage to the hallux adductors, often leading to pathologic hallux valgus and associated pressure ulceration. This problem can be avoided by retaining the proximal metaphysis of the second toe when possible (**Figure 3**).

Ray resection is controversial. Amputation of a single outer (first or fifth) ray leaves a very functional terminal weight-bearing foot. Central ray resection requires prolonged management of a difficult wound; therefore, this procedure generally should be avoided. Removing more than one ray creates a very narrow forefoot that is susceptible to an equinus deformity, most likely related to the muscle imbalance associated with motor peripheral neuropathy. The large calf muscles (and their motor nerves) are less affected than the weaker anterior ankle dorsiflexors.

MIDFOOT AMPUTATION

Shoe wear difficulties associated with the narrow forefoot after multiple ray resection can be avoided by performing a well-contoured amputation at the level of the proximal metaphyses of the metatarsals or at the tarsometatarsal (Lisfranc) level. When performing amputation at the tarsometatarsal level, late ankle equinus can be avoided by performing a percutaneous Achilles tendon lengthening, followed by postoperative use of a below-knee total contact weight-bearing cast for 1 month.

The level of transmetatarsal amputation is controversial. Each centimeter of length retained in the residual metatarsals requires more than twice the length of soft-tissue flap coverage. Retaining increased metatarsal length improves the lever arm at terminal stance phase, but the risk of recurrent plantar transfer lesions or recurrent plantar ulcers underneath the terminal residual metatarsal shaft is appreciably increased. This risk can be avoided by performing the amputation surgery at the level of the proximal metatarsal metaphyses with only a small apparent loss of leverage in terminal stance phase. Long plantar flaps are more durable, but an equal dorsal/plantar flap is preferable to sacrificing bony length, which is beneficial as a lever arm at the terminal stance phase of gait.

HINDFOOT AMPUTATION

Amputation at the Boyd or Chopart levels, which allows the gastrocnemius-soleus complex to be unopposed, is often complicated by a late equinus deformity, even when the Achilles tendon is released (**Figure 4**). Although Bowker recommends this approach, others have not been as successful. Reattaching the anterior tibial tendon to the distal center of the residual foot can assist potential dorsiflexion. Even when successful, the retained lever arm available for push-off produces a gait pattern with a poor push-off capacity. These amputation levels were more popular before the development of the dynamic elastic response (energy-storing) prosthetic feet. Ankle disarticulation amputees appear to have a far more functional gait pattern, with decreased risk for late residual limb ulceration.

ANKLE DISARTICULATION/SYME'S AMPUTATION

Ankle disarticulation provides a durable end-bearing stable residual limb. In both traumatically injured patients and patients with diabetes mellitus, the surgery can be performed in a

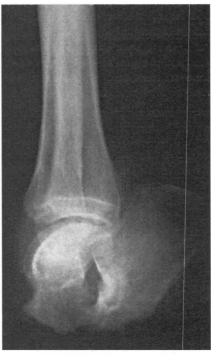

Figure 4 This patient underwent open excision of 1 cm of Achilles tendon and 4 weeks of immobilization in a short leg cast. Once the cast was removed, a severe ankle equinus deformity developed that could not be accommodated with a shoe or an orthotic.

single stage. The normal weight-bearing articular cartilage of the distal tibia should be retained. The medial and lateral malleoli are removed at the joint line. The medial and lateral flares of the distal tibial and fibular metaphyses are also removed in line with the medial and lateral borders of the tibial and fibular shafts. The heel pad then can be secured to the anterior distal tibia with nonabsorbable suture via anterior drill holes. The combination of securing the heel pad anteriorly and adhering of the flap to the exposed metaphyseal distal tibia and fibula prevents the heel pad from migrating.

MIDFOOT/HINDFOOT AMPUTATION VERSUS ANKLE DISARTICULATION

How does the surgeon decide on the amputation level when the available soft tissue will support wound healing

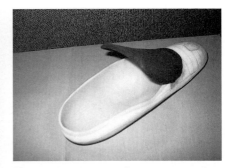

Figure 5 Accommodative custom foot orthosis combined with a toe filler provides a functional prosthesis for a midfoot amputee with diabetes mellitus.

in this region? The patient with diabetes mellitus who is undergoing amputation at this level has a reasonable goal of walking independently. These patients generally are not working at high physical demand occupations, and running or climbing is not an essential requirement. A well-performed midfoot amputation will allow them to walk comfortably with a simple depth inlay shoe and "prosthotic" (combination of accommodative custom foot orthosis and toe filler) (**Figure 5**).

The young person with a traumatic midfoot amputation will have a functional limb but will have decreased stability walking and climbing and a small, short walking platform and decreased lever arm. Patients frequently reject a combination shoe filler and ankle-foot orthosis because of its cumbersome nature. Removal of the talus and calcaneus with ankle disarticulation allows placement of a dynamic elastic response (energy-storing) prosthetic foot, which creates a more stable walking platform and strong lever arm to allow more high-demand activities.

TRANSTIBIAL AMPUTATION

Transtibial amputation is generally performed with a long posterior myofasciocutaneous flap. Although increasing the length of the residual tibia allows a larger surface for weight bearing, increasing the length of the

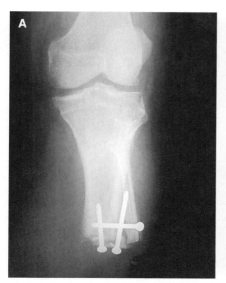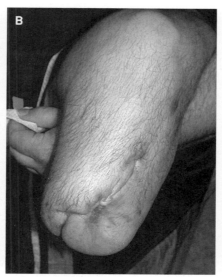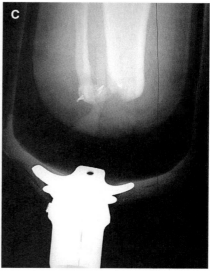

Figure 6 **A,** Immediate bone bridge distal tibiofibular fusion performed at the time of wound closure following traumatic transtibial amputation. **B,** The residual limb 6 months after surgery. Note the square residual limb that is capable of accepting some direct load transfer (end bearing). The small area of wound breakdown is caused by scar tissue that has not yet matured. **C,** The screws were removed when the bone bridge healed, allowing the patient (a carpenter) to return to work.

residual tibia beyond 12 to 15 cm (proximal-middle third junction) does not allow coverage of the distal tibia with muscle. Myodesis (securing the gastrocnemius to the tibia via drill holes or suture to the periosteum and anterior compartment fascia) is mandatory both to create an adequate soft-tissue envelope and to reestablish normal functional muscle tension. The concept of an extended posterior flap has recently been introduced. Instead of creating the myodesis at the anterior distal border of the tibia, the residual muscle belly is secured 1 to 2 cm proximally. This improved cushioning may well prove to be a valuable improvement for load transfer.

The fibula has historically been amputated 1 cm proximal to the tibia. This issue is now very controversial as a result of the renewed interest in bone bridging (fusion of the residual distal tibia and fibula) (**Figure 6**). Many experts now believe that residual limb stability and improved load transfer are enhanced when the fibula is amputated at the same level as the tibia. Bone bridging is currently usually advised only for transtibial

amputation in trauma as a method of providing a larger, more stable surface area for load transfer. Some of these effects can be achieved in amputation of dysvascular tissue when the fibula is amputated at the same level as the tibia.

Author's Preferred Treatment and Rationale

Preservation of the proximal metaphysis of the proximal phalanx of the hallux stabilizes the medial column of the foot by retaining the attachment of the flexor hallucis brevis. If the entire proximal phalanx needs to be removed, patients will have decreased stability at terminal stance, and little difference in function will be observed compared with resection of the entire first ray. When more than one ray needs to be resected, midfoot amputation at the level of the proximal metatarsal metaphyses has produced durable residual limbs with a low incidence of late re-ulceration.

The advent of dynamic elastic response prosthetic feet has supported the use of Syme's ankle disarticulation as a function-sparing amputation

level. I perform the procedure in a single stage, resecting the malleoli at the level of the distal tibial articular surface and removing the metaphyseal flares of the distal tibia and fibula flush with the diaphyseal borders.

Transtibial amputation in the dysvascular patient with diabetes mellitus requires a durable soft-tissue envelope. Securing the gastrocnemius muscle flap over the distal-anterior end of the tibia will provide a more durable soft-tissue envelope. The bone bridge (fusion of the distal tibia and fibula) is currently reserved for the traumatic amputee or the amputee with mechanical residual limb pain. A lesson that has been learned from the bone bridge experience is questioning the length of the residual fibula. It is now felt that the fibula can be resected at the same level (or slightly shorter) as the residual tibia, beveling the anterior-distal tibia only.

Gottschalk's function-sparing adduction flap has greatly enhanced the functional capacity of the transfemoral amputee. A long medial flap allows securing the adductor muscles to the femur. This decreases the risk for the "adductor lurch" that is common to transfemoral amputees and provides a cushioned soft-tissue envelope to enhance prosthetic socket fitting.

Management of Complications

Wound infections and late tissue breakdown in the residual limb initially require basic medical care. Infected and ischemic tissues must be removed. Antibiotic therapy should be based on tissue-specific surgically obtained cultures. Wound healing potential should be optimized by enhancing the patient's nutritional and immune status.

When these issues have been addressed, the surgeon can use the basic principles of load transfer in amputee rehabilitation to plan surgical reconstruction. Bony length must be adequate to accomplish load transfer. The soft-tissue envelope should be composed of mobile muscle and full-thickness skin, capable of dissipating the forces associated with weight bearing and prosthetic use. This will often require bony shortening or a consideration of shortening the limb to the next proximal functional amputation level.

References

Burgess EM, Romano RL, Zettl JH: *The Management of Lower Extremity Amputations.* Washington, DC, US Government Printing Office, 1969.

Pinzur MS: Current concepts: Amputation surgery in peripheral vascular disease. *Instr Course Lect* 1997;46:501-509.

Pinzur MS, Gottschalk F, Smith D, et al: Functional outcome of below-knee amputation in peripheral vascular insufficiency. *Clin Orthop* 1993;286:247-249.

Pinzur MS, Pinto M, Schon L, Smith DG: Controversies in lower extremity amputation. *Instr Course Lect* 2003;52:445-451.

Pinzur MS, Stuck R, Sage R, Hunt N, Rabinovich Z: Syme ankle disarticulation in patients with diabetes. *J Bone Joint Surg Am* 2003;85:1667-1672.

Reiber GE, Lipsky BA, Gibbons GW: The burden of diabetic foot ulcers. *Am J Surg* 1998;176:5S-10S.

Wagner FW Jr: Management of the diabetic neurotrophic foot: Part II. A classification and treatment program for diabetic, neuropathic, and dysvascular foot problems. *Instr Course Lect* 1979;28:143-165.

Coding

ICD-9 CODES

250.7   Diabetes mellitus with peripheral circulatory disorders

440.24   Atherosclerosis, of native arteries of the extremities, atherosclerosis of the extremities with gangrene

CPT CODES

27871   Arthrodesis, tibiofibular joint, proximal or distal

27888   Amputation, ankle, through malleoli of tibia and fibula (eg, Syme, Pirogoff-type procedures), with plastic closure and resection of nerves

28800   Amputation, foot; midtarsal (eg, Chopart-type procedure)

28805   Amputation, foot; transmetatarsal

29345   Application of long leg cast (thigh to toes)

29445   Application of rigid total contact leg cast

Partial and Total Calcanectomy

Douglas G. Smith, MD

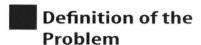

Definition of the Problem

Patient Presentation

Partial and total calcanectomies remain very satisfactory surgical procedures for the treatment of soft-tissue defects around the heel and osseous pathology of the calcaneus. These conditions most frequently present with diabetic heel ulceration and contiguous osteomyelitis. The soft-tissue defect at the heel can occur from pressure during prolonged bed rest, casting, friction of walking, pressure or friction from shoes, and minor trauma.

Partial or total calcanectomy procedures remove the involved bone and excise ulcerations and unsuitable soft tissue. The surgical technique entails removing a very large bony prominence and creating medial and lateral fasciocutaneous flaps from the remaining soft-tissue envelope. With thoughtful planning and careful dissection, fasciocutaneous flaps can be created that will gently rotate and translate, allowing primary closure of the defect. The need for free tissue transfer usually can be eliminated.

Calcanectomy creates both a cosmetic deformity and a functional loss. Some authors have found that describing calcanectomy as an "amputation of the back of the foot" better conveys to the patient and the patient's family the issues of loss and deformity. Furthermore, using the word amputation also conveys the need to replace the heel through proper orthotic management. However, the ankle joint and a substantial amount of function are retained despite loss of calcaneal bone and the new hindfoot shape. In most circumstances this is a much-preferred option to transtibial amputation.

Physical Examination

The typical examination reveals chronic soft-tissue loss resulting from ulceration that is deep or near the bone surface. For the patient to be a candidate for partial or total calcanectomy, the remaining soft-tissue envelope must appear healthy and durable and should be clinically free of cellulitis, induration, and chronic skin changes. The existing literature gives general guidelines as to the size of acceptable defects and indicates that lesions as large as 5 × 7 cm have been addressed successfully using these techniques. Clinical judgment and some expertise are needed to preoperatively determine whether the surrounding soft-tissue envelope can be closed after removal of the posterior process of the calcaneus.

If active infection is present, initial treatment includes débridement, antibiotics, elevation, and alleviation of pressure. Active infection, more than colonization or quiescent osteomyelitis, typically leads to a staged approach. Only after débridement of infected tissue and assessment of the response to initial treatment can it be determined whether salvage with calcanectomy is technically feasible or the extensive nature of involvement requires transtibial amputation.

The vascular status also should be carefully assessed to estimate the potential for successful healing. As with all corrective surgery and partial foot amputation procedures in the diabetic foot, no single test can verify the adequacy of circulation or predict successful healing. All factors including clinical examination, tissue quality, circulation, and nutrition should be considered. The ankle-brachial indices and toe blood pressures can provide some helpful information; low values indicate poor potential for healing. Normal or high values can occur with medial arterial calcinosis and should be interpreted with caution because arterial inflow may be inadequate. Transcutaneous oxygen studies can be helpful in surgical decision making if readings are poor (less than 20 mm Hg) or acceptable (greater than 30 mm Hg). However, most patients have readings that vary or have predictive values that fall in the "gray zone." Unfortunately, there is no optimal study to predict successful healing. Specifically for calcanectomy procedures, posterior tibial circulation appears to be very important for the collateral circulation to the remaining heel tissue. Distal circulation can be assessed with physical examination, duplex ultrasound, or arteriography. It has been suggested that the lack of posterior tibial flow is a contraindication to this procedure, and strong consideration should be given to transtibial amputation.

Differential Diagnosis
- Contiguous osteomyelitis
- Secondary squamous cell carcinoma
- Tumors

Additional Work-up

Imaging studies such as the bone scan, gallium scan, indium-labeled white blood cell scan, and MRI are not always helpful in determining the extent of bone involvement. None of these studies is especially good at differentiating the edema and natural physiologic bone response from infection because they lack sensitivity and specificity. Intraoperative clinical judgment must be based on the direct examination of bone; this information is then used in conjunction with imaging studies. Direct examination and radiographs usually are adequate to determine the extent of bony involvement and make the decision between partial and total calcanectomy.

If squamous cell carcinoma is suspected, a biopsy should be performed. A biopsy of the surrounding hypertrophic rim is much more diagnostic than a biopsy of the necrotic tissue region. In addition, palpable lymph nodes in the popliteal fossa and groin should be identified. If a diagnosis of squamous cell carcinoma is confirmed, lymph node biopsy usually is recommended.

■ The Solutions

Treatment Options and Rationale

Calcanectomy (either partial or total) has a long history. The author of a classic article reported use of a plantar midline incision in the treatment of 11 patients with calcaneal osteomyelitis. After the cortical shell of the calcaneus was split in the sagittal plane, a sequestrectomy was performed by débridement of the soft osteomyelitic cancellous interior of the calcaneus. Open wound treatment yielded satisfactory healing and function in 91% of patients.

Another author reported good results with use of the plantar midline incision for excision of the calcaneus for severe fractures. The advantages of this approach were described as decompression of the swollen foot and preservation of the midtarsal joints. At present, this approach is rarely performed in this straight plantar midline fashion; however, the cortical splitting technique may still have a role in the treatment of children with osteomyelitis.

The literature supports either partial or total calcanectomy in the treatment of people with diabetes mellitus who have heel ulceration and exposed bone. However, most patients are managed with partial calcanectomy. Two reviews that specifically describe patients with a total calcanectomy illustrate the potential for instability of the talonavicular joint. With complete dissection of the anterior portion of the calcaneus, the ligamentous support for the talonavicular area can be weakened, and subluxation may occur. However, the precise incidence of skeletal subluxation or instability is unknown. Therefore, surgeons should be aware that subluxation of the talonavicular joint can occur after total calcanectomy, and attempts should be made to prevent this complication with more substantial orthotic management or closer patient follow-up. If the problem arises, then fusion or higher level amputation may be required.

Another consideration is whether the defect should be closed primarily or if delayed closure or secondary healing should be contemplated. Treatment of patients who do not have active infection includes excision of all involved tissue, thorough irrigation, and primary closure over drains. If erythema, swelling, and warmth from active infection are present, then a staged approach including delayed primary closure should be considered. Secondary healing is not typically a goal of this treatment but is supported in the older literature. If secondary healing is chosen, most of the wound is closed and a small area is treated open and allowed to heal secondarily. This decision would, in part, be based on the finding of gross purulence at the time of surgery.

The possible role of free tissue transfer, complex regional flaps, or skin grafts has been discussed primarily in isolated case reports. The goal of calcanectomy in the patient with diabetes mellitus is to allow direct apposition of the remaining soft-tissue envelope. In general, free flaps and skin grafts have not been seen as long-term, durable solutions for soft-tissue defects on the plantar surface or heel area of the foot.

Occasionally individual authors have proposed internal replacement of the calcaneus with either allograft bone or custom prosthetic implants. Given the good functional results presented with partial and total calcanectomy and primary closure, the risks of implantation of allograft must be weighed against the perceived benefits. Although allograft replacement of the calcaneus may be a rare consideration when the patient has no soft-tissue defect, it is not a consideration in the patient with diabetes mellitus.

Author's Preferred Treatment and Rationale

Although it is difficult to quantify, I assess the location, size, and shape of the cutaneous defect and visualize

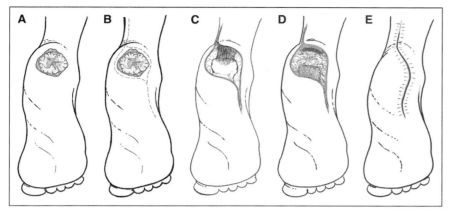

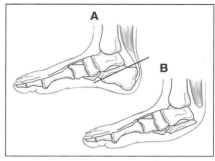

Figure 1 **A,** Heel ulceration with extensive soft-tissue loss and exposed bone; the lesion is round or larger in the longitudinal dimension. **B,** Incision extends proximally off the medial edge of the lesion and distally off the lateral edge of the lesion. **C,** Elevation of flaps to expose the distal Achilles tendon and the calcaneus. **D,** Following osteotomy and excision of the posterior calcaneus. **E,** Flaps translate and slide together to oppose and close the defect with an S-shaped closure. (Courtesy of Prosthetics Research Study, Seattle, WA.)

Figure 3 Preoperative (**A**) and postoperative (**B**) views showing the extent of calcaneal excision and the portion of the Achilles tendon that frequently requires débridement. (Courtesy of Prosthetics Research Study, Seattle, WA.)

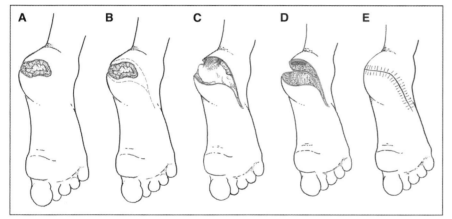

Figure 2 **A,** Heel ulceration with extensive soft-tissue loss and exposed bone; the lesion is larger in the transverse dimension. **B,** Incision extends just off the medial edge of the lesion with long lateral extension toward the calcaneocuboid joint. **C,** Elevation of flaps to expose the distal Achilles tendon and the calcaneus. **D,** Following osteotomy and excision of the posterior calcaneus. **E,** Flaps simply oppose to close the defect. (Courtesy of Prosthetics Research Study, Seattle, WA.)

how the remaining heel pad and surrounding skin will provide an adequate soft-tissue envelope covering for the remaining hindfoot. The largest defect I have treated successfully by partial calcanectomy measured 5 × 7 cm.

The surgical approach is tailored to fit the size and shape of the skin loss. Patients with a more circular ulcer may be treated with a longitudinal approach, but the lesion is not bi-sected by the incision. The proximal and distal limbs of the incision are off-set, one medial and one lateral, to allow better approximation of the skin (**Figure 1**). For some patients with an ulcer that is larger in the transverse dimension, the ulcer margins are excised and the posterior process of the calcaneus is removed through this defect. An extension of the incision can be made either laterally or medially to allow a transverse skin approxima-

tion. The lateral extension is preferred if technically feasible to minimize damage to the collateral circulation (**Figure 2**).

In all patients, the dissection is carried down on the calcaneus, with elevation of full-thickness flaps to protect the remaining viable heel pad, nerves, and vessels. The Achilles tendon is released from the calcaneus, and all necrotic tendon is excised. In most patients with diabetes mellitus, the distal Achilles tendon is involved, and after excision the remaining tendon is allowed to retract.

The posterior process of the calcaneus is excised beginning 1 cm posterior to the edge of the subtalar joint, and an osteotomy is directed to 1 cm posterior to the calcaneocuboid joint (**Figure 3**). After bony excision, all additional necrotic or devascularized tissue is excised. The remaining bone is assessed clinically for a normal trabecular pattern and appearance or the presence of destruction from infection. If the bone does not appear normal, then total calcanectomy is performed. Otherwise, the remaining bone edges are smoothed down to avoid prominence.

The medial and lateral fasciocutaneous flaps are examined and gently rotated to determine the most durable and tension-free closure. With removal of the posterior process of the

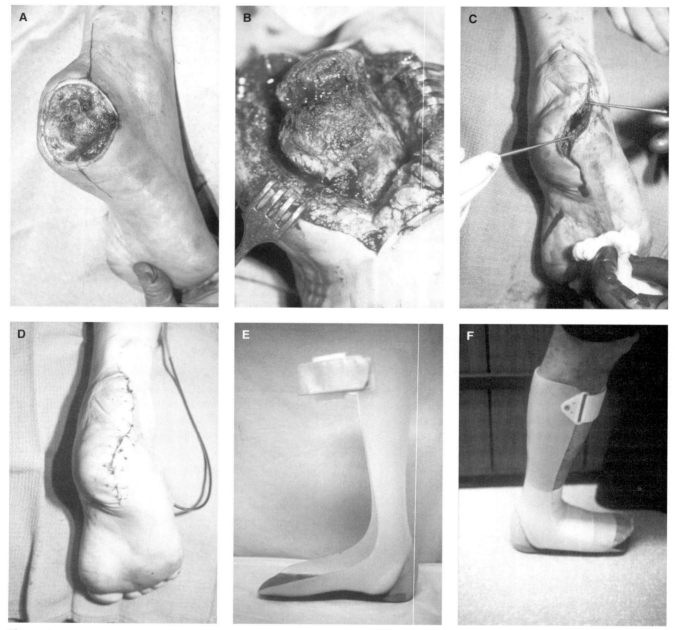

Figure 4 **A,** Longitudinal surgical approach to a large chronic heel ulceration in a patient with diabetes mellitus. **B,** Exposure of the posterior process of the calcaneus. **C,** Offset incision allows approximation of medial and lateral flaps. **D,** Closure over suction drain. **E,** Custom ankle-foot orthosis with a soft inner foam liner and a dense outer foam heel. **F,** Lateral photograph of the patient standing in the custom ankle-foot orthosis. (Reproduced with permission from Smith DG, Stuck RM, Ketner L, Sage RM, Pinzur MS: Partial calcanectomy for the treatment of large ulcerations of the heel and calcaneal osteomyelitis: An amputation of the back of the foot. *J Bone Joint Surg Am* 1992;74:571-576.)

calcaneus, the remaining soft tissue usually is sufficient to facilitate primary closure in layers. If the closure appears to be under tension, excision of more calcaneus should be considered. The flaps are then contoured and inset for closure.

Postoperatively, the foot is stabilized in 30° of equinus using a cast or splints. This position keeps tension off the closure. The wounds are treated with suction drainage if there is primary wound closure in layers. Open wound care can be required for secondary wound healing or if delayed primary closure is planned. The foot is kept splinted, and the patient is not allowed to bear weight for 6 to 8 weeks. The position of the foot is advanced from equinus to neutral after 4 weeks.

Finally, a custom ankle-foot orthosis is constructed with an inner soft foam liner to improve comfort and decrease abrasions and an outer dense foam heel to absorb impact (**Figure 4**). Patients should not ambulate without wearing the protective device.

Management of Complications
Wound healing complications, including infection, dehiscence, and gangrene, can occur. Treatment may consist of secondary healing with intermittent minor wound débridement, revision, and delayed closure, or conversion to transtibial amputa-tion. If subluxation of the talonavicular joint occurs, treatment may include open reduction and arthrodesis.

References

Baumhauer JF, Fraga CJ, Gould JS, Johnson JE: Total calcanectomy for the treatment of chronic calcaneal osteomyelitis. *Foot Ankle Int* 1998;19:849-855.

Broudy AS, Scott RD, Watts HG: The split-heel technique in the management of calcaneal osteomyelitis in children: Report of three cases. *Clin Orthop* 1976;119:202-205.

Crandall RC, Wagner FW Jr: Partial and total calcanectomy: A review of thirty-one consecutive cases over a ten-year period. *J Bone Joint Surg Am* 1981;63:152-155.

Muscolo DL, Ayerza MA, Aponte-Tinao LA: Long-term results of allograft replacement after total calcanectomy: A report of two cases. *J Bone Joint Surg Am* 2000;82:109-112.

Smith DG, Stuck RM, Ketner L, Sage RM, Pinzur MS: Partial calcanectomy for the treatment of large ulcerations of the heel and calcaneal osteomyelitis: An amputation of the back of the foot. *J Bone Joint Surg Am* 1992;74:571-576.

Woll TS, Beals RK: Partial calcanectomy for the treatment of osteomyelitis of the calcaneus. *Foot Ankle* 1991;12:31-34.

Coding

ICD-9 CODES

707.14 Chronic ulcer of skin, Ulcer of lower limbs, except decubitus, Ulcer of heel and midfoot

730.07 Osteomyelitis, periostitis, and other infections involving bone, Acute osteomyelitis, ankle and foot

730.17 Chronic osteomyelitis, ankle and foot

CPT CODES

14020 Adjacent tissue transfer or rearrangement, scalp, arms and/or legs; defect 10 sq cm or less

14021 Adjacent tissue transfer or rearrangement, scalp, arms and/or legs; defect 10.1 sq cm to 30.0 sq cm

14040 Adjacent tissue transfer or rearrangement, forehead, cheeks, chin, mouth, neck, axillae, genitalia, hands and/or feet; defect 10 sq cm or less

14041 Adjacent tissue transfer or rearrangement, forehead, cheeks, chin, mouth, neck, axillae, genitalia, hands and/or feet; 10.1 sq cm to 30.0 sq cm

15738 Muscle, myocutaneous, or fasciocutaneous flap; lower extremity

28120 Partial excision (craterization, saucerization, sequestrectomy, or diaphysectomy) bone (eg, osteomyelitis or bossing); talus or calcaneus

Two-Stage Reconstruction of Diabetic Forefoot Ulcer

John E. McDermott, MD

■ Definition of the Problem

Patient Presentation

A diabetic foot can present the most challenging fracture and wound problems an orthopaedic surgeon must face. The nonhealing diabetic foot ulcer is a complication of the assault of diabetes mellitus on the neurovascular system. Fluctuations in blood glucose result in nerve cell damage, particularly of the sensory nervous system. This phenomenon is aggravated by the effects of the disease on arterial structures, leading to vascular impairment and localized arterial insufficiency of skin, soft tissue, and bone.

Uninfected ulcers are best treated initially by occlusive casting. Recent developments in cast bracing and use of cast boots to unload pressure can provide similar prevention and also allow for localized wound care. Cast boots are as effective as casts in management of diabetic foot ulcers. Following healing by either cast or cast boot, the patient can progress to accommodative shoe wear with custom insoles to ensure further protection and help prevent additional breakdown and recurrence.

Patients with ulcers at Wagner grade II and beyond in whom this program has failed may be candidates for aggressive surgical management as an alternative to regional amputation (see chapter 71).

Physical Examination

The subtleness of neuropathic sensory loss is frustrating to the patient and complicates the orthopaedist's examination. The loss of sensation is not easily identified by sensory wheels or standard pinprick evaluation. Like the other subtle neuropathies of leprosy and syphilis, it can be identified primarily by use of specialized filament testing (Semmes-Weinstein monofilaments).

The neurologic work-up for surgical planning includes sensory mapping using the Semmes-Weinstein monofilaments. A lower extremity vascular examination is done. Most focused diabetic foot services and academic institutions find use of an evaluation sheet most helpful (**Figure 1**). This form allows not only basic documentation for diagnosis but also is useful in measurement of disease progression, treatment outcome, and follow-up planning.

Evaluation of the ulcer itself includes consideration of location. Despite depth and infection, by virtue of their location, certain ulcers respond to specific surgical intervention. The heel ulcer is difficult to protect, and revascularization with skin growth is not usually successful. Ulcers of the arch area secondary to Charcot midfoot collapse usually are resistant to local efforts but respond well to exostectomy.

Differential Diagnosis

- Infective neuropathy secondary to both bacterial and viral disease
- Congenital neurologic disease
- Posttraumatic neuropathy (central or peripheral)
- Senile dementia and neuropathy secondary to central nervous system degeneration
- Venous stasis and arterial insufficiency
- Osteomyelitis
- Vascular compromise/osteonecrosis
- Renal disease and systemic damage of renal dialysis
- Metabolic bone disease with resultant deformity
- Tumor, primary or metastatic

Additional Work-up

The association of vascular compromise with the altered glucose metabolism in diabetes mellitus mandates that the vascular status of the patient with a diabetic foot problem be adequately evaluated. The measurement of ankle-brachial indices, which is standard in patient evaluation, must not be considered definitive because the association of atherosclerotic vascular change leads to false readings in almost half of patients with diabetes. As a result of this unreliability, Doppler ultrasound can provide more reliable information; however, transcutaneous oxygen ($TcPo_2$) determination is the best predictor of wound healing. Although a time-consuming examination, it is readily available as a result of its common use in neonate monitoring. The $TcPo_2$ will indicate the

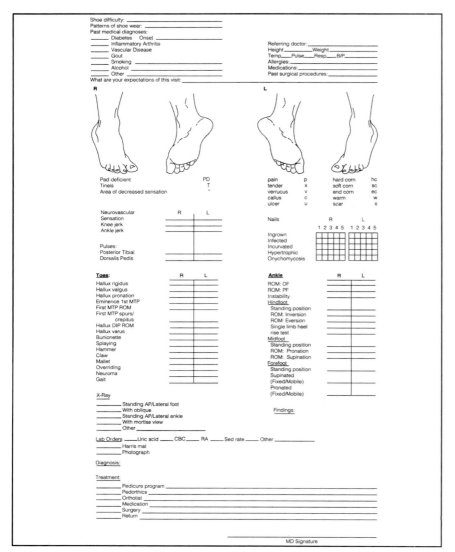

Figure 1 Evaluation sheet for recording findings during evaluation of the diabetic foot. (Courtesy of St. Michael Hospital, Milwaukee, WI.)

likelihood of ulcer healing and also can predict the ability of an incision to heal in these compromised patients.

Preoperative planning includes the use of wound culture and, if indicated, deep tissue biopsy culture for determination of optimum antibiotic coverage. In selected patients, sinogram or MRI should be considered to determine the presence of a deep regional abscess.

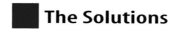

The Solutions

Treatment Options and Rationale
Casting and other wound care efforts are generally tried for several months or, if no real progress is achieved, a shorter period. The ulcerated foot is cleaned, and a dry dressing is applied. This dressing is covered by stockinette padding and a plaster or fiberglass cast is fashioned to protect and allow for unloading of the ulcerated area. This

technique involves repeated changing, usually every 2 weeks and, on occasion, is augmented by wound supplements.

The option of amputation, particularly regional amputation, represents a definitive result. However, the advantages of tissue preservation, foot balance, enhanced gait, and psychological factors, make consideration of reconstructive efforts an attractive alternative. For non–weight-bearing areas, plastic surgery techniques are a consideration.

Exostectomy is relatively easily performed through a medial or lateral approach, allowing direct exploration of the plantar osseous structure deep to the fascial soft-tissue plane and thus deep to and away from the ulcer bed.

Early surgical intervention with localized amputation should be considered for ulcers involving the first metatarsal head region and both the distal and proximal bony prominences of the fifth metatarsal. Ulcers involving the plantar surface of the hallux are best managed with either interphalangeal fusion or tendon balancing procedures. A Jones procedure for metatarsal head elevation and correction of interphalangeal deformity can be considered if the ulcer involves the plantar surface of the interphalangeal region. An interphalangeal fusion may be necessary to achieve appropriate toe position and relieve plantar pressure.

The use of skin grafting is more of an adjunct than an option to facilitate ulcer care. Microvascular tissue transfer may be successful. The use of both free and rotated muscle pedicle flaps to increase local profusion and allow skin coverage is particularly applicable to difficult graft areas such as the medial malleolus. The International Microvascular Research Group study of 493 grafts showed a success rate of 97% in patients with diabetes.

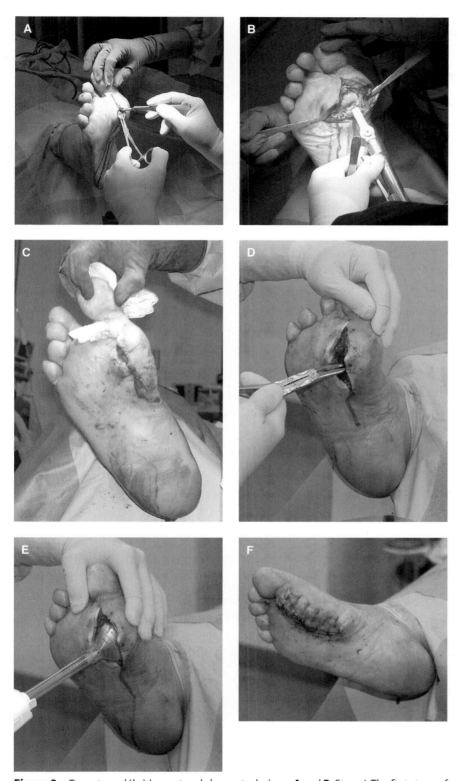

Author's Preferred Treatment and Rationale

The two-stage surgical technique consists of deep surgical resection followed by soft-tissue mobilization and delayed secondary skin closure, which may shorten healing time and improve prognosis (**Figure 2**).

Stage I consists of deep, wide resection and débridement of the ulcer, the underlying soft tissue, and infected or pressure-producing osseous structures such as the metatarsal head. During this stage, cultures and deep biopsies are obtained for laboratory analysis and appropriate antibiotic identification for the subsequent second stage. All necrotic, avascular, and devitalized tissue is sharply excised. Wounds are irrigated, and loose closure performed over adequate drains. Suction and vacuum-type drains may improve tissue viability.

The patient is not allowed to bear weight, and the foot is kept elevated. Antibiotics are given immediately during surgery and are modified 4 to 7 days later, based on cultures.

Stage II consists of a second débridement with pulsatile irrigation. The patient is returned to the operating room for this second procedure. Deep cultures are repeated with adjustment of the antibiotic if indicated, and then the delayed primary closure is performed using retention-type suture technique, a combination of No. 00 wire and No. 000 nonabsorbable synthetic sutures. Following surgery, a protective dressing is applied to the wound, and the patient still is not allowed to bear weight until healing allows. The sutures are often left in for up to 1 month because tissue healing in these patients is extremely compromised and the nature of the surgery itself results in tissue tension and compromised tissue position. The wound is protected with dressings and, if desired, casting.

Figure 2 Two-stage débridement and closure technique. **A** and **B,** Stage I. The first stage of the procedure consists of a deep, wide resection including resection of metatarsal head. **C,** The closure is loose over drains. Cultures and biopsies are submitted for laboratory evaluation. **D** and **E,** Stage II consists of a repeat débridement with pressure irrigation and repeating cultures. **F,** Delayed primary closure with retention sutures is performed.

Management of Complications

The common complications of reconstructive surgery of infected ulcers are failure of wound healing and infection. If an inflammatory response or evidence of sepsis develops following the second stage surgery, a decision must be made to release the retention sutures and re-drain and explore the wound. Repeat cultures of drainage and further antibiotic adjustment may, on occasion, be successful.

I have found tissue immobilization with occlusive or cast boot casting to be beneficial after the second stage. A compressive dressing is used for the first week to 10 days, then the patient is placed in a padded diabetic-type foot cast, which is changed in 10 days. As needed, an additional cast is applied for 2 weeks. If preferred or needed to facilitate wound and dressing needs, a removable cast boot may be used.

If appropriate healing is not achieved, hyperbaric oxygen may augment ulcer healing. Although this modality is controversial, when applied on a 5- out of 7-day basis in a controlled setting at 3 atmospheres with a large chamber to accommodate patient and attendant, I have shown that a 70% successful healing to resolution may be achieved for patients in whom the only other option may be amputation. All such efforts, however, are most effective when done as part of a multidisciplinary, focused, comprehensive wound care and follow-up program. Success requires meticulous attention to perioperative care and reflective thought in surgical planning. Control of the patient's diabetes by appropriate insulin and medication management is required. Follow-up is continued based on the patient's risk factor management or the institution's follow-up program for the diabetic foot.

References

Brodsky JW: Outpatient diagnosis and care of the diabetic foot. *Instr Course Lect* 1993;42:121-139.

Colen LB: Limb salvage in the patient with severe peripheral vascular disease: The role of microsurgical free-tissue transfer. *Plast Reconstr Surg* 1987;79:389-395.

Flynn MD, Tooke JE: Etiology of diabetic foot ulceration: A role for the microcirculation? *Diabet Med* 1992;9:320-329.

Karanfilian RG, Lynch TG, Lee BC, et al: The assessment of skin blood flow in peripheral vascular disease by laser Doppler velocimetry and transcutaneous oxygen tension determination in predicting healing of ischemic forefoot ulcerations and amputations in diabetic and nondiabetic patients. *J Vasc Surg* 1986;4:511-520.

Khouri RK, Cooley BC, Kunselman AR, et al: A prospective study of microvascular free flap surgery and outcome. *Plast Reconstr Surg* 1998;102:711-721.

Kumagai SG, Mahoney GR, Fitzgibbons TC, McMullen JT, Connolly TL, Henkel L: Treatment of diabetic (neuropathic) foot ulcers with two-stage debridement and closure. *Foot Ankle Int* 1998;19:160-165.

Wagner FW Jr: A classification and treatment program for diabetic, neuropathic and dysvascular foot problems. *Instr Course Lect* 1979;28:143-165.

Coding

ICD-9 CODES

707.1   Ulcer of lower limbs, except decubitus

707.13   Ulcer of ankle

707.14   Ulcer of heel and midfoot

707.15   Ulcer of other part of foot

730.07   Acute osteomyelitis, ankle and foot

730.17   Chronic osteomyelitis, ankle and foot

CPT CODES

11041   Debridement; skin, full thickness

11042   Debridement; skin, and subcutaneous tissue

11043   Debridement; skin, subcutaneous tissue, and muscle

11044   Debridement; skin, subcutaneous tissue, muscle, and bone

12041   Layer closure of wounds of feet; 2.5 cm or less

13131   Repair, complex, feet; 1.1 cm to 2.5 cm

CPT copyright © 2003 by the American Medical Association. All Rights Reserved.

Chronic Diabetic Wound Treatment

Christopher E. Attinger, MD

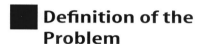

Definition of the Problem

Patient Presentation

A patient with diabetes mellitus presents with a wound on the foot or ankle that is arrested in the inflammatory phase of wound healing. The wound surface is chronically infected and contains an overabundance of proteases that overwhelm local growth factors and prevent them from being effective. Local and systemic factors combine to prevent the conversion of the chronic inflammatory state into an acute wound that can progress through the normal stages of healing.

Foot and ankle wounds usually occur in patients with diabetes because of acute or repetitive trauma in a biomechanically unstable foot. The wound does not heal as a result of persistent biomechanical abnormality in the face of hyperglycemia, neuropathy, infection, inadequate blood flow, ineffective immune system, or poor nutrition. The acute wound then becomes a chronic wound.

In patients with diabetes, healing is seriously affected by poorly controlled blood glucose levels. Glucose levels above 300 mg/dL prevent the white blood cells from effectively destroying invading bacteria and directing the wound healing effort. The high glucose levels also contribute to the stiffening of joints and tendons by binding to collagen and reducing their natural flexibility. Over 60% of diabetic ulcers have insufficient blood flow resulting from peripheral vascular disease. The atherosclerotic disease is usually manifest below the popliteal artery and involves the anterior tibial artery, the posterior tibial artery, and/or the peroneal artery. In addition, blood viscosity in patients with diabetes is increased because high blood glucose binds to the cytoskeleton of red blood cells, rendering them less pliable. The viscosity leads to decreased blood flow through the capillaries and, with it, decreased local tissue oxygenation.

A thorough patient history is obtained from the patient, family and friends, emergency medical technologist, and/or referring physician to help determine the wound's etiology. The origin (usually traumatic) and age of the wound are determined. The trauma usually is related to biomechanical abnormalities causing excessive local pressure during gait, changes in shoe wear, penetrating trauma, or excessive heat (hot water foot baths). The patient's tetanus immunization status is determined, and the patient is inoculated if revaccination is indicated. It is important to ask what topical therapy has been applied to the wound because certain topical agents can contribute to the wound becoming chronic (eg, caustic agents such as hydrogen peroxide, 10% iodine, sodium hypochlorite solution, and so forth).

The medical history should emphasize possible symptoms of atherosclerotic disease in the heart, nervous system, kidneys, eyes, and lower extremities. For patients on dialysis, the onset and type of dialysis is documented. Venous circulation is evaluated by noting abnormalities in blood coagulation, liver disease, heart failure, previous venous thrombi, and pulmonary emboli. The extent of the neuropathy present, including loss of sensation, muscle weakness, and loss of ability to sweat, is then explored. The patient's ability to monitor and treat his or her blood glucose is carefully examined. Finally, nutritional status, including recent weight gain or loss and the quality of the patient's diet, is assessed. The patient's smoking status is documented, and a complete list of medications and drug allergies is obtained.

A social history is then obtained to determine the patient's level of activity, the level of home help available, and the type of work the patient is involved in. This information can help the orthopaedist assess the patient's potential to comply with the treatment regimen because these wounds can involve up to 6 months of inactivity (eg, Ilizarov treatment of a Charcot collapse). Lack of compliance is the single largest cause of postoperative wound complications (> 20%).

One or more of the authors or the departments with which they are affiliated have received something of value from a commercial or other party related directly or indirectly to the subject of this chapter.

Physical Examination

The wound is assessed carefully by measuring its size and depth. The area is obtained by multiplying the length of the longest axis by the width of the widest axis perpendicular to it. Depth is assessed to find what layers of tissue are involved: epidermis, dermis, subdermal fat, fascia, muscle, tendon, joint capsule, joint, and/or bone. A metallic probe is used to assist in the determination of the wound depth. If the probe touches bone, there is an 85% chance that osteomyelitis is present. If tendon is involved, the infection is very likely to have tracked proximally or distally. The orthopaedist should check for bogginess proximally and distally along the potentially involved tendon sheaths. If the suspicion is strong that a distal infection has spread proximally, the dependent proximal areas where the tendon sheaths are readily accessible should also be checked (eg, extensor retinaculum, tarsal tunnel). The wound is then photographed.

If cellulitis is present, the border of the erythema is delineated and dated (hour, day, month) with indelible ink. The spread or retreat of the erythema can then be continuously monitored after deep cultures of the wound are obtained and broad-spectrum antibiotics are started. If, after 4 to 6 hours, the cellulitis has extended beyond the inked boundary, either the antibiotics are inadequate and/or the wound has been inadequately débrided.

It is important to avoid confusing cellulitis with dependent rubor seen in patients with chronic ischemia or chronic wounds. If the erythema disappears when the affected leg is elevated above the level of the heart, then the erythema is a result of dependent rubor. With dependent rubor, inflammation is usually absent, and the skin should have visible wrinkling. If the erythema persists despite elevation, the wound has surrounding cellulitis and needs antibiotic treatment, with or without débridement. Dependent rubor also may often be seen at a fresh surgical site and should not be confused with postoperative cellulitis.

Blood flow to the area is then evaluated by palpation and/or handheld Doppler. The presence of palpable anterior and posterior tibial pulses suggests adequate blood flow. If one of the pulses is absent, then the pulses should be evaluated with a Doppler. A triphasic Doppler signal indicates normal blood flow, biphasic indicates adequate blood flow, and monophasic warrants further investigation. If the quality of flow is questionable, a formal noninvasive arterial Doppler evaluation must be performed. If blood flow is inadequate, the patient should be referred to a vascular surgeon who specializes in distal revascularization.

Sensation must also be assessed. Lack of protective sensation can be established when the patient is unable to feel 10 g of pressure (5.07 Semmes-Weinstein monofilament). This lack of sensation prevents patients from feeling damage that occurs as a result of excessive local pressure (eg, prolonged decubitus position, tight shoes, clothes, or dressings; biomechanical abnormalities; or the presence of foreign bodies).

The biomechanical abnormalities caused by motor dysfunction, skeletal abnormalities, and/or a tight Achilles tendon cause high focal plantar pressures during gait. The local tissue at those sites eventually breaks down under the repetitive stress of normal ambulation (on average, a person takes 10,000 steps a day) if the patient is insensate. The motor neuropathy is most often seen in the intrinsic muscles of the foot, with resultant claw toe formation. Skeletal abnormalities, which may include a prominent metatarsal head and Charcot collapse, are best evaluated by weight-bearing radiographs.

Because the elasticity of the Achilles tendon is affected by diabetes mellitus, it should also be carefully evaluated. The patient's ability to dorsiflex the supinated foot tests the elasticity of the Achilles tendon. If the orthopaedist can dorsiflex the foot more than 15° with the knee extended and flexed, then the tendon has sufficient plasticity. If the foot can be dorsiflexed only when the knee is flexed, then the gastrocnemius portion of the Achilles tendon is tight. If the foot cannot be dorsiflexed when the knee is extended or flexed, then both portions of the Achilles tendon are tight.

Differential Diagnosis

- Ischemia
- Cellulitis versus dependent rubor
- Osteomyelitis
- Biomechanical abnormality

Additional Work-up

Laboratory studies should be obtained. The immediate blood glucose level and chronic glucose level (hemoglobin A_{1C}) should be assessed. A hemoglobin A_{1C} over 6% indicates poor control of blood glucose levels (6% = mean plasma glucose level of 135 mg/dL, 7% = 170 mg/dL, 8% = 205 mg/dL, 9 = 240 mg/dL, 10% = 275 mg/dL, 11% = 310 mg/dL, 12% = 345 mg/dL). High blood glucose in combination with a low hemoglobin A_{1C} can indicate acute infection. The white blood cell and differential blood cell counts are also very helpful in monitoring systemic infection. The numbers, however, can look deceptively normal in renal failure in patients with diabetes mellitus. An erythrocyte sedimentation rate can be helpful as a tracking tool during treatment of an infection. Renal function should be carefully evaluated because many patients may require an angiogram.

Radiography is critical to evaluate the underlying bone architecture. It may not detect acute osteomyelitis, however, because it can take up to 3 weeks for osteomyelitis to appear on plain radiographs. MRI or nuclear medicine scan is usually superfluous if the surgeon plans to evaluate the affected bone during the débridement. However, these studies can be useful when the extent of osteomyelitis in the suspected bone is unclear or when other bones are believed to be involved.

Noninvasive arterial studies are useful adjuncts to help assess the quality of blood flow to the foot. Ankle-brachial indices are inaccurate in patients with diabetes mellitus because their arterial walls calcify, thereby preventing the cuff from compressing the vessel. Because the digital arteries are less likely to calcify, toe pressures higher than 50 mm Hg indicate adequate flow. Tissue oxygen levels can be very useful if the laboratory tests them reliably. Levels lower than 20 mm Hg indicate poor healing potential, levels between 20 and 40 mm Hg indicate possible healing, and levels higher than 40 mm Hg indicate good healing potential.

The Solutions

Treatment Options and Rationale

The goal is to convert the chronic wound into an acute healing wound with wrinkled skin edges, healthy granulation tissue, and neoepithelialization. The reconstruction then usually can be accomplished by simple techniques 90% of the time and complex flap reconstruction 10% of the time. The steps to achieve a healthy healing wound include establishing a correct diagnosis, ensuring a good local blood supply, débriding the wound to a clean base, correcting the biomechanical abnormality, and nurturing the wound until it shows signs of healing. It is important to preserve all possible healthy tissue so that all possible reconstructive options remain.

Given the complexity of issues involved in a chronic diabetic wound,

resolution mandates a team effort. The team should include a diabetologist to bring the blood glucose in control, an infectious disease specialist to optimize antibiotic therapy, a foot and ankle surgeon to address the existing biomechanical abnormalities, a vascular surgeon to improve local blood flow, a wound specialist to convert the chronic wound into a healthy healing wound, and a plastic surgeon to close wounds that require flap reconstruction. Frequently one of the treating physicians possesses two or more of the skill sets necessary to treat diabetic wounds.

In patients with undetermined or inadequate blood flow, débridement should be delayed until blood flow status has been corrected. However, immediate débridement is indicated regardless of the vascular status when wet gangrene, ascending cellulitis from a necrotic wound, or necrotizing fasciitis is present. The wound can then be kept clean with dressing changes until revascularization. If the wound manifests progressive gangrene, maggots should be applied every other day while the patient awaits revascularization to minimize the potential for removing potentially viable tissue. After successful bypass surgery, it takes 4 to 10 days for oxygen in the surrounding tissue to rise to the optimal level. Definitive débridement and aggressive wound care should follow as soon as possible thereafter.

Open or percutaneous release of the Achilles tendon decreases forefoot pressure in the equinovarus foot during gait sufficiently to allow for the rapid healing of plantar forefoot ulcers. Unless correction of the underlying biomechanical abnormality is part of the entire treatment plan, débriding and good wound care may prove futile.

DÉBRIDEMENT

The Role of Débridement in Wound Healing Débridement is critical because necrotic tissue, foreign material,

and infecting bacteria impede wound healing by producing or stimulating the production of proteases, collagenases, and elastases. These substances destroy the building blocks (eg, chemotactants, growth factors, growth receptors, mitogens) necessary for normal wound healing, resulting in an environment in which bacteria can proliferate and further inhibit wound healing. Bacteria produce enzymes that inhibit wound healing, and they consume many of the scarce local resources (oxygen, nutrition, and building blocks) necessary for wound healing. A review of the effect of platelet-derived growth factor on the healing of chronic diabetic wounds led to the seminal observation that wounds healed more successfully when débrided weekly rather than more sporadically. The scheduled removal of wound healing inhibitors allowed the wounds to progress out of the inflammatory phase and into the proliferative phase.

Débriding a wound adequately consists of removing all nonviable tissue until healthy viable tissue is reached. The body itself débrides any necrotic tissue, but this is a slow process with unpredictable results, especially in the setting of chronic wounds. It is usually faster and safer to débride a wound surgically, with maggots and/or with topical agents. The wound should be débrided after the diagnosis has been established, and the steps to improving the local environment are underway. The first step in débriding a wound is to obtain deep tissue cultures so that broad-spectrum antibiotics can be started. Several cultures should be obtained to improve the chances of identifying exactly which organisms are involved. Great care should be taken to avoid contaminating the culture with skin flora. As soon as definite organisms are identified, more targeted antibiotics can be started. Deep tissue cultures should be obtained with every débri-

---

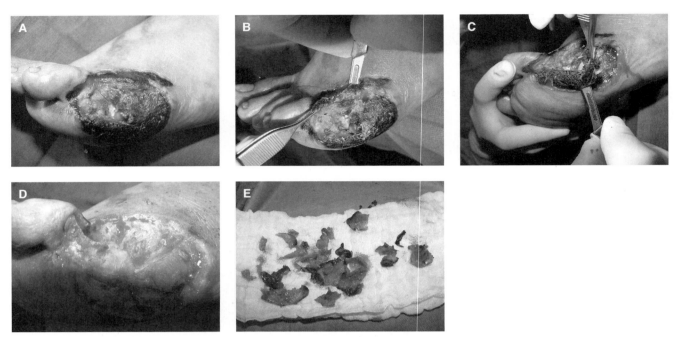

Figure 1 **A,** Wet gangrene over the lateral forefoot of a man with diabetes mellitus. **B,** The best technique for débriding the wound is to slice it serially until healthy tissue appears. **C,** Thinner slices should be taken when getting closer to normal tissue so as to minimize the loss of healthy tissue. **D,** Adequately débrided wound with no necrotic soft tissue remaining. The bone is then addressed in the same way using a sagittal saw until normal bone appears. **E,** The tissue slices removed to reach normal tissue are shown on the towel.

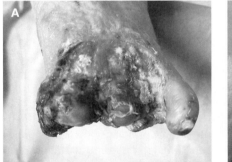
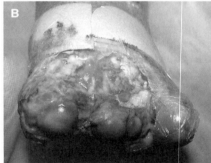
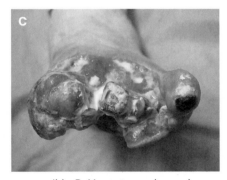

Figure 2 **A,** Maggots are applied to complete the débridement, saving as much normal tissue as possible. **B,** Maggots are changed every 2 days until no further necrotic tissue remains **(C).**

dement to evaluate its effectiveness and that of the antibiotics.

The wound should be débrided as often as necessary until it is deemed clean and ready for reconstruction. The optimal technique consists of taking serial slices of tissue until bleeding tissue is reached (**Figure 1**). The wound is watched closely and débrided repeatedly as long as there is devitalized tissue. Topical débriding agents can be used when a minimal amount

of tissue has to be removed and surgical débridement is poorly tolerated; however, these topical agents can also be painful. The use of biosurgery with maggots is an extremely effective alternative to débriding a wound when the patient cannot tolerate surgery or topical agents (**Figure 2**). The initial problem I have encountered with this method is that of educating other health care professionals to the use of maggots. However, once hospital pro-

tocols have been established and accepted, their use becomes routine. The only caveat to the use of maggots is that on rare occasions septic-like reactions to the maggots have been seen, but these respond quickly to removal of the maggots.

Topical antibiotics can help reduce the bacterial load between débridements; dressings impregnated with silver ions or silver sulfadiazine work well for most wounds. For methicillin-resistant *Staphylococcus aureus* (MRSA), mupirocin is useful, although resistance can develop quickly. For *Pseudomonas* infections, one fourth strength acetic acid, silver ion-containing dressing, or gentamicin ointment works well. For minimally infected wounds, bacitracin is adequate. An alternative dressing consists of placing methylmethacrylate beads impregnated with 1 g of vancomycin (powder) and 2.8 g of tobramycin (powder) on the wound and then covering it with an occlusive dressing or vacuum-assisted closure (VAC) device (KCI, San Antonio, TX). Maggots are the only agent that effectively destroys MRSA or vancomycin-resistant enterococci. Alternatively, the VAC device can be applied after débridement to well-vascularized wounds to help reduce the bacterial flora. The negative pressure applied to these wounds quickly reduces the bacterial load to below 10^5 bacteria per gram of tissue within 4 days.

Patients can develop an allergy to a topical antibiotic, which then should be immediately discontinued. Topical steroids can help treat the allergic skin reaction that may ensue around the ulcer.

WHAT TO DÉBRIDE

The key to débriding soft tissue is to resect back to bleeding tissue. The presence of clotted veins in the subcutaneous tissue signifies that further débridement is necessary (**Figure 3**). The skin edges should have pinpoint bleeding, and the subcutaneous fat should be bright yellow. The best technique is to take serial slices of tissue until normal tissue is reached (**Figure 1**). The closer the surgeon gets to what appears to be normal tissue, the thinner the slices should become to avoid removing healthy tissue.

All stringy and soft tendon or fascia should be débrided back to hard, solid connective tissue. When dealing with large tendons, such as the

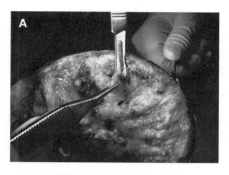

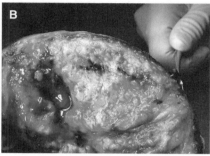

Figure 3 Clotted veins are an excellent marker to indicate that further débridement is necessary.

Achilles tendon, the tendon should be shaved down until glistening tendon fibers appear and the normal hard texture is felt. The soft tissue that overlies the tendon proximally and distally to the ulcer should be explored by making proximal and distal skin incisions to ensure that the entire necrotic tendon has been removed.

Any exposed cartilage at the base of the wound should be removed. However, if fresh healthy cartilage is exposed during the débridement and the wound is to be closed immediately thereafter, then there is no necessity to remove it.

The bone should be burred or cut back to healthy bleeding bone. When dealing with a large bone, it is best to burr it with a cutting burr until punctate bleeding is seen (paprika sign). If débriding smaller long bones, serial cuts with a sagittal saw should be made until there is hard bleeding cortical bone and normal-appearing cancellous bone. Bone sequestra should likewise be removed because they act as a foreign body.

All foreign bodies should be removed from the wound bed if possible. This includes fixation devices, joint implants, stitches, mesh, and synthetic vascular grafts. This may not always be possible when dealing with vascular grafts or orthopaedic fixation. In those cases, the débridement is coordinated with the surgeon who is familiar with the foreign body (ie, a vascular surgeon, orthopaedist).

VACUUM-ASSISTED CLOSURE DEVICE

Once the wound is clean and adequately vascularized, it can then be covered with a VAC device dressing. The VAC device applies negative pressure to a wound by means of a closed suction mechanism. The negative pressure accelerates the formation of granulation tissue, sterilizes the wound, and reduces tissue edema. The mechanisms by which this is accomplished are poorly understood. However, it is believed that the removal of inhibitory wound healing factors, decreased edema, increased blood flow, and alteration of the cellular cytoskeleton play a role in sterilizing the wound and stimulating the rapid formation of new tissue.

The VAC system consists of a polyurethane ether foam sponge with pore sizes ranging from 400 to 600 μm, which is placed directly on the wound surface (**Figure 4**). A noncollapsible evacuation tube with a fenestrated distal end surrounded by an adhesive dressing is placed on the outer surface of the sponge. The fenestrations at the end of the tube establish communication between the lumen of the tube and the foam sponge. Both the sponge and the adhesive dressing are cut to fit the size of the wound. A Mayo scissors is particularly well suited to tailor the shape of the sponge.

The wound, with sponge and evacuation tube in place, is covered with an impermeable adhesive drape that extends 3 to 5 cm over the adjacent skin. The proximal end of the evacuation tube is connected through a drainage canister to an adjustable

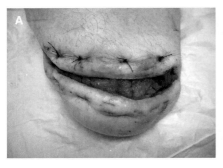

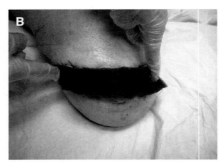

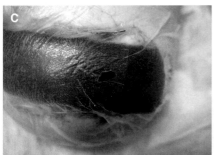

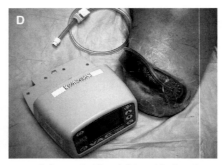

Figure 4 The use of a VAC as a dressing on normal tissue. **A,** The dehisced below-knee amputation was débrided and then the skin edges were reapproximated. The VAC dressing is placed **(B)** and secured **(C),** then attached to the portable VAC device that the patient can take home **(D).**

vacuum pump. The pump creates suction that allows subatmospheric pressure to be applied to the entire wound surface. The open-cell nature of the foam enables equal distribution of the applied suction to the entire surface of the wound. The drainage canister collects any fluid that is expressed from the wound. The subatmospheric pressure can be applied in a constant or intermittent mode with pressures up to 125 mm Hg. The intermittent mode has been found to stimulate the formation of granulation tissue more rapidly because it can constantly maintain an increased level of blood flow compared with constant suction.

If the VAC is being placed over a neurovascular bundle or a tendon, then petroleum-impregnated gauze mesh or silicone mesh should be placed between the wound and VAC sponge to minimize potential damage to the underlying structures. With long-term use of a VAC device, the wound can develop an odor. This can be addressed in one of two ways: (1) a layer of silver ions suspended in a solid sheet or in an absorptive dressing matrix is placed between the wound and the sponge, or (2) the VAC device may be stopped for a day or two while an acetic acid (0.25%) and gauze dressing is applied. If the wound is ischemic or still has necrotic tissue in it, the use of the VAC device is contraindicated. In the former case, it can cause further necrosis of the wound edges; in the latter, further infection can develop.

VAC has changed the way chronic wounds are currently being treated. It is being used to help convert a débrided chronic wound to an acute healing wound. The VAC can be used in almost any kind of wound, providing that the wound is clean and well vascularized. It allows the surgeon to electively plan the reconstruction rather than being rushed because of time limitations. The surgeon may choose to use the VAC device to allow an ulcer to heal by secondary intention rather than use reconstructive techniques. VAC has been shown to be effective in wounds in which there is an exposed fracture or joint. However, I have found that the combination of a local or pedicled flap over the exposed joint or bone and a skin graft over the rest of the wound to be a more effective treatment. The VAC device is then applied as a bolster-type dressing over a skin graft placed on the rest of the wound and on the flap donor sites. This helps ensure a very high take (> 95%) over what are often very irregular surfaces.

DETERMINING WHEN A WOUND IS READY TO CLOSE

When all the abnormal parameters surrounding the wound have been corrected and all signs of inflammation have disappeared, the wound can be allowed to heal by secondary intention or closed by delayed primary closure, skin grafted, or covered with a flap.

The wound itself should have no surrounding erythema. Cellulitis should not be confused with dependent rubor caused by ischemia or recent local surgery. If the surrounding erythema immediately fades with elevation, then the wound has dependent rubor; if it persists, then inflammation still exists. If the wound initially had massive cellulitis that has resolved, there is usually sloughing of the superficial epithelium where the cellulitis had been. Pain should have subsided in a wound with resolving inflammation. Decreasing pain, however, is a less reliable indicator than resolving erythema or induration.

The wound edges should have minimal if any induration. Wrinkled skin lines at the wound edges are reliable signs that inflammation has largely resolved. Induration may be present in patients who lack good immunologic response (ie, patients with renal failure, steroid dependence).

Fresh granulation within the wound shows that there is sufficient blood supply and a hospitable environment for the wound to progress to the proliferative phase of healing. If quantitative bacteria counts are available, then a count of less than 10^5 bacteria per gram of tissue signifies that the wound is ready to successfully be skin grafted. Alternatively, if a xenograft placed on the wound is adherent and pink, then the wound bed is sterile. The presence of new epithelium at the wound edges reflects a healthy wound that is on its way to healing by secondary intention.

CLOSURE TECHNIQUES

Closure techniques include allowing the wound to heal by secondary intention or to close using delayed primary closure, skin graft, local flap, pedicled flap, or free flap. While preparing the wound for closure by débridement and wound healing adjuncts, all possible viable tissue should initially be preserved because it may be useful in the final reconstruction (**Figure 5**).

A healthy granulating wound normally decreases in surface area by at least 10% to 15% per week. A moist dressing (a water-based gel) allows the most rapid epithelialization. The biomechanical abnormality that caused the wound should be addressed. If the wound is on the plantar forefoot, the Achilles tendon and/or hyperextended toe should be corrected and the plantar foot should be unweighted. If the wound is located near a joint surface (ankle), the involved joint should be immobilized. Several

adjuncts can help a wound heal by secondary intention if it fails to respond to dressing changes.

Platelet-derived growth factor has been shown to be effective in diabetic wounds when they are well vascularized, clean, and regularly débrided. The proteinaceous coagulum must be removed from the wound surface before applying the growth factor because the coagulum contains proteases that will digest the applied growth factor before it can affect the wound. Patients are given scrub brushes or soft toothbrushes and are instructed to scrub the wound surface every time before applying the growth factor. Alternatively, if pain is an issue in treating the wound surface aggressively, a topical débriding agent containing collagenase can be used between applications of the growth factor.

Xenograft (pigskin) or allograft (cadaver skin) provides an excellent, inexpensive, temporary moist dressing over clean healthy wounds. This dressing provides a collagen-based scaffolding for new tissue to grow into. If the temporary graft "takes" before the body rejects it, the underlying bed is sterile and vascularized well enough for a split-thickness skin graft to successfully survive. In healthy patients, rejection starts at approximately 9 days. In the immune-compromised patient, it can take up to a month before the temporary skin graft is rejected.

Although cultured skin substi-

tutes are not skin graft substitutes per se, they provide a moist living covering that produces the entire gamut of local growth factors to the underlying wound bed. They are created by allowing live cells to migrate into and populate a collagen scaffolding. This scaffolding can be covered with a layer of epidermis grown separately. These products come in two commercial forms: combined dermal-epidermal grafts or pure dermal grafts. They have been shown to be effective in healing both venous stasis ulcers and diabetic ulcers.

For the cultured skin substitute to work, the wound base should be clean and well vascularized. The skin substitute should be applied and treated like a skin graft. To ensure a good take, no motion should be present at the wound site. The VAC device can be used as a dressing to help decrease the edema and bacterial count, as well as eliminate the periwound fluid. The skin substitute should be changed every 4 to 6 weeks, if necessary. Again, it must be stressed that if the biomechanical problem that led to the ulceration is not addressed initially, the graft will not be very effective.

Hyperbaric oxygen supplies the body with oxygen concentrations at two to three times normal atmospheric pressures for 90 minutes a session. This pressure allows sufficient oxygen to dissolve in the blood plasma to reach the edge of the wound where

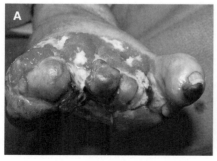 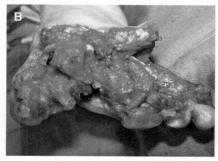 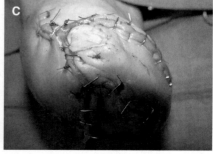

Figure 5 Preparation for transmetatarsal amputation. **A,** The entire wound is débrided. **B,** The metatarsals are cut to create a new metatarsal arcade. **C,** The fifth toe is filleted, the wound is pulse irrigated with saline solution, and all available tissue is used to close the amputation.

hemoglobin may not have a pathway, improving the oxygen concentration at the wound edges and increasing the oxygen gradient between the edge and center of the wound. The higher the gradient, the more effectively the wound healing module functions. The oxygen can then more rapidly promote angiogenesis, collagen synthesis, and neoepithelialization. In addition, hyperbaric oxygen potentiates the ability of the white blood cells to destroy bacteria.

Hyperbaric oxygen is effective only if there is adequate vascular inflow. Before undergoing hyperbaric oxygen treatment, patients should undergo an oxygen challenge test that shows a rise in the local tissue oxygen pressure after the lungs are exposed to increased oxygen content. Breathing in 100% oxygen should lead to at least a 10 mm Hg rise in tissue oxygen levels. Diving in a chamber at two atmospheres should increase the tissue oxygen level to above 300 mm Hg; otherwise, the treatment is unlikely to be effective.

The surgeon should monitor the wound closely for changes to ensure that the treatment is effective. Hyperbaric oxygen and platelet-derived growth factor work synergistically; they are more effective together than

either is alone. Therefore, if the wound is clean and well vascularized and hyperbaric oxygen is chosen to stimulate wound healing, growth factor should probably also be applied for more rapid results.

DELAYED PRIMARY CLOSURE

The wound edges have to be freshly débrided, and the wound should be closed without tension. No blanching should be present at the wound edges. Often the skin edges are too far apart to close primarily (eg, postfasciotomy). Gradual reapproximation of the skin edges is possible by using rubber bands or spring-loaded approximating devices in both wound edges. If reapproximation is done carefully, the skin will relax, and the wound edges can then be primarily closed.

Because the leg consists of circumferential soft tissue around a bone pillar, it is easy to apply excessive circumferential pressure when a wound is closed too tightly. It is important to check distal blood flow with a Doppler if there is any suspicion that a tight closure may have compromised distal blood flow.

Skin Graft This is the simplest of all coverage techniques, provided that the underlying bed has healthy granulation tissue. Split-thickness

skin grafts at 0.015 in are usually sufficient. Skin graft survival is improved if the base of the wound is completely débrided before placement of the skin graft. Survival is further improved if the graft is covered with a nonadherent dressing (silicone or petroleum jelly mesh) and a VAC device for 3 days postoperatively. This procedure ensures maximal contact between the skin graft and the bed while removing excess fluid (**Figure 6**).

For lower leg wounds, an Unna boot dressing allows the patient to ambulate immediately postoperatively. If the area is around a joint or on top of tendon or muscle, then immobilization with a posterior splint or external fixator and non–weight-bearing status for 2 or more weeks is critical for the graft to take successfully. If the graft is on the plantar aspect of the foot, the patient should not bear weight until the skin graft has matured (usually 6 weeks). For plantar wounds, plantar skin grafts from the instep at a thickness of 0.030 in are ideal because these grafts recreate the normal plantar surface. The instep can then heal by secondary intention or be skin grafted with a thin autograft. The plantar skin graft takes longer to heal and weight bearing should not be allowed until the graft has completely healed.

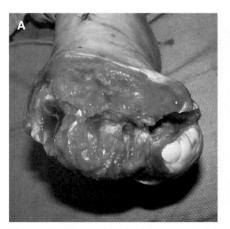 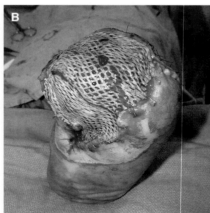 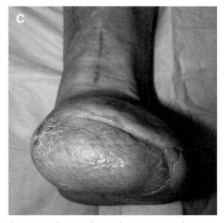

Figure 6 This patient had gangrene of the toes and metatarsophalangeal heads. **A,** When the wound was clean, the metatarsals were trimmed back in a parabola approximately 1 cm shorter than the soft-tissue envelope. **B,** The tissue edges were approximated and a skin graft placed on the denuded tissue. The skin graft was held in position for 3 to 5 days with a VAC device to ensure maximum take. **C,** The wound was healed completely within 6 weeks.

Local Flaps Local flaps are flaps with an unidentifiable blood supply that are designed adjacent to the defect. They come in various shapes (square, rectangular, rhomboid, semicircular, or bilobed) and usually consist of skin and fat or skin, fat, and fascia. The length-to-width ratio is critical for the survival of the tip of the flap. Because the blood flow to the skin is not as well organized as that in the muscle, the length-to-width ratio should not exceed 1:1 or 1:1.5. The viability of such a flap is increased when it is possible, with a Doppler, to identify an arterial signal from a cutaneous perforator at the base of the planned flap.

Local flaps are very useful for the closure of smaller defects. The donor site can often be closed primarily or skin grafted. To increase the size of the flap, the flap has to be delayed for 4 to 10 days. The simplest way to do this is to incise both sides of the flap and undermine it. The incisions are then closed, forcing the blood to flow from the base of the flap toward the tip and vice versa. When the flap has been sufficiently delayed, the tip is incised and the flap is elevated and rotated into position.

Local flaps are especially useful around the ankle to cover exposed bone or joint. The remaining defect can then be skin grafted. It is always safer when a Doppler can be used to identify a perforator at the base of these flaps. The remaining defect can then be skin grafted.

Pedicled Flaps These flaps have identifiable blood vessels feeding the flap via a pedicle. They can be cutaneous, fasciocutaneous, muscle, musculocutaneous, osteocutaneous, or osteomusculocutaneous flaps. These flaps work well if they were not involved in the initial trauma, infection, or radiation field. Otherwise, the flaps are stiff, difficult to dissect out, and difficult to transfer over. In addition, the vascular pedicle is usually very intolerant of any twisting or turning that occurs when the flap is swung into its new position. The complication rate can be as high as 40%.

MICROSURGICAL FREE FLAP

The microsurgical free flap is the most complex reconstruction and, paradoxically, carries the highest success rate (> 95%). There has to be a good recipient artery and vein(s) to which the flap vessels can be anastomosed. Muscle flaps with or without skin work best to cover osteomyelitis and the sole of the foot. Good donor muscles include the gracilis, rectus abdominis, serratus, and latissimus dorsi. Fasciocutaneous and cutaneous flaps work better elsewhere on the non–weight-bearing portions of the foot (dorsum of the foot, ankle). Fasciocutaneous flaps that are frequently used include the radial forearm flap, the lateral arm flap, the lateral thigh flap, and the parascapular flap.

Author's Preferred Treatment and Rationale

My preferred treatment of a diabetic foot ulcer is very much along the lines of what has been described above. The wound is assessed with special attention to blood supply, existing biomechanical abnormalities, depth and spread of the wound, and presence of infection. The medical status of the patient is evaluated. If there is wet gangrene present, the patient is admitted, and the wound is débrided immediately. If the wound is stable, a full work-up is undertaken. The medical and vascular status are optimized. The wound is serially débrided. If the skeleton requires stabilization, an appropriate external frame is applied.

Appropriate wound healing adjuncts are used if the wound fails to convert into a healthy wound. The VAC device, hyperbaric oxygen, growth factors, and cultured skin grafts are some of the options available. Most wounds respond to débridement and application of the VAC device.

When the wound is healthy, then reconstruction of the soft-tissue defect can be performed. The simplest mode of reconstruction available that yields a biomechanically stable foot is chosen. Ninety percent of wounds can be closed by secondary intention, delayed primary closure, skin graft, or local flap. Special care is taken to address any concurrent biomechanical abnormalities. The Achilles tendon is always addressed if its tightness contributed to the wound or may contribute to recurrent wound breakdown. The postoperative dressing is carefully chosen so that the operated-on area is protected from trauma. A non–weight-bearing regimen is instituted, and the patient is followed weekly until the wound is healed. Proper orthoses and shoes are prescribed, and the patient is allowed to start ambulating when the shoes are ready.

Management of Complications

Complications in diabetic foot and ankle reconstruction average 30% to 40% and include dehiscence, infection, and skin graft loss. The principal complication that occurs with diabetic foot reconstruction is dehiscence of the wound edges (20%). This is a result of either inadequate immobilization, noncompliance with a non–weight-bearing regimen, or inadequate blood flow. When patients with diabetes mellitus were monitored as to their ability to continuously wear a removable walker boot, the compliance rate was found to be a dismal 28%. The postoperative dressing and adherence to a non–weight-bearing regimen is critical to minimizing this complication. Reconstructions that are done in the marginally vascularized limb also run the chance of dehiscence because the incision may fail to heal as a result of the insufficient blood supply. This occurs more frequently in patients with renal failure in addition to the diabetes. The patient should be reevaluated by the vascular surgeon for further revascularization. If that is not possible, an amputation at a more proximal level should be attempted. If the wound edges fail to bleed, then the patient runs the risk of limb loss.

Infection is the second most frequent complication seen in diabetic reconstruction. It is for this reason that single-stage débridement and reconstructions should be avoided unless the wound is pristine and without infection at presentation. Otherwise, all reconstructions should be done in two or more stages. Reconstruction should only proceed when the wound shows no signs of inflammation and shows signs of healing. Reaching this stage may require the use of wound healing adjuncts such as the VAC, growth factors, hyperbaric oxygen, and/or cultured skin substitutes. Even

when the wound appears pristine, patients with diabetes mellitus and renal failure remain susceptible to further tissue-edge necrosis because of residual hidden infection. The treatment is aggressive débridement and delayed primary closure.

Poor skin graft take can be a complication that occurs because of residual infection, poor vascular bed, graft shearing, or nonadherence secondary to seroma or hematoma. By preparing an adequate healthy granulating recipient bed and sterilizing it with silver ion dressing, silver sulfadiazine, the VAC device, or a temporary xenograft, the risk of infection is minimized. By meshing the skin graft, there is minimal chance for a he-

matoma or seroma forming under the graft to disrupt it. By placing a VAC device on the skin graft for the first 3 to 5 days postoperatively, the surgeon ensures excellent adherence of the skin graft to the bed and minimizes the risk of shear forces disrupting the graft. In addition, the VAC device removes all excess fluid and keeps the area bacterial load to a subclinical level. Petroleum jelly or silicone gauze should be placed between the sponge and underlying bed to allow for easy removal of the VAC device at the end of the application. The foot should remain protected and immobilized until the graft has matured (3 to 6 weeks).

References

Attinger CE, Cooper P, Blume P, Bulan EJ: The safest surgical incisions and amputations using the Angiosome Concept and Doppler on arterial-arterial connections of the foot and ankle. *Foot Ankle Clin North Am* 2001;6:745-801.

Defranzo AJ, Argenta LC, Marks MW, et al: The use of vacuum-assisted closure therapy for the treatment of lower-extremity wounds with exposed bone. *Plast Recon Surg* 2001;108:1184-1191.

Morykwas MJ, Argenta LC, et al: Vacuum assisted closure: A new method for wound control and treatment: animal studies and basic foundation. *Ann Plast Surg* 1997;38:553-562.

Rodeheaver GT: Wound cleansing, wound irrigation, wound disinfection, in Krasner D, Kane D (eds): *Chronic Wound Care,* ed 2. Wayne, PA, Health Management Publication, 1997, pp 97-108.

Steed DL, Donohoe D, Webster MW, et al: Effect of extensive debridement and treatment on the healing of diabetic foot ulcers. *J Am Coll Surg* 1996;183:61-64.

Coding

ICD-9 CODES

040.0	Gas gangrene
250.4	Diabetes with renal manifestations
250.6	Diabetes with neurological manifestations
250.7	Diabetes with peripheral circulatory disorders
440.22	Atherosclerosis of the extremities with rest pain
440.23	Atherosclerosis of the extremities with ulceration
440.24	Atherosclerosis of the extremities with gangrene
682.6	Other cellulitis and abscess, leg, except foot
682.7	Other cellulitis and abscess, foot. except toes
707	Chronic ulcer of skin
713.5	Arthropathy associated with neurological disorders
730.16	Chronic osteomyelitis, lower leg
730.17	Chronic osteomyelitis, ankle and foot
736.71	Acquired equinovarus deformity
785.4	Gangrene

CPT CODES

11041	Debridement; skin, full thickness
11042	Debridement; skin, and subcutaneous tissue
11043	Debridement; skin, subcutaneous tissue, and muscle
11040	Debridement; skin, subcutaneous tissue, muscle, and bone
13160	Secondary closure of surgical wound or dehiscence, extensive or complicated
15000	Surgical preparation or creation of recipient site by excision of open wounds, burn eschar, or scar (including subcutaneous tissues); first 100 sq cm or each additional one percent of body area of infants and children
15100	Split graft, trunk, arms, legs; first 100 sq cm or less, or one percent of body area of infants and children (except 15050)
15120	Split graft, feet, and/or multiple digits; first 100 sq cm or less, or one percent of body area of infants and children (except 15050)
15121	Split graft, feet, and/or multiple digits; each additional 100 sq cm, or each additional one percent of body area of infants and children, or part thereof (List separately in addition to code for primary procedure)
15240	Full thickness graft, free, including direct closure of donor site, feet; 20 sq cm or less
15241	Full thickness graft, free, including direct closure of donor site, feet; each additional 20 sq cm (List separately in addition to code for primary procedure)
15342	Application of bilaminate skin substitute/neodermis; 25 sq cm

Coding

15343   Application of bilaminate skin substitute/neodermis; each additional 25 sq cm (List separately in addition to code for primary procedure)

15738   Muscle, myocutaneous, or fasciocutaneous flap; lower extremity

27606   Tenotomy, percutaneous, Achilles tendon (separate procedure); general anesthesia

27687   Gastrocnemius recession (Strayer procedure)

27880   Amputation, leg, through tibia and fibula

27882   Amputation, leg, through tibia and fibula; open, circular (guillotine)

27886   Amputation, leg, through tibia and fibula; re-amputation

28001   Incision and drainage, bursa, foot

28002   Incision and drainage below fascia, with or without tendon sheath involvement, foot; single bursal space

28003   Incision and drainage below fascia, with or without tendon sheath involvement, foot; multiple areas

28005   Incision, bone cortex (eg, osteomyelitis or bone abscess), foot

28110   Ostectomy, partial excision, fifth metatarsal head (bunionette) (separate procedure)

28111   Ostectomy, complete excision; first metatarsal head

28112   Ostectomy, complete excision; other metatarsal head (second, third, or fourth)

28113   Ostectomy, complete excision; fifth metatarsal head

28114   Ostectomy, complete excision; all metatarsal heads, with partial proximal phalangectomy, excluding first metatarsal (eg, Clayton type procedure)

28118   Ostectomy, calcaneus

28120   Partial excision (craterization, saucerization, sequestrectomy, or diaphysectomy) bone (eg, osteomyelitis or bossing); talus or calcaneus

28122   Partial excision (craterization, saucerization, sequestrectomy, or diaphysectomy) bone (eg, osteomyelitis or bossing); tarsal or metatarsal bone, except talus or calcaneus

28124   Partial excision (craterization, saucerization, sequestrectomy, or diaphysectomy) bone (eg, osteomyelitis or bossing); phalanx of toe

28140   Metatarsectomy

28800   Amputation, foot; midtarsal (eg, Chopart type procedure)

28805   Amputation, foot; transmetatarsal

28810   Amputation, metatarsal, with toe, single

28820   Amputation, toe; metatarsophalangeal joint

28825   Amputation, toe; interphalangeal joint

29515   Application of short leg splint (calf to foot)

Forefoot Neuropathic Ulcers

Heidi Multhopp Stephens, MD, MBA

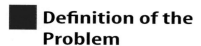 Definition of the Problem

Patient Presentation

Forefoot ulcers are frequently encountered in patients with significant neuropathy. The most common cause of neuropathy in the United States is diabetes mellitus; however, other causes include myelodysplasia, Lyme disease, alcohol, drug-related neuropathy, and leprosy. Typically, the patient has a history of minor trauma that he or she associates with the development of the ulcer. Patients commonly report changes in shoe wear, minor trauma from stepping on a foreign object, or pulling off a piece of skin with tape. The ulcer usually has been present for weeks-to-months at the time of presentation, and it is not uncommon for the ulcer to have existed for years. Normally the ulcer is painless unless it is associated with underlying osteomyelitis, proximal cellulitis, or infection. The ipsilateral calf generally is swollen, and the swelling may give the appearance of a deep venous thrombosis. Significant foot infection may manifest as calf pain in a patient with dense neuropathy in the foot. Patients will often report having been on antibiotics, either oral or intravenous, for an episode of cellulitis. There is rarely a limp, and patients often present in regular shoes. A foot ulcer may lead to a diagnosis of previously unrecognized diabetes mellitus.

Physical Examination

The patient is typically ambulatory without a limp while wearing regular shoes. Sensory examination reveals lack of protective sensation as determined by examination with a 5.07 Semmes-Weinstein monofilament. Pulses are palpable unless the diabetes is of long duration. Motor neuropathy leads to intrinsic muscle wasting and clawing of the toes as an early finding. Later motor changes associated with ascending neuropathy lead to extrinsic muscle imbalance. The tibialis anterior, a major dorsiflexor, may be affected early. The result is relative overpull of the gastrocnemius-soleus and peroneus longus, which can lead to static or dynamic equinus contracture of the ankle. Ankle range of motion should be assessed to determine the contribution of gastrocnemius-soleus contracture to the forefoot ulceration. Two other dynamic contractures may also contribute to the development of forefoot ulcers. Relative overpull of the flexor hallucis longus results in a typical plantar hallux ulcer of the interphalangeal joint. This ulcer may also be present with structural hallux rigidus, so passive dorsiflexion of the first metatarsophalangeal (MTP) joint should be assessed. Relative overpull of the peroneus longus will contribute to the formation of an ulcer beneath the first metatarsal head-sesamoid region.

Ulcers beneath the lesser metatarsal heads occur when one metatarsal is anatomically longer or more plantar than the others. Clawing of the toes from the intrinsic wasting shifts the metatarsal fat pad and increases the plantar pressure beneath the metatarsal head. Clawing may lead to ulcers at the tip of the toe or dorsally over the proximal interphalangeal (PIP) joint region. Frank dislocation of the MTP joint dramatically increases the pressure beneath the involved metatarsal head and is very highly correlated with plantar ulceration. Forefoot neuropathic ulcers occur not only on the more typical plantar aspect of the foot but also between the toes or between the toes and shoes where pressure occurs.

The diameter and depth of the ulcer are measured. The nature of the wound bed may be granulation, slough, or eschar. Wagner grading of the ulcer is helpful for both treatment and prognosis (**Table 1**). Ulcers graded Wagner 0 to 1 often can initially be treated nonsurgically, whereas ulcers graded Wagner 3 or higher are almost always treated surgically. The approach to treating Wagner grade 2 wounds depends on factors such as location, tissue necrosis, and infection.

The diagnostic work-up of a foot with a forefoot ulcer begins with evaluation of healing potential. If pulses are not palpable, significant ischemia may exist. The toe pressure is an indicator of healing potential related to arterial inflow in the forefoot. If the toe pressure is greater than 50 mm Hg, arterial inflow is adequate for healing in a patient with diabetes. With a toe pressure less than 30 mm

Table 1 Wagner Grading System

Grade	Description
0	Foot has intact skin. There may be multiple foot deformities and hyperkeratotic areas. Hypoesthesia or hyperesthesia of neuropathy may be present.
1	Superficial ulcer in the skin only
2	Deeper ulcer that includes tendon, bone, ligament, or joint
3	Still deeper lesion that includes abscess and/or osteomyelitis
4	Gangrenous area of some portion of the forefoot
5	Gangrenous area over the greater percentage of the foot

(Reproduced with permission from Wagner FW: Management of the diabetic-neurotrophic foot *Instr Course Lect* 1979;28:143-165.)

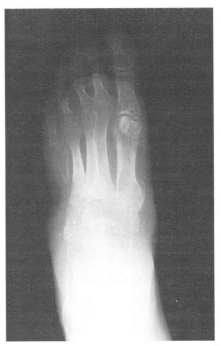

Figure 1 AP radiograph shows the defect in the lateral midfoot soft tissue seen with a significant ulcer.

Hg, healing is highly unlikely. When the pressure is between 30 and 50 mm Hg, the healing potential is questionable. Any patient with a toe pressure lower than 50 mm Hg should undergo formal vascular evaluation before surgical treatment. Further work-up would include noninvasive vascular studies, an arteriogram, and, possibly, vascular intervention. An elevated erythrocyte sedimentation rate may indicate the presence of osteomyelitis. If the ulcer can be probed to bone, osteomyelitis is considered present until proven otherwise.

Weight-bearing AP and lateral radiographs with a marker placed at the location of the ulcer help to locate the bony prominence associated with increased pressure. Osteomyelitis may be noted as well. A sesamoid view is helpful for ulcers beneath the first metatarsal head area to diagnose sesamoid osteomyelitis. Gas may be seen in the soft tissues when an ulcer is present (**Figure 1**). It is important to differentiate air seen in the soft-tissue void, which is a normal finding when an ulcer is present, from the speckled appearance of the soft tissues seen in gas gangrene (**Figure 2**). Emergency surgical débridement is imperative with gas gangrene as this condition can be limb- or life-threatening.

Differential Diagnosis
- Diabetes mellitus (most common cause in the United States)
- Leprosy (most common cause worldwide)
- Myelomeningocele
- Lyme disease
- Alcoholism
- Toxic exposures (chemotherapy, heavy metals)
- Central nervous system injuries (stroke, partial spinal cord injury)
- Peripheral vascular disease
- Venous stasis disease (trauma, burns, frostbite)

Additional Work-up
Other imaging techniques are of limited benefit because of a high rate of false-positive studies. MRI is useful primarily to visualize an abscess in the area of an ulcer or a septic MTP joint. There is almost always edema in the bony process associated with an ulcer as a result of hyperemia, and this edema is poorly correlated with osteomyelitis and leads to false-positive findings. Triple-phase technetium Tc 99m bone scans have a similar high false-positive rate for osteomyelitis because of generalized hyperemia to the local area. Combining a technetium Tc 99m bone scan with an indium-labeled white blood cell scan

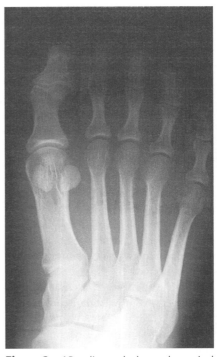

Figure 2 AP radiograph shows the typical speckled soft-tissue pattern associated with gas gangrene. (Reproduced with permission from Stephens HM: The diabetic plantar hallux ulcer: A curative soft tissue procedure. *Foot Ankle Int* 2000;22:954-955.)

may help confirm the presence of osteomyelitis. This dual scanning, however, is time consuming and costly. Often in these patients, resection or biopsy of the suspected bone is more helpful. Deep cultures may be obtained, and the bony pressure point resected.

———————■

■ The Solutions

Treatment Options and Rationale

The primary treatment of a forefoot ulcer is highly dependent on the grade of the ulcer. Initial treatment of Wagner grade 1 or 2 ulcers is directed at off-loading the involved area and wound care. Grade 2 ulcers may require débridement if necrotic or infected tissue is present. Treatment of grade 3 ulcers may vary depending on the chronicity of the osteomyelitis. Surgical resection of the involved bone is often necessary. Grade 4 and 5 ulcers are treated with some type of amputation.

Wound care with neuropathic ulcers is highly controversial. The primary goal is to achieve a clean, viable wound bed that is kept moist. Enzymatic débriding agents may be used to remove slough, but in some instances these agents may be too aggressive and deepen the ulcer. Judicious bedside surgical débridement is probably the most reliable way to maintain a viable wound bed and remove surrounding callus. Antibiotic ointment is excellent for maintaining a moist ulcer bed. If the surrounding area is macerated, then the ulcer is too moist, and dressing changes should be more frequent or less ointment should be used. The plantar wound should not be packed excessively because the packing will act as an additional pressure irritant. A flat dressing will absorb drainage and

not add to the local pressure phenomenon.

Grade 1 ulcers are treated initially with off-loading techniques. It is not reasonable to simply tell patients to avoid weight bearing and to use crutches, a walker, or wheelchair. The poor strength and general medical condition of many of these patients, combined with the lack of pain sensation, make compliance with non–weight-bearing status virtually impossible. A custom-molded insole (with relief for the area of the ulcer) in an extra-depth, extra-wide shoe is often adequate to heal superficial ulcers. Total contact casting or a total contact open cell foam-lined ankle-foot orthosis (TCAFO or healing boot) may also be used for more recalcitrant ulcers. A grade 1 ulcer treated nonsurgically with off-loading may heal, but it may progress to grade 2 if pressure is not adequately decreased or if there is ischemia or osteomyelitis. It is important to check ankle dorsiflexion. A gastrocnemius recession or Achilles tendon lengthening may be successfully combined with nonsurgical off-loading techniques to decrease forefoot pressure.

In grade 2 ulcers off-loading techniques are attempted but successful healing is less likely. After a reasonable attempt at off-loading (4 to 6 weeks) more aggressive intervention is considered. The surgical treatment is highly dependent on the location of the ulcer. For ulcers in the web space between two toes, a condylectomy of the involved condyles of one or both toes is indicated. An ulcer at the tip of the toe or dorsal PIP region may require correction of the toe deformity. A flexible toe may only need a flexor digitorum longus release but a rigid deformity may be treated with a PIP arthroplasty and MTP release.

If the ulcer is beneath a metatarsal head, treatment may depend on the pathoanatomy. If there is no clawing or dislocation of the metatarsal head with a plantar ulcer, the treatment

should be plantar condylectomy of the metatarsal from a dorsal approach. If clawing of the MTP joint and a plantar ulcer are present, treatment should include extensor tendon lengthening or tenotomy, dorsal capsulotomy, collateral ligament release, and plantar condylectomy. If the MTP joint is dislocated and there is a plantar ulcer, treatment may include a metatarsal head resection with resection of the proximal phalangeal base with extensor tendon lengthening or tenotomies. It is very important not to overtreat these ulcers with too much bony resection because a transfer-lesion ulcer may occur under an adjacent metatarsal.

Ulcers beneath the first metatarsal head usually follow the same algorithm as described above for the lesser metatarsals. The sesamoids are sometimes the cause of the ulceration. The weight-bearing AP radiograph with a marker is helpful in identifying the exact pressure point. If the sesamoid appears to be the offending prominence, sesamoidectomy is the preferred procedure. The plantar plate must be kept intact to prevent medial, lateral, or dorsal deviation of the hallux. The sesamoid is shelled out subperiosteally with repair of the plantar plate defect. If the forefoot ulcer is associated with limited dorsiflexion of the ankle, a gastrocnemius recession or Achilles tendon lengthening may be indicated.

Grade 3 ulcers involve infection of the underlying bone. They usually are best treated with resection of the bony prominence causing the ulcer. Bony resection is dictated by the extent of infection as well as that of the bony prominence. The surgeon uses the appearance of viability of the bone as a guide. Deep surgical cultures are done to guide the choice of postoperative antibiotic treatment. In patients who have minimal bony involvement at the time of surgery and in whom a susceptible bacteriologic agent is identified, an oral antibiotic may be adequate. For most patients, an intravenous course of antibiotic is required to treat the infection postoperatively.

Grade 4 and 5 ulcers are treated with amputation, the level of which is typically dictated by the margin of soft-tissue viability. Often these conditions have vascular insufficiency. If there are no palpable pulses, a vascular surgery consultation is indicated.

Author's Preferred Treatment and Rationale

In grade 1 or 2 ulcers without osteomyelitis, it is essential to consider soft-tissue releases or procedures. There are several distinct circumstances in which a simple soft-tissue procedure is often sufficient to off-load an ulcer in a certain location. The best known of these procedures is Achilles tendon lengthening for a forefoot ulcer. Achilles tendon contracture is a prevalent condition in patients with previous transmetatarsal amputation. A flexor digitorum longus tendon release may be effective for end calluses and ulcers in the lesser toes. Personal experience has shown that release of the peroneus longus tendon is frequently effective at off-loading the plantar first metatarsal head area as long as osteomyelitis of the sesamoids is not present. There is an analogous role for release of the posterior tibial tendon for a plantar ulcer at the fifth metatarsal base. I believe that these lower risk soft-tissue procedures may be tried before bony resection. The patient should be advised about the possible need for a bony procedure if the lesser procedure fails.

I follow these general principles when operating on neuropathic feet with ulcers: (1) These patients are excellent candidates for regional blocks for surgical anesthesia. (2) Beware of transfer lesions (ulcers). If too much of a bony prominence is removed, another may manifest in the form of a new ulcer. (3) Surgical cultures are advised. Many patients return postoperatively with cellulitis or wound infection. The cultures will guide the choice of antimicrobials. (4) If wound closure is indicated, use robust closure on the skin. Nonneuropathic patients will not bear weight because of pain, but neuropathic patients may be walking on their freshly operated-on foot even before leaving the hospital. Staples and robust retention sutures may help hold the wound together and minimize late night calls. (5) Leave skin closure in for at least 3 weeks.

Management of Complications

Surgical intervention may be complicated by infection, wound dehiscence, and transfer lesions. The use of broad-spectrum postoperative antibiotics is strongly recommended. Wound closure requires strong subcutaneous suture and skin. Staples and retention suture on the skin are also advised.

------■

References

Birke JA, Pavich MA, Patout CA Jr, Horswell R: Comparison of forefoot ulcer healing using alternative off-loading methods in patients with diabetes mellitus. *Adv Skin Wound Care* 2002;15:210-215.

Lin SS, Lee TH, Wapner KL: Plantar forefoot ulceration with equinus deformity of the ankle in diabetic patients: The effect of Tendo-Achilles lengthening and total contact casting. *Orthopedics* 1996;19:465-475.

Stephens HM: The diabetic plantar hallux ulcer: A curative soft tissue procedure. *Foot Ankle Int* 2000;21:954-955.

Coding

ICD-9 CODES

250.8   Diabetes with other specified manifestation

718.47   Contracture of joint, ankle and foot

730.27   Unspecified osteomyelitis, ankle and toe

735.4   Acquired deformities of toe, hammer toe

735.5   Acquired deformities of toe, claw toe

735.8   Other acquired deformities of toe

CPT CODES

27685   Lengthening or shortening of tendon, leg or ankle; single tendon (separate procedure)

27687   Gastrocnemius recession (eg, Strayer procedure)

28001   Incision and drainage, bursa, foot

28114   Ostectomy, complete excision; all metatarsal heads, with partial proximal phalangectomy, excluding first metatarsal (eg, Clayton type procedure)

28124   Partial excision (craterization, saucerization, sequestrectomy, or diaphysectomy) bone (eg, osteomyelitis or bossing; phalanx of toe

28230   Tenotomy, open, tendon flexor; foot, single or multiple tendon(s) (separate procedure)

28232   Tenotomy, open, tendon flexor; toe, single tendon (separate procedure)

28270   Capsulotomy; metatarsophalangeal joint, with or without tenorrhaphy, each joint (separate procedure)

28288   Ostectomy, partial, exostectomy or condylectomy, metatarsal head, each metatarsal head

28315   Sesamoidectomy, first toe (separate procedure)

SECTION 9
Neurologic Problems

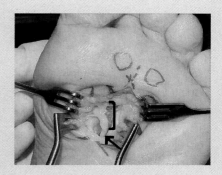

Glenn B. Pfeffer, MD
Editor

Complex Nerve Problems of the Foot and Ankle

John S. Gould, MD

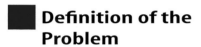

Definition of the Problem

Patient Presentation

Nerve problems in the foot and ankle are extensive and typically a result of injury directly to the nerves, injury to the tissues surrounding nerves, and complications following surgical intervention. Problems also are caused by various diseases, entrapments, and traction phenomena as well as failed surgical interventions for these conditions. This chapter describes posttraumatic and iatrogenic nerve injuries and failed nerve surgery, including unsuccessful repairs, Morton's neuromas, and tarsal tunnel syndrome.

Injury to a nerve may occur by laceration, varying degrees of direct pressure on the nerve, a sudden blow or crush, traction, electrical current, and neurotoxins. The nerve may be completely intact anatomically but have a temporary conduction block (the mildest type of neurapraxia), it may have internal anatomic damage of varying degrees (neurapraxia, loss of Schwann cells, or axonotmesis), or it may be partially or completely structurally divided (neurotmesis) with or without a reparable distal component. Many nerve injuries consist of combinations of these levels. As a result of an injury to the extremity, a nerve may be bound in external scar, which restricts its normal gliding motion with movement of the extremity; it may be swollen in certain areas as a result of specific constriction sites; or it may have internal neuromas and intraneural fibrosis.

Nerve injuries may result in loss of sensibility, loss of motor function, autonomic changes, pain, and various combinations of these findings. The surgeon must delineate the parameters of the problem, determine the options for treatment, develop a recommended plan of action, and be prepared to discuss these options with the patient. Unfortunately, few surgical options guarantee a full recovery or perfect result. Consequently, the surgeon must know both the literature's and personal statistics on outcomes of prospective surgery and disclose them in the discussion with the patient. Contingency plans are also needed in the event that the first or even second procedure is unsuccessful. Nonsurgical measures, physical and pharmacologic, also enter into any plan to complement, if not to substitute for, the surgery. Finally, the surgeon must be technically capable of performing the surgical options.

Physical Examination

Assessing nerve injury requires a good history and a careful physical examination. The type of trauma is important; for example, a crush injury typically causes nerve injury or entrapment from edema and scarring, even without concomitant fractures and dislocations. Patients often give a history of such trauma, describing a visit to an emergency department at which time they were told that the radiograph was nega-

tive for fractures and that the injury was only a bruise. However, the patient is still in pain, and no one can determine why. Therefore, the history of the chief report of pain is essential. When does the patient have the pain (mechanical or rest); how does the patient characterize it (sharp, shooting, aching, burning), where is it located anatomically, and what relieves it? Such information may suggest nerve-type pain or essentially rule it out.

The physical examination demonstrates neurologic deficits and should differentiate a patient's report of numbness from an area of actual sensory loss. An area or point of tenderness over or along a nerve or a Tinel's sign may be an important clue. Special tests may be as simple as using a paper clip to identify areas of sharp and dull or two-point discrimination (more important in the hand than in the foot) and using Semmes-Weinstein monofilaments to evaluate pressure threshold sensibility or as complicated as performing electrodiagnostic testing, which may require the services of a neurologist or physiatrist. In the foot, two-point discrimination is not particularly helpful because the normal ability to discriminate between one of two points approaches 20 mm on the great toe, but monofilament testing can be very valuable to show some objective evidence of a nerve deficit.

When pain is the presenting symptom, there may be little objective evidence for the diagnosis other than subtle autonomic changes such as skin color. Also, the presentation may be dynamic, in that movement or weight bearing may aggravate the neural component, as in tarsal tunnel syndrome, making static testing potentially less likely to be positive.

Differential Diagnosis

- Neurogenic injury
- Vasogenic injury
- Mechanical injury
- Inflammation
- Oncologic condition

Additional Work-up

No additional studies are necessary for a definitive diagnosis.

——————■

■ The Solutions

Treatment Options and Rationale

There currently are specific options for treatment of each nerve problem. In general, however, there is a variety of potential options for treating injured nerves. They may require repair; repair with grafting; neurolysis with or without barrier materials; excision with or without redirection into a minimal contact area; excision with nerve, vein, or other conduits; and implantation of electrical stimulators, both locally and at the spinal cord level. Finally, mechanical devices may be implanted to administer medications directly to painful nerves.

Because this chapter focuses primarily on failed nerve surgery and its remedies, each of these approaches will find a place and be an option in one diagnosis or another. Treatment of an injured nerve usually is governed by that nerve's functional importance and its historic response to certain modalities. In general, sensory nerves can be discarded or excised when they are painful because the sen-

sory deficit created may be small as a result of adjacent nerve overlap, or it gradually becomes smaller as a result of a phenomenon known as "peripheral sprouting" as the territory of the adjacent nerve expands. However, it is important to preserve motor components, and hence mixed motor and sensory nerves are usually treated to preserve function.

There are exceptions. For example, in the upper extremity, the superficial radial nerve does not do well with excision alone, which results in major problems with painful neuromas. Consequently, if the distal end is available, most surgeons make every attempt at repair, including grafting, when there is a laceration. The equivalent nerve in the lower extremity, the superficial peroneal, does not have such a problem.

Author's Preferred Treatment and Rationale

All of the sections below reflect my preferred treatment. I believe this is very specific, and I have avoided discussing options except as a progressive algorithm.

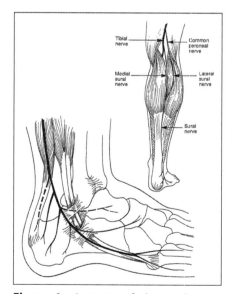

Figure 1 Anatomy of the sural nerve (Adapted with permission from Miller SD: Sural nerve injury and entrapment. *Foot Ankle Clin* 1998;3:462).

NERVE INJURIES USUALLY REQUIRING EXCISION OR REEXCISION ONLY

Sural Nerve Traumatic neuromas and severe crush injuries to the sural nerve occur with calcaneal fractures and fifth metatarsal base fractures, and iatrogenic injury occurs during the surgical repair of these fractures (**Figure 1**). The sural nerve also is injured with Achilles tendon surgery (particularly a small branch of the nerve that runs along the lateral border of the tendon), gastrocnemius recession, peroneal tendon procedures, and reconstructions of the lateral ligament of the ankle.

The usual treatment of choice for sural nerve injuries is excision of the nerve. The sensory deficit is small and recedes with time. The diagnosis often is missed when pain exists after lateral ankle ligament surgery, Achilles tendon surgery, or an otherwise successfully repaired fifth metatarsal fracture; however, a careful history should reveal the diagnosis. The main nerve lies midway between the lateral edge of the Achilles tendon and the posterior border of the lateral malleolus (except for the branch along the lateral border of the tendon) and travels proximally toward the posterior midline with the short saphenous vein, ending in the midline on the aponeurosis of the gastrocnemius as Kaplan's "white line." Simply excising the nerve proximally usually eliminates pain caused by an injured sural nerve, except for the few patients who have an aberrant accessory nerve branch. Another reason for failure of simple excision is that the nerve has not been excised proximally enough.

Saphenous Nerve Orthopaedic surgeons usually do not think of injuries to this insignificant nerve that runs with the greater saphenous vein in the foot and ankle. It usually is injured during vein harvesting for coronary artery bypass surgery; the patient presents to the orthopaedic surgeon with pain in the anteromedial ankle and tenderness between the anterior edge of the medial malleolus and the crest of the tibia. The saphenous nerve also may be injured in distal tibial fractures and their treatment, in open fractures when a crush injury requires a flap or graft, and when the saphenous vein is taken for vein wrapping procedures (**Figure 2**). Simple excision is curative, and failure, when it occurs, is usually a result of scarred anatomy and failure to find the nerve, which is remedied by finding the vein or its original location more proximally and excising its fellow traveler, the nerve.

Superficial Peroneal Nerve The superficial peroneal nerve commonly is injured iatrogenically during surgery on the lateral ligament of the ankle and during ankle arthroscopy because of the proximity of the nerve branches to the anterolateral portal and the anterolateral approaches to ankle and syndesmosis injuries. At the ankle, the nerve divides into the medial and intermediate cutaneous nerves of the foot; the sural nerve becomes the lateral cutaneous nerve of the foot, dividing into plantar and dorsal branches. The medial cutaneous nerve crosses the dorsum of the foot superficially and obliquely, crossing the tarsometatarsal joint of the great toe to lie along the dorsomedial border of the first metatarsal and metatarsophalangeal joint and terminating in the medial skin of the great toe. Thus, it is extremely vulnerable to injury in bunion surgery.

If the medial cutaneous nerve alone is damaged, it should be excised just proximal to the first tarsometatarsal joint. When an intermediate nerve branch is injured, simple excision is usually sufficient. However, when the neuromas resulting from these procedures are painful and do not respond to conservative measures, more proximal excision is warranted. This nerve emerges anterolaterally from under the muscle fascia at the junction of the middle and distal thirds of the leg, midway between the crest of the tibia

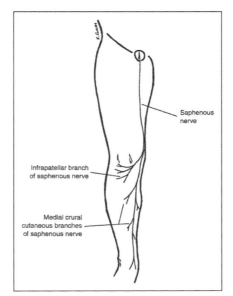

Figure 2 Anatomy of the saphenous nerve in the leg (Adapted with permission from Curry EE, Gould JS: Entrapment syndrome or damage to the saphenous nerve. *Foot Ankle Clin* 1998;3:447.)

and the anterior edge of the fibula. Locating the nerve at this point of emergence, cutting it, and allowing the proximal end to retract under the fascia is usually sufficient to relieve symptoms after an injury at a lateral arthroscopy portal site and, particularly, after a crush injury to the dorsum of the foot.

Deep Peroneal Nerve This nerve, which runs with the dorsalis pedis artery, can be located easily under the extensor hallucis brevis. It runs distally with the dorsalis pedis artery and then with the first dorsal metatarsal artery to the first web space where it is injured during first web space surgery for bunion reconstruction. Distal excision often is insufficient; excision under the extensor hallucis brevis muscle is more successful.

NERVE INJURIES OFTEN REQUIRING REDIRECTION AND/OR CONDUITS
Intermetatarsal and digital nerves may be injured during metatarsal fractures and osteotomies, hammer toe surgery, and sesamoid fractures and excisions (hallucal nerve). Treatment of Mor-

ton's neuroma, a traction irritation of the intermetatarsal and proximal digital branches on the distal edge of the intermetatarsal ligament, can also be problematic.

Simple excision is often successful except for excision of the medial hallucal nerve, which notoriously fails to respond. Morton's neuroma usually is approached initially with a linear dorsal incision in the second or third web space, extending from the proximal edge of the commissure to the level of the metatarsal heads. The metatarsal heads are separated by a retractor, and the ligament is divided, taking care not to injure the intrinsic tendon. The nerve is separated from the artery, and after traction is applied, the nerve is divided. For recurrence of a Morton's neuroma, a repeat dorsal approach is difficult and often futile. A plantar incision at the interval between the metatarsal heads, extending proximally, easily exposes the proximal end of the intermetatarsal nerve and the neuroma just under the plantar fascia. Searching more deeply, perhaps at the tendon level, will cause the surgeon to miss the nerve, which is more superficial.

The hallucal nerves, which are managed in the same manner as a recurrent neuroma of the intermetatarsal (or failed Morton's neuroma), are exposed in a similar manner. A low medial sagittal incision will expose the medial hallucal nerve plantar to the abductor hallucis muscle, and a plantar approach in the first web, following the skin lines, will reexpose the lateral hallucal nerve, which lies just plantar to the fibular sesamoid.

Redirection After excision of the neuroma, the intermetatarsal nerve is repositioned to a relatively quiet area where there is less likelihood of either direct pressure or adjacent moving structures. There are no large, relatively immobile muscles to put the nerve into, implantation into bone has not been reliable, and silicone nerve caps have not been dependable. Consequently, I place the nerve into the midmetatarsal space, essentially halfway between the dorsum and plantar aspects of the foot. I use a hemostat to bluntly tunnel through the intermetatarsal space from the plantar surface to the dorsum, taking a route that follows a natural plane for the nerve and will not twist it across or entrap it around a tendon or muscle. When the dorsal skin is tented by the end of the hemostat, a counterincision long enough to visualize the dorsal anatomy is made on the dorsum. A second hemostat, identical in size to the first, grasps the opened first hemostat, following the same curvature of the opening and then is pushed from dorsal to plantar, emerging into the plantar wound. A No. 4-0 bioabsorbable suture is attached to the distal end of the nerve, and the small noncutting needle is placed into the open hemostat, which closes over its point. The hemostat, needle, suture, and nerve are then drawn dorsally while the path of the nerve is observed from the plantar side. To avoid accidentally suturing a moving tendon or a superficial sensory nerve, the suture is attached to superficial myofascia without drawing the nerve up to this level and without any tension on the nerve, thereby suspending the nerve in its new "quiet" location. The lateral plantar nerve is positioned the same way in the first web space, and the medial plantar nerve is redirected in the same manner to the first web space.

Vein Conduits When redirection is unsuccessful or the nerve resection level has reached a branching point, proximal interfascicular dissection to obtain separation and length is not adequate. If I do not want to sacrifice the adjacent nerve, my next recourse is a vein conduit. (As a result of numerous interfascicular interconnections, extensive separation of fascicles will lead to hypersensitive, painful nerves.) This procedure originated with the use of nerve graft conduits

after neuroma excision to lead a nerve end out of a distal area in which a place to hide the nerve ending, and anticipated neuroma, was nonexistent or limited. Although this technique is successful, it requires taking an autogenous nerve; it also risks a new site for a painful neuroma and is a common cause of generalized nerve hypersensitivity in patients who already have a painful nerve, particularly in the same extremity.

Autogenous veins seem to work well as a substitute for nerves for this purpose. There seems to be two effects: (1) The end of the nerve neuroma is enclosed and protected from attaching to other moving structures, and (2) the nerve regenerates no more than 1 cm into the vein and then tends to stop regenerating rather than form a neuroma, apparently from a lack of neurotropic effect as is found from reattachment to a distal nerve end, even with a graft. This "nerve graft to nowhere," as I have termed it, is particularly effective in this salvage situation. I usually harvest a 6- or 7-cm long piece of the greater saphenous vein or a branch thereof, depending on the size of the nerve involved, marking the proximal end of the vein with a hemostat indicating that blood would flow toward that direction. Vein branches are ligated or cauterized. The vein is dilated mechanically, flushed with a local anesthetic solution, and then a suture passer is placed down the vein from the proximal or hemostat marked end to emerge through the distal opening. A nylon suture is passed through the nerve end and fed though the suture passer loop; the passer is withdrawn from the vein, pulling the nylon and the nerve inside the vein. The nerve is pulled into the vein in such a direction that as it regenerates, it will not be impeded by a valve.

Approximately 1 cm of the nerve is covered by the vein, and the vein lumen edge is sutured to the nerve epineurium with No. 8-0 nylon inter-

rupted sutures, using loupe magnification. The nylon stitch is then withdrawn. A nonpermanent suture is attached to the end of the vein, and it is led to a new deeper location, often the intermetatarsal space as described above for redirection maneuvers.

MIXED NERVES REQUIRING NEUROLYSIS, OFTEN WITH BARRIER MATERIALS: POSTERIOR TIBIAL NERVE AND BRANCHES (TARSAL TUNNEL)

The posterior tibial nerve, medial and lateral plantar nerves, and various branches, such as the first branch of the lateral plantar to the abductor digiti minimi and the calcaneal branches from the main nerve, are vulnerable to trauma to the hindfoot and ankle, to surgical procedures around the posteromedial ankle and plantar aspect of the foot, to tumors such as neurilemmomas, and to tarsal tunnel syndrome. Except for the calcaneal branches, these nerves are mixed motor and sensory, supplying the intrinsic muscles of the foot as well as the sensibility of the plantar aspect of the foot. Failure of decompression or neurolysis of these nerves may result from a lack of appreciation of the anatomy and potential points of entrapment. The "classic" tarsal tunnel syndrome is believed to be secondary to space-occupying lesions behind the laciniate ligament or posteromedial flexor retinaculum. This situation is relatively rare, whereas a traction neuritis often related to chronic plantar fasciitis or posterior tibial tendon dysfunction is much more common. In this situation, the more distal edge of the deep fascia of the abductor hallucis, the medial edge of the plantar fascia, and the underlying superficial fascia of the quadratus plantae are the culprits and require release (**Figure 3**).

When evaluating a failed surgery in this area, I first determine from the skin incision if the release was likely to be complete. At surgery, in a repeat situation, I am concerned whether

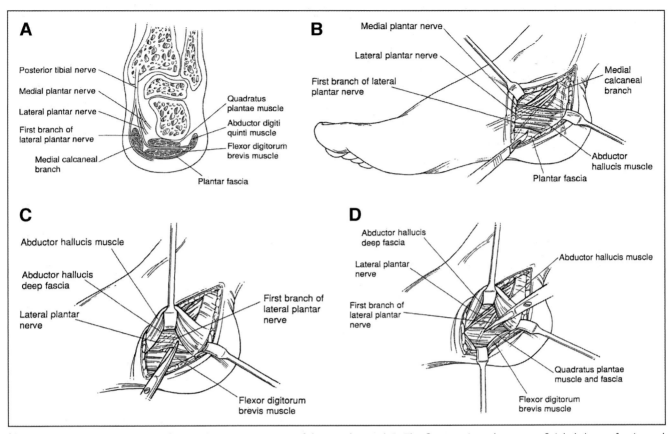

Figure 3 Tarsal tunnel, plantar fascia release. **A,** Anatomy of the tarsal tunnel. **B,** The flexor retinaculum, superficial abductor fascia, and plantar fascia are released. **C,** The deep fascia of the abductor hallucis is released. **D,** The fascia of the quadratus plantae under the lateral plantar nerve is released. (Adapted with permission from DiGiovanni F, Gould JS: Tarsal tunnel syndrome and related entities. *Foot Ankle Clin* 1998;3:405-426.)

there was an incomplete release, significant external scar compressing the nerve, or internal nerve damage with either neuromas or intraneural fibrosis. If the release was incomplete, I do a complete release and fully expose the nerve and its branches by releasing the laciniate ligament, the entire abductor hallucis, the entire plantar fascia, and possibly a part of the flexor digitorum brevis. The quadratus plantar fascia underlying the lateral plantar nerve is released. By ligating crossing arterial and venous branches of the posterior tibial artery and vein, the posterior tibial nerve, the medial and lateral plantar nerves, the calcaneal branches, and the branch to the abductor digiti quinti can be fully and easily visualized using loupe magnification. If there is a neuroma of a cal-

caneal branch, I may use a vein conduit for it, leading it deeply, possibly into the retrocalcaneal space. If there is clear evidence of external scar around the nerve or minimal intrinsic nerve damage, I will add a vein wrapping. If there is significant intrinsic nerve damage or a vein wrapping has failed, I recommend the use of a peripheral nerve or dorsal column stimulator.

Vein Wrapping Reports of successful salvage with both autogenous and allograft vein have been optimistic. Glutaraldehyde-preserved umbilical vein is used as an allograft. Its advantage is accessibility without the need for and morbidity of an autogenous donor site. It is, however, a large thick tissue that is somewhat unwieldy for a smaller nerve, and some

patients have had an adverse reaction to the material. Autogenous greater saphenous vein is readily available, more sheer and easy to work with, accommodating to large or small nerves, and never rejected. However, there is a limit to its quantity, its harvest and preparation add significant time to the procedure, and it deprives a patient who may someday be a candidate for coronary artery bypass surgery of a valuable component of that procedure, at least from one leg.

To wrap a nerve the size of the main posterior tibial, the length of vein needed is about three times the length of nerve to be covered. The branches require more of a 1:1 ratio. The vein is harvested starting anterior to the medial malleolus and extending proximally no more than one half to

477

three fourths of the way up the leg. I never go above the knee. Branches are ligated, and the vein is dilated and flushed with a local anesthetic. It is then slit longitudinally to create a ribbon of vein. The vein, with the intimal side facing the nerve, is then wrapped around the involved nerve like the stripes on a barber pole. The proximal and distal ends of the vein are anchored in the soft tissue to avoid constriction at the ends of the wrap. A No. 7-0 suture is used with interrupted stitches to connect the coils of vein. The wrap is well contoured, but the nerve is not tightly wrapped, and the closure is not watertight. Calcaneal branches are allowed to emerge through generous openings in the wrap.

In the typical situation, the wrap starts on the posterior tibial nerve and continues along the lateral plantar nerve until the nerve is pristine. The medial plantar nerve is wrapped with a separate piece of vein, if needed, until it passes under the abductor hallucis. Patients are placed in a soft dressing and follow non–weight-bearing regimes for a month but are encouraged to move the foot and ankle to promote gliding of the nerve and vein in the soft tissues. A gliding plane has been noted to develop between the vein and surrounding tissues, as well as between the nerve and the vein. The patient is then allowed to bear weight with an orthotic device that supports the longitudinal arch but has a nerve relief channel under the nerve path posteromedially.

Implanted Nerve Stimulators I have used implanted nerve simulators for intrinsically damaged painful nerves, but I am less enthusiastic about their use at this time than I once was. The nerve is exposed in a normal area proximal to the damaged area. The silicone paddle that contains the electrodes is placed on or under the nerve and connected by silicone-covered wires to an implanted generator-stimulator. For the posterior tibial nerve, the generator, which has a typical life span of no more than 5 years is usually placed in the medial thigh. It is a simple matter to replace the generator periodically. Alternatively, the generator may be replaced with a receiver, and this device is activated by an externally worn battery pack instead of being fully internal. The implanted device may be programmed to vary the stimulation signal and to cycle it on and off. The patient has a device that he or she can use to turn the device on and off and to vary the intensity of the stimulation.

Because the electrode paddle tends to move (ie, pitch, roll, and yaw), attaching it to the adventitia of the nerve is important. Problems with these devices include (1) movement of the electrode paddle with loss of contact, (2) scarring under the paddle, (3) surges of stimulation caused by external sources (eg, electronic scanners in stores and at security checkpoints), (4) electrical leakage at connectors, and (5) premature draining of power from the generators. Dorsal column stimulators have been somewhat more successful for chronic pain relief, providing broader coverage of the extremity and fewer of the problems mentioned above.

Management of Complications

Nerve regeneration in the proximal and distal lower extremities tends to be dysesthetic. As a result, the surgeon tends to repair only essential nerves, using excision and redirection techniques judiciously. For the most part, I repair the posterior tibial and the medial and lateral plantar nerves. Intrinsic loss can be improved with tendon transfer (flexor to extensor), but the large plantar sensory deficits are a significant impairment. If a prior attempt to repair such a nerve has failed, I redo it with a nerve graft using single or multiple strands of graft material. I usually use a microscope and use the contralateral sural nerve as my graft to avoid increasing the sensory deficit on the affected side. Alternative reconstruction includes neurocutaneous flaps for the plantar aspect of the foot to provide at least protective sensation. Where this is not possible, the patient is coached, like a patient with peripheral neuropathy, to use "occulocutaneous" sensation, frequently inspecting the plantar foot visually, and using protective shoe inserts. When a nerve tumor of these plantar nerves destroys a portion of the nerve, I also graft the defect in the nerve. In a late situation, I assess the functional deficit and pain to determine the best course of action, which again may be a segmental nerve graft for all or part of the nerve.

———————————————■

References

Cohen BE, Gould JS: Peripheral nerve stimulation as a treatment modality of painful nerves in continuity. *Foot Ankle Clin* 1998;3:537-544.

DiGiovanni BF, Gould JS: Tarsal tunnel syndrome and related entities. *Foot Ankle Clin* 1998;3:405-426.

Gould JS: Autogenous vein wrapping for painful nerves in continuity. *Foot Ankle Clin* 1998;3:527-536.

Gould JS: Nerve problems of the foot and ankle. *Foot Ankle Clin* 1998.

Mackinnon SE, Dellon AL: (eds): *Surgery of the Peripheral Nerve* New York, NY, Thieme, 1988.

Seddon HJ: Three types of nerve injuries. *Brain* 1943;66:237-288.

Sunderland S: A classification of peripheral nerve injuries producing loss of function. *Brain* 1951;74:491-516.

Coding

ICD-9 CODES

355.5	Tarsal tunnel syndrome
355.6	Lesion of plantar nerve
355.7	Other mononeuritis of lower limb

CPT CODES

20926	Tissue grafts, other (eg, paratenon, fat, dermis)
20926-59	Tissue grafts, other (eg, paratenon, fat, dermis); distinct procedural service
64575	Incision for implantation of neurostimulator electrodes; peripheral nerve (excludes sacral nerve)
64590	Incision and subcutaneous placement of peripheral neurostimulator pulse generator or receiver, direct or inductive coupling
64590-59	Incision and subcutaneous placement of peripheral neurostimulator pulse generator or receiver, direct or inductive coupling
64708	Neuroplasty, major peripheral nerve, arm or leg; other than specified
64708-22	Neuroplasty, major peripheral nerve, arm or leg; other than specified, unusual procedural services
64782	Excision of neuroma; hand or foot, except digital nerve
64784	Excision of neuroma; major peripheral nerve, except sciatic
64787	Implantation of nerve end into bone or muscle (list separately in addition to neuroma excision)

Recurrent Interdigital Neuromas

James L. Beskin, MD

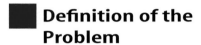 Definition of the Problem

Patient Presentation

Failure to achieve the desired result is a potential consequence of any surgery. It can be particularly disquieting if after satisfactorily completing the straightforward task of removing a Morton's neuroma the patient experiences similar or even worse symptoms. The physician is then obligated to completely reassess whether there was a correct preoperative diagnosis or whether the failure was caused by a technical error or an anomalous healing process.

Nerve pain is a complex problem that warrants careful consideration in even the most straightforward Morton's neuroma. Postoperative complications are best prevented by accurate assessment of the original problem. Disappointment after surgery is often the result of failure to recognize the correct source of the nerve pain. Several diseases can cause symptoms manifested by the interdigital nerve. This indirect, or secondary nerve pain should be distinguished from the symptoms of a primary Morton's neuroma. Indirect nerve pain can be divided into two main categories: (1) referred pain from nerve dysfunction, such as neuropathy or radiculopathy, that is not related to the interdigital nerve; (2) and interdigital nerve pain secondary to a pathologic process, such as synovitis or bursitis in the adjacent tissues, that directly affects the digital nerve.

With a recurrent neuroma, patients often report improvement for several months after surgery before the new problem develops. This improvement presumably occurs during the time it takes the regenerative axons to migrate into the adjacent tissues. Symptoms may increase as the nerve tissues approach the weight-bearing areas of the forefoot. The discomfort is typical of nerve pain and usually is similar to that of the original Morton's neuroma: diffuse, poorly defined, often aching pain. Footwear issues are less consistent than with primary neuromas because the problem is a true neuroma rather than an entrapment neuropathy. However, as with primary Morton's neuromas, weight bearing usually increases symptoms.

A percentage of patient problems are confirmed to be a result of technical failures to remove the nerve. Nerve removal cannot always be discerned from the surgical note, but a review of the pathology report may provide more information on the quality and quantity of nerve tissue removed. Most authors advocate resection as far proximal as possible to prevent a symptomatic stump neuroma. This resection entails cutting the plantar skin branches with at least 2 to 3 cm of nerve proximal to the bifurcation to reduce the risk of nerve regrowth to the weight-bearing area of the forefoot.

The communicating branch between the medial and lateral plantar nerves from the second to the third interspace will also contribute to a percentage of failures. When a dorsal approach is used, this branch, which is present 25% to 30% of the time, may not be resected proximally enough to avoid a weight-bearing stump neuroma.

Occasionally, the discomfort after neurectomy is not from a stump neuroma but instead results from new problems. Late, recurrent pain that occurs more than 1 year after surgery is often from an unrelated source. An adjacent neuroma should be considered as its occurrence has been reported in at least 5% of patients. When more than the three central toes are involved, other sources of nerve pain should be investigated. Pain involving the entire foot should lead to an evaluation of peripheral neuropathy, tarsal tunnel syndrome, complex regional pain syndrome, or radicular nerve pain sources.

Physical Examination

The most consistent finding on physical examination of a patient with a stump neuroma is tenderness to palpation over the affected site. Swelling or other changes in the appearance of the foot are not typical. Closer scrutiny of the patient's response to the examination will often give clues to a neurogenic origin. Many patients describe a tingling or electric sensation produced by direct pressure over the neuroma site. Often, the symptomatic stump neuroma has developed under the weight-bearing part of a metatarsal head that can serve as a landmark for future localization. Gentle tapping will frequently produce a positive nerve percussion response similar to a Tinel's sign. Recording the precise location of the maximal area of sensitivity will help with planning subsequent treatment such as injections or surgical exploration.

A basic neurologic examination will also help identify any relevant proximal nerve pathology evidenced by reflex, motor, or sensory changes beyond what would be expected from digital nerve involvement. If neurectomy was accomplished at the primary surgical procedure, some diminished sensory perception in the affected web space is expected and should be confirmed. Patients with diffuse hyperesthesias and color and temperature changes should also be examined for sympathetic nervous system dysfunction.

Differential Diagnosis
- Adjacent primary neuroma
- Symptomatic stump neuroma
- Complex regional pain syndrome
- Tarsal tunnel syndrome
- Peripheral neuropathy
- Lumbar radiculopathy
- Metatarsophalangeal synovitis
- Stress fracture
- Freiberg's infraction

Additional Work-up
Laboratory and radiographic studies are helpful when the clinical history and examination are less than straightforward. Radiographs can add information about the condition of the adjacent joints and bone structure but are not diagnostic for nerve pathology. Ultrasound has been reported to be helpful for visualizing primary Morton's neuromas, as well as postoperative stump neuromas, but depends on experienced technical and radiologic staffing. MRI has an emerging role in assessing difficult problems

and can be used to identify abnormal thickening of the nerves associated with Morton's neuroma and postoperative neuromas. Perhaps more importantly, MRI can identify other occult conditions of the joints or tendons that could be contributing to the symptoms.

Neurophysiologic studies, including nerve conduction velocity studies and electromyography, may also provide additional information when atypical pain is evident on the clinical examination. These studies are useful in identifying other sources of nerve dysfunction, including neuropathy, radiculopathy, or proximal entrapment lesions, that produce symptoms in the forefoot.

■ The Solutions

Treatment Options and Rationale
For a significantly symptomatic Morton's neuroma, surgical resection has been the standard practice since the 1940s. However, a stump neuroma is the expected outcome of every surgical neurectomy. The literature suggests that 10% or more of these remain symptomatic. It is logical to assume that even with a perfect procedure, some will recur as a result of the natural healing variability among patients.

Nonsurgical management is appropriate but often of limited value for a stump neuroma. Nonnarcotic analgesics may provide temporary relief. Anticonvulsants, including gabapentin, caramazepine, and phenytoin, as well as some antidepressants such as amitriptyline, can have a temporizing effect but are less desirable long-term solutions.

Orthotics to reduce pressure at the neuroma site may be helpful, but these require specific measures. The typical metatarsal lift will actually increase pressure at the site of symp-

toms in most patients and should be avoided. Recession of the orthotic material under the area of involvement is more likely to be effective.

Local injection with bupivicain and a steroid is a useful diagnostic and potentially therapeutic maneuver. Careful placement at the site of symptoms can confirm the origin of the pain because temporary relief is provided by the local anesthetic and potentially longer improvement by the steroid. However, multiple, repeated injections should be avoided to reduce complications from fat-pad atrophy.

In most patients, a significantly symptomatic stump neuroma will require revision surgery to obtain a satisfactory result. After the surgeon has carefully assessed the potential causes of failure and excluded radicular and other neuropathic sources for the symptoms, a plan to identify and revise the stump neuroma is reasonable.

It is important to determine what will be done differently to avoid a similar result when the nerve is re-resected. If the surgeon determines that the primary procedure was inadequate as a result of a limited nerve resection, simply revising the nerve to an appropriate level, usually 2 to 3 cm above the metatarsal heads, will suffice. If the surgeon determines that the primary resection was adequate but the nerve has regenerated, a different approach is advised. In some nerves the axons are capable of growing several centimeters, enabling

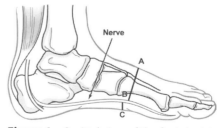

Figure 1 Sagittal view of the foot depicting the relationship of the plantar nerves relative to the dorsal and plantar surfaces. Note the difference in the dissection between a dorsal approach (line AB) and a plantar approach to the nerves (line CB).

them to return to the weight-bearing portion of the forefoot despite a satisfactory proximal resection. In these circumstances, the nerve should be rerouted or the nerve end buried, and proximal replacement should be planned.

There are two surgical approaches, dorsal and plantar. Although a dorsal incision simplifies healing an uncomplicated primary Morton's neuroma, a plantar approach for revision surgeries is advantageous. As the need to move proximally into virgin tissue increases, the capacity to do so from a dorsal incision is greatly limited by the converging anatomy of the metatarsals. Further difficulty arises because the sagittal diameter of the foot increases with proximal dissection (**Figure 1**). However, plantar incisions must be placed carefully to avoid bony prominences. These incisions significantly improve exposure of the nerves. Patients with hyperkeratosis or keloids may be at higher risk of skin complications and need individual consideration.

Author's Preferred Treatment and Rationale

SINGLE SPACE RECURRENT STUMP NEUROMA

A plantar incision is centered between the appropriate metatarsal heads, extending proximally 4 to 5 cm into the arch (**Figure 2**). Loupe magnification is helpful. The dissection is deepened carefully through the fat pad to the plantar fascia septae. The initial dissection is started proximally in virgin tissue to identify the common digital nerve branch just deep to the level of the plantar fascia. Visualization of the lumbrical or interossei tissues reveals that the dissection is too deep. Once the nerve is identified, it is traced distally to the metatarsal head area where the neuroma typically is found. If normal-appearing nerve tissue is found up to or beyond the metatarsal heads, resection probably was inadequate at the index proce-

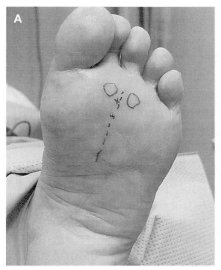 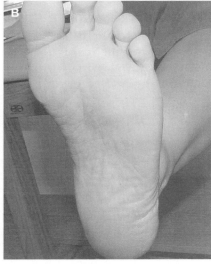

Figure 2 A, Plantar incisions are placed longitudinally between the metatarsal heads. **B,** The usual benign healing at this area.

dure. Further resection to the proximal corner of the wound, allowing the stump to retract into unaltered tissue, usually will suffice. It is essential that the new nerve end be located in a non–weight-bearing portion of the foot. At the third interspace, any communicating nerve branches from the second interspace between the medial and lateral plantar nerves should be sought and addressed.

When a long segment of regenerative nerve is encountered (**Figure 3**), burying the nerve deep into muscle will lessen the chance of a symptomatic weight-bearing stump neuroma. The distal nerve is mobilized, maintaining length for replacement deep into the intrinsic musculature of the midfoot, by resecting the neuromatous bulb, placing a bioabsorbable No. 4-0 suture into the nerve end, and bringing it into the intrinsic musculature by direct repair or by using Keith needles to pull temporary sutures through the dorsal midfoot. Check to see that the nerve stays buried while the ankle is brought through its range of motion. The foot should be splinted, and the patient should not bear weight for 2 weeks after surgery.

RECURRENT NEUROMA WITH ADJACENT INTERDIGITAL NERVE SYMPTOMS

Occasionally recurrent pain or persistent pain at the primary procedure site is determined to be associated with an additional adjacent Morton's neuroma. Under these circumstances, it is prudent to address both nerves simultaneously through a plantar incision.

The same longitudinal incision used to expose the recurrent neuroma can be used to expose the adjacent nerve. If necessary, the proximal end of the incision can be directed either medial or lateral in an "L" or "J" shape to facilitate exposure. After addressing the recurrent neuroma, the adjacent unal-

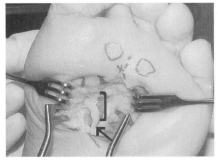

Figure 3 The normal nerve is shown by the arrow. The bracket highlights the regenerative nerve tissue that has extended to the weight-bearing area of the forefoot.

tered nerve is identified in the next interspace between the plantar fascia septae. Several centimeters of nerve should be resected and the proximal end allowed to retract into normal tissue. It is not necessary to dissect out or remove the distal bifurcation area unless a pathologic specimen of the Morton's neuroma is desired.

If a significant amount of regenerative tissue is found at the recurrent neuroma site, indicating that an adequate resection had been performed but a long segment of regenerative neuromatous tissue was produced, burying both the primary and recurrent nerve ends as described in the previous section may reduce the risk of recurrent pain.

When revision surgery is planned properly, 70% to 80% of patients experience improvement. However, a significant percentage of patients will have some degree of residual discomfort.

Management of Complications
Surprisingly few wound or skin problems are associated with properly placed plantar incisions. Occasionally, a scar develops over a weight-bearing area, and orthotic, or rarely, surgical intervention is needed to revise the scar or remove an underlying bony prominence.

In some patients the regeneration and formation of symptomatic stump neuromas seem extraordinary. The value of tertiary revisions depends on the surgeon's knowledge of what was accomplished at the secondary procedure and an honest evaluation of what additional benefit could be hoped for in the next procedure. If simple resections resulted in several months of good relief before relapse, revising the nerves with stump burial deep into muscle tissue should be considered.

If symptoms are believed to be related to neuropathic pain and not amenable to nerve resection, the surgeon is faced with the difficult task of pain management, which often requires a multidisciplinary approach. However, a patient with neuropathic pain who has a clear stump neuroma may still benefit from surgical excision.

————————————■

References

Amis JA, Siverhus SW, Liwnicz BH: An anatomic basis for recurrence after Morton's neuroma excision. *Foot Ankle* 1992;13:153-156.

Beskin JL, Baxter DE: Recurrent pain following interdigital neurectomy: A plantar approach. *Foot Ankle* 1988;9:34-39.

Johnson JE, Johnson KA, Unni KK: Persistent pain after excision of an interdigital neuroma: Results of reoperation. *J Bone Joint Surg Am* 1988;70:651-657.

Richardson EG, Brotzman SB, Graves SC: The plantar incision for procedures involving the forefoot: An evaluation of one hundred and fifty incisions in one hundred and fifteen patients. *J Bone Joint Surg Am* 1993;75:726-731.

Wolfort SF, Dellon AL: Treatment of recurrent neuroma of the interdigital nerve by implantation of the proximal nerve into muscle in the arch of the foot. *J Foot Ankle Surg* 2001;40:404-410.

Coding

ICD–9 CODES

355.6   Mononeuritis of lower limb, Lesion of plantar nerve; Morton's metatarsalgia, neuralgia, or neuroma

729.2   Neuralgia, neuritis, and radiculitis, unspecified

956.4   Injury to peripheral nerve(s) of pelvic girdle and lower limb; Cutaneous sensory nerve, lower limb

CPT CODES

28080   Excision, interdigital (Morton) neuroma, single, each

64787   Implantation of nerve end into bone or muscle (list separately in addition to neuroma excision)

CPT copyright © 2003 by the American Medical Association. All Rights Reserved.

Equinovarus Deformity

Michael J. Botte, MD

▇ Definition of the Problem

Patient Presentation

Equinovarus deformity develops frequently in adults with acquired spasticity from disorders including traumatic brain injury (TBI), cerebrovascular accidents (CVA), and spinal cord injury. As a result of muscle imbalance, the patient has a deformity consisting of plantar flexion of the ankle and/or midfoot (equinus) and inversion of the hindfoot or midfoot (varus) (**Figure 1**). Toe flexion deformities often coexist (**Figure 1**, *A* and *B*). The equinus component is caused mainly by spasticity of the gastrocnemius and soleus, with additional contributions from the tibialis posterior, flexor hallucis longus, and flexor digitorum longus. In patients with TBI and CVA, the varus component is most commonly caused by spasticity of the tibialis anterior. In congenital spasticity, such as the child with cerebral palsy, the varus is more commonly caused by spasticity of the tibialis posterior. Toe flexion deformities result from spasticity of the extrinsic and intrinsic toe flexors. Secondary soft-tissue contractures from lack of motion contribute to the stiffness of the deformity and can result in a rigid deformity. Ipsilateral spastic hip flexion and adduction and knee flexion deformities often develop (**Figure 1**, *D* and *E*). Planovalgus, cavus, toe extension, and other foot deformities are rare but do occur as a result of atypical muscle imbalance. Because sensory pathways to the brain also can be disrupted, the patient may have varying loss of limb sensibility. Cognition often also is affected.

Following the neurologic insult, the deformities may initially improve in varying degrees as a result of neurologic recovery. Recovery occurs over a 6-month period in CVA, a 12-month period in incomplete spinal cord injury, and over 18 months or more in TBI. Knowledge of these recovery times is important because corrective surgical procedures are usually delayed until the patient has reached a plateau in improvement.

Chronic equinovarus with toe flexion deformities produces several problems: (1) functional deficits in ambulation or limb stance for transfers; (2) painful callosities on the lateral plantar foot from concentrated pressure beneath the fifth metatarsal head or styloid process; (3) inability to obtain a comfortable foot position on a wheelchair platform; and (4) difficulty with shoe wear or use of orthotic devices. Severe varus can result in maceration and breakdown within the skin folds

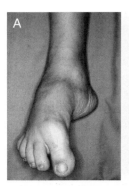
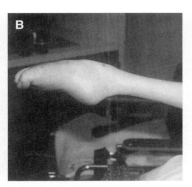
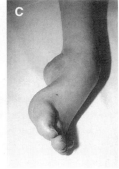
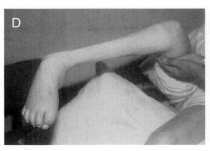
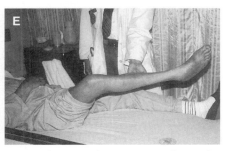

Figure 1   **A-E**, Equinovarus deformities in patients with acquired spasticity. Toe flexion deformities are also present in *A* and *B*. Concomitant knee flexion and hip flexion contractures are also present in *D* and *E*.

of the medial foot. Pain often accompanies these deformities because of the continuous muscle activity and from passive stretch against myostatic contractures when the limb is used to lift or position patients. Callosities develop on the tips of the toes from toe flexion deformities where the toes press against the floor. Callosities may also develop on the dorsum of the proximal interphalangeal joints where extension at the metatarsophalangeal joint and/or acute flexion of the proximal interphalangeal joint results in increased shoe pressure.

Physical Examination
Evaluation of motor impairment includes assessment of muscle tone, the presence of patterned reflexes or volitional control, and the development of clonus, rigidity, or fixed contractures. Motor strength, muscle phasic activity, degree of flexibility, and active and passive range of motion are assessed. If spasticity is mild, muscle strength can be evaluated quantitatively using appliances such as the Cybex (Cybex International, Medway, MA) or MedX (MedX, Ocala, FL) apparatuses.

Dynamic electromyography (EMG) will provide information on muscle activity. During ambulation, the test shows the presence of normal muscle activity (phasic), overactive muscles (spasticity), minimally active or weak muscles (paresis), and/or no muscle activity (paralysis). Dynamic EMG is particularly useful to evaluate the activity of muscles difficult to assess by physical examination alone. It helps identify which muscles are contributing to a deformity, especially in atypical deformities or when multiple muscles may be involved.

Sensibility of the foot is evaluated with touch, pinprick, two-point discrimination, monofilament testing, and proprioception. Assessment may be difficult in the patient with cognitive deficits.

Associated problems, such as impaired ambulation or standing, painful callosities, skin maceration or breakdown, positioning, and pain

from contractures, are evaluated. Both the ability to and comfort in wearing a brace or orthosis are noted, and resulting benefits are assessed. The brace is examined for fit, function, and structural and mechanical condition.

The patient's potential to ambulate is assessed. Requirements include (1) voluntary hip flexion to about 30°, (2) adequate standing balance, and (3) limb stability. Following CVA, 20% to 30% of patients will regain normal ambulation, and 75% will return to some level of ambulation.

Differential Diagnosis
- Equinus or varus from other types of muscle contracture or imbalance (ischemic contracture, crush injury with contracture from myonecrosis)
- Posttraumatic deformity (fracture malunion, burns, skin contracture)
- Equinus or varus from loss of antagonist muscles (peroneal weakness, tendon insufficiency or rupture, paresis from postpolio disorder)
- Equinus or varus from residual congenital deformity (cerebral palsy, clubfoot)

Additional Work-up
Standard radiographs of the foot (AP, lateral, and oblique views) and ankle (AP, lateral, and mortise views) are usually obtained to rule out other skeletal causes of the equinovarus and to demonstrate and document the degree of deformity. Radiographs (but rarely CT) are indicated if the patient has a rigid deformity, has had prior surgical procedures, or has sustained previous skeletal trauma. Arteriograms of the limb are obtained if integrity of the posterior tibial or dorsalis pedis artery is in question, especially if the patient has a history of previous trauma or surgical procedures.

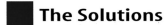

The Solutions

Treatment Options and Rationale
Initial treatment is usually nonsurgical, especially if the patient is in the recovery phase of the neurologic insult. Nonsurgical treatment consists of a comprehensive rehabilitation program that can include physical therapy, splinting, serial casting, muscle relaxants, and nerve blocks. Muscle relaxants commonly used to treat spasticity are baclofen, dantrolene sodium, and diazepam.

Serial lidocaine or bupivacaine tibial nerve blocks can be given to temporarily relax spastic muscles (and allow passive mobilization during physical therapy sessions). For longer acting muscle relaxation, phenol motor nerve blocks or botulinum toxin intramuscular injections can be given. Dilute phenol (3% to 5% solution), injected into the motor branches of the tibial nerve, produces a nerve block that lasts for weeks or months, thereby decreasing equinovarus and toe flexion spasticity. Intramuscular botulinum toxin injections also provide muscle relaxation for weeks or months and have the advantage of not requiring precise motor nerve injection.

When nonsurgical treatment fails to prevent problematic equinovarus, surgical management can be offered. Significant hip and knee deformities usually are addressed first to allow easier positioning of the foot during the later surgical correction of equinovarus. Additional relative indications for foot and ankle reconstruction include (1) a deformity that is so severe that an ankle-foot orthosis (AFO) cannot be fitted, (2) a residual deformity that interferes with ambulation despite use of an AFO, or (3) a mild deformity that is correctable with an AFO in a patient who may become brace-free following reconstruction. Cosmesis alone usually is not an indication for surgical intervention unless function, hygiene, or positioning is impaired as well. Surgical reconstruction also should be considered in the nonambulatory patient in whom correction may produce a plantigrade foot that can be placed on the wheelchair platform or allow dressing and protective shoe wear and prevent skin breakdown. Reconstructive surgery is not, in general, indicated for patients who continue to show improvement in a comprehensive therapy program, especially if still in the neurologic recovery phase.

Goals and expectations of surgery include improved function, improved fit or use of orthotic devices, relief of pain from chronic spasticity or contracture, prevention or treatment of painful foot callosities, improved hygiene, positioning, dressing, and prevention of pressure sores. Some ambulatory patients may become brace-free. In the nonambulatory patient, goals include improved use of orthotic devices, better shoe wear, improved hygiene, easier foot positioning, and prevention of callosities or pressure sores.

Equinovarus deformity in acquired spasticity is surgically treated with Achilles tendon lengthening (TAL) combined with transfer of the tibialis anterior tendon. Toe flexion is addressed with release of the intrinsic and extrinsic toe flexors. These three procedures are usually performed during the same surgical procedure.

The equinus component is caused by overactivity of the gastrocnemius and soleus with additional contributions from the flexor hallucis longus, flexor digitorum longus, and tibialis posterior. This component is corrected by TAL (usually combined with release of the toe flexors for concomitant toe flexion deformity). Several methods, including the percutaneous triple hemisection tenotomy, open Z-lengthening, fractional lengthening at the myotendinous junction, or recession of the origins of the gastrocne-

mius and/or soleus, can be used to lengthen the Achilles tendon.

In the adult with acquired spasticity, the varus component is usually from the tibialis anterior, whereas in the child with cerebral palsy, the varus component is from the tibialis posterior. In acquired spasticity, the extrinsic toe flexors and the tibialis posterior also contribute to varus. Because of these differences in contributing muscles, surgical procedures in the adult with TBI or CVA more commonly involve transfer of the tibialis anterior, whereas procedures in the pediatric population usually involve lengthening or transfer of the tibialis posterior. If needed, preoperative EMGs help identify specific muscles responsible for the varus deformity.

Author's Preferred Treatment and Rationale
CORRECTION OF EQUINUS

For TAL, the triple hemisection tenotomy as popularized by Waters and associates is safe and reliable and requires minimal incisions (**Figure 2**). It is effective for first-time lengthening and is sufficient when both the gastrocnemius and soleus are involved. Open lengthening is preferable if the deformity has recurred after previous lengthening because the previous lengthening can produce adhesions that interfere with percutaneous lengthening. The use of an open procedure in these patients allows precise control of the lengthening.

ACHILLES TENDON LENGTHENING BY PERCUTANEOUS TRIPLE HEMISECTION TENOTOMY

Tenotomy cuts are made with a No. 11 pointed scalpel placed through small stab incisions. The distal and proximal incisions are located medially to help correct any accompanying varus. Approximately half of the tendon is incised at each incision. The foot is passively dorsiflexed to 5°, causing the tenotomy incisions to gap open and the tendon to lengthen. Care is taken

to prevent overcorrection that may lead to a calcaneal gait. In addition, the toe flexors are released as needed to prevent toe flexion deformity that is caused by the tenodesis effect with tight extrinsic toe flexors and is increased when the ankle dorsiflexes.

Postoperative management includes immobilization in a short leg cast for 6 weeks. If the procedure is performed in combination with split anterior tibialis tendon transfer (SPLATT), protection is continued with a locked AFO and night splinting for an additional 4.5 months.

ACHILLES TENDON LENGTHENING USING AN OPEN PROCEDURE

An 8-cm longitudinal incision is placed along the lateral or medial aspect of the Achilles tendon. The sural nerve, located posteriorly and laterally, should be identified and protected from injury. The sheath of the Achilles tendon is opened. A Z-step incision is placed in the tendon with adequate length for correction. Because of the twisting orientation of the tendon, the anterior two

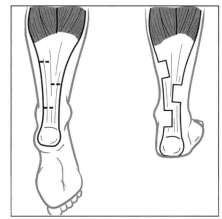

Figure 2 Triple hemisection tenotomy for TAL. Three percutaneous incisions are placed (two on the medial aspect and one on the lateral aspect), each incising approximately 50% of the tendon. The foot is then passively dorsiflexed to about 5°, and gaps are created in the tendon to provide lengthening. (Reproduced with permission from Waters RL, Perry J, Garland D: Surgical correction of gait abnormalities following stroke. *Clin Orthop* 1978;131:54-63.)

thirds of the tendon can be incised distally near the insertion, followed by dividing the medial two thirds of the tendon at a level approximately 8 cm proximally. The knee is extended, and the foot is gently dorsiflexed passively to a corrected position as the tendon slides to an appropriate length. In a tendon that has adhesions from previous lengthening, the entire incision of the Z-step cut is made with a scalpel. The tendon is repaired at the corrected length with No. 2-0 or 3-0 nonabsorbable suture. Overlengthening is avoided to prevent calcaneal deformity. Postoperatively, the foot is immobilized in a corrected position with a well-padded short leg cast applied in the operating room. Cast immobilization is continued for 6 weeks. Additional protection with an AFO for 4.5 months is indicated if the lengthening is performed in combination with the SPLATT.

CORRECTION OF VARUS AND TOE FLEXION

The tibialis anterior is transferred either by SPLATT or by transfer of the entire tendon to the dorsum of the foot. With SPLATT, the lateral half to two thirds of the tibialis anterior is transferred to the cuboid or third cuneiform, converting the deforming force to a corrective force (**Figures 3** and **4**). Overcorrection is prevented by the remaining nontransferred portion of the tendon. It is usually combined with a TAL to correct an equinovarus deformity and with toe flexor release (TFR) to correct toe flexion deformity (**Figure 5**).

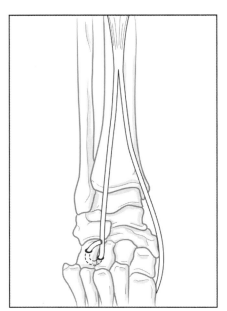

Figure 3 SPLATT. The tibialis anterior tendon is split, transferred to the lateral aspect of the foot, and sutured into place through a drill hole in the cuboid. (Reproduced with permission from Waters RL, Perry J, Garland D: Surgical correction of gait abnormalities following stroke. *Clin Orthop* 1978;131:54-63.)

SPLIT ANTERIOR TIBIALIS TENDON TRANSFER

The procedure is performed through three incisions: (1) one over the base of the first metatarsal to detach the portion of the tibialis anterior; (2) a second approximately 8 cm proximal to the ankle to pass and redirect the transferred tendon; and (3) a third incision over the cuboid and third cuneiform to reattach the tendon. The tendon insertion is identified in the first incision. The lateral half to two thirds of the tendon is detached from its insertion. A heavy

tagging suture is placed in the end of the detached tendon. A long clamp is passed subcutaneously from the second (tibia) incision to the first incision. The clamp grasps the suture in the tendon, and the suture and attached split tendon are pulled to the second incision, further splitting the tendon longitudinally along its fibers. (A uterine forceps works well for the clamp.) The tendon is redirected laterally and passed subcutaneously to the third incision. It then is attached to the lateral aspect of the foot through a 4-mm drill hole in the cuboid or third cuneiform. The tendon is sutured to itself with the foot held in a corrected position.

TOE FLEXOR RELEASE

A 2-cm longitudinal incision is placed at the proximal flexion crease of each toe. The neurovascular bundles are protected, and the flexor tendon sheath is opened. A small right angle retractor is used to retrieve the tendon, pulling it more superficially for the tenotomy. The flexor digitorum brevis is identified first and usually consists of two tendon slips. If the incision was placed distally in the region of the middle phalanx, the flexor digitorum brevis tendons may be located at the medial and lateral margins of the larger, more centrally located flexor digitorum longus. A 1-cm portion of each tendon is excised.

Although the tibialis posterior usually is not the predominant varus deforming force in the patient with acquired equinovarus, it may become secondarily tight (from myostatic

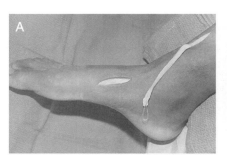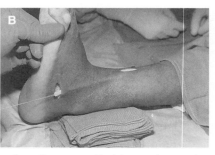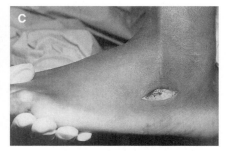

Figure 4 SPLATT. **A,** The tendon is split and transferred to a second incision on the anterior aspect of the calf. **B,** The tendon is transferred to a third incision over the lateral aspect of the cuboid. **C,** The tendon is sutured into place through a drill hole.

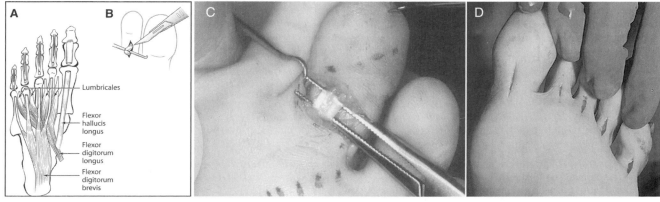

Figure 5 TFR. **A,** The intrinsic and extrinsic toe flexor tendons are released through incisions placed on the plantar aspect of the toes. **B,** The probe is holding the tendon in preparation for incision. (Reproduced with permission from Keenan MA, Gorai AP, Smith CW, et al: Intrinsic toe flexion deformity following correction of spastic equinovarus deformity in adults. *Foot Ankle* 1987;7:333-337.) **C,** Tendon isolation before release. **D,** After release of tendons, showing incisions used.

contracture) and may prevent full correction. If necessary, the tendon is lengthened by Z-lengthening or by fractional lengthening. It can be lengthened through the same posteromedial incision used for open TAL. Tibialis posterior lengthening can also be used in the patient with cerebral palsy, in which the tibialis posterior often is responsible for most of the varus component.

Z-LENGTHENING OF THE TIBIALIS POSTERIOR

The tibialis posterior is approached along the medial aspect of the ankle. The tendon is incised in the standard Z-fashion to obtain adequate length for correction. With the foot placed in a corrected position, the tendon is repaired without slack using braided No. 2-0 or 3-0 nonabsorbable suture. The foot is immobilized for 6 weeks to allow tendon healing in a corrected position.

FRACTIONAL LENGTHENING OF THE TIBIALIS POSTERIOR

The tibialis posterior is approached above the medial malleolus in the distal third of the leg immediately posterior to the tibia. The deep fascia is incised to expose the muscle at the myotendinous junction. For fractional lengthening, two or three inci-

sions are placed in the tendinous portion at the myotendinous junction, leaving the muscle portion intact. The foot is gently manipulated out of varus into a corrected position, thereby opening the gaps in the tendinous incisions and lengthening the muscle. The foot is immobilized for 6 weeks to allow muscle healing in a corrected position.

Following TAL, SPLATT, and TFR (with or without lengthening of the tibialis posterior), the foot and ankle are immobilized in a cast for 6 weeks followed by continued protection in an AFO for an additional 4.5 months. By approximately 6 months after surgery, patients progress in therapy to a brace-free status if physically able. Although TAL, SPLATT, and TFR are well-established procedures to correct equinovarus and toe flexion, approximately 60% to 70% of patients still require an AFO because of residual gastrocnemius-soleus weakness, which is most apparent during late stance phase when the body mass is anterior to the ankle joint. Additional transfer of the long toe flexors to the calcaneus will augment strength of the gastrocnemius-soleus group and help stabilize the ankle. This procedure results in a 40% increase in brace-free patients. Others have indicated that anterior transfer of

the long toe flexors to the dorsum of the foot may provide additional correction.

If there is a severe, long-standing fixed hindfoot varus deformity, soft-tissue procedures such as SPLATT and TAL may not be adequate for correction. Subtalar arthrodesis with a lateral closing wedge osteotomy will help correct a fixed soft-tissue or bone deformity. This procedure may be combined with a posteromedial soft-tissue release, possibly including a TAL, posterior ankle capsulotomy, medial talonavicular joint capsulotomy, and tibialis posterior Z-lengthening.

SUBTALAR ARTHRODESIS WITH LATERAL CLOSING WEDGE

The subtalar joint is approached through a long lateral incision for adequate exposure of the lateral aspects of the calcaneus and talus. The peroneal tendons are retracted, and the subtalar joint capsule is incised. A small power saw is used to resect bone from both the talar and calcaneal surfaces, creating a lateral closing wedge at the joint surface. Cannulated cancellous screws or multiple pins are used for fixation. Bone graft from the iliac crest is used as needed. The hindfoot is immobilized in a cast for 8 to 12 weeks or until adequate consolidation is complete.

If the calcaneus is deformed with

a varus component, and the subtalar joint appears relatively normal and without degenerative changes, a calcaneal osteotomy is considered.

CALCANEAL OSTEOTOMY FOR FIXED HINDFOOT VARUS DEFORMITY

The calcaneus may be osteotomized using a lateral closing wedge, a sliding osteotomy of the tuberosity, or a crescentic osteotomy through the tuberosity and body. The specific technique should be individualized according to the shape and deformity of the calcaneus. The calcaneus is approached through a lateral incision placed along the tuberosity. Care is taken to avoid injury to branches of the sural nerve or to the peroneal tendons. A lateral closing wedge can be placed diagonally across the tuberosity to bring the weight-bearing portion of the calcaneus laterally. Cannulated screws or multiple pins are used for fixation. Bone graft is used as needed. The foot is immobilized until consolidation is complete, usually for 12 weeks.

Management of Complications

Problems associated with equinovarus reconstruction include rupture of transferred or lengthened tendons, recurrence of deformity, inadequate correction, and overcorrection. Tendon ruptures are rare if the foot is protected postoperatively as outlined above. During the initial 6 weeks of casting, the wounds are checked frequently, and it is imperative that the foot be held continuously in the corrected position during the cast changes. Treatment of transferred tendon rupture is surgical repair.

Recurrence of deformity or inadequate correction is rare if adequate correction is obtained initially. Following TAL, the foot should be able to be dorsiflexed passively to 5°. Following transfer of the tibialis anterior, the foot should be able to be held in a corrected position in neutral varus and valgus. Recurrence is managed initially nonsurgically (eg, physical therapy, passive muscle stretching, serial casting) as outlined above. If correction remains inadequate, repeat surgical reconstruction can be considered.

Overlengthening of the Achilles tendon is a problematic outcome. The tendon initially should be conservatively lengthened so that the foot dorsiflexes passively only to about 5°. Overlengthening results in loss of ankle stability and can precipitate a calcaneal and crouch gait in which the ankle dorsiflexes and the knee flexes to accommodate the ankle. This complication is avoided with judicious lengthening of the Achilles tendon. Management is with bracing of the ankle to stabilize dorsiflexion. Surgical correction is difficult.

References

Botte MJ, Bruffey JD, Copp SN, Colwell CW: Surgical reconstruction of acquired spastic foot and ankle deformity. *Foot Ankle Clin* 2000;5:381-416.

Hoffer MM, Reiswig JA, Garret AM, Perry J: The split anterior tibial tendon transfer in the treatment of spastic varus hindfoot of childhood. *Orthop Clin North Am* 1974;5:31-38.

Keenan MA, Creighton J, Garland DE, Moore T: Surgical correction of spastic equinovarus deformity in the adult head trauma patient. *Foot Ankle* 1984;5:35-41.

Keenan MA, Gorai AP, Smith CW, Garland DE: Intrinsic toe flexion deformity following correction of spastic equinovarus deformity in adults. *Foot Ankle* 1987;7:333-337.

Keenan MA, Lee GA, Tuckman AS, Esquenazi A: Improving calf muscle strength in patients with spastic equinovarus deformity by transfer of the long toe flexors to the os calcis. *J Head Trauma Rehabil* 1999;14:163-175.

Perry J, Waters RL, Perrin T: Electromyographic analysis of equinovarus following stroke. *Clin Orthop* 1978;131:47-53.

Waters RL, Perry J, Garland D: Surgical correction of gait abnormalities following stroke. *Clin Orthop* 1978;131:54-63.

Coding

ICD-9 CODES

718.47   Other derangement of joint, Contracture of joint, ankle and foot

754.51   Certain congenital musculoskeletal deformities, Varus deformities of feet, Talipes equinovarus

CPT CODES

27685   Lengthening or shortening of tendon, leg or ankle; single tendon (separate procedure)

27690   Transfer or transplant of single tendon (with muscle re-direction or rerouting); superficial (eg, anterior tibial extensors into midfoot)

28230   Tenotomy, open, tendon flexor; foot, single or multiple tendon(s) (separate procedure)

28300   Osteotomy; calcaneus (eg, Dwyer or Chambers type procedure), with or without internal fixtion

28725   Arthrodesis; subtalar

Pes Cavus

Ian J. Alexander, MD

▪ Definition of the Problem

Patient Presentation

Pes cavus can be a challenging condition to treat. The spectrum of involvement ranges from mild elevation of the longitudinal arch in patients who are completely functional to rigid deformities in patients with secondary arthritis, stress fractures, profound weakness, and ligamentous insufficiency. Moreover, many patients with a cavus foot have an underlying progressive neurologic disorder. In these individuals, the dynamic nature of the problem can result in late loss of correction after what initially appeared to be a successful, well-conceived procedure. Two thirds of patients who seek treatment of a painful high arch will have an underlying neurologic problem; half of these will have Charcot-Marie-Tooth disease, an inherited degenerative disorder of the central and peripheral nervous system that causes muscle atrophy and loss of proprioception. Unilateral involvement is rare in progressive inherited polyneuropathies. True unilateral pes cavus is often a result of poliomyelitis, spina bifida, or trauma. Deep posterior compartment syndrome and crush injuries to the foot with intrinsic muscle ischemia are the most common causes of traumatic pes cavus.

Cavus foot deformity associated with neurologic disorders is caused by muscle imbalance. The overpull of one muscle relative to its weak antago-

nist eventually results in progressive deformity, which, although initially flexible, may ultimately become rigid. As the neurologic problem progresses the muscle that initially caused the deformity may weaken, making it difficult for the orthopaedist who sees the patient at a single point in a gradually progressive disorder to explain the reason for the observed malalignment.

The prevalence of neurologic disorders in patients with a cavus foot makes it imperative to elicit factors that might clarify the origin of the problem when obtaining a history. A relatively detailed developmental history, a history of the progression of the deformity, and a history of balance problems when the patient is in the dark or standing with his or her eyes closed should be elicited. Family history is also important, and the patient should be questioned about neurologic disorders and whether any family members have a high arch and calf muscle wasting.

Physical Examination

Pes cavus is a biomechanically complex condition; to treat it effectively, the treating physician must understand the pathomechanics of each case. This understanding is particularly important in making decisions regarding surgical intervention; it depends on a thorough assessment by a clinician competent in biomechanical evaluation of the foot who is able to address the following questions: (1) Is the deformity unilateral or bilateral

and is involvement symmetric? (2) Is the deformity primarily anterior or posterior? (3) Does the forefoot cavus deformity involve all metatarsals or predominantly the first ray? (4) Is the associated hindfoot varus deformity fixed or flexible and, if flexible, does it passively correct completely? (5) Is gait affected? (6) Are the claw toes passively correctable? (7) What is the current status of muscle involvement? (8) How profound is the sensory impairment?

Distinguishing anterior from posterior pes cavus has significant treatment implications. Calcaneocavus, or posterior pes cavus, is usually associated with weakness of the gastrocnemius-soleus complex. Anterior pes cavus is generally either idiopathic or associated with inherited polyneuropathy. Calcaneocavus deformity is recognized on physical examination by a foreshortened hindfoot and malleoli that are relatively high and posterior. Radiographically, calcaneocavus deformity is characterized by a vertically oriented and often foreshortened calcaneus with, on lateral radiographs, a calcaneal pitch angle (the measurement of the angle between the tangent of the plantar aspect of the calcaneus and the floor) of greater than 30° (**Figure 1**). Because the deformity usually occurs early in life and is most frequently observed in individuals with marked weakness of the gastrocnemius-soleus complex, growth of the calcaneus is not influenced by the pull of the

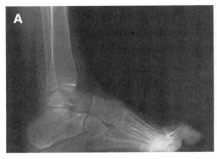

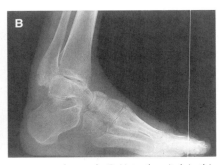

Figure 1 Calcaneal pitch angle. **A**, The line demonstrates the angle. **B**, Note the pitch in this calcaneocavus foot.

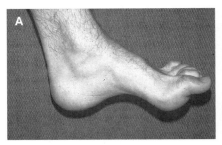

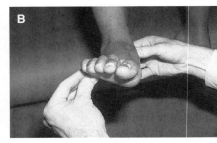

Figure 2 Cavus foot with forefoot valgus. **A**, Medial view. **B**, Tangential forefoot view.

Achilles tendon, and the calcaneus is usually short and wide. Common neurologic conditions resulting in this malformation include poliomyelitis and spina bifida and its associated spinal cord anomalies. Because profound neurologic involvement is not unusual, many of these children, if ambulatory, are brace dependent.

Anterior or forefoot cavus is also frequently related to an underlying neurologic disorder. The shape of the foot in these children or adolescents is quite different from that of those with a calcaneocavus foot. Because the gastrocnemius-soleus complex is usually one of the last muscle groups to become weak in the progressive neuropathies, calcaneal shape and orientation are usually normal. The calcaneal pitch angle is almost invariably less than 30°, and the origin of the cavus deformity appears to be primarily in the midfoot, with relative plantar flexion of the metatarsals. On radiographs, the arch is high, and plantar angulation originates at or between the transverse tarsal (calcaneocuboid

and talonavicular) and tarsometatarsal joints.

In global metatarsus equinus all of the metatarsals are plantar flexed symmetrically, and the forefoot plane (judged by a line tangential to the plantar aspect of the first and fifth metatarsal heads) is perpendicular to the central axis of the heel. This, in mechanical terms, is defined as forefoot neutral. As a result, the hindfoot, when the foot is flat on the floor, is vertically oriented or in slight valgus as in a normal individual. The forefoot in the transverse plane is neither adducted nor abducted. The relative alignment of the talar head and the anterior process of the calcaneus is normal on the AP radiograph, and the navicular is centrally located on the talar head.

Cavus foot with associated forefoot valgus, or plantar flexion of the first ray relative to the fifth, is commonly associated with neurologic disorders including diastematomyelia, spinal cerebellar degeneration, and a variety of inherited polyneuropathies,

the most common of which is Charcot-Marie-Tooth disease. The more recent terminology for this array of conditions is hereditary sensory motor neuropathies (**Figure 2**). With these peripheral neuropathies, age of onset varies, and common characteristics include autosomal dominant inheritance, muscle atrophy, weakness, and foot deformity. Unsteady gait and balance problems are related to weakness and proprioceptive impairment. In approximately 70% of patients the condition is steadily progressive, in 23% it will ultimately arrest completely, and in 7% the associated problems manifest intermittently. In general, X-linked recessive and autosomal recessive forms have an earlier onset (first and second decades, respectively) and are more rapidly progressive; severe involvement is usually present within a decade of the appearance of the first symptoms. Patients with recessive forms of Charcot-Marie-Tooth disease are often more disabled with more proximal muscle group involvement and more extensive loss of upper extremity function. Loss of hand intrinsics is common in both dominant and recessive inheritance. Scoliosis is seen in more severely involved patients with recessive inheritance.

Although forefoot valgus (plantar flexed first ray) usually can be seen with the patient in a sitting position, the best way to evaluate relative forefoot and hindfoot position is with the patient prone. The position of the forefoot coronal (or frontal) plane with respect to the central access of the heel is most relevant clinically. To measure forefoot position, evaluate the acute angle formed by the perpendicular to the central access of the heel and the forefoot coronal plane. In the cavus foot, this ranges from 0° to as much as 45° of valgus, with the acute angle opening laterally and the plantar aspect of the forefoot facing away from the midline (**Figure 3**).

The examiner should also assess

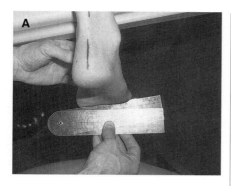

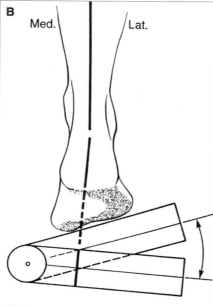

Figure 3 Clinical photograph (**A**) and diagram (**B**) demonstrating how to measure forefoot valgus.

the patient's gait, looking particularly for evidence of a steppage gait, a varus roll of the hindfoot, and reversal of the toe-touch sequence, with the great toe descending first followed by each more lateral toe in sequence. A steppage gait indicates marked weakness of the ankle dorsiflexors or a drop foot, and varus hindfoot roll and reversal of the toe-touch sequence suggest forefoot valgus with compensatory hindfoot varus.

The rigidity of the deformities has significant treatment implications. The examiner should evaluate, by passive manipulation, the rigidity of the toe deformities, plantar flexion of the first ray relative to the second and more lateral rays, and subtalar motion. The Coleman lateral block test is useful in assessing rigidity of the hindfoot varus deformity.

Muscle testing is critical. Each motor unit acting across the ankle as well as on the toes should be assessed, graded, and documented for later reference as involvement is likely to change over time and may have a significant influence on planned surgical procedures. It is important for the examiner to demonstrate the muscle weakness

to the patient or the parent during the examination and to make it clear that progressive muscle weakness with time is likely if an inherited polyneuropathy is the basis of the problem.

Although the relationship between specific muscle weakness and deformity is not always completely clear, there do seem to be some relatively common muscle imbalances that relate to the characteristic deformities. The following discussion focuses on the cavus and forefoot valgus deformity, but it is also important to mention the contribution to the observed clawing of the lesser toes of weak foot intrinsics and relative overpull of long toe extensors working hard to compensate for a weak tibialis anterior.

Forefoot valgus is caused by an imbalance of muscle groups. The tibialis anterior muscle, which normally elevates the first ray, is usually involved early in the disease. Although the peroneus brevis is also weak early on, the peroneus longus is believed to remain strong and, as a significant antagonist of the weak tibialis anterior, it plantar flexes the first ray without resistance. With time, the forefoot val-

gus alignment becomes rigid. Weakness of the tibialis anterior relative to its other antagonist, the gastrocnemius-soleus complex, results in a drop foot that is manifested in a steppage gait. This probably is the most disturbing problem, from a cosmetic point of view, for adolescents.

Along with the gastrocnemius-soleus complex, the tibialis posterior is usually one of the last muscles to be affected. With its antagonist, the peroneus brevis, becoming weak early, relative overpull of the tibialis posterior further aggravates the varus malalignment of the hindfoot, which already has been passively induced by the forefoot valgus. To understand how forefoot valgus induces compensatory hindfoot varus, the foot needs to be visualized as a tripod having three primary contact points: the first metatarsal head, the center of the heel, and the fifth metatarsal head. If the forefoot is in a valgus position with a plantar flexed first ray, the only way the lateral limb of the tripod (the fifth metatarsal head) can come into contact with the floor is by shifting the hindfoot into a varus posture. Initially, this varus posture is dynamic with varus hindfoot roll occurring with each step. The associated sensation of instability at the ankle joint is magnified by the weakness of the peroneus brevis, the primary dynamic lateral hindfoot stabilizer, and the overpull of the tibialis posterior. Ultimately, the varus position of the hindfoot will become fixed. Identification of this fixed varus is important because it significantly influences both surgical and nonsurgical treatment.

The rigidity of the hindfoot varus is best determined by manual assessment of subtalar range of motion and the Coleman lateral block test. To perform this test, blocks that usually are used to assess limb-length discrepancy are placed under the heel and the lateral border of the foot, allowing the first ray to drop to the floor. Supporting the lateral forefoot eliminates the influence of forefoot valgus on the hindfoot. By observing the posted foot from the rear, the orthopaedist can assess the alignment of the heel. If heel alignment corrects to neutral or slight valgus, the patient has a flexible hindfoot (**Figure 4**).

Differential Diagnosis

- Pes cavus secondary to muscle imbalance as a result of inherited polyneuropathy, trauma, poliomyelitis, spina bifida, or diastematomyelia
- Idiopathic pes cavus

Additional Work-up

The work-up should include an evaluation by a neurologist and, if suspicion of an inherited disorder is high enough, genetic testing. Confirming a genetic basis for the condition will help in genetic counseling if the patient ultimately plans a family and will be helpful in advising other family members. Electromyography (EMG) and nerve conduction velocity studies usually show slow sensory and motor conduction and selective muscle degeneration. Since the advent of genetic testing, EMG and nerve conduction

velocity studies are rarely necessary as confirmative tests. Particularly with patients in whom there does not appear to be a definite genetic basis to the problem, and perhaps in all patients, spinal radiographs should be obtained to evaluate for diastematomyelia. If physical findings or plain radiographs suggest diastematomyelia, CT and/or MRI of the spine is advisable, and surgically addressing the tethered cord may be helpful in preventing progressive foot deformity.

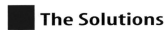

■ The Solutions

Treatment Options and Rationale
CALCANEAL CAVUS

Many patients with calcaneal cavus deformity have severe muscle involvement and, if ambulatory, require either an ankle-foot orthosis (AFO) or a knee-ankle-foot orthosis. For patients with milder calcaneal cavus in whom stabilizing the foot is not as critical,

some type of accommodative or cushioning foot orthosis may be helpful, particularly if plantar heel pain or plantar breakdown in the insensate foot is a problem. The indications for surgical intervention include pressure ulcer under the heel or metatarsal heads and failure of orthotic management. One surgical procedure that might be considered is a dorsal closing wedge osteotomy of the calcaneus between the posterior facet and the posterior superior apex of the calcaneus. For patients in whom this interval is extremely short, a crescentic osteotomy from the superior calcaneus posterior to the posterior facet to the plantar cortex distal to the tubercles may be preferable. This osteotomy is made with the concavity on the apical side of the tuberosity. A simple plantar fascia release is essential to allow the apical fragment to be displaced superiorly. A partial tenodesis of the Achilles tendon to the tibia to block unrestricted passive dorsiflexion may be performed early without the osteotomy or, in patients with more advanced deformity, with the osteotomy.

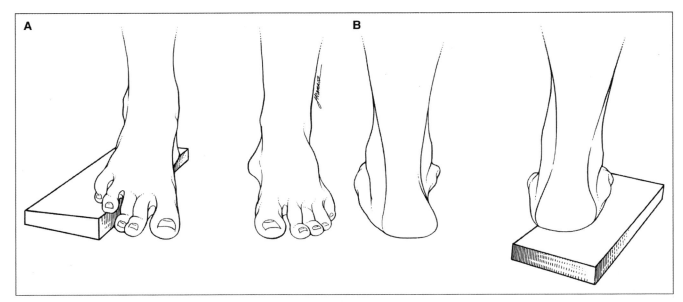

Figure 4   Coleman lateral block test. **A**, Anterior view. **B**, Posterior view.

GLOBAL METATARSUS EQUINUS

Patients with global metatarsus equinus tend to function relatively well so surgical intervention is not usually necessary. These patients lack the hindfoot instability associated with forefoot valgus and tend not to have a progressive problem. They may have problems with metatarsalgia as a result of prominence of the metatarsal heads and clawing of the toes. Patients with metatarsalgia and irritation of the toes are best treated with an orthosis made of a combination of thermal moldable cork to transfer weight bearing to the metatarsal shafts and PPT (Langer Biomechanics Group [UK] Ltd, Staffordshire, England) to cushion the metatarsal heads in a shoe with a deep toe box that accommodates the deformed toes.

Surgery to correct alignment can be performed at the base of the metatarsals or through the midfoot. I prefer to perform multiple basal metatarsal dorsiflexion osteotomies as described by Swanson, although this surgery can result in a "bayonet"-shaped foot. It is important to remember to release the plantar fascia to allow closure of these osteotomies. Several midfoot osteotomies have also been described, including the tarsal-metatarsal truncated wedge osteotomy described by Jahss, which is performed at the tarsal-metatarsal level; the midfoot wedge osteotomy of Cole, which is performed through the middle of the navicular, cuneiforms, and cuboid; and the Japas V-osteotomy. These procedures carry considerable risk of late midfoot degenerative changes, as well as the possibility of nonunion, which is greatest after a dorsal midfoot wedge osteotomy. Dorsal closure usually requires simultaneous release of the plantar fascia with any of these osteotomies.

PES CAVUS WITH FOREFOOT VALGUS

Treatment of Very Early Cases

Treating the cavus foot with associated forefoot valgus and compensa-tory hindfoot varus is a complex undertaking; preoperative assessment of the mechanics of the deformity, including which components are rigid as well as the strength of extrinsic and intrinsic muscles, is critical in surgical planning. Children with early minimal muscular involvement often have a flexible hindfoot with minimal varus hindfoot alignment and a plantar flexed but relatively flexible first ray. Often, if a child is observed over time, the first ray plantar flexion becomes progressively more rigid, and hindfoot varus becomes apparent and gradually more severe. These children usually have demonstrably weak ankle dorsiflexion and foot eversion. Drop foot is rarely a significant problem in the early stages of the deformity. Orthotic treatment consists of mild lateral forefoot posting, extended to the hindfoot region if necessary, to block the hindfoot varus roll and eliminate the associated feeling of ankle instability that often occurs. Parents should be taught to stretch the child's Achilles tendon with the forefoot held in valgus. While holding the forefoot in valgus, hindfoot alignment will remain neutral during stretching, maximizing gastrocnemius stretching and minimizing further attenuation of a gastrocnemius that may already be pathologically elongated. When asked about strengthening exercises for weak muscles, the orthopaedist needs to explain that the muscle lacks nerve stimulation and that a strengthening program likely will not make much difference. Despite this, it is not advisable to discourage parents, especially in the early stages. Appropriate stretching exercises to prevent contractures should be the principal objective in the child with early involvement.

If progressive forefoot valgus is apparent as the child is followed over the first year, transfer of the peroneus longus to the peroneus brevis may be especially helpful in slowing or stopping progression. If the peroneus longus is still active, this transfer will re-duce the tendency to forefoot valgus by eliminating the plantar flexion motor on the first ray, and it will help stabilize the hindfoot because the active peroneus longus will help restrain the roll into a varus position. This procedure was recommended in the early nineteenth century with reported good results and resolution of early cavus in many patients. Restoring its popularity may help reduce the need for late bony procedures such as osteotomies and arthrodesis.

Rigid Forefoot Valgus With Flexible Hindfoot Varus Once a rigid forefoot deformity is established and relatively severe, a laterally posted orthosis may be very helpful in maintaining hindfoot flexibility and preventing hindfoot varus malalignment. It may also spare the lateral ankle structures that tend to become stretched over time with recurrent inversion and prevent a fifth metatarsal stress fracture, a secondary problem seen in some of these patients.

If hindfoot flexibility is maintained and is correctable to neutral but the forefoot valgus is rigid, the best surgical approach is a dorsiflexion osteotomy of the first metatarsal and, if necessary, the second and third metatarsals. To close these osteotomies, it is necessary to also perform a plantar fascia release. The first metatarsal osteotomy can be performed through a direct medial approach, removing a dorsally based wedge at least 1 cm distal to the first tarsometatarsal joint. The amount of wedge excised depends on the amount of correction to be achieved. Enough bone must be removed to ensure alignment of the first and fifth metatarsals in the same plane perpendicular to the center of the calcaneus. This alignment can be assessed using the two thumb test in which pressure is evenly applied to the plantar aspect of the first and fifth metatarsals (**Figure 5**). With the calcaneus in the same sagittal line as the lower leg, the plane between the surgeon's thumbs should be perpendicu-

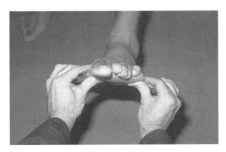

Figure 5 Two thumb test.

lar to the axis of the leg. Fixation of the osteotomy with crossed Kirschner wires is usually adequate, but postoperative immobilization in a non–weight-bearing cast for 6 weeks is also recommended.

The prominence of the second and third metatarsals relative to the first metatarsal head is then assessed. If the second metatarsal feels prominent relative to the first, an incision can be made on the dorsum of the foot between the bases of the second and third metatarsals. The second metatarsal then is osteotomized, removing a wedge sufficient to make it palpably level with the first metatarsal head. Once the second metatarsal is level with the first metatarsal, it also is fixed with crossed Kirschner wires, and the position of the third metatarsal is assessed relative to the second. If the third metatarsal head is prominent relative to the second, it also should be osteotomized. An osteotomy of the fourth and fifth metatarsals is not necessary in a patient with a forefoot valgus deformity. If the basal first metatarsal growth plate is still open and the child is not close to the end of his or her adolescent growth spurt, I perform the peroneal transfer and defer the metatarsal osteotomy until growth is complete, if it is still necessary. If the patient also has problems with ankle dorsiflexion, it may be worth considering a transfer of the tibialis posterior tendon to the dorsum of the foot through the interosseous membrane to reduce or eliminate a drop foot. The results of this procedure are

somewhat unpredictable, however, and the patient and parents should be advised of the significant chance that this procedure may not permanently correcting the drop foot problem.

Rigid Forefoot Valgus and Hindfoot Varus In patients who have retained hindfoot motion but have a hindfoot that is not correctable to neutral, a lateral closing wedge osteotomy of the calcaneus (Dwyer type) may be considered to correct the hindfoot alignment. In this procedure the skin incision and line of the osteotomy extend from the dorsal aspect of the calcaneus midway between the posterior facet and the posterosuperior aspect of the tuberosity to the plantar aspect of the calcaneus just anterior to the tubercles. If, however, subtalar motion is significantly restricted or absent, triple arthrodesis may be a more reliable long-term procedure that allows for some correction of forefoot valgus through the transverse tarsal joint.

Correction of forefoot valgus is absolutely essential when performing a triple arthrodesis to improve hindfoot alignment. If the forefoot is left in a rigid valgus position while the hindfoot is corrected, the ankle joint will predictably run into problems postoperatively. The reason for this can be appreciated by revisiting the tripod effect described by Coleman and Paulos. With the tripod effect, to allow the foot to become plantigrade (ie, the fifth metatarsal to come to the floor) in the presence of rigid forefoot valgus, the hindfoot must roll into a varus position. Because the hindfoot is now fused in a neutral position, the only way the hindfoot can become plantigrade is through varus tilting of the talus in the mortise with every step. This position causes significant asymmetric surface loading in the ankle joint. In younger patients, it may result in a ball-and-socket ankle, further compromising hindfoot stability. In skeletally mature patients, progressive degeneration of the ankle joint with medial joint space loss is the result

due to repetitive overloading of the medial mortise. Progressive attenuation of the lateral ligament further aggravates asymmetric loading. Reports of degenerative arthritis of the ankle joint following triple arthrodesis for pes cavus reflect a failure in both understanding the underlying mechanics and correcting the forefoot valgus with medial metatarsal osteotomies. I believe that forefoot position needs to be evaluated after the triple arthrodesis using the two thumb test described previously. When performing the intraoperative two thumb test after triple arthrodesis, it is important to directly observe that the talus is sitting squarely in the mortise during the test. In the presence of lateral ligament attenuation, the surgeon may incorrectly think that the forefoot is neutral if the talus is tilting in the mortise while the test is being performed. In case of lax lateral ligaments, I have gone as far as temporarily pinning the talus square in the mortise while doing the test. If lateral ligamentous laxity is so severe, I have performed a Broström-type repair to stabilize the ankle, but this step is of little value without having first corrected the faulty mechanics through osteotomies or arthrodesis.

Postoperative Bracing AFOs play an important role, even in patients with surgically corrected alignment. If drop foot is a persistent problem, a dorsiflexion-assisted AFO can be beneficial. AFOs are also helpful to stabilize the weak foot, to prevent inversion injuries, and to slow the development of deformity in patients with progressive weakness. It is difficult to manage the foot with fixed forefoot valgus and fixed hindfoot varus in an AFO alone because malalignment results in considerable friction against the brace, which may lead to skin breakdown and poor patient tolerance. In general, if treating severely malaligned feet nonsurgically, the most success will be achieved in high-top shoes that contain a custom orthosis. In very severe cases a custom-fitted boot may be the only alternative for those who refuse surgery.

Author's Preferred Treatment and Rationale

Global metatarsal equinus is generally best treated with basal metatarsal osteotomies as this surgery results in less loss of foot motion and chance of late arthritic change osteotomies performed through the tarsal bones of the midfoot. Preoperative lateral weight-bearing radiographs can be traced to assess the effects of removing dorsally based wedges from the metatarsal bases. The major downside of correction through basal metatarsal osteotomies is a bayonet-shaped foot, which probably is the result of overzealous wedge resection. Preoperative drawings simulating the wedge resection can be helpful in estimating the width of the base of the wedge, but it is always best to be conservative on the first wedge resection, to assess the degree of correction achieved, and to resect further bone if necessary. Remember that plantar fascia release will be necessary.

There is no single solution to the variety of clinical presentations of pes cavus with forefoot valgus. Key to effective therapy is careful preoperative evaluation, with particular attention to the patient's physical findings, distinguishing rigid and flexible deformities, recognizing muscle contractures, and assessing residual muscle strength. In the case of flexible deformities, osteotomies in combination with tendon lengthening or transfer and plantar fascia release are most appropriate when attempting to retain as much motion as possible. However, with these motion-sparing procedures, patients with an underlying neurologic problem and their families must be cautioned about the progressive nature of the condition and that further muscle deterioration may, in the long term, compromise what initially appears to be a good surgical outcome. The approach to rigid deformities is much more likely to include corrective arthrodesis in an attempt to provide more reliable long-term correction. Release of contractures and/or tendon transfers may be used in combination to improve the functional range of motion and stability of unfused joints, particularly the ankle.

Management of Complications

The most common complications are, in the short term, inadequate initial correction and, in the long term, recurrent or progressive deformity and late arthritis. All that can be done in these situations is a reevaluation of mechanics followed by attempts at bracing or in some cases repeat surgical intervention.

———————■

References

Coleman SS, Chestnut WJ: A simple test for hindfoot flexibility in the cavovarus foot. *Clin Orthop* 1977;123:60-62.

Jahss MH: Tarsometatarsal truncated-wedge arthrodesis for pes cavus and equinovarus deformity of the fore part of the foot. *J Bone Joint Surg Am* 1980;62:713-722.

Levitt RL, Canale ST, Cooke AJ Jr, et al: The role of foot surgery in progressive neuromuscular disorders in children. *J Bone Joint Surg Am* 1973;55:1396-1410.

Paulos L, Coleman SS, Samuelson KM: Pes cavovarus: Review of a surgical approach using selective soft-tissue procedures. *J Bone Joint Surg Am* 1980;62:942-953.

Coding

ICD-9 CODE

736.73 Other acquired deformities of ankle and foot, Cavus deformity of foot

CPT CODES

27685 Lengthening or shortening of tendon, leg or ankle; single tendon (separate procedure)

27690 Transfer or transplant of single tendon (with muscle redirection or rerouting); superficial (eg, anterior tibial extensors into midfoot)

28008 Fasciotomy, foot and/or toe

28300 Osteotomy; calcaneus (eg, Dwyer or Chambers type procedure), with or without internal fixation

28308 Osteotomy, with or without lengthening, shortening, or angular correction, metatarsal; other than first metatarsal, each

28309 Osteotomy, with or without lengthening, shortening, or angular correction, metatarsal; multiple (eg, Swanson type cavus foot procedure)

Forefoot Equinus Deformity

Richard J. Claridge, MD, FRCS

■ Definition of the Problem

Patient Presentation

Patients present with symptoms ranging from painful plantar callosities to hindfoot instability. The cause of the plantar callosities is clear, whereas the cause of the hindfoot instability is less so. In the normal foot at midstance, the hindfoot and the forefoot are aligned in the horizontal plane. If the foot is considered a tripod with the calcaneus as one leg and the first and fifth metatarsal heads as the other legs, all three are in the same plane in midstance (**Figure 1**). Commonly, the first metatarsal is elevated relative to the fifth. This situation is defined as forefoot varus and is common in patients with pes planus but otherwise normal feet. In order for the first metatarsal to contact the ground, the hindfoot must evert or pronate.

If the first metatarsal is flexed relative to the fifth, forefoot valgus re-

sults. The first ray contacts the ground first. Before the lateral border of the foot can bear weight, the hindfoot must invert, placing the hindfoot in varus at midstance (**Figure 2**). These patients initially have a flexible hindfoot varus that can become fixed with time. The varus attitude of the hindfoot at midstance places the center of gravity of the hindfoot more medial than usual, predisposing the patient to inversion sprains of the hindfoot. Often the presenting symptoms in these patients are ankle instability and recurrent ankle sprains. The varus hindfoot produces a more rigid foot as a result of the divergence of the axis of the talonavicular and calcaneocuboid joints. The foot is less flexible, placing more stress on the metatarsal heads and exacerbating the metatarsalgia. This lack of flexibility and reduced plantar weight-bearing surface make these patients unable to tolerate long periods of standing or walking. Many athletic activities are precluded because of the foot's inability to withstand repetitive loads.

Patients with forefoot equinus often have a neurologic imbalance as the underlying cause. Charcot-Marie-Tooth disease is the most common accompanying neurologic disorder. There are three inheritance patterns (autosomal dominant, recessive, and X-linked) with variable expression from generation to generation, making these patients common in any foot and ankle practice. When interviewing these patients it is important to ask about their relatives' feet and even to

casually examine any accompanying relative's feet.

In the Charcot-Marie-Tooth disease tibialis anterior is more commonly affected than the other anterior compartment muscles, and the peroneus brevis is more commonly affected than the peroneus longus. The subsequent weakness of ankle extension leads to recruitment of the toe extensors, producing metatarsophalangeal (MTP) hypertextension and claw toe deformities. This MTP hyperextension exacerbates the metatarsalgia caused by the metatarsal equinus. In addition, a first interphalangeal (IP) flexion deformity develops as a result of overpull of the extensor hallucis longus leading to a tightening of the flexor hallucis longus. The relative preservation of peroneus longus muscle strength compared with that of the peroneus brevis leads to weakness of hindfoot eversion and exacerbates the equinus of the first metatarsal, producing forefoot valgus.

Other neurologic conditions, such as polio, cerebral palsy, vertebral abnormalities, and spinal cord trauma, can also produce forefoot equinus as a result of long-standing muscle imbalance. The exact anatomy of the deformity varies with the specifics of the muscle imbalance. There is no treatment formula that will apply to every patient.

Physical Examination

Following an adequate history, a thorough physical examination is re-

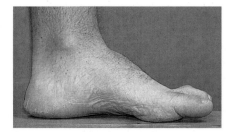

Figure 1 Standing lateral view of a patient with forefoot equinus. Note the prominence of the midfoot, the high arch, and the varus attitude of the hindfoot.

quired. The examination begins by observing the patient walk barefoot with adequate exposure of the lower extremities. A steppage gait with a wide stance and poor balance indicates poor proprioception. The examiner should observe how the foot goes from heel strike to foot flat, looking for the normal movement of the calcaneus from varus to valgus and back to varus at toe-off. The next step is a brief examination of the spine, pelvis, and upper extremities, looking for the scoliosis, muscle weakness, spinal stigmata, pelvic obliquity, and limb-length discrepancy that may accompany many neurologic disorders.

Once these areas have been cleared, the examiner can focus on the foot and ankle, observing whether the hindfoot lies in slight valgus at foot flat and, if the hindfoot is in varus, using the Coleman block test to determine whether the deformity is fixed or flexible (**Figure 3**). With a 1-in block under the fifth metatarsal head, a flexible deformity will correct; a fixed de-

formity will not. The single-stance heel rise test is used to confirm the function of the posterior tibial tendon. With the patient sitting comfortably on the examining table, ankle range of motion (with the knee flexed and extended) is assessed to identify any subtle equinus deformity. The hindfoot must be held in varus, locking the midtarsal joint to eliminate any midfoot contribution to extension. The examiner should determine the range of hindfoot eversion and inversion; normally there is more inversion than eversion. The plantar fascia is palpated to determine if it is excessively tight, and the forefoot is examined for corns and callus from toe deformities and metatarsalgia. Other questions the examiner needs to answer include (1) Are the MTP joints fixed in extension? (2) Does the first MTP joint have a normal range of motion? (3) Is there a fixed contracture of the great toe IP joint?

The examiner should observe the foot end-on to identify forefoot

valgus (**Figure 4**). If the hindfoot is held in a neutral varus-valgus position with one hand and the ankle is brought to neutral flexion-extension by gently pushing the forefoot to neutral with the other hand, the metatarsal heads should be in the same horizontal plane as the hindfoot as the examiner looks along the axis of the foot. The examination is completed by palpating for pulses, assessing muscle strength (particularly eversion and inversion), and measuring reflexes and vibration sense (128-cps tuning fork).

Differential Diagnosis

- Charcot-Marie-Tooth disease
- Friedreich's ataxia
- Poliomyelitis
- Spinal disraphism
- Cerebral palsy
- Muscular dystrophy
- Brain injury
- Congenital disorders (clubfoot residual, arthrogryposis)
- Compartment syndrome
- Crush injury

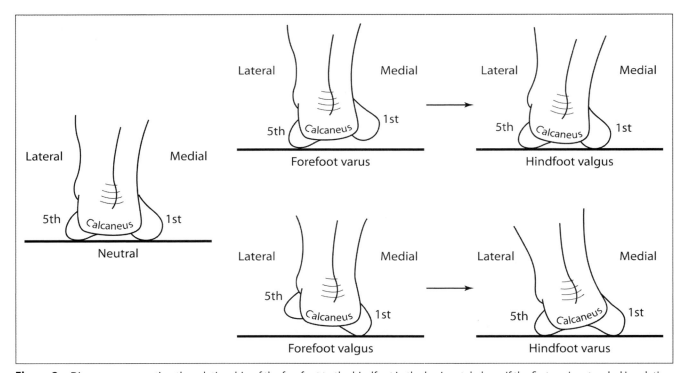

Figure 2   Diagram representing the relationship of the forefoot to the hindfoot in the horizontal plane. If the first ray is extended in relation to the lesser metatarsals, hindfoot valgus results. If the first ray is flexed in relation to the lesser metatarsals, hindfoot varus results.

Additional Work-up

Weight-bearing radiographs of the ankle and foot are required, the importance of which can be seen in **Figure 5**. Referral to a neurologist for prognosis and family counseling should be considered for patients with newly diagnosed Charcot-Marie-Tooth disease. Gait analysis with electromyographic monitoring can be helpful in selected patients, particularly when tendon transfers are being considered.

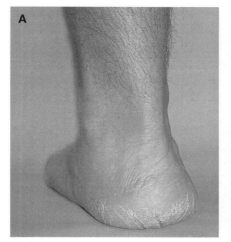 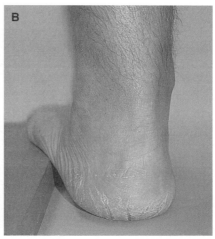

Figure 3 The Coleman block test. **A,** The hindfoot lies in varus. **B,** A 1-in block placed under the lateral portion of the forefoot compensates for the plantar prominence of the first ray, allowing the hindfoot to move into valgus; this indicates flexible hindfoot varus.

■ The Solutions

Treatment Options and Rationale

The typical patient with forefoot equinus has Charcot-Marie-Tooth disease with forefoot valgus. Depending on the severity and longevity of the problem, the hindfoot deformity may be fixed or flexible. If the hindfoot deformity is fixed, initial treatment should be directed at restoring normal hindfoot alignment with osteotomies, fusions, or tendon transfers. Once hindfoot balance has been restored, treatment can focus on the forefoot equinus deformity.

Nonsurgical options include a stretching program to keep the foot as supple as possible, custom orthotics to relieve the metatarsalgia, and appropriate bracing to help counteract any significant muscle weakness. A custom ankle-foot orthosis is very useful in maintaining a plantigrade foot. Footwear must be accommodative and shock absorbing, such as a good quality athletic shoe. The patient requires regular review to ensure that these measures are satisfactory and that the deformity does not require surgical correction.

Surgical options depend on the severity and characteristics of the de-

formity. With forefoot valgus, the first metatarsal is flexed in excess of the other metatarsals. If the deformity is mild, pain and tenderness in the first metatarsal are often major symptoms. A Jones procedure alone is indicated to correct the first MTP joint hyperextension and correct the flexion deformity of the IP joint. The extensor hallucis longus is transferred to the neck of the first metatarsal, and the IP joint is fused. In more severe deformities, an extension osteotomy of the first metatarsal is required to level the tread and bring the first metatarsal head into the same plane as the other metatarsal heads.

Less commonly the forefoot equinus also involves the lesser metatarsals. This involvement occurs most often in patients who have had poliomyelitis. The plantar fascia is contracted as well. Because the apex of the deformity is usually in the tarsus, a dorsal closing wedge midtarsal osteotomy provides better correction with less residual deformity than multiple metatarsal osteotomies. Lengthening of the plantar fascia is required. A Steindler stripping works well in this situation. The plantar fascia is incised just distal to the calcaneus, and the short flexors are released from the

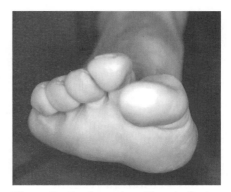

Figure 4 Forefoot valgus. Note the flexion of the first metatarsal exceeds that of the others.

calcaneus, reducing any contribution from intrinsic muscle contracture.

In an attempt to improve ankle extensor strength, the long flexor tendons can be transferred into the lateral cuneiform (Hibbs procedure). This procedure will also reduce MTP joint overpull and help correct any accompanying toe deformity.

Metatarsal head excision must be avoided if at all possible. The metatarsalgia can be relieved and the metatarsal heads saved using osteotomies and tendon transfer. Many patients with this problem are young, often in laboring occupations. Metatarsal head excision will

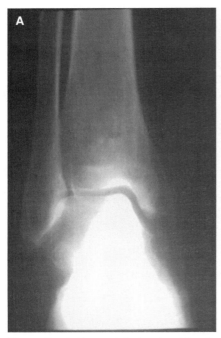 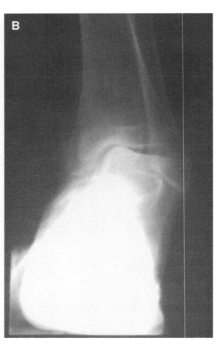

Figure 5 **A,** Non–weight-bearing AP radiograph of the ankle in a 68-year-old woman with long-standing Charcot-Marie-Tooth disease. **B,** Weight-bearing AP view of the ankle obtained 2 weeks later reveals marked varus deformity secondary to medial joint space loss.

often prevent them from returning to the laboring work force.

Author's Preferred Treatment and Rationale

The most common presentation of forefoot equinus is forefoot valgus and flexible hindfoot varus. In the absence of hallux MTP joint hyperextension, extension osteotomy of the first ray will restore forefoot alignment. The base of the first metatarsal is exposed through a dorsal incision. A Synthes mini-fragment T plate (Synthes USA, Paoli, PA) is templated just distal to the first MTP joint, and the two proximal holes are drilled. An osteotomy is marked out just distal to the cross of the T and made perpendicular to the shaft, leaving the plantar cortex intact. A second osteotomy is made 2 mm distal to the first (more if more extension is needed). A small wedge of bone

is removed, and the osteotomy is closed. The goal is to place the first ray in the same horizontal plane as the lesser metatarsal heads. The plate is fixed to the proximal fragment with two screws and to the distal fragment under compression while the osteotomy is reduced. Occasionally the second metatarsal may need to be extended as well.

If hallux hyperextension is a problem, a Jones procedure can be added at this time. It consists of transfer of the extensor hallucis longus to the neck of the first metatarsal, dorsal MTP capsulotomy, and IP fusion.

In an attempt to rebalance the foot, the peroneus longus is transferred into the tendon of peroneus brevis using a Pulver-Taft weave, thereby removing it as a deforming force and augmenting hindfoot eversion. Occasionally, judicious lengthening of the tibialis posterior tendon is also required. If

the plantar fascia is too tight, a Steindler stripping is indicated.

Postoperative care includes a non–weight-bearing cast for 6 weeks followed by splinting for several months, usually with a custom ankle-foot orthosis.

Management of Complications

Residual deformity is the most common complication. Residual hindfoot deformity requires calcaneal osteotomy or hindfoot arthrodesis. Arthrodesis is required if joint degeneration has resulted from a long-standing deformity.

Residual forefoot equinus may require a midtarsal osteotomy, usually in combination with a Steindler stripping. If the deformity is confined to the first ray, repeat extension osteotomy combined with a Jones procedure may solve the problem. Care should be taken to avoid excessive extension of the first metatarsal.

Other complications include nonunion or malunion of the first IP arthrodesis. Malunion can result in a plantar prominence at the IP joint that is a result of hyperextension. Revision with care to slightly flex the IP joint will solve this problem. Nonunion is rare with adequate screw fixation and is usually asymptomatic.

Injury to the sural nerve can occur from the peroneal tendon transfer. If symptoms are minimal no treatment is required. If symptoms are very bothersome, neurolysis or neurectomy may be required. Fortunately, the medial and lateral plantar nerves are rarely damaged during Steindler stripping. Injury to the medial calcaneal branch can be avoided by making the incision oblique (dorsal proximal to plantar distal) and distal to the calcaneal fat pad.

References

Brewerton DA, Sandifer PH, Sweetnam DR: Idiopathic pes cavus: An investigation into its aetiology. *Br Med J* 1963;5358:659-661.

Hsu JD, Mann DC, Imbus CE: Pes cavus, in Jahss MH (ed): *Disorders of the Foot and Ankle*, ed 2. Philadelphia, PA, WB Saunders, 1991, pp 872-891.

Ingram AJ: Anterior poliomyelitis, in Edmonson AS, Crenshaw AH (eds): *Campbell's Operative Orthopaedics*, ed 6. St Louis, MO, CV Mosby, 1980, pp 1435-1442.

Mann RA: Pes cavus, in Mann RA, Coughlin MJ (eds): *Surgery of the Foot and Ankle*, ed 6. St Louis, MO, Mosby, 1993, pp 785-801.

Coding

ICD-9 CODES

356.1   Hereditary and idiopathic peripheral neuropathy, Peroneal muscular atrophy, Charcot-Marie-Tooth disease

736.73   Other acquired deformities of foot and ankle, Cavus deformity of foot

754.71   Certain congenital musculoskeletal deformities, Other deformities of feet, Talipes cavus, Cavus foot (congenital)

CPT CODES

27690   Transfer or transplant of single tendon (with muscle redirection or rerouting); superficial (eg, anterior tibial extensors into midfoot)

27692   Transfer or transplant of single tendon (with muscle redirection or rerouting); each additional tendon (List in addition to code for primary procedure)

28250   Division of plantar fascia and muscle (eg, Steindler stripping) (Separate procedure)

28304   Osteotomy, tarsal bones, other than calcaneus or talus

28306   Osteotomy, with or without lengthening, shortening or angular correction, metatarsal; first metatarsal

28308   Osteotomy, with or without lengthening, shortening or angular correction, metatarsal; other than first metatarsal, each

28760   Arthrodesis, with extensor hallucis longus transfer to first metatarsal neck, great toe, interphalangeal joint (eg, Jones type procedure)

Index